T0201333

A Practical Approach to Special Care in Dentistry

A Practical Approach to Special Care in Dentistry

Edited by

Pedro Diz Dios, MD, DDS, PhD, EDiOM, FDSRCS (Edin)
Special Care Dentistry Unit, School of Medicine and Dentistry,
University of Santiago de Compostela & Galician Health Service (SERGAS),
Santiago de Compostela, Spain

Navdeep Kumar, BDS, FDSRCS (Eng), PhD, Cert RDP, Cert Surg & Pros Implantology
Royal National Ear, Nose and Throat & Eastman Dental Hospitals,
University College London Hospitals NHS Foundation Trust/University
College London, London, United Kingdom

Content Editors

Stephen Porter, BSc, MD, PhD, FDSRCS (Eng), FHEA
UCL Eastman Dental Institute
London, United Kingdom

Jacobo Limeres Posse, DDS, MSc, PhD
Special Care Dentistry Unit, School of Medicine and Dentistry, University of Santiago de Compostela
Santiago de Compostela, Spain

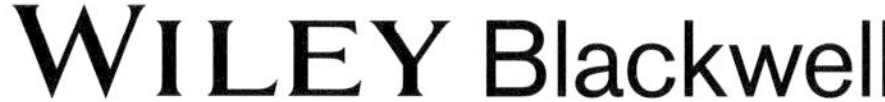

This edition first published 2022

Registered Offices
John Wiley & Sons, Inc., 111 River Street, Hoboken, NJ 07030, USA
John Wiley & Sons Ltd, The Atrium, Southern Gate, Chichester, West Sussex, PO19 8SQ, UK

Editorial Office
9600 Garsington Road, Oxford, OX4 2DQ, UK

For details of our global editorial offices, customer services, and more information about Wiley products visit us at www.wiley.com.

Wiley also publishes its books in a variety of electronic formats and by print-on-demand. Some content that appears in standard print versions of this book may not be available in other formats.

Library of Congress Cataloging-in-Publication Data Applied for

[Hardback ISBN 9781119600046]

Cover Design: Wiley
Cover Image: © Pedro Diz Dios

Set in 9.5/12.5pt STIXTwoText by Straive, Pondicherry, India

Printed in Singapore
M098778_241121

Contents

About the Authors

Dr Pedro Diz Dios
MD, DDS, PhD, EDiOM, FDSRCS (Edin)
Professor, Consultant and Head of the Special Needs Unit at the School of Medicine and Dentistry, Santiago de Compostela University (Spain). He is a member of the International Association of Disability & Oral Health (IADH) Curriculum Working Group and IADH Scientific Committee, and Honorary Visiting Professor at the UCL-Eastman Dental Institute (UK). He has written and edited 10 books, over 40 book chapters and over 220 papers cited on MEDLINE. He is the Editor in Chief of *Special Care Dentistry Journal*, an Associate Editor of *Oral Diseases Journal* and of *Medicina Oral Cirugía Oral Patología Bucal*, and an Editorial Board Member of the *Journal of Disability and Oral Health*.

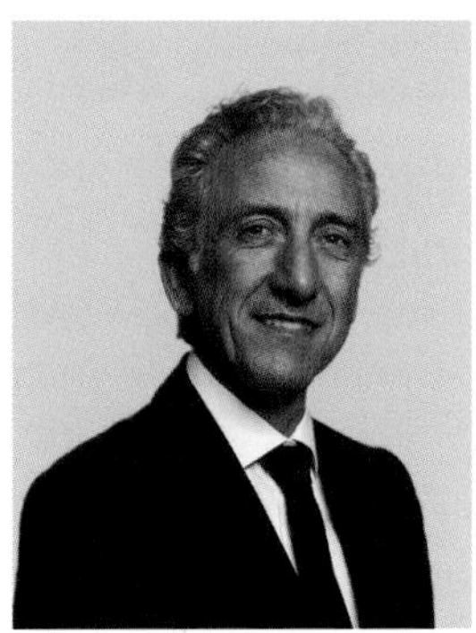

Dr Navdeep Kumar
BDS, FDSRCS (Eng), PhD, Cert RDP, Cert Surg & Pros Implantology
Consultant in Special Care Dentistry, Honorary Senior Lecturer and Divisional Clinical Director RNENT & EDH, at the University College London Hospitals NHS Foundation Trust. Over the last 20 years Dr Navdeep Kumar has been committed to special care dentistry (SCD) and has acquired an extensive range of clinical, teaching and research experience in the area to ensure the delivery of high-quality oral care for people with an impairment or disability. She has considerable expertise in the clinical management of the medically compromised patient and the management of oral complications of systemic diseases. She has an integral role in training others with an interest in SCD, examining in this field, and is actively involved in the promotion of oral care for this vulnerable cohort, contributing to the development of national and international guidelines and numerous publications in this area.

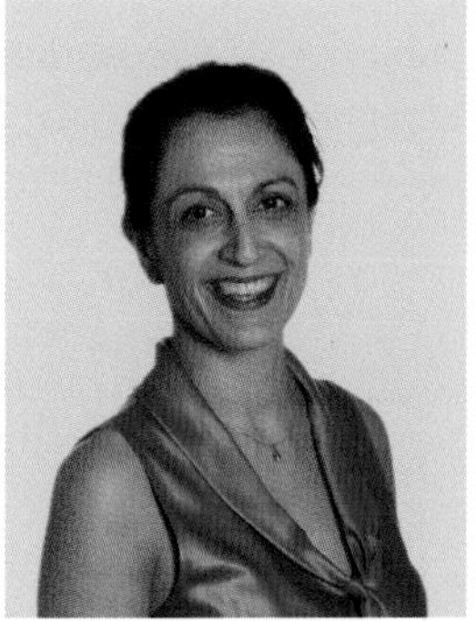

List of Contributors

Fatima Al Sarraf
BDS (Hons)-NUI, MFDS (RCSI), KBAGD, MGDS (RCSI), MSC (SCD), FGDS (RCSI)
Advanced General and Special Care Dentistry, Ministry Of Health Kuwait, Kuwait City, Kuwait

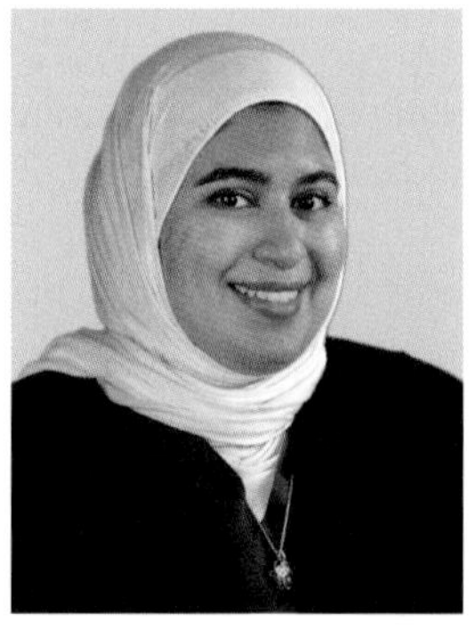

Lim Guang Xu David
BDS, MSc, PGDip, ACLP, MFDS (RCS Ed)
Tzu Chi Free Clinic, Buddhist Compassion Relief Tzu Chi Foundation, Geriatric and Special Needs Dentistry Clinic, National Dental Centre Singapore, Oral Health Therapy, Nanyang Polytechnic, Singapore

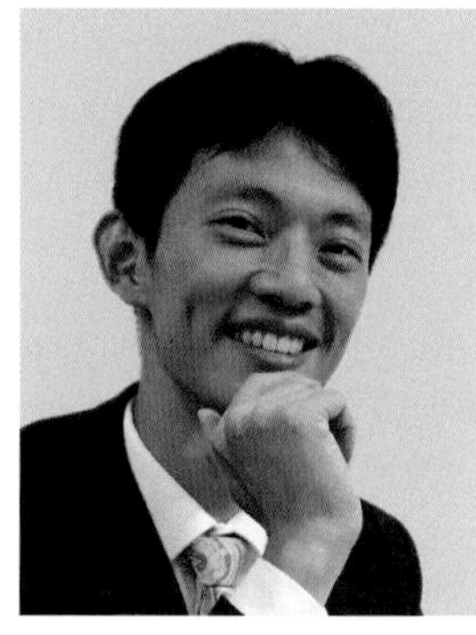

Sofia Bonvallet Commentz
BSD, PgDip, MSc
University of Valparaiso & Valparaiso San Antonio Health Service, Valparaiso, Chile

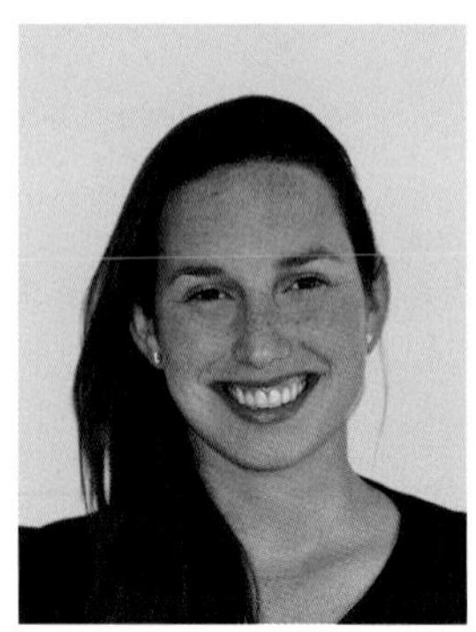

Javier Fernández Feijoo
MD, DDS, MSc, PhD, PCD
Special Care Dentistry Unit, School of Medicine and Dentistry, University of Santiago de Compostela, EOXI Santiago de Compostela, Galician Health Service (SERGAS), Santiago de Compostela, Spain

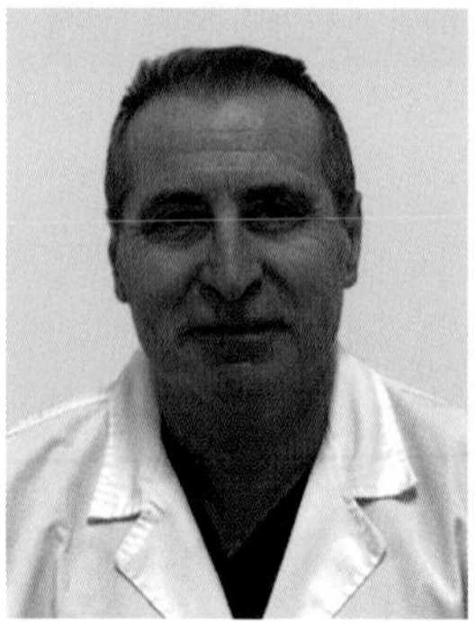

Márcio Diniz Freitas
DDS, MSc, FDS, PhD
Special Care Dentistry Unit. School of Medicine and Dentistry, University of Santiago de Compostela, Santiago de Compostela, Spain

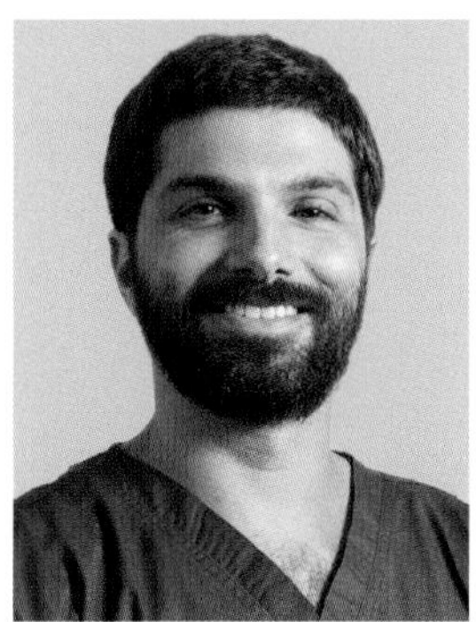

Jee-Yun Leung
BDSc (Hons), MSc (SCD), DSCD (RCS Eng)
Adelaide Dental School, The University of Adelaide, Special Needs Unit, Adelaide Dental Hospital, SA Dental, Adelaide, Australia

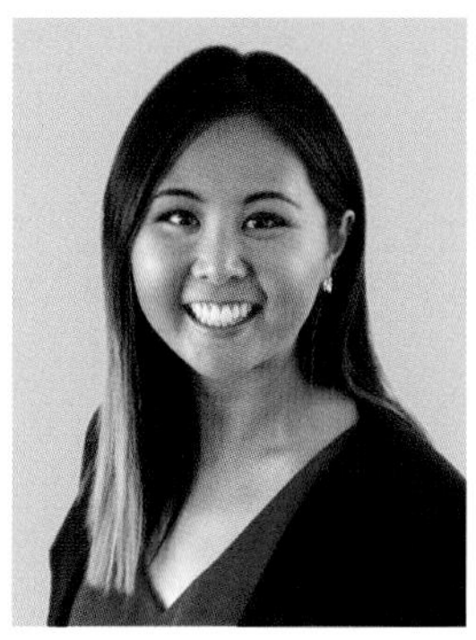

Emma Vázquez García
DDS, MSc, PhD, PCD
EOXI Pontevedra-Salnés, Galician Health Service (SERGAS), Pontevedra, Spain

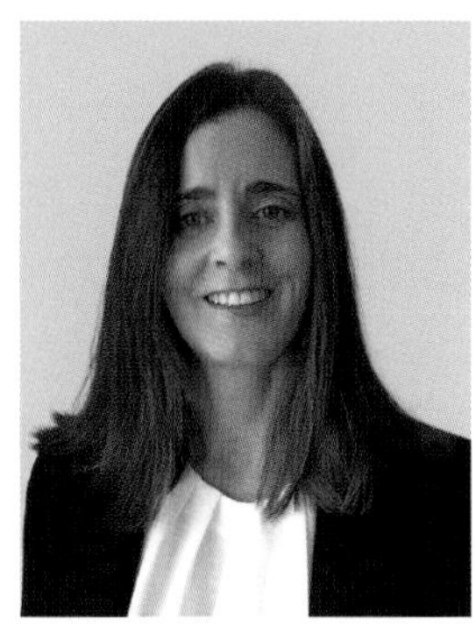

Lucía Lago Méndez
DDS, MSc, FDS, PhD, PCD
EOXI Santiago de Compostela, Galician Health Service (SERGAS), Santiago de Compostela, Spain

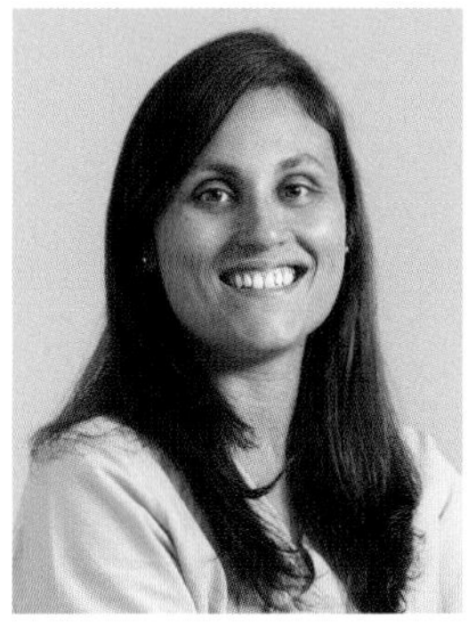

María Consuelo Cousido González
MD, PhD, BDS, BDM, PCD
EOXI Coruña-Cee, Galician Health Service (SERGAS), La Coruña, Spain

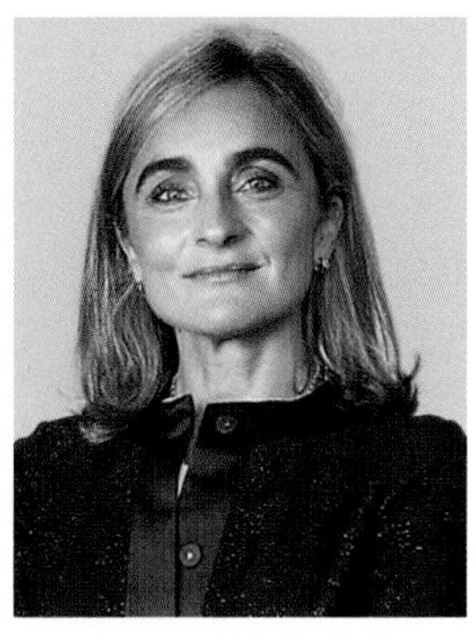

Ricca Mae Roco-Bernardino
DMD, MSc (SCD)
The Medical City and Philippine Children's Medical Center, Metro Manila, Philippines

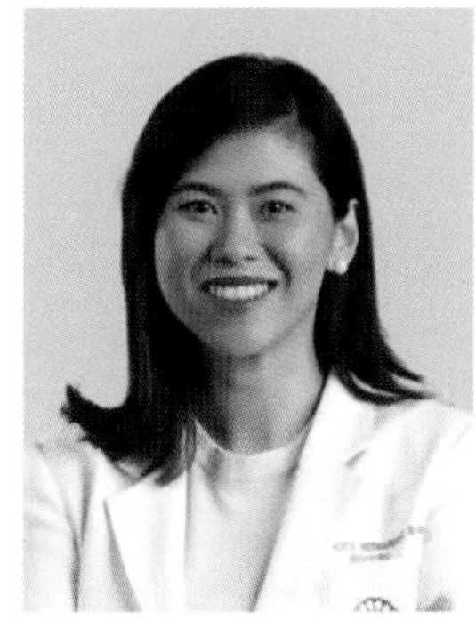

Preface

Special Care Dentistry (SCD) was previously defined by patient characteristics, such as their medical condition or behavioural issues. However, it has changed in recent decades to reflect the complexity of providing holistic oral care for patients with multiple comorbidities which may lead to physical and/or intellectual, sensory, mental or social impairment. Although it commonly relates to adults, in some countries it also includes the oral care of children with disabilities.

There is a significant geographical variation in access to SCD related to lack of training, appropriate infrastructure and financial factors. Nevertheless, it is rapidly growing due to increased demand and is now acknowledged as an essential field of dentistry across the world. Dramatic improvements in medicine, mainly in areas related to early diagnosis and new therapeutic approaches, have resulted in increased life expectancy and the quality of life of chronically ill patients and individuals with severe disability. Hence, individuals requiring care are not limited to hospitalised patients and more commonly include those living in the community, either independently or with support.

As a consequence, it is essential that undergraduates, postgraduates and general dental practitioners acquire specific knowledge in the field of SCD, so that they can integrate this discipline into their daily practice. To enable this, we have created this book, which contains 61 topics based on clinical cases from across the world, reflecting the most common clinical conditions which may present in general dental practice. This scenario-based approach enables the application of elements of problem-based learning and structured clinical reasoning, allowing the reader to appreciate that patients rarely present with a single medical condition or risk factor, and that multiple factors must be taken into consideration when providing care.

Each case includes the application of a risk assessment framework of medical, social and dental risk factors. This allows the systematic consideration of appropriate modifications that should be implemented prior to commencement of dental treatment, thereby reducing complications and treatment planning errors.

Subsequently, the main oral findings and the specific considerations for dental management for each condition/disease are discussed. The ACCESS mnemonic is utilised to ensure that six domains which address different aspects of care are considered:

1) **A**ccess
2) **C**ommunication
3) **C**onsent
4) **E**ducation
5) **S**urgery
6) **S**pread of infection

Lastly, each chapter concludes with background information on each condition/disease, with updated medical content on their definition, aetiopathogenesis, clinical presentation, diagnosis, treatment and prognosis.

In 2006, under the guidance of Professor Crispian Scully, we published the book entitled *Special Needs in Dentistry (Handbook of Oral Healthcare)*. A few years later, in December 2015, we received an email announcing that 'The Special Care Dentistry book will be 10 years old next year! I am intent on producing something that focuses on the younger generations and that can be regularly updated'. The tragic and premature loss of Professor Scully deprived us of his academic guidance, editorial experience and enormous knowledge. We have therefore put all our efforts into this new publication, which launches today thanks to the contribution of a group of relevant collaborators. We hope it will serve as a tribute to our master, mentor and friend.

Pedro Diz Dios and Navdeep Kumar

1

Physical Disability

1.1 Cerebral Palsy

Section I: Clinical Scenario and Dental Considerations

Clinical Scenario

A 24-year-old patient attends your dental practice with acute pain from a lower right molar tooth. Two courses of antibiotics prescribed by the general medical practitioner have been ineffective. She attends alone and has used a private taxi that has been able to accommodate her wheelchair.

Medical History
- Spastic cerebral palsy
- Degenerative disc disease and spondylosis of the cervical spine
- Adjustment disorder (presented after divorce; undergoing follow-up by psychiatry)

Medications
- Trihexyphenidyl hydrochloride
- Baclofen
- Bromazepam
- Lormetazepam
- Mirtazapine
- Omeprazole

Dental History
- Irregular dental attender – avoided attending as she is anxious that dental treatment will make her gag
- No experience of local anaesthesia to enable dental treatment in the dental clinic setting
- Previous dental treatment provided under general anaesthesia on 2 occasions, when she was a child
- Good level of co-operation
- Brushes her teeth regularly herself, although she admits difficulty accessing the posterior teeth due to her gag reflex and involuntary movements

Social History
- Lives alone and is not currently working
- Divorced and does not have a good relationship with her ex-husband's family; no children or close family
- A caregiver visits every morning to help with basic activities of daily life
- Wheelchair user (Figure 1.1.1)
- Limited financial resources

Oral Examination
- Involuntary movements of the jaw
- Moderate sialorrhoea – saliva does not spill over the vermilion border
- Pronounced gag reflex
- Mouth in very poor condition, with numerous carious teeth and deposits of calculus (Figure 1.1.2)
- Caries: #11, #15, #17, #21, #22, #25, #26, #27, #35, #37, #41, #42, #44, #45 and #48
- Tenderness on palpation: #48; no associated swelling
- Missing teeth: #36, #46 and #47

Radiological Examination
- Orthopantomogram – artefacts due to the patient's movement
- Supplemented by long-cone periapical radiography anteriorly
- Endodontic treatment of #11 and #21 (obturation satisfactory; no periapical radiolucent areas)
- Extensive, deep and unrestorable caries in #15 and #48 (with pulpal involvement)
- Restorable caries in #17, #22, #25, #26, #27, #35, #37, #41 and #44
- Recurrent caries associated with the dental fillings in #16, #42 and #45
- Missing teeth #36, #46 and #47

A Practical Approach to Special Care in Dentistry, First Edition. Edited by Pedro Diz Dios and Navdeep Kumar.

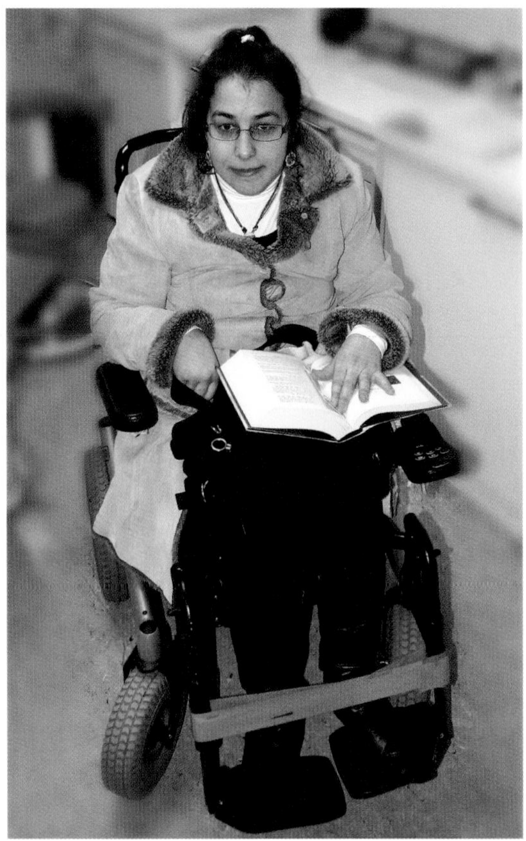

Figure 1.1.1 Patient with spastic cerebral palsy and preserved intellectual ability in the dental practice.

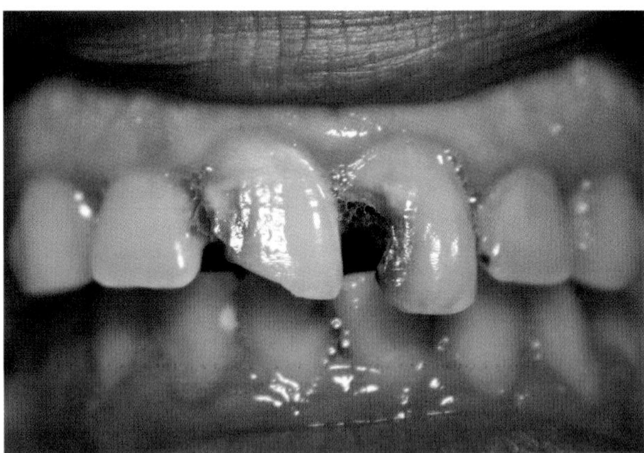

Figure 1.1.2 Extensive caries upper central incisors.

Structured Learning

1) The #48 is painful on palpation and you suspect periapical periodontitis. The patient's temperature is not elevated and there is no associated lymph node enlargement. What emergency management would you propose and why?
   - It is important to treat the dental infection urgently to reduce the risk of significant morbidity and life-threatening sequelae, including Ludwig's angina
   - However, within the last 20 years, antimicrobial resistance has become a significant issue with prescribed antibiotics/dosages being ineffective
   - Hence it is important to remove the source of infection, establish drainage and prescribe analgesics
   - Further effective antibiotics may also enable successful dental intervention at a later date, namely effective local anaesthesia followed by removal of the infected pulpal contents or by extraction of the tooth
   - Drainage of an associated abscess should also be considered if swelling develops
2) The patient has received appropriate and high-dose antibiotics and requests that you attempt to extract the tooth the same day. Although she has no previous experience with local anaesthesia, she appears to be co-operative and has capacity. What would you discuss with her?
   - Extraction of #48 is the preferred treatment option as:
     - The use of rotary instrumentation for caries removal is associated with increased risk due to the posterior position of the tooth, uncontrolled movements and increased gag reflex
     - There is limited access to allow for endodontic treatment (e.g. due to difficulties accessing the posterior sections of the mouth)
     - The patient struggles to access her posterior teeth for cleaning
   - As this is an urgent procedure, the dental extraction can be attempted in the dental chair
   - Given her considerable dental treatment needs, this can be followed up by the provision of non-urgent procedures (e.g. restorations) provided in a hospital setting under general anaesthesia
   - Prosthetic rehabilitation and subsequent follow-up/treatment sessions should be performed in the dental clinic, if possible
3) What factors are considered important in assessing the risk of managing this patient?
   - Social
     - Lack of available escort
     - Transport difficulties when attending dental clinic/hospital
     - Limited financial means
   - Medical
     - Neck position compromised by the dental chair and by problems in the cervical spine; consider the option of treating the patient in her wheelchair

  - Risks associated with general anaesthesia may be increased in patients with cerebral palsy (hypothermia, hypotension)
  - Adjustment disorder may reduce compliance and manifest as increased anxiety/tearfulness
- Dental
  - Local stimuli and stress can increase involuntary movements
  - Gag reflex
  - Limited access to the oral cavity
  - Sialorrhoea compromises operatory field isolation
  - Poor self-cleansing of the oral cavity
  - Unsupervised oral hygiene habits

4) The patient requests premedication/sedation. What do you need to consider when selecting the correct approach?
   - The patient is already taking oral benzodiazepines
   - Hence, a medical consultation is required before proceeding, given the risk of synergy with some of the drugs the patient is taking, i.e. the effects can be increased when midazolam is combined with bromazepam
   - Given the absence of chronic respiratory problems, nitrous oxide may be used
5) The patient requests oral prosthetic rehabilitation after her teeth are extracted/stabilised. What options would you discuss?
   - If oral hygiene improves:
     - Removable prostheses can be difficult to insert and, with oral dyskinesias, are more unstable, potentially causing injuries to the mucosa/obstruction of the airway if dislodged
     - Fixed implant-supported or tooth-supported prostheses are preferable; these can be limited to the anterior/aesthetic zones to allow for improved appearance and easier access for cleaning
     - The cost of these options needs to be considered
   - If oral hygiene remains poor and the dental caries risk remains high:
     - It may be preferable to accept the gaps rather than compromise further teeth
     - Alternatively, a removable dental prosthesis may be attempted as this is reversible and can be removed to allow access for cleaning
     - Furthermore, teeth can be added to the partial denture, if further dental extractions become necessary
     - This may be better than implant-supported measures if there are financial limitations
6) Drooling (sialorrhoea) is a common consequence of cerebral palsy among patients with difficulties swallowing saliva. What medication is this patient taking that could be of benefit?
   - Trihexyphenidyl hydrochloride is an anticholinergic drug and hence reduces saliva production
   - This medication may also be effective for reducing dystonia or improving upper arm function in patients with cerebral palsy
7) What are the most widely used therapeutic modalities for sialorrhoea?
   - Physiotherapy for swallowing and postural re-education
   - Drugs: anticholinergic agents (scopolamine, atropine, glycopyrrolate) or botulinum toxin
   - Surgery: Wharton's duct relocation, excision of a submandibular gland or selective neurectomy

General Dental Considerations

Oral Findings

- Delayed eruption of primary dentition
- Enamel hypoplasia
- Bruxism and abnormal dental attrition
- Gingivitis and periodontal disease
- Anterior tooth trauma due to falls
- Spontaneous dislocation or subluxation of the temporomandibular joint
- Malocclusion (anterior open bite and Angle class II-1) (Figure 1.1.3a)
- Sialorrhoea/drooling, promoted by the head position and difficulties swallowing saliva (Figure 1.1.3b)

Dental Management (Figure 1.1.4)

- The dental treatment plan is determined more by the disease severity (e.g. severity of the spasticity) and its comorbidities (e.g. respiratory impairment) than by the type of cerebral palsy (Table 1.1.1)
- Dental manipulation and stress can intensify the uncontrolled movements

Section II: Background Information and Guidelines

Definition

Cerebral palsy is a group of permanent disorders of the development of movement and posture, resulting from non-progressive disturbances (structural abnormalities) that occurred in the developing foetal or infant brain. It is the most common form of chronic motor disability in childhood, with an estimated prevalence of 2.0–3.5 cases per 1000 live births in developed countries.

(a)

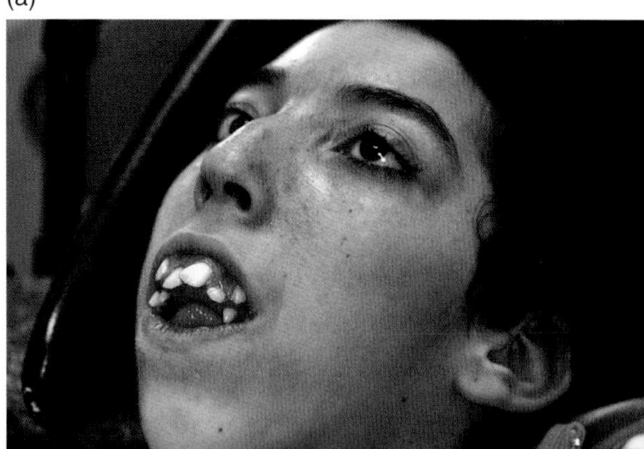

(b)

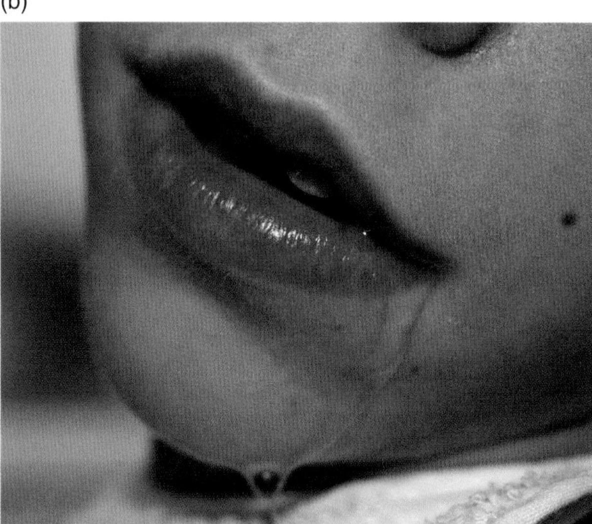

Figure 1.1.3 (a) Severe malocclusion with anterior open bite. (b) Sialorrhoea/drooling.

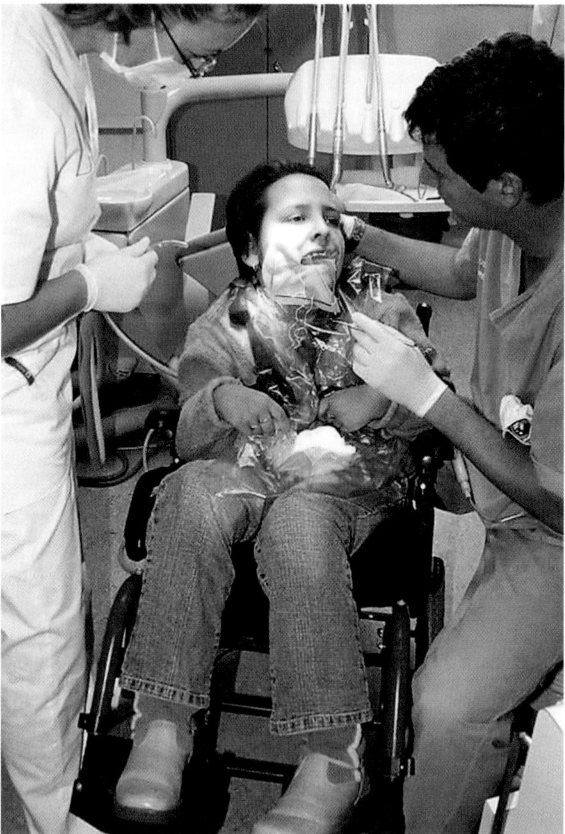

Figure 1.1.4 Patients who present in wheelchairs may have treatment provided without transfer.

- In over 50% of patients, it is accompanied by disturbances of sensation (visual and auditory defects), perception, cognition, communication and behaviour
- Epilepsy and musculoskeletal problems may also be present

Aetiopathogenesis
- The condition is attributed to structural brain abnormalities and hypoxia due to cerebrovascular insufficiency
- This may occur during the prenatal, perinatal or postnatal periods
  - Prenatal: infections, exposure to toxins and multiple pregnancies
  - Perinatal: traumatic births and prematurity (especially for infants weighing less than 2500 g)
  - Postnatal: infections, intracranial haemorrhages and kernicterus

Clinical Presentation
- Cerebral palsy is subdivided into spastic, dyskinetic (including dystonic) and ataxic forms, depending on the area of the brain that is mainly involved (Table 1.1.2; Figure 1.1.5)

Diagnosis
- There are no specific tests to confirm or eliminate the diagnosis of cerebral palsy
- The suspected diagnosis is based on clinical findings and the failure to reach appropriate developmental milestones for the patient's age
- There is general consensus of an upper age limit of 2 years for the onset of the non-progressive brain disturbance and five years for a clinical or developmental diagnosis
- Diagnostic brain imaging tests, including computed tomography and magnetic resonance imaging, can be of use
- An electroencephalogram, genetic analysis and metabolic tests may also be undertaken

Management
- Physical therapy and occasionally orthopaedic surgery

Table 1.1.1 Considerations for dental management.

Risk assessment	• Involuntary movements and contractions – these can increase further with stress and local stimuli • Abnormal gag/bite reflex • Abnormal swallowing and cough reflex • Aspiration risk • Epilepsy
Criteria for referral	• Referral to a specialised clinic or hospital centre is determined by: – Factors related to the severity of the patient's general condition (e.g. respiratory distress, uncontrolled seizures) – Factors that significantly limit access for dental procedures (e.g. pathological reflexes and uncontrolled movements)
Access/position	• Patients who present in wheelchairs may have treatment provided without transfer, particularly if there is a wheelchair platform available (Figure 1.1.4) • If they are transferred to the dental chair, the patients will need to be stabilised with pillows • Consider safe immobilisation of the head using vacuum cushions/supports with consent
Communication	• Frequent difficulties in verbal communication • Non-verbal language might sometimes need to be interpreted • The level of comprehension can be normal • Concentration may be poor
Consent/capacity	• Capacity may be intact • Do not make assumptions due to the physical signs/symptoms or impaired verbal communication • Clinical holding may be required (e.g. to reduce involuntary arm movements) – this must be appropriately risk assessed, undertaken by trained staff, consented and documented • Regular medication may be sedative and hence impair capacity
Anaesthesia/sedation	• Local anaesthesia – Not contraindicated, although involuntary movements may make delivery challenging • Sedation – Conscious sedation can help control anxiety, nausea and lingual dystonia – Medical consultation is recommended if the patient takes neuroleptics, is already taking benzodiazepines or has respiratory difficulties • General anaesthesia – May be indicated if the movements are uncontrollable or there is a lack of co-operation (the risk/benefit should be assessed)
Dental treatment	• Before – The need for conscious sedation should be anticipated and consent for any intervention undertaken prior to this – Orthodontic treatment planning should consider the impact of increased muscle tone • During – Consider the use of atraumatic mouth openers, protective thimbles and stainless steel/plastic mirrors (involuntary contractions) – Fixed prostheses are generally preferable over removable prostheses (due to difficulties inserting the prosthesis, involuntary movements and the risk of fracture in patients with epilepsy) • After – Close follow-up after completion of orthodontic therapy as relapse is more frequent
Drug prescription	• Consider the associated systemic complications and concurrent medications • Caution with the use of benzodiazepines if the patient is already taking sedation medication
Education/prevention	• Involve the relatives and caregivers where possible • An electric or adapted manual toothbrush should be considered • Regular oral prophylaxis/calculus removal • Fluoride treatment • Dietary counselling

Table 1.1.2 Classification and characteristics of cerebral palsy.

Type (lesion location)	Frequency	Clinical presentation	Subtype/area involved
Spastic (upper motor neuron)	70–80%	Muscle hypertonia Contracture Hyperreflexia	• Monoplegic: one extremity • Paraplegic: legs • Hemiplegic: one arm and one ipsilateral leg • Double hemiplegic: all extremities but more in the arms • Diplegic: all extremities but more in the legs • Tetraplegic: all extremities
Athetoid (basal ganglia)	15%	Vermiform movements Muscle hypertonia	• Chorea (restless, fidgety, dancing movement): face, chest and extremities • Athetosis (slow, writhing movement): hands and feet • Choreoathetosis: generalised
Ataxic (cerebellum)	10%	Abnormal equilibrium and gait	

- Drug treatment for tone/movement disorders, including baclofen, trihexyphenidyl, gabapentin, diazepam, clonidine and botulinum toxin
- Neurosurgical interventions, including selective rhizotomy and electrode implantation in the basal ganglia
- Epilepsy control, speech therapy and hearing and vision support
- Special education and occupational therapy

Prognosis

- The life expectancy for cerebral palsy may be reduced in relation to the number and severity of the associated disabilities
- If gross and fine motor functioning, independent feeding, mental and visual capacities are severely impaired, survival to 40 years of age may be as low as 40%
- Causes of early death may include pulmonary aspiration and pneumonia, accidents, associated disorders (e.g., congenital heart disease) and delayed recognition of illness

A World/Transcultural View

- The prevalence of cerebral palsy is estimated at 1.9/1000 live births in China, 2.1/1000 in Europe and 3.6/1000 in the US. This variability is probably an expression of the predominant aetiological factors. For exam-

(a)

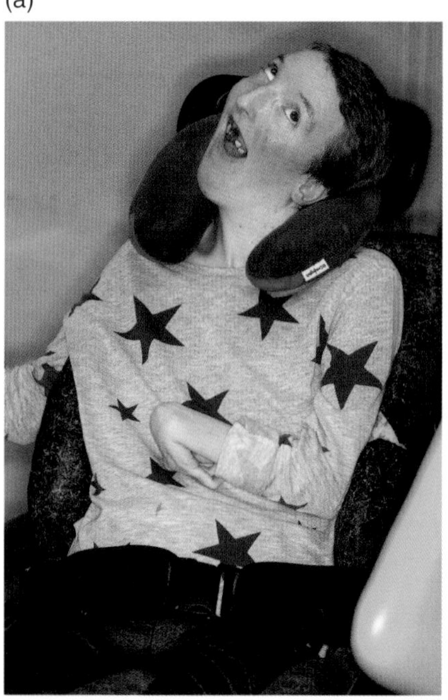

(b)

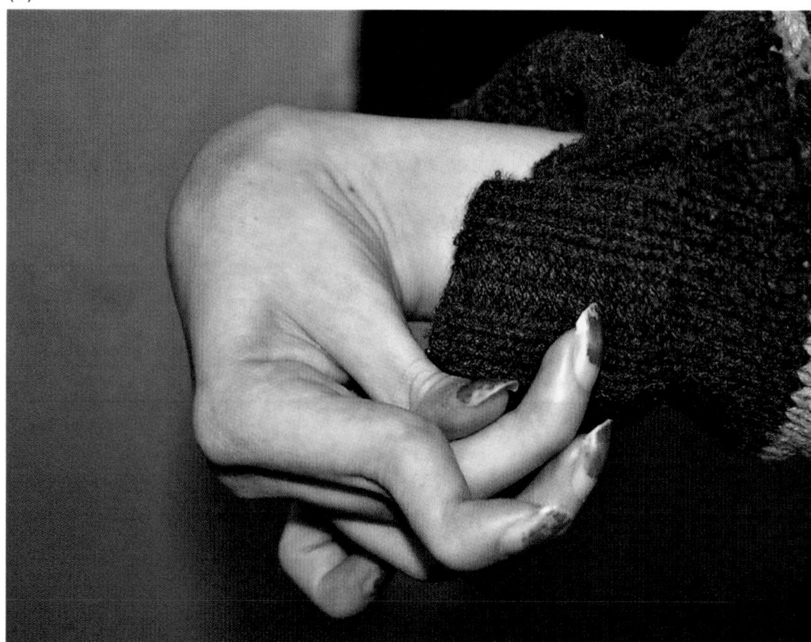

Figure 1.1.5 (a) Spastic cerebral palsy. (b) Hand deformity calls for adaptive tools (e.g. adapted toothbrush handle).

ple, cerebral palsy among the Jewish population is due mostly to premature births, while among the Arab population, the condition is especially attributed to consanguinity and genetic factors
- In low- and medium-income countries such as India, there are educational and healthcare deficiencies in terms of the principles of the International Classification of Functioning, Disability and Health, while in higher-income countries such as Canada, the parents of children with cerebral palsy perceive a more conducive environment and express a more social outlook on their children's health

Recommended Reading

Abeleira, M.T., Outumuro, M., Diniz, M. et al. (2016). Orthodontic treatment in children with cerebral palsy. In: *Cerebral Palsy – Current Steps* (ed. M.K. Gunel), 129–140. Rijeka, Croatia: Intech.

Bensi, C., Costacurta, M., and Docimo, R. (2020). Oral health in children with cerebral palsy: a systematic review and meta-analysis. *Spec. Care Dentist.* 40: 401–411.

Cahlin, B.J., Lindberg, C., and Dahlström, L. (2019). Cerebral palsy and bruxism: effects of botulinum toxin injections-a randomized controlled trial. *Clin. Exp. Dent. Res.* 5: 460–468.

Cardoso, A.M.R., de Medeiros, M.M.D., Gomes, L.N. et al. (2018). Factors associated with health and oral health-related quality of life of children and adolescents with cerebral palsy. *Spec. Care Dentist.* 38: 216–226.

Colver, A., Fairhurst, C., and Pharoah, P.O. (2014). Cerebral palsy. *Lancet* 383: 1240–1249.

Jan, B.M. and Jan, M.M. (2016). Dental health of children with cerebral palsy. *Neurosciences.* 21: 314–318.

Rai, T., Ym, K., Rao, A. et al. (2018). Evaluation of the effectiveness of a custom-made toothbrush in maintaining oral hygiene and gingival health in cerebral palsy patients. *Spec. Care Dentist.* 38: 367–372.

Vpk, V., Mohanty, V.R., Balappanavar, A.Y. et al. (2020). Effectiveness of different parenting interventions on oral hygiene of cerebral palsy children: a randomized controlled trial. *Spec. Care Dentist.* 40: 335–343.

1.2 Epilepsy

Section I: Clinical Scenario and Dental Considerations

Clinical Scenario

A 17-year-old female presents to an emergency hospital department following facial trauma experienced during an epileptic seizure (Figure 1.2.1). She complains of pain and mobility in the maxillary central incisors. Your dental opinion is sought.

Medical History
- Refractory epilepsy (3–5 seizures a day with variable presentation, including generalised tonic–clonic seizures). The patient is awaiting assessment for inserting a vagus nerve stimulator
- Delayed psychomotor development
- Intellectual disability (moderate)

Medications
- Ethosuximide
- Lamotrigine
- Clonazepam
- Sodium valproate

Dental History
- Seizures resulting in repeated trauma in the orofacial region – deciduous and permanent dentition affected
- Limited co-operation – only dental examinations possible in the past; no previous dental radiographs or dental treatment undertaken
- Patient brushes her teeth twice a day, supervised by her mother

Social History
- Lives with her parents and a younger sibling
- During the day, the patient attends an occupational therapy centre
- Patient requires help for basic activities of daily life

Oral Examination
- Mucosal scarring from previous seizure-related trauma
- Displacement, proclination and significant mobility of the maxillary central incisors (Figure 1.2.2)
- Localised areas of gingival enlargement

Radiological Examination

- Not performed due to lack of co-operation

Structured Learning

1) The decision was made to undertake a detailed examination and deliver any required dental treatment under general anaesthesia in a hospital setting. Why?
   - The patient's epilepsy is not under control
   - The patient's degree of co-operation is limited due to intellectual impairment
2) What factors are important to consider when assessing the risk of managing this patient?
   - Social
     - Availability of escorts/family to accompany the patient (younger sibling requires supervision)
     - Capacity assessment required: if the patient is assessed as lacking capacity in relation to the proposed procedure, a best interest decision will be required; this should involve family members, social services, any health and social care professionals involved with the adult's care, carers
     - Deprivation of Liberty standards cannot be applied if the patient is admitted as she is below the age of 18 years old
     - Financial means (insurance coverage) to cover the costs of treatment in a hospital setting under general anaesthesia (varies between countries)
   - Medical
     - Increased risks in general associated with general anaesthesia

A Practical Approach to Special Care in Dentistry, First Edition. Edited by Pedro Diz Dios and Navdeep Kumar.

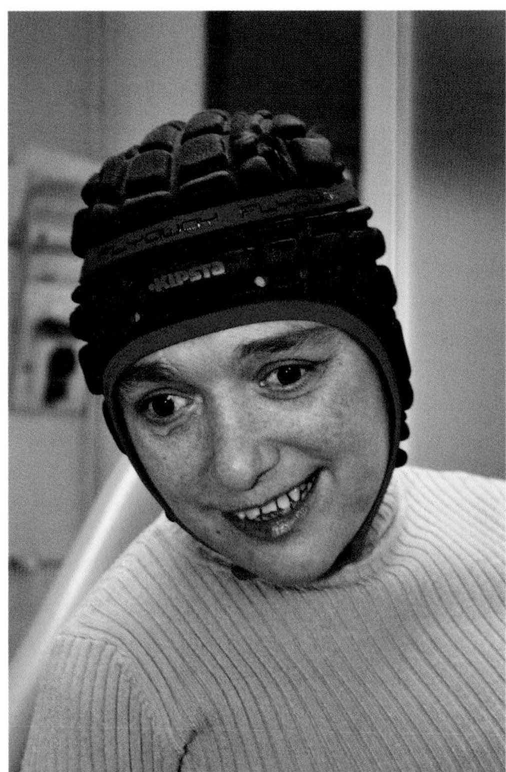

Figure 1.2.1 Patient with uncontrolled epilepsy wearing a protective headgear.

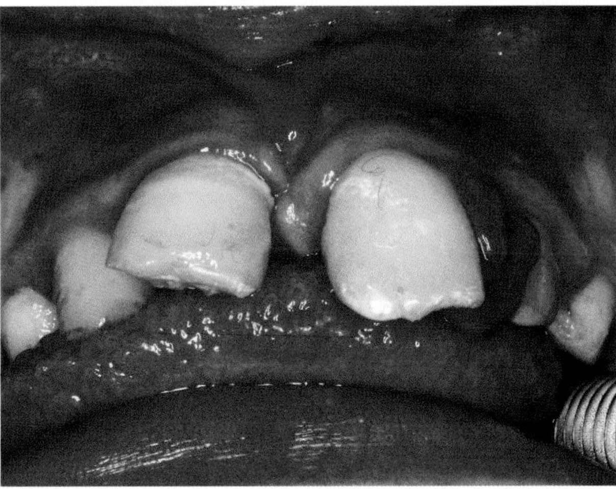

Figure 1.2.2 Severe displacement of the maxillary central incisors following facial trauma.

  - High risk of seizures perioperatively due to the refractory epilepsy; hence inpatient bed and neurology support needed during admission
- Dental
  - Urgency of dental treatment (due to pain/mobility of anterior teeth) – cannot be delayed until the patient may be more stable after the vagus nerve stimulator is placed
  - High risk of further dental trauma
  - Risk of caries related to the oral dryness induced by the anticonvulsant drugs
  - Limited efficacy of brushing exacerbated due to the gingival enlargement (secondary to ethosuximide, sodium valproate, lamotrigine)
  - Potential bleeding tendency (sodium valproate)
  - Difficulty following up the patient due to her lack of co-operation

3) You determine that it is likely the displaced incisors will need extraction. Why is a full blood count and coagulation test advisable prior to this?
   - Routine preoperative full blood count testing for patients undergoing general anaesthesia is mandatory in most countries
   - The patient is taking sodium valproate: this can cause blood dyscrasias, including thrombocytopenia, aplastic anaemia, pure red cell aplasia, macrocytosis, neutropenia, and bleeding disorders (coagulation defects)
4) During the best interest discussion, the patient's family insists that prosthetic rehabilitation is performed during the same general anaesthetic session as any dental extractions. Why is this not recommended?
   - There is a high risk of dental prosthetic fracture due to further trauma
   - It is advisable to delay this procedure until the epilepsy is controlled (at least wait until the efficacy of the vagus nerve stimulator has been observed)
   - It is also preferable to wait until the remodelling of the bone crest is complete and to rule out damage of the contiguous teeth
5) During the intraoperative examination, a comminuted fracture of the external table of the maxillary bone is discovered. What is the ideal approach?
   - Attempt to preserve the alveolus and maintain the integrity of the bone crest
   - Consider applying bone regeneration techniques (with bone or filling biomaterials and barrier membranes) (Figure 1.2.3)
   - The risk of delayed healing and exposure of the membrane should be assessed prior to proceeding
6) What antibiotic should be prescribed after completing the surgical procedure?
   - The recommendation is for beta-lactams, lincosamides and macrolides
   - Metronidazole and quinolones should be avoided (risk of triggering seizures)

General Dental Considerations

Oral/Perioral Findings

- As the result of trauma during seizures

(a)

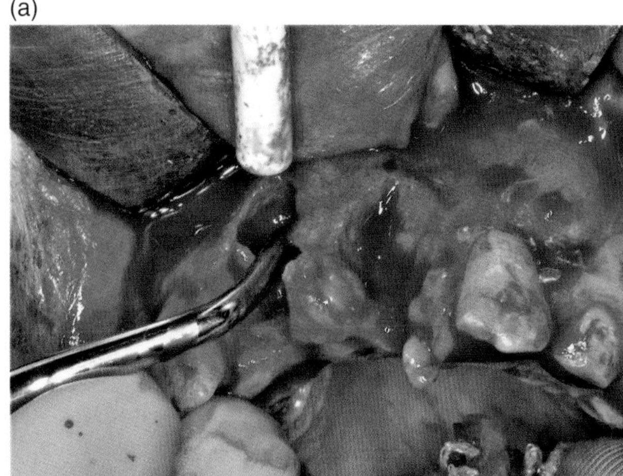

(b)

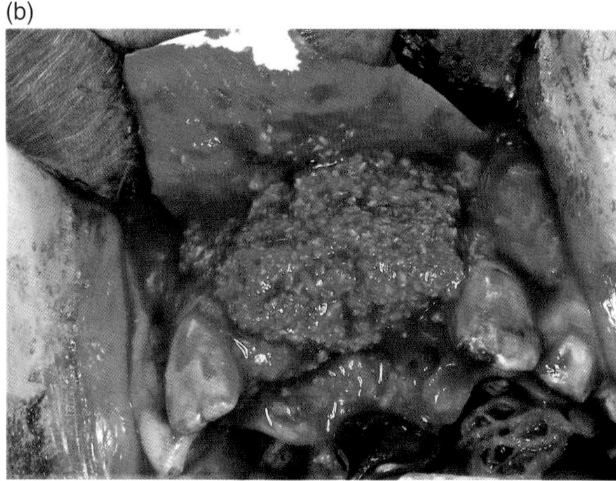

Figure 1.2.3 (a) Tooth extraction and removal of maxillary bone fragments. (b) Bone regeneration techniques application.

(a)

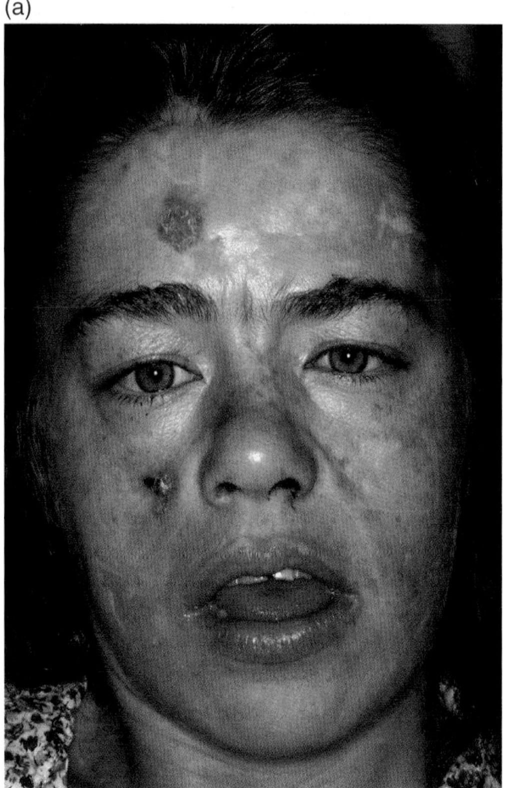

(b)

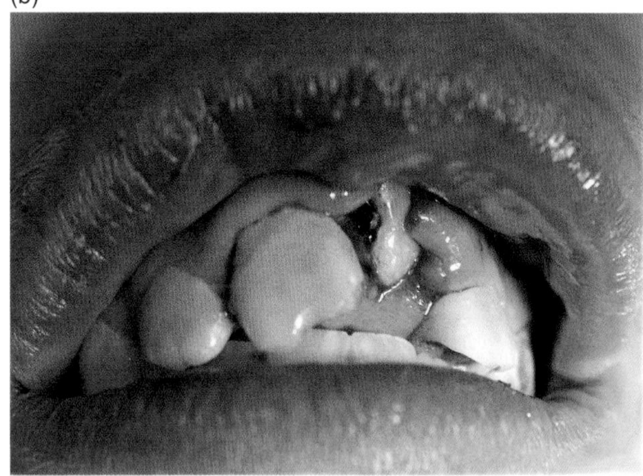

Figure 1.2.4 (a) Sequelae of repeated facial injuries secondary to epileptic seizures. (b) Tooth intrusion as a result of oral trauma during a seizure.

  - Facial trauma (Figure 1.2.4a)
  - Tooth fractures, luxation or avulsion (Figure 1.2.4b)
  - Temporomandibular joint subluxation
  - Lacerations of the tongue or oral mucosa
- Adverse effects of antiepileptic drugs
  - Gingival enlargement (phenytoin, sodium valproate, phenobarbitone, vigabatrin, primidone, mephenytoin and ethosuximide) (Figure 1.2.5)
  - Ulcers (carbamazepine)
  - Petechiae and gingival bleeding (carbamazepine, phenytoin and valproate)
  - Xerostomia (carbamazepine)
  - Dental abscesses (phenytoin, carbamazepine and valproate)
  - Delayed healing (phenytoin, carbamazepine and valproate)
  - Rashes (lamotrigine)
  - Hyperpigmentation (phenytoin)
  - Stevens–Johnson syndrome (carbamazepine, lamotrigine)

Dental Management

- As with many other neurological diseases, the dental treatment plan will be determined more by the degree of disease control than by the type of disease (Table 1.2.1)

- The dental team should be trained to provide emergency management of epileptic seizures in a dental setting; this is particularly important as typical stimuli in the dental clinic (stress, lights, noise) can trigger an epileptic attack (Table 1.2.2)

Section II: Background Information and Guidelines

Definition

Epilepsy is a neurological disorder in which there is recurrent, paroxysmal abnormal brain activity, causing seizures and/or periods of unusual behaviour, sensations and sometimes loss of awareness. Approximately 50 million people worldwide have epilepsy, making it one of the most common neurological diseases globally.

Aetiopathogenesis

- Epilepsy is idiopathic in almost two-thirds of cases and typically presents in childhood
- The disease has also been associated with cerebral hypoxia, infections, trauma, stroke and other neurological diseases, brain tumours and some genetic disorders
- The triggers include food and sleep deprivation, hormonal changes, metabolic disorders, sensory stimuli and a number of legal and illicit drugs
- The pathogenesis of epilepsy includes an imbalance between excitatory (glutamate) and inhibitory activity (gamma-aminobutyric acid) within a neuronal network

Table 1.2.1 Considerations for dental management.

Risk assessment	• Seizures may be triggered by stress, bright lights (including polymerisation lights), fatigue, vibration (electric toothbrushes) • Patient may appear confused and tired if they present for care after a recent seizure • Increased risk of trauma, including dental trauma • Antiepileptic drugs have been associated with adverse effects on the coagulation system – carbamazepine, phenytoin and valproic acid can cause thrombocytopenia
Criteria for referral	• Patients with poorly controlled/intractable epilepsy should be treated in a hospital setting • Medical advice is recommended for patients wearing vagus nerve stimulators
Access/position	• Perform dental treatment during a stable phase when seizure frequency is controlled (preferably at least 6 months without seizures) • Avoid the time of day when seizures are more frequent • Consider minimising stress with pharmaceutical sedation taken by the patient prior to the dental visit (may be prescribed by the doctor) • If protective headgear is worn by the patient, do not remove it • Consider the use of thimble protectors if seizures are associated with mouth clenching
Communication	• Some patients might have associated cognitive impairment • Anticonvulsants can cause bradypsychia, hinder speech and hence impede the ability to understand
Consent/capacity	• Capacity may be impaired by the use of sedative medications taken to reduce stress/anxiety • Following a recent seizure, patients may feel tired and experience memory loss
Anaesthesia/sedation	• Local anaesthesia – Lidocaine may have proconvulsant effects, particularly if administered in large amounts or if inadvertently injected intravenously – It has been suggested that electronic dental analgesia should be avoided • Sedation – It has been suggested that midazolam and nitrous oxide should be avoided • General anaesthesia – Sevoflurane, enflurane, etomidate, methohexital and ketamine should be employed with care

(*Continued*)

Table 1.2.1 (Continued)

Dental treatment	• Before – Ensure antiseizure medication has been taken as prescribed – Minimise seizure triggers (e.g. reduce stress and anxiety by explaining procedures before starting, keep bright light out of patient's eyes and provide dark glasses for the patient to wear) – For patients who take valproate or phenytoin, the results of a full blood count/coagulation screen should be requested before performing an invasive procedure – Patients wearing a vagus nerve stimulator should have a protocol in place preoperatively and attend with the supplied magnet • During – Gingivectomy may be necessary for treating gingival enlargement – Avoid diathermy devices in patients wearing vagus nerve stimulators (bipolar systems are strongly preferred) – Fixed prostheses with a metal structure are recommended although anterior surfaces can be made of resin to facilitate repairs – If a removable prosthesis is chosen, it should be made of radiopaque material, with metal bases or at least acrylic reinforced with a metallic mesh; the design should also take into account the choking hazard – Consider the construction of a bilaminate mouthguard if there is a history of repeated trauma to the teeth • After – Prior to discharge, confirm that the patient is well with no evidence of seizure onset
Drug prescription	• The following drugs should be avoided (interfere with anticonvulsants and/or increase their adverse effects): aspirin, tramadol, metronidazole, quinolones, azole antifungals
Education/prevention	• Avoid electric toothbrushes if vibrations are known to be a trigger for seizures • Good oral hygiene and periodic calculus removal reduce the rate and severity of gingival enlargement • If drug-associated gingival enlargement is recurrent, the physician should be consulted regarding changing the antiepileptic drug • Modification of the brushing technique may be required if there is increased bleeding as a side-effect of some antiepileptic medication

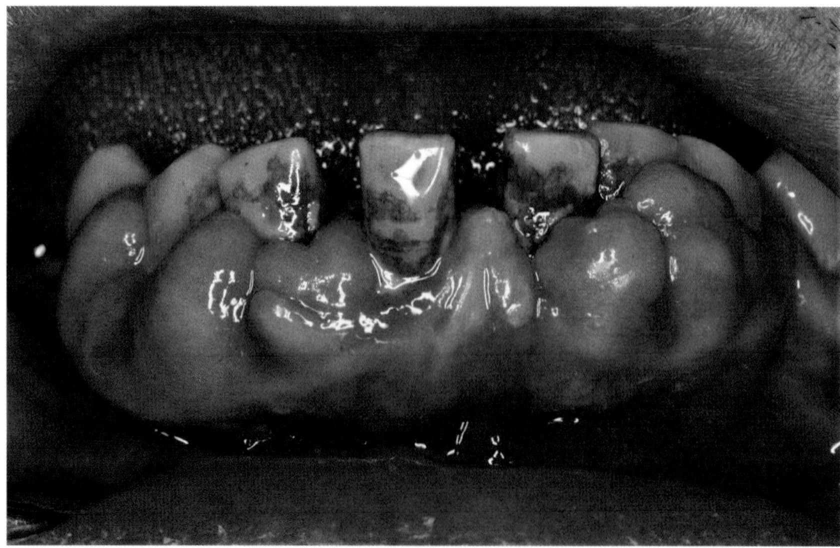

Figure 1.2.5 Severe gingival hyperplasia in a patient on phenytoin.

Table 1.2.2 Management of epileptic seizure in the dental clinic.

Recommendations	Not recommended
• Discontinue the dental treatment • Remove the instrumentation from the mouth • The patient should remain in supine decubitus • Manual application of the vagus nerve stimulation magnet may be helpful • Loosen the patient's clothing and tight fittings • Keep the airway patent, and place the head laterally to prevent aspiration • Time the seizure • Contact medical assistance if the seizure lasts longer than 5 min/is repeated (more than 3 in an hour) • Administer oxygen (10–15 L/min) • Administer midazolam (route/dose varies according to national guidelines; 10 mg buccal midazolam generally recommended for adults; alternatively, 10 mg diazepam intramuscularly or rectally is recommended in some countries) • Assess transferring the patient to a hospital	• Sit the patient up • Transfer the patient to the floor • Place patient in lateral decubitus • Restrict their movements • Put your fingers in their mouth • Insert a mouth opener or similar • Administer benzodiazepines at the start of the seizure (should wait up to 5 min; national guidelines vary) • Give food and drink if they have not fully recovered • Send all patients to a hospital (not required for a patient with known epilepsy who has a self-terminating seizure with normal fit activity, and has recovered well, is accompanied and orientated)

Clinical Presentation

- In March 2017, the International League Against Epilepsy (ILAE), a group of the world's leading epilepsy professionals, introduced a new method to group seizures (Table 1.2.3). The main changes are:
  - 'Partial' becomes 'focal'
  - 'Awareness' is used as a classifier of focal seizures
  - The terms dyscognitive, simple partial, complex partial, psychic and secondarily generalized are eliminated
  - New focal seizure types include automatisms, behaviour arrest, hyperkinetic, autonomic, cognitive and emotional
  - Atonic, clonic, epileptic spasms, myoclonic and tonic seizures can be of either focal or generalised onset
  - Focal to bilateral tonic–clonic seizure replaces secondarily generalised seizure
  - New generalised seizure types are absence with eyelid myoclonia, myoclonic absence, myoclonic–atonic, myoclonic–tonic–clonic
  - Seizures of unknown onset may have features that can still be classified
- In view of this, seizures are divided into 3 main groups depending on:
  - Site of onset in the brain: focal/generalised/unknown
  - Level of awareness: aware/impaired
  - Presence of other symptoms: motor/non-motor
- This is summarised in Table 1.2.4

Diagnosis

- The diagnosis is established mainly based on clinical findings and electroencephalograms (EEGs) (Figure 1.2.6)

Table 1.2.3 New classification of epilepsy.

Type of seizure	Type of epilepsy (EEG activity)	Aetiology
• Focal • Generalised • Unknown	• Focal • Generalised • Generalised and focal	• Structural • Genetic • Infectious • Metabolic • Immune • Unknown

Source: Adapted from Scheffer, I.E., Berkovic, S., Capovilla, G. et al. (2017). ILAE classification of the epilepsies: Position paper of the ILAE Commission for Classification and Terminology. *Epilepsia* 58: 512–21.

Table 1.2.4 Clinical presentation of seizures.

Type of seizure	Characteristics	Signs/symptoms
Focal onset (may affect one lobe or a large part of one hemisphere)	• Focal aware or focal impaired awareness • Motor onset or non-motor onset • Can be followed by a bilateral tonic–clonic seizure	**Motor symptoms** • Automatisms (lip-smacking, chewing movements, running, cycling, kicking, repeatedly picking up objects or pulling at clothes) • Loud cry or scream • Twitching, jerking or stiffening movements of a body part • Sudden loss of muscle tone or limbs suddenly becoming stiff **Non-motor symptoms** • Changes in sensation, emotions, experiences • Feeling of déjà vu (feeling like you have been here before) • Unusual smell or taste • Sudden intense feeling of fear or joy • Numbness or tingling • Visual disturbances (coloured/flashing lights or hallucinations)
Generalised onset	• Motor (tonic–clonic/other) or non-motor (absence)	**Tonic–clonic** • Typically last 1–3 min • At the start of the seizure: – The person becomes unconscious – Body goes stiff and they may fall – May cry out – May bite their tongue or cheek • During the seizure: – Jerk and shake as their muscles relax and tighten rhythmically – Breathing might be affected and become difficult or sound noisy – Skin may change colour and become very pale or bluish – Incontinence may occur • After the seizure: – Often feel tired, confused, have a headache or want to sleep **Absence** • More common in children • Can be frequent • Last a few seconds • Typical absences: 'daydreaming', blank, unresponsive, may be missed • Atypical: start and end more slowly, can last longer, may also include reduced muscle tone
Unknown onset	• Motor (tonic/clonic/epileptic spasms) or non-motor	• Variable symptoms as described above
Unclassified	• Due to inadequate information/inability to place in the above categories	

Source: Adapted from Scheffer, I.E., Berkovic, S., Capovilla, G. et al. (2017). ILAE classification of the epilepsies: Position paper of the ILAE Commission for Classification and Terminology. *Epilepsia* 58: 512–521.

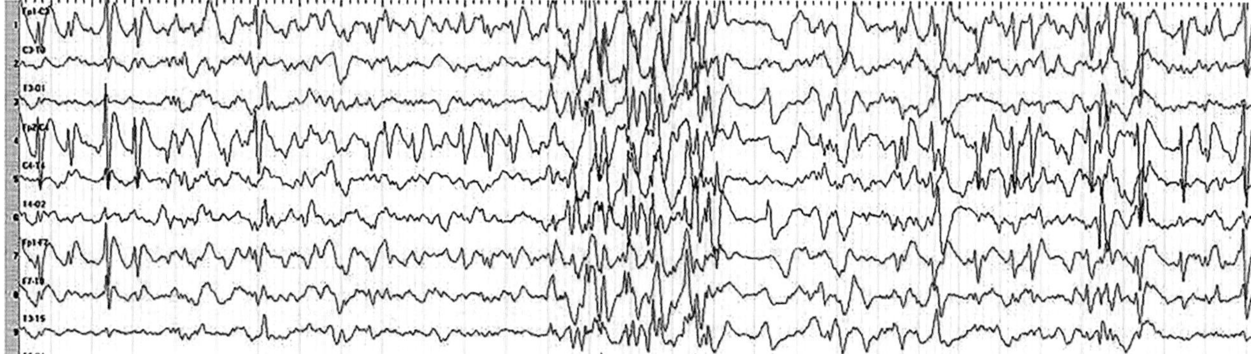

Figure 1.2.6 Electroencephalogram (EEG) showing epileptiform activity.

- High-resolution structural images (high-field magnetic resonance) and functional radionuclide imaging (positron emission tomography/single-photon emission computed tomography) can be useful (Figure 1.2.7)
- Genetic testing has gained importance in diagnosing some forms of epilepsy

Management

- Drug treatment with glutamate inhibitors (e.g. carbamazepine, lamotrigine, phenytoin and topiramate)
- Gamma-aminobutyric acid enhancers (e.g. barbiturates, benzodiazepines, gabapentin, primidone, tiagabine, valproate and vigabatrin)
- Surgery for drug-resistant focal epilepsy (resection or disconnection of a circumscribed cerebral area, or vagal nerve stimulation)

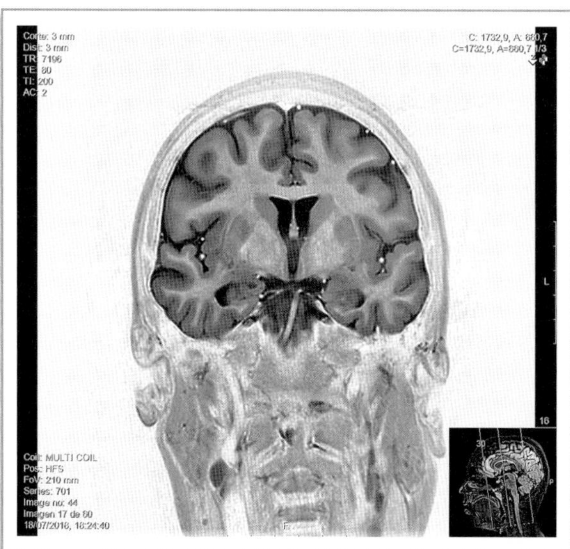

Figure 1.2.7 Magnetic resonance imaging (MRI) can identify structural changes in the brain that may cause seizures.

Prognosis

- The prognosis is determined by the underlying disease, the extent of the brain damage and the severity and frequency of the seizures
- The estimated mortality of status epilepticus (generalised tonic–clonic seizures that last more than 5 minutes) is approximately 20%
- The risk of premature death in people with epilepsy is up to 3 times higher than for the general population

A World/Transcultural View

- Approximately 80% of people with epilepsy live in low- and middle-income countries
- Unfortunately, 75% of people with epilepsy living in low-income countries do not receive the treatment they need
- In many parts of the world, people with epilepsy and their families suffer from stigma and discrimination
- The religious beliefs prevalent in some countries have resulted in a portion of the population still believing that epilepsy is caused by supernatural possession, resorting to religious healing for its treatment
- In Africa, Asia and Latin America, alternative therapies such as medicinal herbs are often used to treat epilepsy (e.g. rhizomes of *Acorus calamus* and leaves from the *Bacopa monnieri* plant), most of which have not been pharmacologically evaluated
- The socio-economic and cultural environment significantly affects accessibility to drug treatment, which can jeopardise access for 75–90% of individuals with potentially treatable epilepsy in low-income countries

Recommended Reading

Aragon, C.E. and Burneo, J.G. (2007). Understanding the patient with epilepsy and seizures in the dental practice. *J. Can. Dent. Assoc.* 73: 71–76.

Cornacchio, A.L., Burneo, J.G., and Aragon, C.E. (2011). The effects of antiepileptic drugs on oral health. *J. Can. Dent. Assoc.* 77: b140.

Davidson, G.T., Eaton, M., and Paul, S.P. (2016). Childhood epilepsy: a clinical update. *Community Pract.* 89: 25–29.

Fiske, J. and Boyle, C. (2002). Epilepsy and oral care. *Dent. Update* 29: 180–187.

Morgan, H.I., Abou, E.F.R.K., Kabil, N.S., and Elagouza, I. (2019). Assessment of oral health status of children with epilepsy: a retrospective cohort study. *Int. J. Paediatr. Dent.* 29: 79–85.

Robbins, M.R. (2009). Dental management of special needs patients who have epilepsy. *Dent. Clin. North Am.* 53: 295–309.

Schöpper, M., Ludolph, A.C., and Fauser, S. (2016). Dental care in patients with epilepsy: a survey of 82 patients and their attending dentists and neurologists in southern Germany. *Int. Dent. J.* 66: 366–374.

Thijs, R.D., Surges, R., O'Brien, T.J., and Sander, J.W. (2019). Epilepsy in adults. *Lancet* 393: 689–701.

1.3 Muscular Dystrophy

Section I: Clinical Scenario and Dental Considerations

Clinical Scenario

A 15-year-old patient is referred by the Ear, Nose and Throat (ENT) specialist for an orthodontic assessment. There is concern that the patient's palatal morphology may be responsible for his chronic nasal respiratory distress (Figure 1.3.1).

Medical History

- Child of a primiparous mother who had Steinert myotonic myopathy (also known as myotonic dystrophy type 1)
- Patient diagnosed with myotonic muscular dystrophy, confirmed during the first days of life
- Hypertrophic cardiomyopathy
- Recurrent respiratory infections
- Obstructive sleep apnea
- Kyphoscoliosis
- Hypermetropia (long-sightedness)

Medications

- Atenolol
- Prednisone

Dental History

- Good level of co-operation
- Regular dental attender (yearly)
- No previous dental treatment received
- Patient brushes his teeth on a regular basis without supervision

Social History

- Mother deceased as a result of complications relating to the myopathy
- Father estranged
- Lives with his elderly grandparents, who are his primary care-givers and are very protective of him
- Requires specially arranged hospital transport to attend his appointments with both of his grandparents attending with him
- Mild intellectual disability
- Attends a public school

Oral Examination

- Fair oral hygiene
- Caries in #36 and #46
- High-arched/pointed (ogival) palate
- Anterior open bite (Figure 1.3.2)

Radiological Examination

- Orthopantomogram – confirmed the clinical findings (Figure 1.3.3)
- Pattern of vertical mandibular growth (lateral cephalogram)

Structured Learning

1) What factors are considered important in assessing the risk of managing this patient?
   - Social
     - Transport arrangements to attend dental appointments
     - Excessive protectiveness by his guardians (the grandparents have already lost their daughter to the disease)
   - Medical
     - Myotonic dystrophy type 1-associated myotonia and multiorgan damage; muscle weakness, sleep disorders
     - Diagnosis confirmed at birth is generally associated with a poor prognosis
     - Risk resulting from cardiomyopathy and respiratory impairment
     - Position in the dental chair compromised by the kyphoscoliosis

A Practical Approach to Special Care in Dentistry, First Edition. Edited by Pedro Diz Dios and Navdeep Kumar.

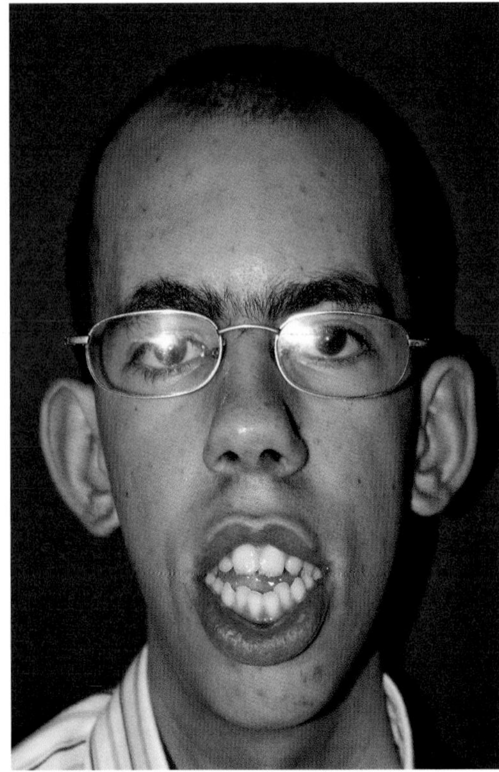

Figure 1.3.1 Facial myopathy with severe open mouth.

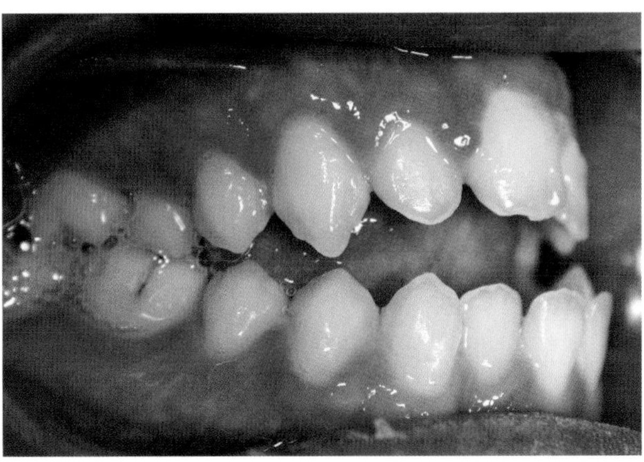

Figure 1.3.2 Anterior open bite.

- Dental
  - Risk of aspiration during the dental procedure
  - Unsupervised oral hygiene habits
  - Follow-up difficulties due to social situation

2) The patient is taking prednisone at a dose of 20 mg/day. What are the implications of this when performing an invasive dental procedure?
   - Delayed healing

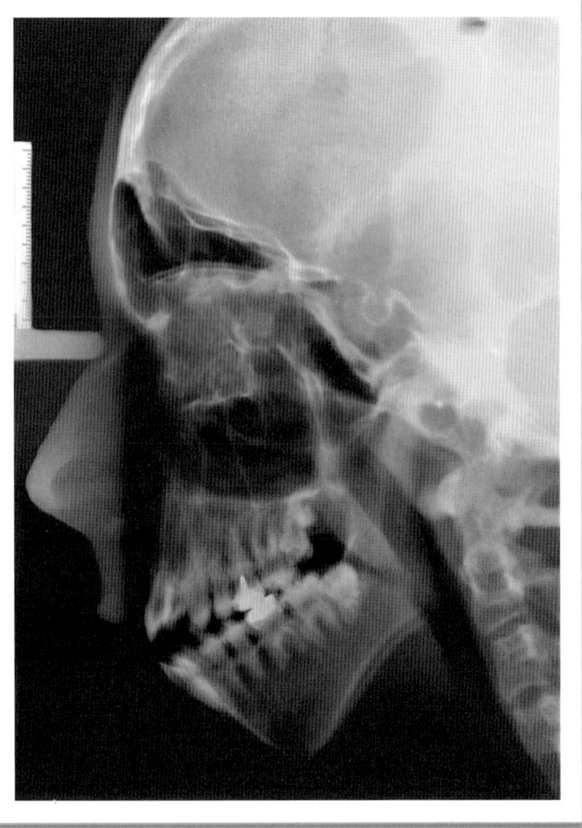

Figure 1.3.3 Lateral cephalogram showing a dolichocephalic growth pattern (relatively long skull).

   - Increased risk of significant infection
   - Adrenal crisis may be triggered by surgical interventions due to chronic hypothalamic–pituitary–adrenal axis suppression – a corticosteroid supplementation protocol is required to prevent this (see Chapter 12.1)
3) What precautions should be undertaken in view of the patient's history of hypertrophic cardiomyopathy?
   - Limit the administration of anaesthetics containing adrenaline and avoid intravascular injections
   - Some cardiologists may disagree with international consensus guidelines, and hence recommend that these patients should receive antibiotic prophylaxis to prevent bacterial endocarditis if an invasive dental procedure is planned
   - A number of drugs, such as atenolol, can cause orthostatic hypotension
4) The patient's grandparents are insistent that an orthodontic appliance should be fitted as they feel that the palate is becoming more arched. What requirements should the patient satisfy before proceeding with orthodontic treatment?

- The oral hygiene should be extremely good
- The dentition should be stabilised, including restoration of #36 and #46
- The patient should be able to accept and tolerate both the intraoral and extraoral appliances
- Close liaison with the medical team is required in order to evaluate the risk/benefit of proceeding, taking into account the progression of the muscular dystrophy

5) What type of appliances are recommended?
   - In general, functional orthodontic devices are not recommended because the biological muscle forces are usually impaired
   - Devices that may be prescribed for this patient include a palatal expander, multibracket appliances (for tooth alignment), a transpalatal bar with a stimulator/lingual pearl and/or a tongue guard and extraoral appliances such as a vertical traction chinguard
   - However, due to the age of this patient, they may not be effective
6) What is the prognosis of the orthodontic treatment?
   - The prognosis for the open bite and vertical mandibular growth is poor
   - The defect cannot be corrected in many patients, and the recurrence rate is high
7) Why are prevention and periodic follow-up especially important for this patient?
   - The patient will have increasing difficulty performing mechanical oral hygiene techniques
   - Physiological mouth cleaning will worsen with time
   - The bacterial load of the oral cavity can promote respiratory infections
   - Managing the patient in the dental clinic will become increasingly complex

(a)

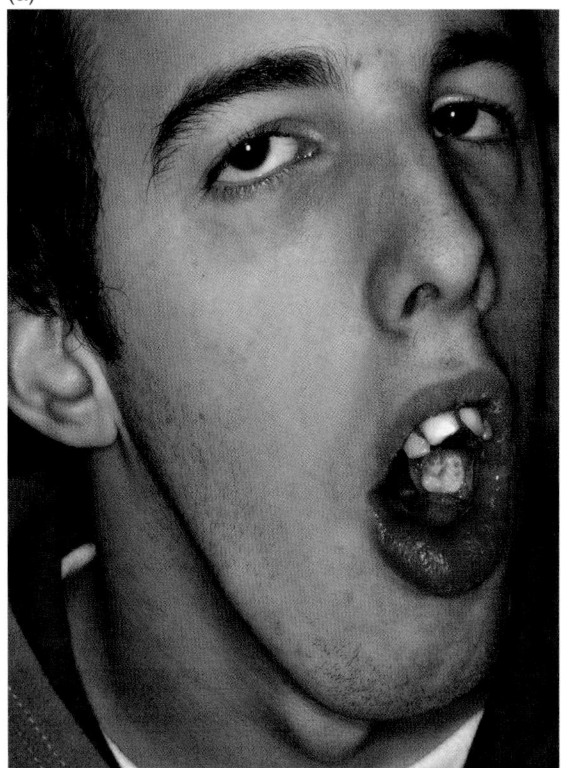

(b)

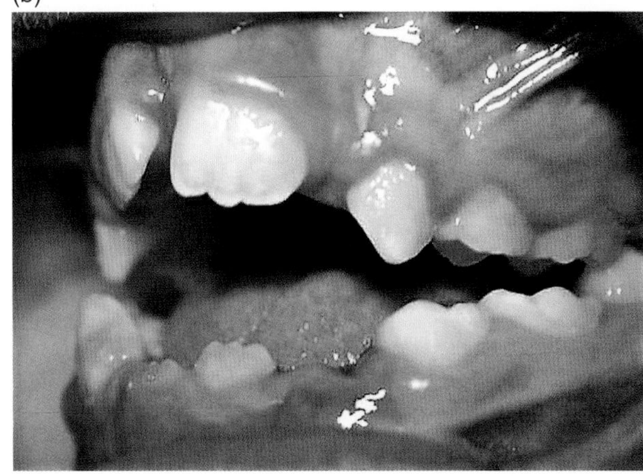

Figure 1.3.4 (a) Facial myopathy (hypotonia, dolichocephaly and open mouth). (b) Malocclusion with anterior open bite.

General Dental Considerations

Oral Findings

- Difficulties in chewing, swallowing and phonation
- Facial myopathy (hypotonia, dolichocephaly, open mouth) (Figure 1.3.4a)
- Malocclusion with anterior open bite, posterior crossbite and tendency to Angle class III (Figure 1.3.4b)
- Labial incompetence, mouth breathing, macroglossia and lingual protrusion
- Tooth eruption delay
- Agenesis, microdontia and hypoplasia, typically of the premolars
- Accumulation of dental plaque and calculus, leading to gingivitis
- Bone disorders of the temporomandibular joint, limited mouth opening and occasional joint subluxation
- Oral manifestations secondary to drugs such as corticosteroids, antiarrhythmic agents, tricyclic antidepressants, benzodiazepines and calcium antagonists

Dental Management

- The dental treatment plan will be determined by the muscle groups involved, the disease severity and the patient's life expectancy (Table 1.3.1)
- Prevention is the key focus because the difficulties in performing dental procedures in these patients tend to worsen with time

Section II: Background Information and Guidelines

Definition

Muscular dystrophy consists of a heterogeneous group of hereditary diseases characterised by progressive weakness and impairment of skeletal muscles. These diseases are the main degenerative diseases in childhood. Duchenne muscular dystrophy is the most prevalent type, with 1 case per 3500 births, with no geographical or ethnic preferences.

Aetiopathogenesis

- It has been suggested that muscular dystrophy is the result of a mutation in the genes that program critical proteins for muscle integrity, such as dystrophin
- Dystrophin is found not only in skeletal muscle but also in the smooth and cardiac muscles, and also in the brain
- The pattern of inheritance is variable:
  - Sex-linked muscular distrophies – Duchenne, Becker, Emery–Dreifuss
  - Autosomal dominant – facioscapulohumeral, distal, ocular, oculopharyngeal
  - Autosomal recessive – limb-girdle form

Clinical Presentation

- There are more than 30 different types of muscular dystrophy, which vary in symptoms and severity
- There are nine different categories used for diagnosis (Table 1.3.2)
- The clinical manifestations are determined by the type of muscular dystrophy

Table 1.3.1 Considerations for dental management.

Risk assessment	• Progressive deterioration/poor prognosis (depending on the subtype) • Comorbidities may be present (e.g. cardiomyopathy, arrhythmia, hypoventilation and neuropsychiatric disorders) • Aspiration risk due to the loss of protective reflexes • Pressure ulcers (decubitus) may be present • Long-term use of corticosteroids can result in adrenocortical suppression • Risk of rhabdomyolysis associated with general anaesthesia
Criteria for referral	• Patients can often be treated in a conventional dental clinic, especially during the initial stages of the disease • Referral to a specialised clinic or hospital centre is determined by the patient's general condition (e.g. respiratory distress, severe heart disease and highly advanced stages of the disease) • Patients with severe muscle contractures and/or medical complications should typically be treated in a hospital setting
Access/position	• Physical assistance for the transfer • Orthopaedic devices may be worn • Wheelchair use is common • Short sessions (frequent changes in position) • Dental chair positioned at 45° • In advanced phases of the disease, emergency dental care may be provided in a home (domiciliary) or hospital setting
Communication	• A consultation with the patient's doctor is advisable to determine the degree of disease control and the presence of complications • Occasionally, the disease is accompanied by intellectual disability • Verbal communication may be impeded due to dysarthria among their manifestations (e.g. oculopharyngeal muscular dystrophy)
Consent/capacity	• In most cases, capacity is not impaired • Inform the patient that the dental treatment plan will need to consider the expected progression and life expectancy in relation to the muscular dystrophy

(*Continued*)

Table 1.3.1 (Continued)

Anaesthesia/sedation	• Local anaesthesia – Caution is advised when using local anaesthesia with vasoconstrictors in patients with cardiomyopathy and arrhythmias • Sedation – Avoid opioids and benzodiazepines for conscious sedation (respiratory depression) • General anaesthesia – May be contraindicated in cases of cardiomyopathy or severe respiratory disease – Endotracheal intubation can be challenging (due to kyphoscoliosis or neck flexion) – Neuromuscular blockers and some inhaled anaesthetics produce respiratory depression – Succinylcholine administration in patients with Duchenne and Becker muscular dystrophies is associated with life-threatening rhabdomyolysis and hyperkalaemia – Risk of regurgitation, prolonged hypoventilation and aspiration pneumonia post intubation
Dental treatment	• Before – Assess the requirement for corticosteroid supplementation – Assess the need for mouth props – Orthodontic therapy to improve the chewing function and the airway may be considered – Rehabilitation with tooth-supported and implant-supported prostheses may be considered (isolated cases have been published) • During – If mouth opening is impaired, consider careful use of mouth props (exercise increased caution as protective reflexes may be lost) – Use rubber dam (decreased protective reflexes) – Use a high-volume suction to prevent aspiration • After – Ensure that the oral cavity is clear of all debris
Drug prescription	• Consider drug interactions with medications used to treat comorbidities (e.g. selective serotonin reuptake inhibitors inhibit several families of hepatic enzymes, which may delay the biotransformation of codeine to its active metabolite)
Education/prevention	• Difficulties maintaining good mechanical oral hygiene • Dietary counselling • Consider the use of topical fluoride and fluoride varnish • Fissure sealants may be considered • Establish regular check-up visits to control plaque/tartar – increase frequency as muscular control deteriorates

- Duchenne muscular dystrophy is the most common amongst children and is characterised by:
  - Inheritance (linked to the X chromosome)
  - Onset in the first years of childhood
  - Involvement of all muscles (generalised muscle weakness)
  - Muscle pseudohypertrophy (enlargement)
  - Pelvic girdle muscle impairment
  - Difficulty standing up (Gowers sign)
  - Severe lumbar lordosis and peculiar gait ('duck-like')
  - Confined to wheelchair before puberty
  - Cardiomyopathy
  - Respiratory impairment
  - In some cases, intellectual impairment may be present
  - Death in the first years of the adult stage

Diagnosis

- The initial diagnosis is based on clinical findings (e.g. generalised muscle weakness)

Table 1.3.2 Classification and characteristics of muscular dystrophy.

Type	Sex	Age at onset	Muscles involved	Associated complications	Life expectancy
Duchenne muscular dystrophy	Males	3–5 years	All	Cardiomyopathy Intellectual disability	Die at the end of adolescence
Becker muscular dystrophy	Males	10–20 years	All	Cardiomyopathy (uncommon)	Normal
Emery–Dreifuss muscular dystrophy	Males	<10 years	All	Cardiomyopathy (severe)	Die at 30–50 years
Limb-girdle muscular dystrophy	Both sexes	15–20 years	Pelvic girdle and shoulders	Cardiomyopathy	Variable
Facioscapulohumeral muscular dystrophy	Both sexes	15–20 years	Face and shoulders	Cardiomyopathy (uncommon)	Normal
Myotonic muscular dystrophy – types 1 and 2	Both sexes	20–30 years	All	Cardiomyopathy Cutaneous dystrophy Ocular disorders Intellectual disability	Die at 30–50 years (earlier for type 1)
Congenital muscular dystrophy	Both sexes	Birth	All	Respiratory distress Intellectual disability	Variable
Oculopharyngeal muscular dystrophy	Both sexes	40–50 years	Upper eyelids, pharynx, tongue	Vision problems Dysphagia Cardiomyopathy	Normal
Distal muscular dystrophy	Both sexes	40–60 years	Distal	Respiratory distress (in advanced phases)	Normal

- Blood tests: serum levels of creatine phosphokinase (CPK), aspartate transaminase (AST) and lactate dehydrogenase (LDH)
- Electromyography
- Muscle biopsy (histopathological and immunological analysis of the muscle) (Figure 1.3.5)
- In some types of muscular dystrophy, genetic analysis may be of value

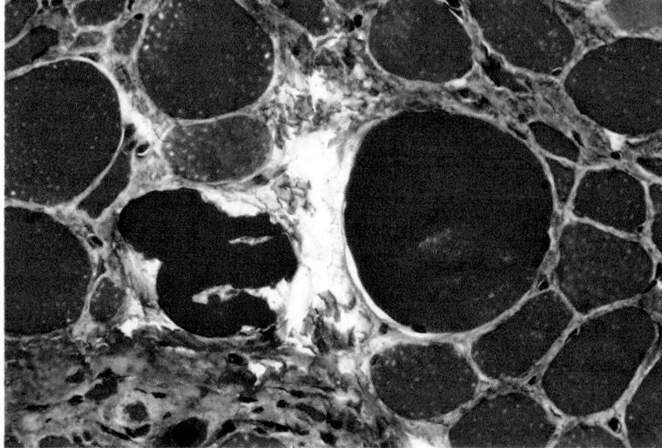

Figure 1.3.5 Diagnostic muscle biopsy showing random variation in fibre size, increase in fibrosis and degeneration of muscle fibres (Masson trichrome staining, ×20).

Management

- Physical therapy
- Occasionally orthopaedic surgery to help correct the shortening of muscles or to improve scoliosis (Figure 1.3.6)

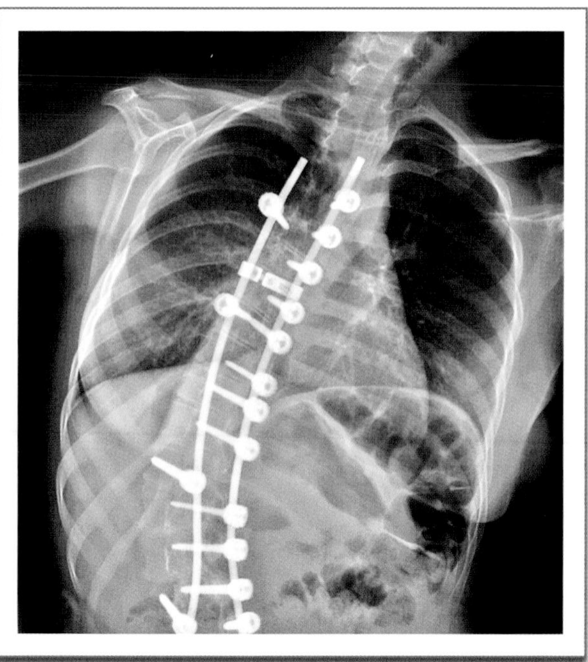

Figure 1.3.6 Orthopaedic surgery to improve scoliosis.

- Additionally, cardiac surgery and/or surgery to repair cataracts may be required
- Corticosteroids, cardioprotective agents, antidepressants, ventilation with positive non-invasive pressure
- Although there is no known cure, there has been notable progress in correcting the underlying genetic mutations

Prognosis

- The prognosis for muscular dystrophy depends on the type and severity of symptoms
- However, most individuals do lose the ability to walk and eventually require a wheelchair
- Life expectancy is reduced if there is pulmonary dysfunction and/or cardiac involvement
- In most cases, the patients die at the end of adolescence or at the start of adulthood, as the consequence of pneumonia or cardiopulmonary failure

A World/Transcultural View

- There are major differences between countries in terms of the prevalence of muscular dystrophy. For example, the rate of Duchenne muscular dystrophy in South Africa is estimated at 1 case/100 000 males compared with approximately 17 cases/100 000 males in Sweden
- The survival of individuals with some varieties of muscular dystrophy has increased significantly in countries with access to corticotherapy, cardiac medical treatment and mechanical ventilation

Recommended Reading

Balasubramaniam, R., Sollecito, T.P., and Stoopler, E.T. (2008). Oral health considerations in muscular dystrophies. *Spec. Care Dentist.* 28: 243–253.

Flanigan, K.M. (2014). Duchenne and Becker muscular dystrophies. *Neurol. Clin.* 32: 671–688.

Goiato, M.C. (2016). Duchenne muscular dystrophy and the stomatognathic system. *Dev. Med. Child Neurol.* 58: 650.

Mielnik-Błaszczak, M. and Małgorzata, B. (2007). Duchenne muscular dystrophy – a dental healthcare program. *Spec. Care Dentist.* 27: 23–25.

Morinushi, T. and Mastumoto, S. (1986). Oral findings and a proposal for a dental health care program for patients with Duchenne type muscular dystrophy. *Spec. Care Dentist.* 6: 117–119.

Symons, A.L., Townsend, G.C., and Hughes, T.E. (2002). Dental characteristics of patients with Duchenne muscular dystrophy. *ASDC J. Dent. Child.* 69: 277–283.

Waldrop, M.A. and Flanigan, K.M. (2019). Update in Duchenne and Becker muscular dystrophy. *Curr. Opin. Neurol.* 32: 722–727.

2

Cognitive Impairment

2.1 Attention Deficit and Hyperactivity Disorder (ADHD)

Section I: Clinical Scenario and Dental Considerations

Clinical Scenario

A 13-year-old male presents to the dental clinic with his mother. She is concerned about her son's teeth, stating that 'they are discoloured, and keep falling out'. Other dentists have been unable to examine her son and have refused to provide care.

Medical History

- Attention deficit and hyperactivity disorder (ADHD) diagnosed at the age of 5 years old
- Self-harm predominantly associated with stress
- Mild learning disability
- Dental anxiety

Medications

- Methylphenidate

Dental History

- Managed to have a single amalgam filling placed in a deciduous tooth when he was 9 years old
- Last dental visit was 18 months ago when repair of a fractured incisal tip was attempted; the tooth is asymptomatic at present
- Mother reports this was a traumatic experience for her son as the dental nurse held her son down to allow the dentist to examine the tooth
- Dentists have since declined to provide care as the patient has refused to co-operate with examination and treatment
- Now an irregular attender
- Only brushes his teeth once a day or when he remembers and refuses help

Social History

- Lives with parents
- Youngest of five siblings
- Only member of the family with a learning disability and ADHD
- Attends a special education school
- Poor dietary habits, snacks frequently on biscuits and sweets, consumes fizzy drinks daily

Oral Examination

(performed within 2 desensitisation visits)

- Generalised plaque, calculus, gingival inflammation and spontaneous bleeding
- Enamel demineralisation at gingival margins most pronounced on the buccal aspect of the upper teeth
- Fractured incisal tip of tooth #21 – simple without pulp exposure, no mobility (Figure 2.1.1)
- Caries: #54, #53, #65, #75, #84 and #85 (Figures 2.1.2 and 2.1.3)
- Stained fissures: #16 and #26
- Maxillary canine bulge can be palpated buccally on both sides

Radiological Examination

- Patient required acclimatisation appointments to enable bite-wing radiographs (Figure 2.1.4)
- Hence #54 and #65 present in clinical images but missing in the radiographic images as they had exfoliated naturally by the time the images were taken
- Patient did not accept orthopantomogram, hence further evaluation not possible

Structured Learning

1) What factors may be impacting on this patient's poor oral health and increased caries risk?
   - Compliance issues in daily life
   - Lack of perceived need
   - Cognitive difficulties due to learning disability
   - Motor problems due to hyperactivity

A Practical Approach to Special Care in Dentistry, First Edition. Edited by Pedro Diz Dios and Navdeep Kumar.

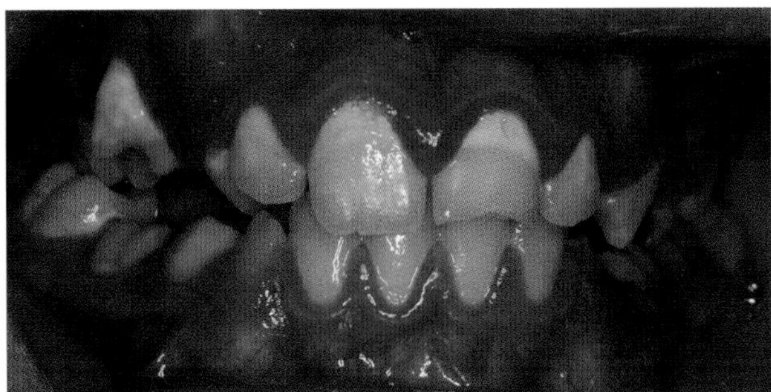

Figure 2.1.1 Dentition: generalised plaque, calculus and gingival inflammation, fracture of the incisal tip of tooth # 21.

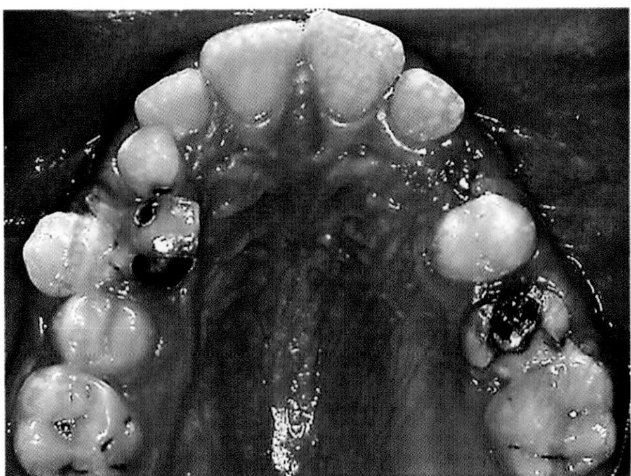

Figure 2.1.2 Maxilla: caries in teeth #54, #53, #65, stained fissures in #16 and #26.

- Poor oral health habits and diet
- Irregular dental check-ups due to dental anxiety and lack of access
- Oral dryness due to methylphenidate
- Changes in oral health behaviour during adolescence

2) How would you manage the dental caries?

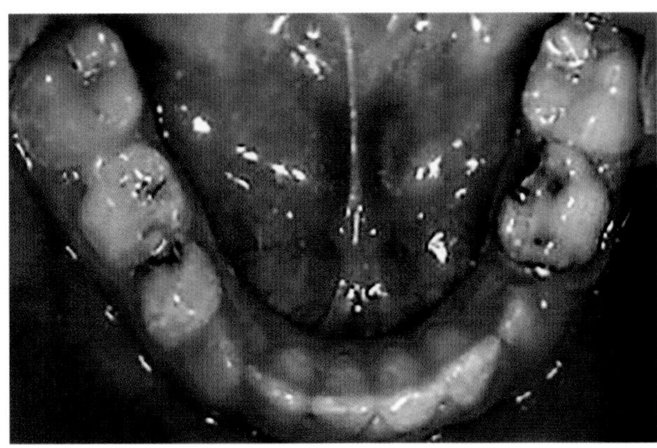

Figure 2.1.3 Mandible: caries in teeth #75, #84 and #85; calculus on the lingual aspect of lower incisors; buccal enamel demineralisation.

- Reduce caries risk – dietary analysis, educate parents, reinforce oral hygiene, consider fluoride supplementation
- Acclimatise the patient further – he has already demonstrated improved compliance by allowing bitewing radiographs
- Reattempt an orthopantomogram and consult with an orthodontist as the patient is at a mixed dentition stage
- If compliance is limited, plan to allow deciduous teeth to exfoliate if they are asymptomatic and focus on the permanent dentition
- Place fissure sealants and attempt restorations (temporary restorations can be recommended and any local anaesthetics avoided for the patient to get used to)

3) The patient asks you to repair the fractured incisal tip #21 as he does not like its appearance. What factors would you need to consider?

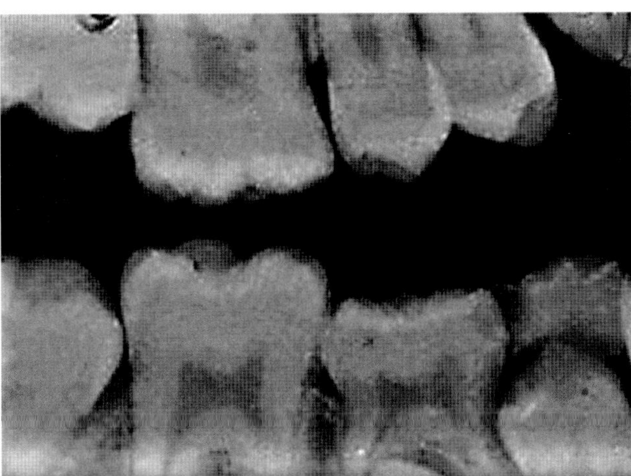

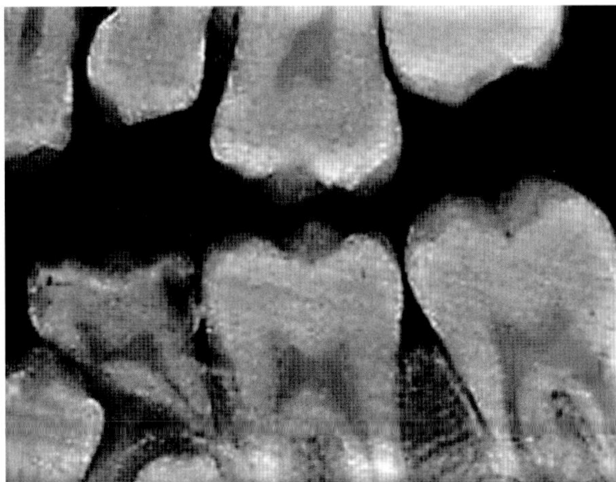

Figure 2.1.4 Right and left bitewing radiographs: mixed dentition; caries in #75, #84 and #85.

- Further information regarding how and when the fracture occurred, and any related symptoms
- Capacity of the patient to understand what is planned
- In relation to previous successful dental filling placement at the age of 9 years old:
  - Where and how it was carried out?
  - How co-operative was the patient?
  - What behavioural modification tools were used?
- In relation to unsuccessful treatment a year ago:
  - Why was clinical holding used, i.e. was it to assist with uncontrolled movements?
  - Was it agreed and consent in place?
  - Why did it go wrong?
- With this information, confirm the modified plan

4) The patient's mother has also noticed that her son makes a loud noise with his teeth predominantly at night – what could be the cause and why?
   - Sleep and day bruxism has been linked to ADHD
   - It may also be a side-effect of the medications used to manage the condition, including methylphenidate
5) What other factors could be contributing to tooth surface loss?
   - Xerostomia due to methylphenidate
   - Dietary acid/erosion due to high sugar and acid intake
6) What factors are considered important in assessing the risk of managing this patient?
   - Social
     - Irregular attender, dental anxiety
     - Learning disability, poor compliance and tolerance
     - Self-injurious behaviour
     - Availability of escort
   - Medical
     - Potential side-effects associated with methylphenidate include headache or nausea
     - Signs of trauma/self-harm
   - Dental
     - Bruxism leading to tooth surface loss
     - Increased risk of caries due to xerostomia induced by methylphenidate
     - High caries rate
     - Cariogenic diet
     - History of dental trauma

General Dental Considerations

Oral Findings

- Poor oral hygiene due to reduced attention span and compliance for tooth brushing
- Increased caries and periodontal disease
- Bruxism
- Higher risk for dental/oral trauma due to inattention, impulsivity
- Adults are at potentially high risk for periodontal disease and oral cancer due to high rates of smoking
- Medication-related side-effects including xerostomia, dysphagia, dysgeusia, bruxism, angio-oedema, glossitis and orofacial dyskinesias

Dental Management

- Compliance for the delivery of dental care can vary (Table 2.1.1)
- Treatment should be modified based on reassessment of the patient on the day of the appointment

Section II: Background Information and Guidelines

Definition

ADHD, once called hyperkinesis or minimal brain dysfunction, is a disorder that interferes with the ability to persist in a task and to exercise age-appropriate inhibition. It affects 3–5% of children and is twice as common in boys as in girls. It often continues into adolescence and adulthood.

Aetiopathogenesis

- The main cause is unclear
- Physical triggers: hyperkinetic syndrome, brain damage, low intelligence, anxiety states, drug abuse, high intake of refined sugar and food additives (e.g. tartrazine sensitivity)
- Social triggers: child–parent relationship, rejection or overprotection, inconsistent discipline, lack of parental love, marital disharmony, depression, institutionalised, excessive demands from school
- Evidence for familial predisposition

Clinical Presentation

- ADHD is characterised by inattention and hyperactivity and/or impulsivity, which are excessive, long-term and pervasive
- Signs of inattention include:
  - Becoming easily distracted by irrelevant sights and sounds
  - Failing to pay attention to details and making careless mistakes
  - Rarely following instructions carefully and completely

Table 2.1.1 Considerations for dental management.

Risk assessment	• Inappropriate behaviour with uncontrolled movements or aggression • Lack of attention with tendency to stand up suddenly and explore surroundings/leave the clinic room • This may cause distress and potential injury for staff and the patient • Contamination of surfaces may occur as the patient explores and examines the contents of surgery and cupboards • Dental treatment may be considered an exhausting experience for both the patient and the dental team • Potential interaction of dental local anaesthetics with medications used to manage ADHD
Criteria for referral	• Patients with very disruptive behaviour who may require pharmacological adjuncts to enable dental treatment to be undertaken safely may be treated in specialist dental services
Access/position	• Ensure an appropriate escort is available • Consult parents/escort as to the most suitable time of day to arrange an appointment • Do not interrupt meals or prescheduled activities • Appointments need to be short with no waiting time before the patient is seen
Communication	• Ensure that language and sentences are kept short and simple • Use visual aids such as pictures or videos so that parents can run 'training sessions' at home regarding the process of visiting the dentist • Psychological support from the patient's care team may also be available
Capacity/consent	• Explanation of the planned procedure should be provided using simple terminology and short sentences • Parents/guardians (for children)/appropriate escorts should be involved in the consent process
Anaesthesia/sedation	• Local anaesthesia – The administration of local anaesthesia solutions containing vasopressors, such as levonordefrin, epinephrine or norepinephrine, to patients receiving tricyclic antidepressants or monoamine oxidase inhibitors should be avoided if possible as it may produce severe, prolonged hypertension and tachycardia – In situations when concurrent therapy is necessary, careful patient monitoring is essential – Patient may need manageable reassurance – 'Tell–show–do' may be of value especially when applied by a dentist trained in child psychology – If cannot be given safely, alternative approaches should be considered • Sedation – Orally administered agents, such as diazepam, should be avoided as they exacerbate rather than depress overactivity – Relative analgesia using nitrous oxide and oxygen may be useful – Although intravenous sedation may be used, the success of sedation is unpredictable, the outcome of previous sedations being the best prognosis indicator • General anaesthesia – Patients requiring complex dental treatment and those uncontrolled with sedation may be treated with general anaesthesia – Admission to hospital may be problematic and a single side room may be required
Dental treatment	• Before – Ensure that a risk assessment has been completed and the team has been briefed regarding any disruptive/aggressive behaviour – If appropriate, consent and arrangements for safe and approved clinical holding need to be formally recorded and reviewed on the day of treatment – Remove all equipment and items from the surgery which are not needed • During – Additional caution when performing invasive procedures – Terminate treatment if the patient becomes distressed or there are safety issues • After – Give positive reassurance – Re-evaluate next steps
Drug prescription	• Idiosyncratic reactions to diazepam and midazolam have been observed

(*Continued*)

Table 2.1.1 (Continued)

Education/prevention	• Most patients need assistance to brush their teeth • Electronic toothbrushes are often not well tolerated due to the vibration and sound • Implement fluoride supplementation in line with dental caries risk • Dietary advice to reduce caries risk • More regular reviews and shorter recall intervals advisable

  - Losing or forgetting things such as toys, pencils, books and tools needed for the task
- Signs of hyperactivity and impulsivity include:
  - Persistent motion and seem unable to curb their immediate reactions or think before they act
  - Feeling restless
  - Often fidgeting with hands or feet
  - Squirming
  - Running
  - Climbing
  - Leaving a seat when situations where sitting and quiet behaviour are expected
  - Blurting out an answer before hearing the question
  - Difficulty waiting in a queue or for a turn
- Commonly associated disorders may include:
  - Oppositional defiant disorders
  - Developmental language disorders
  - Motor and co-ordination difficulties
  - Learning disability
  - Tourette syndrome – an inherited neurological disorder characterised by repeated and involuntary body movements (tics) and uncontrollable vocal sounds and words (coprolalia)
  - Epilepsy; ~20% of children with epilepsy have ADHD
  - Non-restorative sleep due to insomnia, sleep apnoea, circadian rhythm disturbances, restless leg syndrome and parasomnias
- Although parents frequently describe their child as 'overactive', the term should be limited to those who demonstrate gross behavioural abnormalities, including uncontrolled activity, impulsiveness, impaired concentration, motor restlessness and extreme fidgeting
- These activities are seen particularly when orderliness is required – for example, in a waiting room or surgery

Diagnosis

- The diagnosis is mainly established on clinical findings
- In DSM-V, ADHD is included in the section on neurodevelopmental disorders, rather than being grouped with the disruptive behaviour disorders – this change better reflects the way ADHD is currently conceptualised
- DSM-V has also revised the age of onset criteria to 'several inattentive or hyperactive-impulsive symptoms present prior to 12 years' (5 years later than the 7-year-old marker set by DSM-IV)
- Furthermore, there is no longer the requirement that the symptoms create impairment by age 12, just that they are present
- ADHD subtypes include:
  - Predominantly inattentive
  - Predominantly hyperactive–impulsive
  - Combined subtype
- It may be further classified as mild, moderate or severe

Management

- Behavioural therapy, emotional counselling, specialised educational help and practical support along with parental education are required
- Medication (Table 2.1.2)
  - The selection of drugs to manage ADHD depends on the presenting features
  - Stimulants are the most effective treatment in both children and adults
  - Sedatives and tranquillisers should be avoided as they may impair any associated learning ability or cause a paradoxical reaction such as aggressive behaviour
  - In some cases, antidepressants and antihypertensive agents have also been successfully administered

Prognosis

- ADHD can have a serious and long-lasting impact on a person's life
- By the age of 25, an estimated 15% of people diagnosed with ADHD as children still have a full range of symptoms, and 65% still have some symptoms that affect their daily lives
- When symptoms are effectively managed, the quality of the person's life improves – this in turn leads to increased confidence and motivation to continue a healthy pathway towards a meaningful and fulfilling life
- Untreated ADHD is very disruptive to a person's day-to-day functioning and can cause negative consequences at home, work and school
- Adults with untreated ADHD are more likely to develop a substance abuse disorder as they depend on legal and illegal drugs to control their symptoms

Table 2.1.2 Medical management of attention deficit and hyperactivity disorder.

Symptom	Medication	Systemic side-effects	Oral side-effects
Hyperactivity, inattention, impulsivity	**Stimulants** • Amphetamine • Dextroamphetamine • Methylphenidate • Dexmethylphenidate	Tachycardia Increase in blood pressure Motor tics Dyskinesias Erythema multifome	Xerostomia Dysgeusia Bruxism
	Non-stimulants • Atomoxetine	Tachycardia Increase in blood pressure	Xerostomia
	Antihypertensives • Clonidine • Guanfacine	Drowsiness Dizziness	Xerostomia Dysgeusia Dysphagia
Hyperactivity, inattention and repetitive behaviours	**Atypical antidepressants** • Bupropion	Suicidal risk Angio-oedema	Xerostomia Dysgeusia Dysphagia Bruxism Stomatitis Glossitis
	Tricyclic antidepressants (TCAs) • Amitriptyline • Desipramine • Imipramine	Blurred vision Constipation Weight gain Tachycardia Suicidal risk	Xerostomia Dysgeusia Stomatitis Sialadentitis
Aggressive behaviours	**Antipsychotics** • Olanzapine • Risperidone • Paliperidone	Stiffness Restlessness Weight gain Constipation	Xerostomia Sialorrhoea Dysphagia Dysgeusia Stomatitis Tongue dyskinesia
	Anticonvulsants • Carbamazepine • Valproate • Lamotrigine	Nausea Vomiting Dizziness Angio-oedema	Xerostomia Dysgeusia Stomatitis Glossitis

- Impulsive behaviours cause workplace, financial and legal challenges
- There is a positive association between ADHD and suicidality in both sexes and in all age groups

A World/Transcultural View

- The concept of ADHD first emerged in the USA and from there it spread to all parts of the world during the late 1950s, to be become a global phenomenon
- Recent studies have concluded that the global rate of ADHD is approximately 5%
- However, there are significant differences in how ADHD has been diagnosed and the support that is available in different countries and regions. This is largely due to variable cultural factors and how conditions associated with behavioural and educational challenges are viewed across the globe

Recommended Reading

Bimstein, E., Wilson, J., Guelmann, M., and Primosch, R. (2008). Oral characteristics of children with attention deficit hyperactivity disorder. *Spec. Care Dentist.* 28: 107–110.

Blomqvist, M., Holmberg, K., Fernell, E. et al. (2006). Oral health, dental anxiety, and behavior management problems in children with attention deficit hyperactivity disorder. *Eur. J. Oral Sci.* 114: 385–390.

Broadbent, J.M., Ayers, K.M., and Thomson, W.M. (2004). Is attention deficit hyperactivity disorder a risk factor for dental caries? A case control study. *Caries Res.* 38: 29–33.

Friedlander, A.H., Yagiela, J.A., Mahler, M.E., and Rubin, R. (2007). The pathophysiology, medical management and dental implications of adult attention-deficit/hyperactivity disorder. *J. Am. Dent. Assoc.* 138: 475–482.

Kemper, A.R., Maslow, G.R., Hill, S., et al. Attention Deficit Hyperactivity Disorder: diagnosis and treatment in children and adolescents. Report No. 18-EHC005-EF. Rockville, MD: Agency for Healthcare Research and Quality. (2018).

Kerins, C.A., McWhorter, A.G., and Seale, N.S. (2007). Pharmacologic behavior management of pediatric dental patients diagnosed with attention deficit disorder/attention deficit hyperactivity disorder. *Pediatr. Dent.* 29: 507–513.

Souto-Souza, D., Mourão, P.S., Barroso, H.H. et al. (2020). Is there an association between attention deficit hyperactivity disorder in children and adolescents and the occurrence of bruxism? A systematic review and meta-analysis. *Sleep Med. Rev.* 53: 101330.

Weibel, S., Menard, O., Ionita, A. et al. (2020). Practical considerations for the evaluation and management of Attention Deficit Hyperactivity Disorder (ADHD) in adults. *Encephale* 46: 30–40.

2.2 Autism Spectrum Disorders

Section I: Clinical Scenario and Dental Considerations

Clinical Scenario

A 28-year-old patient presents to your dental clinic due to self-injury to the palate using a fork; he is accompanied by his mother. She suspects toothache as the trigger, as her son had previously been putting his fingers into the corner of his mouth and slapping his face on the right side.

Medical History

- Autism spectrum disorder
- Chronic sleep disorder
- Self-harm episodes
- Avoidant/Restrictive food intake disorder (ARFID)
- Surgery as a child to correct an aortic stricture

Medications

- Haloperidol
- Levomepromazine
- Biperiden

Dental History

- Dental treatment under general anaesthesia 10 years earlier
- No previous dental treatment provided with local anaesthesia
- Patient brushes his teeth himself 3 times a day (supervised/assisted by his mother twice daily, namely morning and at night)
- Still uses the same brand of children's toothpaste as he finds adult toothpastes too strong in taste

Social History

- Lives with his parents
- His mother is highly involved in taking care of him
- During the day, the patient attends a specialised centre and participates in craft workshops
- Non-verbal – uses pictograms for communication
- Avoids eye contact
- Does not like loud sounds or vibrations
- Only eats 'white food', predominantly bread, rice, white fish, milk – sugar added to all food as he finds the taste of salt and spices unpleasant

Oral Examination

- Co-operation facilitated with the use of pictograms (Figure 2.2.1)
- Good oral hygiene
- Fracture of the incisal edge of the crown of #11 and cusp fractures in #14, #24, #26, #27 and #44 (Figure 2.2.2)
- Coronary fracture due to extensive, deep and non-restorable caries in #47; tender on palpation
- Restorable caries: #17, #18, #35 and #45
- Missing teeth: #16

Radiological Examination

- Orthopantomogram successfully undertaken
- In addition to the clinical findings, recurrent caries through noted in #37 and #38 and deep caries with likely pulpal involvement in #47

Structured Learning

1) What factors may have contributed to the high caries rate?
   - Lack of access to regular dental care
   - High sugar content of food
   - Still using a children's toothpaste – fluoride content not optimal for an adult
   - Oral dryness secondary to medication (levomepromazine and biperiden)
2) What could be the cause of the incisal/coronal dental fractures in this patient?
   - Bruxism
   - Self-harm
   - Pica (e.g. lithophagy/ingesting stones)

A Practical Approach to Special Care in Dentistry, First Edition. Edited by Pedro Diz Dios and Navdeep Kumar.

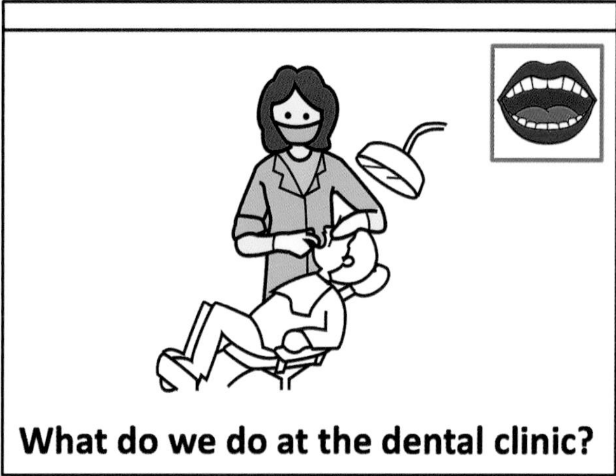

Figure 2.2.1 Oral examination was carried out with the help of pictograms.

(a)

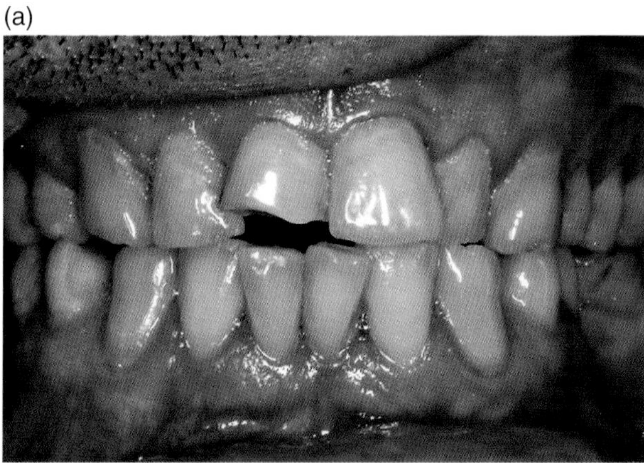

(b)

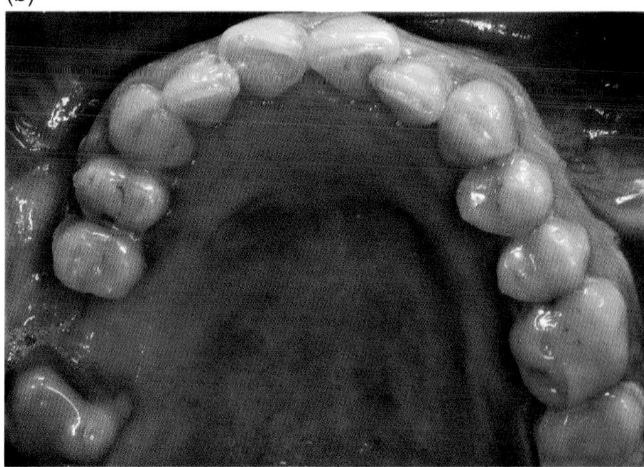

Figure 2.2.2 (a) Fracture of the incisal edge of the crown of tooth #11. (b) Multiple cusp fractures.

3) What factors are considered important in assessing the risk of managing this patient?
   - Social
     - Communication challenges (non-verbal and verbal)
     - Limited co-operation which can be worsened by unfamiliar environments or loud noises
     - Self-harm
   - Medical
     - Aortic stricture corrected should not impact on delivery of dental treatment
     - Vomiting/nausea as a potential side-effect of biperiden
     - Dizziness, lightheadedness, headache as a side-effect of haloperidol
   - Dental
   - Urgent dental treatment required for #47
     - Local stimuli (e.g. rotary instrumentation noise) and stress can negatively impact behaviour
     - Pain tolerance unknown
     - Tooth surface loss/bruxism
     - Increased likelihood of further/recurrent caries due to the highly cariogenic diet and suboptimal fluoride levels in the toothpaste
4) Following a course of antibiotics to manage the acute infection associated with #47, the patient returns for extraction of this tooth. What would you consider?
   - Although this patient has no previous experience with local anaesthesia, it may be possible to attempt more urgent procedures (e.g. extraction of #47) in the dental clinic; acclimatisation visits should be arranged, with appropriate adjustments in place (minimise loud noises, use pictograms)
   - Given the considerable dental treatment needs and depending on the patient's ability to co-operate with treatment under local anaesthesia, this may be followed by comprehensive dental treatment under general anaesthesia session in a hospital setting where available – this will avoid the repeated trigger of vibration/noise from the dental drill
   - Successive follow-up/treatment sessions should be attempted in the dental clinic to ensure regular dental reviews are in place
5) What should you consider when arranging dental visits for assessment and acclimatisation?
   - It may be helpful to create a story book with pictograms to anticipate what's going to happen
   - Keep the appointments in the same time slot/day of the week, ensuring that they do not interfere with the specialised centre visits or important activities for the patient (e.g. going to the swimming pool)
   - Always implement the same study routine (e.g. meeting place, progressive exposure to the setting and instrumentation)
   - Do not change dental treatment rooms or dental chairs

- Always recruit the professional team (both dentist and support staff)
- Do not change attire (e.g. work uniform colour)

6) If the patient needs to be sedated, what technique would you use?
   - Patients with autism often do not tolerate the nasal facemask for applying nitrous oxide/may not accept physical contact on parts of their face (although this can be trained in some cases)
   - Due to the risk of synergy with the antipsychotic drugs the patient is taking, a medical consultation opinion should be accessed if sedatives (e.g. benzodiazepines) are being considered
   - Paradoxical reactions to drug sedation are common
7) After completing the extraction, you note that there is extensive purulent discharge from the socket and prescribe an analgesic and an antibiotic. Which should you avoid?
   - Any nonsteroidal anti-inflammatory analgesic may be prescribed
   - Do not administer opioid analgesics (e.g. codeine or tramadol) due to potential interactions with the antipsychotic drugs
   - Avoid azithromycin because of the interaction with levomepromazine (risk of QT interval prolongation)

General Dental Considerations

Oral Findings

- Prevalence of caries and periodontal disease similar to the general population
- Bruxism more common
- Traumatic lesions often observed
- Dry mouth and occasionally hypersalivation of pharmacological origin
- Enamel erosion due to gastroesophageal reflux disease is not uncommon

Dental Management

- Poor communication and interpersonal skills may be misinterpreted as disruptive behaviour
- Pharmacological adjuncts may be required, with some patients requiring general anaesthesia to deliver dental treatment safely
- An individualised approach is required to enable delivery of dental care (Table 2.2.1; Figures 2.2.3 and 2.2.4)

Table 2.2.1 Considerations for dental management.

Risk assessment	• Variable behaviour/presentation (requires an individualised approach) – Stereotypy/uncontrolled movements – Repetitive routines/activities – Self-aggression, particularly when distressed – Intolerance for physical contact, noise, vibration, bright lights, strong taste/smells • High sensitivity to pain (may not respond when testing for pain/pulp vitality)
Criteria for referral	• Many patients can be treated in a conventional dental clinic, although they generally need several prior desensitisation sessions • Referral to a specialised clinic or hospital centre is indicated mainly by the degree of co-operation and hence pharmacological adjuncts required, and/or the extent of the treatment needs
Access/position	• The presence of a family member/carer is desirable to give the patient reassurance and to also give guidance to the dentist • Arrange acclimatisation visits, ensuring that a predictable routine is followed with the same dental clinic and dentist • Minimise waiting time • Short sessions
Communication	• In many cases, both verbal and non-verbal communication is impaired • Keep language and sentences simple – avoid metaphors, humour may be misunderstood • Allow extra time to process information • Desensitisation in school or at home with visual and manual support may be helpful – Use of pictograms – Simulation of procedures – Repetition of orders • Tell–show–do and immediate positive/negative reinforcement techniques can be useful

(Continued)

Table 2.2.1 (Continued)

Consent/capacity	• Capacity assessment is required as some patients can make informed decisions (e.g. Asperger syndrome) • If capacity is confirmed as being impaired, a best interest decision is required, involving the patient's parents or guardians • The consent process/best interest discussion should include the possibility of unexpected reactions to certain stimuli (e.g. pain and noise)
Anaesthesia/sedation	• Local anaesthesia – Pain tolerance may be present and local anaesthesia may be avoided in some procedures (e.g. some filings) – Acclimatisation with the same process being repeated may be effective – If local anaesthesia cannot be given safely, alternative approaches should be considered • Sedation – The effectiveness of conscious sedation is unpredictable (paradoxical effect may occur) – Inhalational sedation with nitrous oxide and oxygen may not be accepted due to use of the nasal hood/contact with the face • General anaesthesia – May be required for patients needing complex dental treatment and those where sedation is not effective – A single side room rather than a bed on an open ward is preferable – A day-stay modality is desirable
Dental treatment	• Before – Individualised risk assessment required to identify potential triggers that can cause distress – Consider the possibility of pain insensitivity • During – In the event of intolerance to the noise of the rotary instrumentation, chemical–mechanical caries removal techniques may be employed – headphones may also help – The dental chair light may also not be tolerated – dark patient glasses may help; alternatively, consider fibreoptic handpieces and/or smaller light sources – Terminate the appointment if the patient demonstrates signs of anxiety/stress as this can quickly escalate to challenging behaviour • After – Arrange another appointment, ideally at the same time, with the same dentist and in the same dental office
Drug prescription	• Patients taking selective serotonin reuptake inhibitors (SSRIs) may not experience adequate pain relief from codeine or its derivatives (SSRIs inhibit several families of hepatic enzymes, which may delay the biotransformation to the active metabolite of codeine)
Education/prevention	• Involve the relatives and caregivers where required • Use pictograms • Consider that some patients cannot tolerate electric toothbrushes due to the noise and vibration • Consider the use of flavour-free/mild-flavoured toothpastes and mouthwashes; non-foaming toothpastes may also be better accepted • Dietary counselling

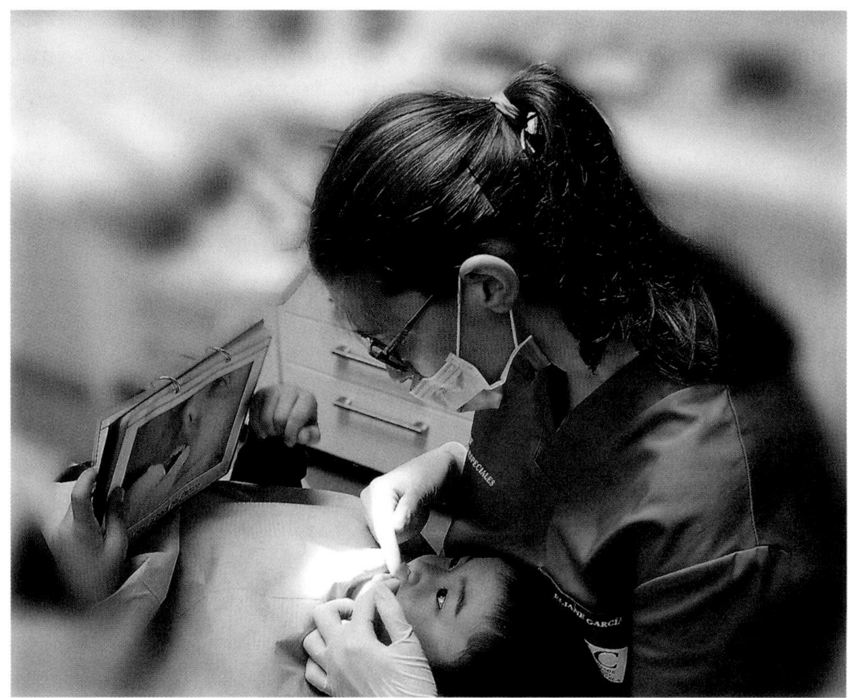

Figure 2.2.3 Desensitisation with visual support may be helpful.

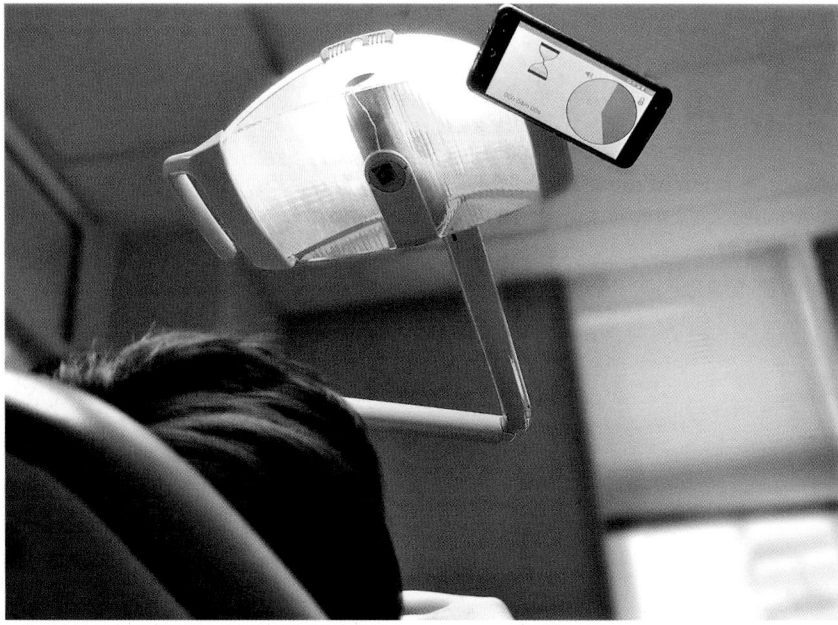

Figure 2.2.4 A visual timer may improve co-operation.

Section II: Background Information and Guidelines

Definition

Autistic spectrum disorders are a heterogeneous series of developmental disorders characterised by poor social skills, lack of interpersonal relationships, restricted interests and compulsive or ritualistic behaviour with repetitive stereotyped activities. Their estimated prevalence in the general population is 1%, preferentially affecting males, and 70% of patients have other comorbidities.

Aetiopathogenesis

- The cause is unknown
- Several risk factors have been identified, including advanced maternal age (increased incidence of germinal mutations) and gestational factors that affect neurodevelopment (including infections, vitamin deficiencies and exposure to chemical agents during pregnancy)
- It has also been suggested that autism is an expression of atypical neuronal connectivity, in which certain genetic abnormalities have been implicated (mainly of genes located in chromosomes 5 and 7)

Clinical Presentation

- Isolated in their own world (fascinated by some inanimate object, Figure 2.2.5a)
- Antisocial behaviour
- Difficulty communicating (avoid visual contact, speech disorders may be present)
- Obsessive resistance to change
- Repetitive actions (hand movements, flapping, body balance)
- Lack of response to external stimuli
- Ritualistic or compulsive behaviour (Figure 2.2.5b)

Table 2.2.2 Common concurrent conditions in the autism spectrum disorders.

Categories	Examples of conditions
Developmental abnormalities	Intellectual disability (70%) Hyperactivity and attention deficit disorder (35%) Tics (25%) Motor deficits (75%)
Medical disorders	Epilepsy (25%) Sleep disorders (65%) Gastrointestinal diseases (40%)
Psychiatric disorders	Anxiety (50%) Depression (40%) Obsessive–compulsive disorder (25%)
Behavioural problems	Aggressiveness (60%) Self-harm (50%) Pica (30%)

(a)

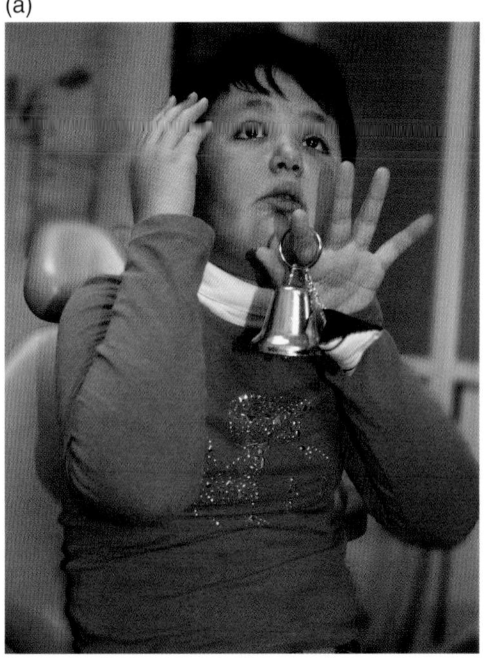

(b)

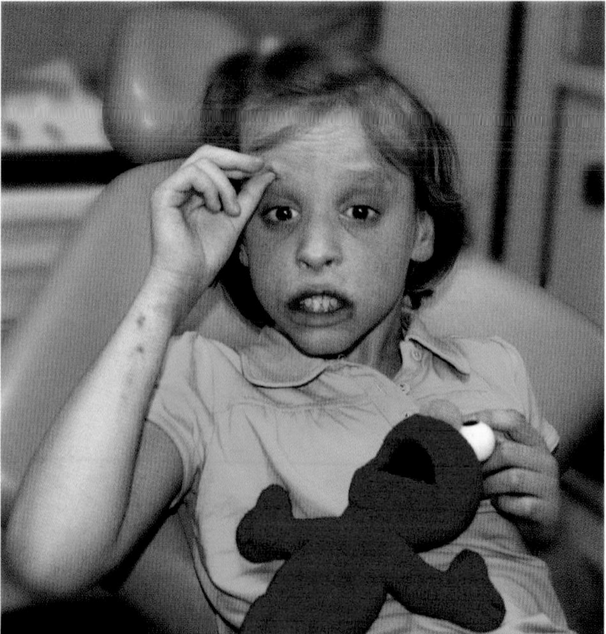

Figure 2.2.5 (a) Fascination by an inanimate object. (b) Ritualistic behaviour and fixation with a toy.

- Hypersensitive to sensory stimuli (but occasionally insensitive to pain and cold)
- Common concurrent conditions (Table 2.2.2)

Diagnosis

- There are no specific genetic, medical or laboratory diagnostic tests
- Diagnosis based on clinical findings suggestive of deficiencies in the area of communication, socialisation or restricted behaviour

Management

- Behavioural interventions and support
- Special education programmes
- Antipsychotic drugs (e.g. risperidone), selective serotonin reuptake inhibitors (e.g. fluoxetine) and stimulants (e.g. methylphenidate)

Prognosis

- The mortality risk is 2.8-fold higher than in the general population of the same age and sex, mainly due to the coexistence of other medical determinants

A World/Transcultural View

- In the US, children of racial ethnic minorities, of low-income families and/or non-English speakers with autism spectrum disorders are diagnosed later than white children, and have greater difficulty accessing healthcare facilities
- Autistic traits and their descriptors are not universal due to cultural differences. For example, asking whether the patient 'enjoys social events' has an excellent predictive value in the United Kingdom and Japan but is not applicable in India

Recommended Reading

Chandrashekhar, S. and Bommangoudar, J.S. (2018). Management of autistic patients in dental office: a clinical update. *Int. J. Clin. Pediatr. Dent.* 11: 219–227.

Corridore, D., Zumbo, G., Corvino, I. et al. (2020). Prevalence of oral disease and treatment types proposed to children affected by autistic spectrum disorder in pediatric dentistry: a systematic review. *Clin. Ter.* 171: e275–e282.

Delli, K., Reichart, P.A., Bornstein, M.M., and Livas, C. (2013). Management of children with autism spectrum disorder in the dental setting: concerns, behavioural approaches and recommendations. *Med. Oral Patol. Oral Cir. Bucal* 18: e862–e868.

Lai, M.C., Lombardo, M.V., and Baron-Cohen, S. (2014). Autism. *Lancet* 383: 896–910.

Limeres-Posse, J., Castaño-Novoa, P., Abeleira-Pazos, M., and Ramos-Barbosa, I. (2014). Behavioural aspects of patients with Autism Spectrum Disorders (ASD) that affect their dental management. *Med. Oral Patol. Oral Cir. Bucal* 19: e467–e472.

Nelson, T., Chim, A., Sheller, B.L. et al. (2017). Predicting successful dental examinations for children with autism spectrum disorder in the context of a dental desensitization program. *J. Am. Dent. Assoc.* 148: 485–492.

Rouches, A., Lefer, G., Dajean-Trutaud, S., and Lopez-Cazaux, S. (2018). Tools and techniques to improve the oral health of children with autism. *Arch. Pediatr.* 25: 145–149.

2.3 Down Syndrome

Section I: Clinical Scenario and Dental Considerations

Clinical Scenario

A 48-year-old patient attends the dental clinic complaining that his removable upper partial denture is unstable and 'does not work when eating'. The patient has been given several dentures in recent years but none of them has been successful

Medical History

- Down syndrome
- Atrial septal defect corrected in childhood
- Recurrent respiratory infections
- Mild hearing loss
- Gastroesophageal reflux
- Chronic anaemia
- Hyperuricaemia

Medications

- Budesonide
- Theophylline
- Allopurinol
- Lansoprazole
- Iron and folic acid

Dental History

- Regular dental attender
- Previous dental treatment with local anaesthesia tolerated on numerous occasions without the need for pharmacological adjuncts (calculus removal, extraction, fillings, endodontics, non-surgical periodontal treatment and prosthetic rehabilitation)
- Three years ago, the patient underwent excision of a maxillary odontogenic cyst (5 × 2.5 cm) under general anaesthesia
- The patient brushes his teeth independently twice a day using a fluoride toothpaste (without supervision)

Social History

- Parents deceased; lives with one of his sisters
- Independent for activities of daily life
- Attends a centre where he participates in cognitive stimulation and craft workshops

Oral Examination

- Very co-operative
- Lip fissures
- Fissured tongue
- Fair oral hygiene
- Microdontia
- Dental spacing
- Missing maxillary teeth: #14, #15, #16, #17, #21, #22, #23, #24, #25 and #26
- The remaining maxillary teeth have significant gingival recession with cervical exposure and grade 1–2 mobility
- Missing mandibular teeth: #32, #35, #42 and #45 (possibly due to agenesis, based on the findings of previous radiographs)
- Irregular alveolar bone crest in the upper left quadrant, with a considerable bone defect as sequela of the cystectomy (intact mucous coating with a normal appearance) (Figure 2.3.1a)
- Unstable upper partial denture (Figure 2.3.1b)

Radiological Examination

- Orthopantomogram and cone beam computed tomography (Figure 2.3.2) undertaken
- No radiological evidence of recurrence of the odontogenic cyst, but there is loss of bone mineral density
- The only available bone volume for the direct insertion of dental implants identified in positions corresponding to teeth #14 and #26

A Practical Approach to Special Care in Dentistry, First Edition. Edited by Pedro Diz Dios and Navdeep Kumar.

(a)

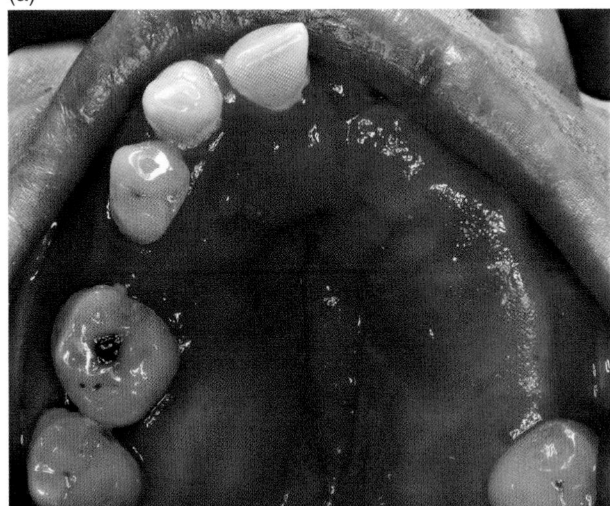

(b)

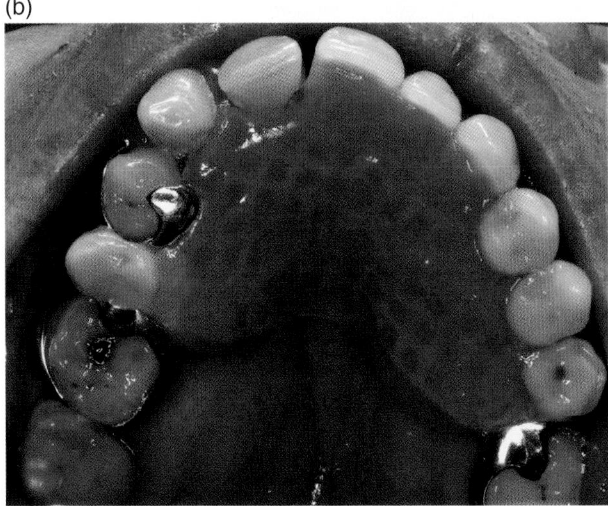

Figure 2.3.1 (a) Irregular palate, with erythema of the denture bearing mucosa (clinically suggestive of candidiasis). (b) Unstable upper partial denture.

Structured Learning

1) What are lip fissures and what causes them?
   - Lip fissures are a frequent finding in patients with Down syndrome (>25%), especially among men, with a peak prevalence in the third decade, and occur preferentially in the lower lip
   - Their aetiology is unknown (embryological defects, mandibular prognathism and lip eversion have been implicated)
   - In most patients, the lesions coexist with angular cheilitis and are colonised by *Candida albicans*
2) What factors are considered important in assessing the risks of managing this patient?
   - Social
     - Favourable family environment
     - Hearing impairment
     - Complications can arise due to other comorbidities associated with Down syndrome (e.g. premature ageing and cognitive impairment)
   - Medical
     - Respiratory dysfunction
     - Fatigue/reduced tolerance for treatment in relation to anaemia
     - Corrected atrial septal defect is not associated with risk when delivering dental intervention
   - Dental
     - Multiple failed attempts at providing removable partial dentures
     - Oral hygiene could be improved
     - Multiple missing teeth but low caries rate; chronic periodontal disease likely cause of tooth loss
     - Prognosis of the remaining teeth guarded
     - Implication for success of osseointegrated dental implants
     - Gastroesophageal reflux-related risk of dental erosion
     - Anaemia-related oral side-effects (pale mucosa, glossitis, oral ulceration)
3) What factors determine the prognosis of the dental implants in this patient (Figure 2.3.3)?
   - The available bone volume is limited
   - Osteopenia
   - Susceptibility to infections (potential defects in neutrophil chemotaxis due to Down syndrome)
   - Sub-optimal oral hygiene and a history of periodontal disease can favour the onset of peri-implantitis. Ongoing oral hygiene/periodontal support provided due to variable compliance
   - Observed higher failure rate: in patients with Down syndrome, 1 in every 5 dental implants fails
4) If considering the use of dental premedication/sedation to place dental implants, what additional factors should be taken into account?
   - Benzodiazepines should not be prescribed for patients with severe respiratory dysfunction or hypotonia (musculoskeletal effect of Down syndrome)
   - Theophylline reverses the sedative effect of benzodiazepines
5) Is administering antibiotic prophylaxis before a surgical procedure such as implant insertion justified?
   - The corrected atrial septal defect does not justify the prescription of antibiotic prophylaxis for the prevention of bacterial endocarditis
   - However, the immunological defects observed in Down syndrome may constitute an indication for administering antibiotics prior to the surgical procedure and for maintaining them in the postoperative period

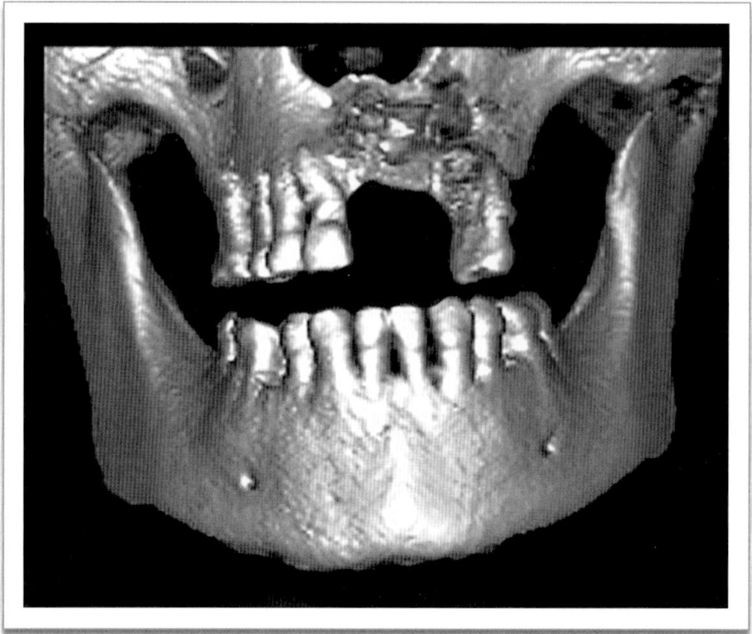

Figure 2.3.2 Cone beam computed tomography showing a bone defect in the upper left quadrant.

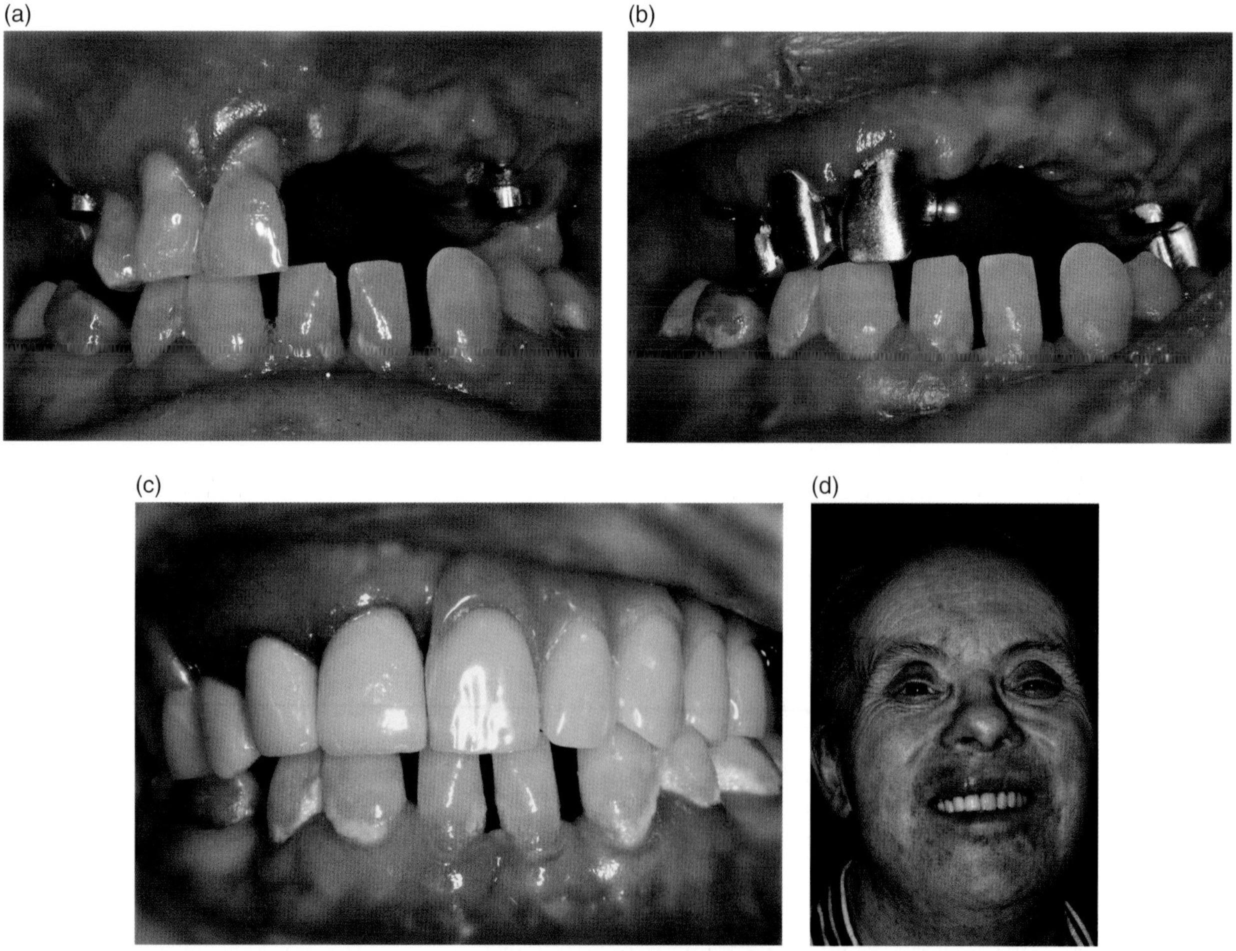

(a) (b) (c) (d)

Figure 2.3.3 (a–d) Prosthodontic rehabilitation with a new upper dental prosthesis supported on the remaining teeth and 2 osseointegrated implants.

6) What antibiotics should be avoided for this patient?

- The toxicity of theophylline increases with macrolide antibiotics and quinolones

General Dental Considerations

Oral Findings

- Orofacial muscle hypotonia
- Poor labial seal/open mouth posture (may lead to xerostomia)
- Lip fissures (Figure 2.3.4a)
- Macroglossia or pseudomacroglossia (Figure 2.3.4b)
- Lingual protrusion
- Fissured tongue
- Increased incidence of gag reflex
- Dental agenesis (especially of the maxillary lateral incisors)
- Tooth eruption delayed
- Tooth morphology abnormalities (microdontia, enamel hypoplasia and hypocalcification)

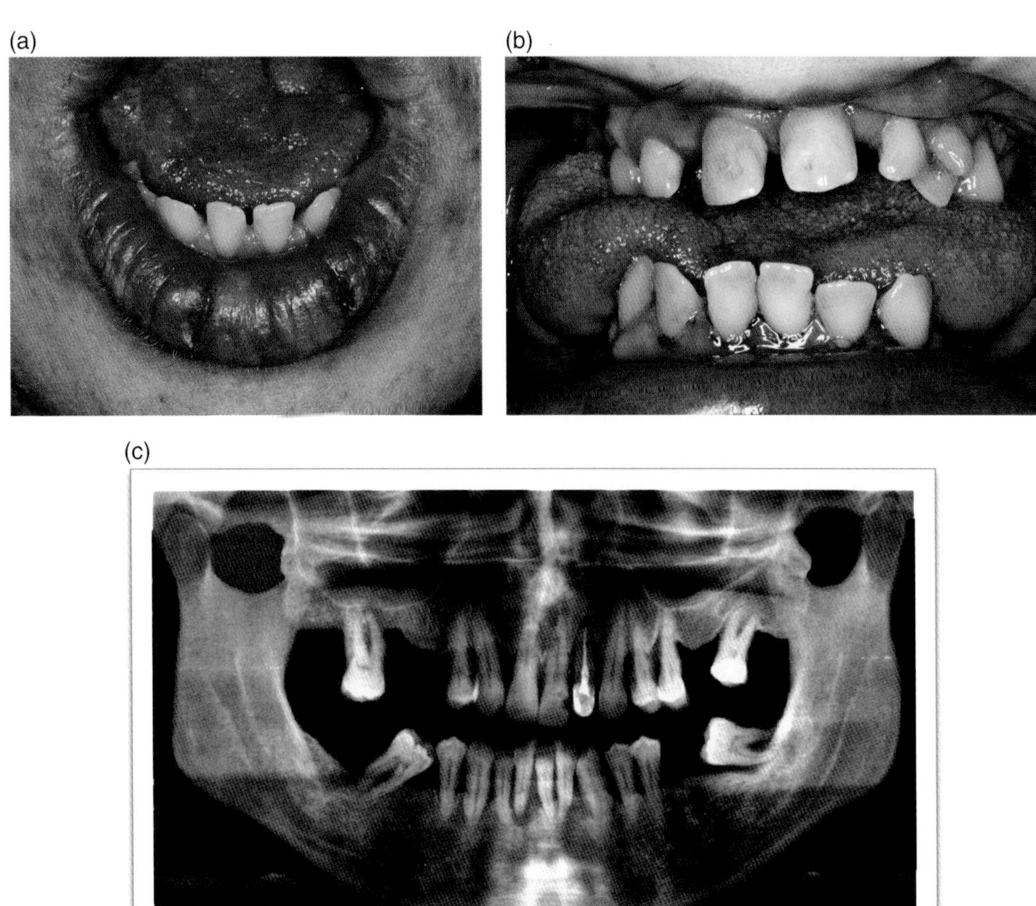

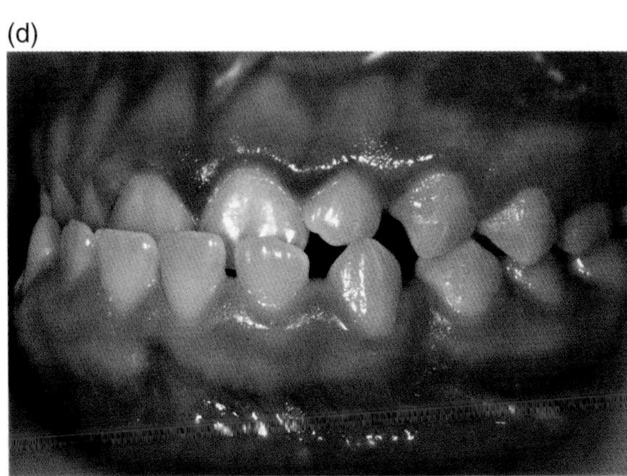

Figure 2.3.4 (a) Lip fissures. (b) Dental agenesis, microdontia and macroglossia. (c) Severe periodontal disease. (d) Angle class III malocclusion.

- Low prevalence of caries
- Severe periodontal disease (Figure 2.3.4c)
- Early tooth loss (compromised immune system and teeth with short conical roots lead to early loss of teeth from periodontal disease)
- Bruxism
- Hypoplasia of the middle third of the face, with Angle class III malocclusion and posterior cross-bite (Figure 2.3.4d)

Dental Management

- The treatment plan will be determined by the patient's oral manifestations, degree of co-operation and the presence of comorbidities (Table 2.3.1; Figure 2.3.5)
- Orthodontic therapy can be performed in selected cases

Section II: Background Information and Guidelines

Definition

Down syndrome is a congenital disorder of chromosomal origin characterised by intellectual disability, systemic abnormalities and a particular phenotype. The estimated prevalence is 1 case per 800 live births.

Aetiopathogenesis

- The mother's age (>35 years) is considered a risk factor
- In 95% of cases, the syndrome is due to the presence of an additional copy of chromosome 21 in all cells ('trisomy 21')

Table 2.3.1 Considerations for dental management.

Risk assessment	• Postoperative infections (immunological deficiencies) • Risk of bacterial endocarditis (congenital heart disease) • Variable co-operation • Speech disorders and intelligibility • Hearing loss • Atlantoaxial instability
Criteria for referral	• Most patients can be treated in a conventional dental clinic • Referral to a specialised clinic or hospital centre is determined mainly by the patient's co-operation and extent of comorbidities (e.g. severe heart disease)
Access/position	• Prevent neck hyperextension (atlantoaxial instability) • Access to the teeth may be impeded by lingual protrusion • Minimise waiting time • Consider shorter sessions
Communication	• Adapt in relation to cognition • If hearing aids are worn, ensure these are present and switched on at the dental appointments
Consent/capacity	• Capacity assessment is required (should be decision specific) • Discussion of risks should include those related to comorbidities (e.g. predisposition to infections) and the level of oral hygiene • Dementia may occur at an early age and have an additional impact on reducing capacity
Anaesthesia/sedation	• Local anaesthesia – This may be challenging to administer in relation to patient co-operation, altered anatomy and lingual protrusion • Sedation – The nasal hood used for inhalational sedation may not fit well due to hypoplasia of the mid-third of the face – Associated comorbidities should be assessed, including the degree of hypotonia, associated cardiac disease and respiratory dysfunction • General anaesthesia – Difficulties in endotracheal intubation (hypoplasia of the middle third of the face, short neck, adenoid hypertrophy, atlantoaxial subluxation) – Increased risk due to cardiac complications (due to underlying heart disease and/or anaemia), respiratory dysfunction and infections (increased susceptibility)

(Continued)

Table 2.3.1 (Continued)

Dental treatment	• Before – Early periodontal treatment and the use of adjuvant antimicrobial mouthwashes are effective in improving periodontal health – Pulpal treatments in primary dentition are not recommended – The prognosis for orthodontic therapy is determined by the patient's degree of collaboration, the level of oral hygiene, the presence of parafunctions and the state of the periodontium – Rehabilitation with fixed prosthesis can be performed if the oral hygiene is optimal, the dental morphology is appropriate and the periodontal state is acceptable; otherwise, opt for a removable prosthesis (not always well accepted by patients) – Stimulating palatal plaques combined with orofacial physical therapy and speech therapy exercises improves muscle tone and orofacial abnormalities • During – Consider the use of tongue guards, supplemented by high-volume suction to improve vision/access to the dentition • After – Orthodontic treatments, with both removable and fixed multibracket appliances, usually take longer than in the general population (slow activation rhythm), and complications are more frequent (particularly traumatic ulcers) – The prognosis for dental implants in these patients is poorer than in the general population, with an estimated failure rate of 20% (generally, the losses occur before completing the prosthetic rehabilitation)
Drug prescription	• Consider drug interactions with medications used to treat comorbidities (e.g. avoid macrolide antibiotics for patients taking antihypertensives such as verapamil/diltiazem)
Education/prevention	• Oral hygiene education • Involve the relatives and care-givers • Increased frequency of reviews (every 3 months) to closely monitor periodontal disease • Periodic calculus removal • Dietary counselling

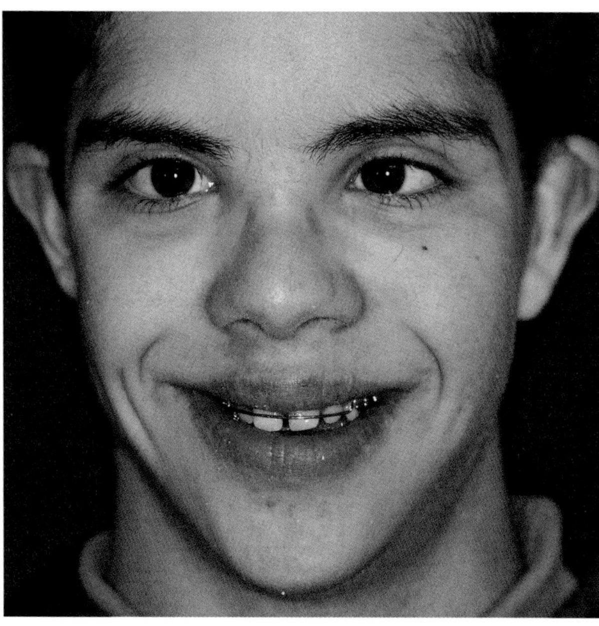

Figure 2.3.5 Orthodontic therapy can be successfully performed in selected patients.

- In 5% of the remaining cases, the syndrome expresses a translocation or mosaicism

Clinical Presentation

Apart from the classic facial characteristics (85%), multiple systems may be affected in Down syndrome (Table 2.3.2)

Diagnosis

- Suspected prenatal diagnosis (imaging techniques and invasive tests) is confirmed with the study of foetal cell DNA
- In newborns, the diagnosis is suspected based on the phenotypic characteristics and is confirmed with karyotyping

Management

- Physical therapy to combat hypotonia
- Early stimulation programs (including speech therapy)
- Treatment of comorbidities
- Special education and occupational therapy

Prognosis

- Median age of death has increased from 25 years in the 1980s to 55 years, with many living into their 60s and 70s
- Mortality by infectious diseases, especially pneumonia, is 12-fold greater than in the general population

A World/Transcultural View

- There is racial disparity in the mortality of patients with Down syndrome; this may be related to healthcare access, for example early referral to cardiology to allow timely surgical intervention
- Social acceptance of the phenotypic appearance is variable: parents surveyed in sub-Saharan Africa demonstrated favourable attitudes towards plastic surgery for their children with Down syndrome, although they admitted their lack of knowledge about the procedure
- Even after several decades, the use of orofacial stimulation therapy has not become widespread and is applied on a regular basis only in a number of South American and northern European countries

Table 2.3.2 Most common systemic conditions in Down syndrome.

Systems	Conditions
Cardiac	• Congenital heart defects are common (40–50%) • Endocardial cushion defect (43%) • Ventriculoseptal defect (32%) • Secundum atrial septal defect (10%) • Tetralogy of Fallot (6%) • Isolated patent ductus arteriosus (4%)
Haematological	• The risk of leukaemia is 1–1.5%, much higher than the general population (10–15 times increased risk) • 65% of newborns have transient myelodysplasia
Immunological	• Abnormal IgA levels • Abnormal T-cell function • Dysfunctional and short-lived neutrophils
Infections	• Increased risk (×12) of developing infectious diseases, including: – Respiratory (pneumonia) – Gastrointestinal – Mucosal – Dermal – Oral infections (periodontal disease, candidal infection, acute necrotising ulcerative gingivitis)
Gastrointestinal	• Gastro-oesophageal reflux disease (GORD) • Vomiting • Duodenal atresia or stenosis, associated with annular pancreas in 2.5% of cases • Oesophageal atresia • Hirschsprung disease (blockage of colon) • Imperforate anus • Coeliac disease (5–16-fold increase compared to general population)
Endocrine	• Hypothyroidism (~15%) • Increased incidence diabetes • Decreased fertility
Reproduction	• Women with Down syndrome are fertile and may become pregnant • Nearly all males with Down syndrome are infertile due to an impairment of spermatogenesis

(Continued)

Table 2.3.2 (Continued)

Systems	Conditions
Neuropsychiatric disorders	• Intellectual disability (100%) • Average prevalence of dementia 50% (7–50%); risk increases when the person is over the age of 35 • Tonic–clonic seizures • Psychiatric disorders: – Obsessive–compulsive disorder – Autism – Attention deficit hyperactivity disorder – Tourette syndrome – Depressive disorder
Skeletal	• Short stature (85%) • Increased joint flexibility (80%) • Spine – Atlantoaxial instability (14%), with excessive mobility of the atlas (C1) and axis (C2); may lead to subluxation of the cervical spine/spinal cord compression – Pelvic dysplasia (70%) • Skull – Brachycephaly (80%), microcephaly, sloping forehead – Large fontanelles with late closure, patent metopic suture – Absence of frontal and sphenoid sinuses – Hypoplasia of maxillary sinuses, hypoplastic midface with relative prognathia • Nose – Hypoplastic nasal bone and flat nasal bridge are typical characteristics • Hands – Short and broad hands – Clinodactyly of the fifth fingers (45%) – 'Simian' single flexion crease (20–40%) • Feet – Wide gap between 1st and 2nd toes
Muscles	• Hypotonia (80%)
Eyes	• Up-slanting palpebral fissures, bilateral epicanthal folds • Brushfield spots (35–90%) • Refractory error (35–76%) • Strabismus (25–57%) • Nystagmus (18–22%) • Cataract (5% of newborns)
Ears	• Small ears with overfolded helices • Hearing loss (75%) • Otitis media • Increased risk of retinoblastoma
Skin	• Psoriasis • Eczema • Palmoplantar hyperkeratosis • Seborrheic dermatitis
Others	• Obstructive sleep apnoea • Hypotonia • Premature ageing • Obesity • Fine, soft hair

Recommended Reading

Abeleira, M.T., Pazos, E., Limeres, J. et al. (2016). Fixed multibracket dental therapy has challenges but can be successfully performed in young persons with Down syndrome. *Disabil. Rehabil.* 38: 1391–1396.

Ferreira, R., Michel, R.C., Greghi, S.L. et al. (2016). Prevention and periodontal treatment in Down syndrome patients: a systematic review. *PLoS One* 11: e0158339.

Hickey, F., Hickey, E., and Summar, K.L. (2012). Medical update for children with Down syndrome for the pediatrician and family practitioner. *Adv. Pediatr.* 59: 137–157.

Limeres Posse, J., López Jiménez, J., Ruiz Villandiego, J.C. et al. (2016). Survival of dental implants in patients with Down syndrome: a case series. *J. Prosthet. Dent.* 116: 880–884.

Mubayrik, A.B. (2016). The dental needs and treatment of patients with Down syndrome. *Dent. Clin. North Am.* 60: 613–626.

Nóvoa, L., Sánchez, M.D.C., Blanco, J. et al. (2020). The subgingival microbiome in patients with Down syndrome and periodontitis. *J. Clin. Med.* 9: 2482.

Outumuro, M., Abeleira, M.T., Caamaño, F. et al. (2010). Maxillary expansion therapy in children with Down syndrome. *Pediatr. Dent.* 32: 499–504.

Roizen, N.J. and Patterson, D. (2003). Down's syndrome. *Lancet* 361: 1281–1289.

3

Sensory Impairment

3.1 Visual Deficit

Section I: Clinical Scenario and Dental Considerations

Clinical Scenario

A 9-year-old girl attends your dental clinic for an oral examination. You observe that she has low insertion and thickening of the upper labial frenum in the interincisal region. This is associated with a midline diastema which the patient's mother wants corrected.

Medical History

- Sphenoidal encephalocele repaired at birth
- Blindness (complete loss of vision), panhypopituitarism and diabetes insipidus suspected to be postsurgical sequelae
- Patent foramen ovale (resolved percutaneously at birth)
- Bacterial meningitis at 3 months of age

Medications

- Desmopressin
- Hydrocortisone
- Levothyroxine
- Somatropin
- Vitamin D3

Dental History

- Regular dental attender
- No history of previous dental treatment given using local anaesthesia
- The previous dentist had noted the upper labial frenum was low/thickened but had recommended observation only
- Patient brushes her teeth 3 times a day (supervised by her mother in the morning and evening)

Social History

- Lives with her parents and her brother (3 years older than her, with no medical issues)
- Family history: the patient's mother aborted a previous pregnancy as the foetus had severe heart disease
- Mother is a nurse and is highly motivated to support and protect her daughter
- Attends a mainstream school; assisted by a support teacher

Oral Examination

- Excellent co-operation during the oral examination
- Mixed Angle class III malocclusion (hypoplasia of the superior maxilla and mandibular prognathism)
- Thickened upper labial frenulum (Figure 3.1.1)
- Upper midline, interincisal diastema
- Excellent oral hygiene
- Incipient/early caries in #36 and #46 (require restoration)
- Deep caries in #85

Radiological Examination

Cone beam computed tomography confirms a fusion defect in the superior maxilla, associated with the presence of a cleft palate that had previously been undetected (Figure 3.1.2)

Structured Learning

1) Although the patient's blindness is likely to be a sequela of the surgery, what other causes should be excluded in liaison with the patient's physician?
   - Following detection of the cleft palate, it is important to consider the presence of an underlying hereditary syndrome
   - Underlying syndromes are identified in ~20% of cases of cleft lip and ~40% of cases of isolated cleft palate
   - Furthermore, an associated syndrome, such as poly-malformative syndrome, may be responsible for some of the patient's other conditions, including visual impairment

A Practical Approach to Special Care in Dentistry, First Edition. Edited by Pedro Diz Dios and Navdeep Kumar.

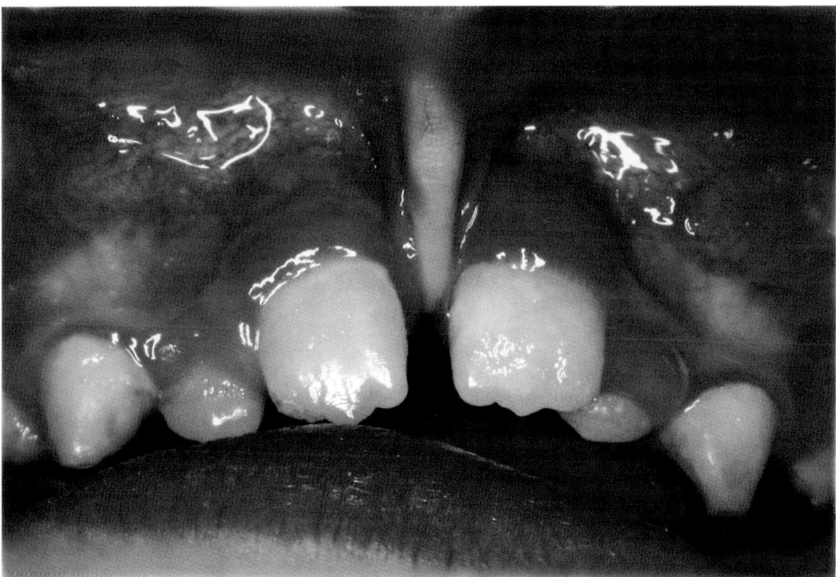

Figure 3.1.1 Thickened upper labial frenulum.

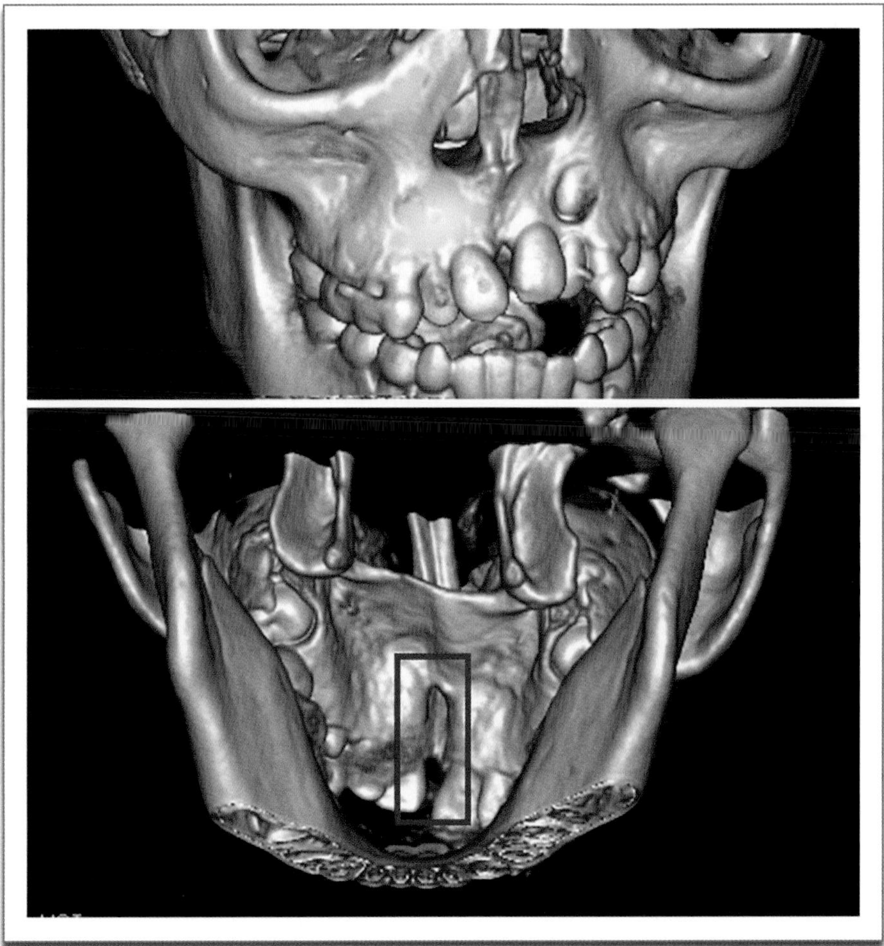

Figure 3.1.2 Cone beam computed tomography showing a considerable isolated cleft palate.

2) The patient's mother insists that her daughter's midline diastema should be corrected. What should you determine when deciding whether to proceed?
   - Is the patient aware of the diastema (in view of her visual impairment) or is it more of a concern to her mother who is very involved in her care?
   - What are the patient's wishes – although she is 9 years old, any elective/cosmetic treatment should be discussed with her to determine her view
   - The patient's age: she is still in the mixed dentition stage
   - The size of the diastema and if it is increasing in size
   - Treatment options in relation to the patient's compliance (frenectomy, orthodontics, restorative treatment)
3) What dental considerations are there for this patient in relation to her underlying diabetes insipidus?
   - Diabetes insipidus and diabetes mellitus are different entities; although both can present with constant thirst and polyuria, central diabetes insipidus is an antidiuretic hormone deficiency caused by damage to the hypothalamus or, as in this case, the pituitary gland
   - Some patients can present with dental fluorosis (due to excessive intake of fluoride in drinking water) and/or dry mouth (due to excessive fluid loss)
   - These patients are susceptible to episodes of orthostatic hypotension
4) What factors are considered important in assessing the risk of managing this patient?
   - Social
     - Impaired communication due to loss of vision; may be further impaired due to the cleft palate (can lead to unclear speech, hearing problems due to middle ear infections)
     - Potential for overprotection due to the mother's professional background
   - Medical
     - Acute complications resulting from panhypopituitarism and diabetes insipidus (e.g. hypoglycaemia, hypotension, agitation)
     - The congenital heart disease has resolved and hence does not require further consideration in relation to planned dental treatment
   - Dental
     - Cleft palate may be associated with malalignment of the teeth and/or nasal regurgitation
     - Complexity of orthodontic treatment and surgery necessary to address the cleft palate
5) You decide to undertake the dental fillings before attempting a frenectomy. After an injection of local anaesthetic, the patient begins to cry and becomes anxious. What would be your approach?
   - The pain threshold for children with blindness can be significantly lower than that of children without blindness
   - Stop and undertake acclimatisation appointments, allowing the patient to feel and touch equipment (with sharp components/needle removed)
   - Ensure you explain what you are going to do at each stage of treatment and acknowledge that this is necessary for all steps as the patient is blind
   - Consider adjuncts to reduce the discomfort associated with local anaesthesia infiltrations (e.g. computer-controlled local anaesthetic delivery)
   - Consider the use of sedation
6) When attempting restoration of the #85, the dental caries is more extensive than previously thought. The tooth is not restorable and requires extraction. The patient is taking 20 mg of hydrocortisone a day. What corticosteroid supplementation regimen should be administered to prevent an adrenal crisis (see Chapter 12.1)?
   - Hydrocortisone is a short-acting glucocorticoid
   - The equivalent dose for 20 mg of hydrocortisone is 5 mg of prednisone or prednisolone (intermediate-acting)
   - Therefore, no supplementation regimen is needed

General Dental Considerations

Oral Findings

- It has been suggested that children with severe visual deficits have more caries, more dental trauma and, in general, poorer oral health compared with children without visual deficits
- However, in most controlled studies with a favourable socio-economic setting and close supervision from parents/carers/dental teams, the oral health of patients with blindness or severe visual deficits is similar to that of the general population, except for a greater accumulation of dental plaque and a higher prevalence of gingivitis
- In general, levels of dental plaque are determined by the degree of visual deficit and are lower in patients with acquired blindness than those with congenital blindness
- Adults and elderly individuals with blindness sometimes have better oral hygiene practices than the general population and achieve similar oral hygiene indices but are incapable of detecting oral diseases early

Dental Management

- Many patients with visual deficit have complained of shortcomings in the availability of accessible oral health services
- The visual deficit can jeopardise oral hygiene and the success of certain procedures (e.g. the insertion/withdrawal of removable dental prostheses and the cleaning of interdental spaces in fixed prostheses)
- A targeted approach is required to ensure appropriate adaptations are in place for dental management (Table 3.1.1)
- Orthodontic treatment can be performed for selected patients (Figure 3.1.3)

Section II: Background Information and Guidelines

Definition

A patient is considered to have a visual deficit if they have considerable difficulty differentiating objects at a distance of 40 cm even when using the best correction possible. Blindness is defined as the complete absence of vision or slight light perception but not in the form of objects (visual acuity less than 3/60). It is estimated that 124 million individuals worldwide have a severe visual deficit (2% of the population) and that 37 million have blindness (0.6% of the population).

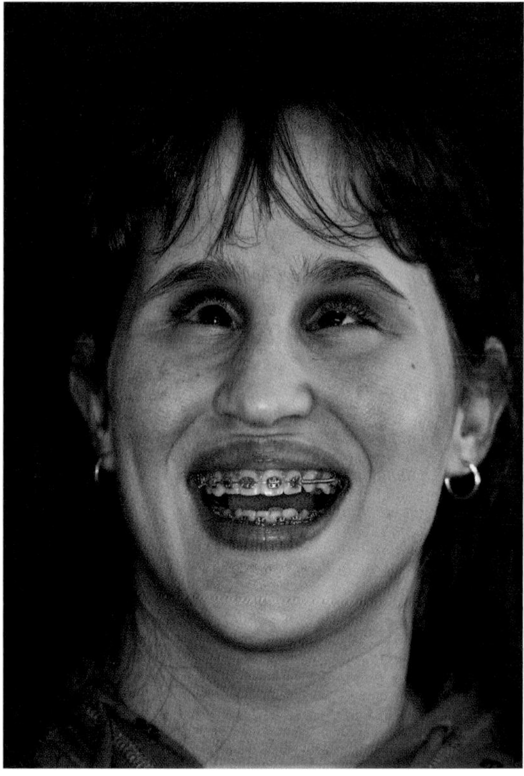

Figure 3.1.3 Orthodontic treatment for a patient with visual impairment.

Aetiopathogenesis

- In industrialised countries, the main causes of visual deficit among adults are age-related macular degeneration,

Table 3.1.1 Considerations for dental management.

Risk assessment	• Consider risks associated with a related underlying disease (e.g. polymalformative syndromes and diabetes) • Unexpected contact, noise, vibration and light can startle the patient and cause unexpected movements • Children with blindness may have a significantly lower pain threshold
Criteria for referral	• Referral to a specialised clinic or hospital centre is rarely required and will be determined by the degree of patient co-operation or the presence of significant comorbidities (e.g. poorly controlled diabetes)
Access/position	• Avoid overprotectiveness • Ask before offering assistance (do not attempt to touch the patient without permission) • When guiding a patient with blindness, walk half a step in front of them to allow them to hold onto your arm if required (optionally, they can hold onto your shoulder or wrist), on the side opposite to the one holding the cane • A patient who uses a guide dog should be asked whether they want to hold on to you or would prefer to follow you (the dog may enter the dental room) • While walking to the dental office, information can be provided on the surroundings • Under no circumstance should the patient's cane or clothing be held, nor should the patient be pushed from behind

(Continued)

Table 3.1.1 (Continued)

Communication	• Talk to the patient while looking them in the face • Directly address the individual with visual deficit and not their companion • Use the patient's name so that they are clear you are talking to them • Introduce yourself so that they know who is talking to them • Let them know if there are other individuals present in the room • Talk in a normal tone, slowly and clearly; do not shout or raise your voice • Be precise in the messages • Do not use gestures as a substitute for spoken words • Consent should be written in large font (ideally in Braille for those patients who have complete blindness)
Consent/capacity	• Patients of legal age can generally sign the informed consent personally • It is essential that this form be printed in sufficiently large type or even have a Braille version • If the patient cannot read, a close family member/friend acting as a witness can read it for them (in some countries, the presence of this witness is mandatory)
Anaesthesia/sedation	• Local anaesthesia – Some patients have poor pain tolerance (increased tactile sensitivity) • Sedation – In the event of glaucoma, benzodiazepines should not be employed to induce conscious sedation • General anaesthesia – For patients with glaucoma who require general anaesthesia, avoid using atropine
Dental treatment	• Before – Consider the use of audio aids which the patient can access at home to remind them of the planned treatment – Allow the patient to touch the chair and equipment – Explain all the dental procedures that will be performed – The 'tell–feel (physical contact)–do' technique can be useful – Before planning rehabilitation with a removable prosthesis, ensure that the patient is sufficiently able to recognise, insert and remove the prosthesis – When planning for prostheses, consider that some patients with visual deficit do not tolerate muco-supported prostheses well – For selected patients, orthodontic treatments can be performed (including multibracket appliances) to improve function and aesthetics if this is a concern • During – Warn the patient if you need to leave the dental office and when you will return – Throughout the procedure, warn the patient of each manoeuvre that will be performed, explaining in advance anticipated contact, noise, vibration and light – Exercise particular caution with rotary instrumentation and injections – Reinforce positive behaviours • After – The success of fixed prostheses can be affected by poor oral hygiene – Reinforce positive behaviours – Postoperative instructions should be written in large font (ideally in Braille for complete blindness) or provided in an audio format
Drug prescription	• For patients with glaucoma, anticholinergic agents (such as atropine, scopolamine and glycopyrrolate, which are prescribed to control drooling), carbamazepine, diazepam, corticosteroids and tricyclic antidepressants are contraindicated
Education/prevention	• Audio, tactile and supervised training techniques and instructions in Braille are useful for improving the oral hygiene of those with visual deficits (whose motivation is usually magnified) • These modified approaches to educational programmes on oral health promotion have demonstrable efficacy • Electric toothbrushes can be more effective than manual toothbrushes as long as the vibration is tolerated

glaucoma and diabetic retinopathy; paediatric blindness is mainly due to retinopathy of prematurity
- In developing countries, the most common causes are cataracts and trachoma; in children, congenital cataracts appear frequently in the context of a polymalformative syndrome (a recognisable pattern of congenital anomalies that are known or thought to be causally related)

Clinical Presentation
- The clinical manifestations depend on the location of the injury causing the visual impairment (e.g. optic nerve injuries are usually irreversible) and its aetiology (e.g. congenital cataracts can be associated with epilepsy)
- The most suggestive symptoms of visual deficit include the following:
  - Visual adaptation problems in dark settings
  - Difficulty focusing on near or distant objects
  - Excessive light sensitivity
  - Eye redness or inflammation
  - Sudden eye pain
  - Double vision
  - Sudden vision loss in one eye
  - Onset of a dark spot in the centre of the visual field
  - Loss of peripheral vision
  - Sudden blurred vision

Diagnosis
- Visual acuity tests include the Snellen test (ability to perceive the forms of objects and to distinguish their details)
- Visual field and peripheral vision tests (ability to perceive objects placed outside the central vision area)
- Ophthalmoscopy/fundoscopy (retinal examination)
- Other: e.g. tonometry, slit-lamp, photometers

Management
- Cataract surgery
- Prescription glasses for correcting refractive errors
- Drugs for age-related macular degeneration
- Support measures include braille (a tactile reading and writing system), electronic methods for identifying colour and, in extreme cases, guide dogs (Figures 3.1.4 and 3.1.5)
- There is speculation as to the future possibility of curing blindness with stem cells

Prognosis
- Life expectancy can be affected by the coexistence of an underlying disease (e.g. polymalformative syndromes, diabetes)

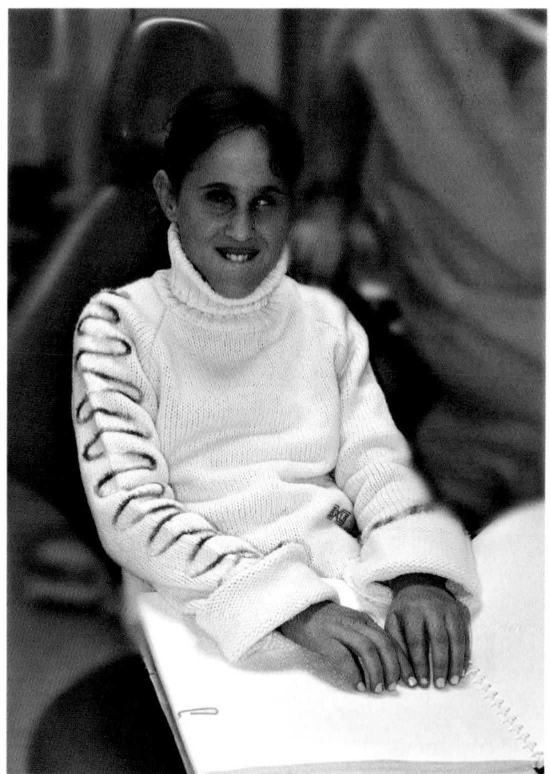

Figure 3.1.4 Braille is a useful communication tool mainly for complete blindness patients.

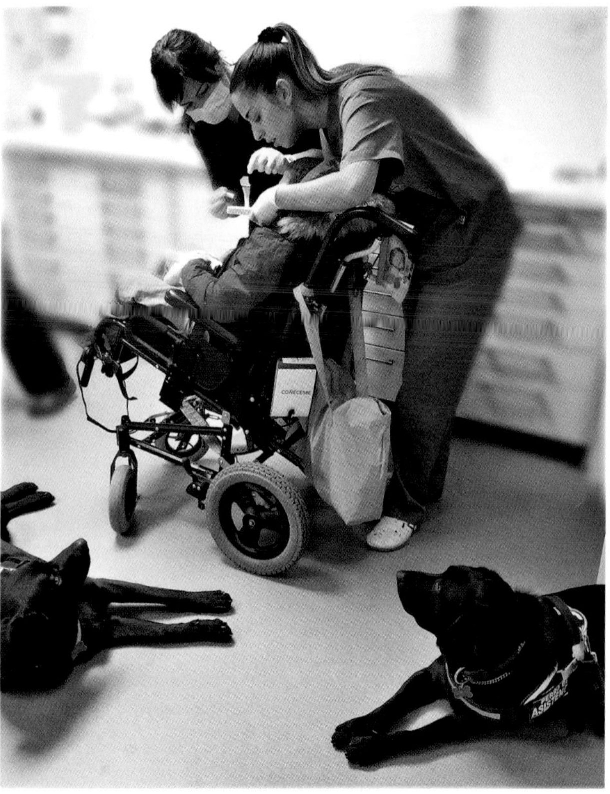

Figure 3.1.5 When the blind patient uses a guide dog, avoid interfering with the dog.

A World/Transcultural View

- About 75% of the population with visual deficits live in the poorest regions of Asia and Africa
- Among the lowest income countries, the proportion of children with blindness but caries free ranges from 53.2% in Sudan to 1.5% in India; paradoxically, studies in India have confirmed the efficacy of various preventive programmes based on promoting adapted oral hygiene techniques

Recommended Reading

GBD 2019 Blindness and Vision Impairment Collaborators; Vision Loss Expert Group of the Global Burden of Disease Study (2020). Causes of blindness and vision impairment in 2020 and trends over 30 years, and prevalence of avoidable blindness in relation to VISION 2020: the right to sight: an analysis for the global burden of disease study. *Lancet Glob. Health*: S2214-109X(20)30489-7.

Hidaka, R., Furuya, J., Suzuki, H. et al. (2020). Survey on the oral health status of community-dwelling older people with visual impairment. *Spec. Care Dentist.* 40: 192–197.

Jain, A., Gupta, J., Aggarwal, V., and Goyal, C. (2013). To evaluate the comparative status of oral health practices, oral hygiene and periodontal status amongst visually impaired and sighted students. *Spec. Care Dentist.* 33: 78–84.

Lee, S.Y. and Mesfin, F.B. (2020). Blindness. www.statpearls.com/

Schembri, A. and Fiske, J. (2001). The implications of visual impairment in an elderly population in recognizing oral disease and maintaining oral health. *Spec. Care Dentist.* 21: 222–226.

Shivanna, V., Jain, Y., Valluri, R. et al. (2019). Estimation of dental anxiety levels before and after dental visit in children with visual impairment using modified dental anxiety scale in Braille text. *J. Int. Soc. Prev. Community Dent.* 10: 76–84.

Tiwari, B.S., Ankola, A.V., Jalihal, S. et al. (2019). Effectiveness of different oral health education interventions in visually impaired school children. *Spec. Care Dentist.* 39: 97–107.

Watson, E.K., Moles, D.R., Kumar, N., and Porter, S.R. (2010). The oral health status of adults with a visual impairment, their dental care and oral health information needs. *Br. Dent. J.* 208: E15.

3.2 Auditory Deficit

Section I: Clinical Scenario and Dental Considerations

Clinical Scenario

A 6-year-old girl presents to your dental clinic with her foster mother who requests management of the patient's dental crowding.

Medical History

- Foetal alcohol syndrome (her biological mother had a drug and alcohol addiction, and is deceased)
- Bilateral mixed hypoacusis/hearing impairment due to sensorineural damage and eustachian tube dysfunction; auditory thresholds of 90 dB in the right ear and 80 dB in the left ear; has worn hearing aids from the age of 8 months but finds these difficult to tolerate
- Pigmentary retinopathy and optic nerve hypoplasia resulting in partial visual impairment
- Osteopenia in the lumbar vertebrae
- Overall growth retardation, with mild intellectual deficit
- Behavioural issues, with occasional aggressive episodes

Medications

- Risperidone
- Vitamin D3

Dental History

- No previous dental visits
- No chewing or swallowing problems
- Patient brushes 3 times a day, supervised by her foster mother

Social History

- Lives with a foster family
- Lack of spoken language but communicates through sign language
- Schooled since the age of 4 years (has a specialised support teacher for deaf-blind children)

Oral Examination

- Good oral hygiene
- Bimaxillary compression resulting in a narrow, pointed/ogival arched palate (Figure 3.2.1)
- Posterior cross-bite; edge-to-edge occlusion of anterior teeth
- Anterior tooth crowding, both maxillary and mandibular
- Delayed tooth eruption
- No caries detected

Radiological Examination

- An orthopantomogram was performed (poor quality due to lack of patient co-operation)
- Demonstrated delay in dental development and tooth eruption of approximately 18–24 months
- Agenesis of #34, #35, #44 and #45

Structured Learning

1) Why is the hypoacusis/loss of hearing in this patient particularly significant?
   - The patient has mixed bilateral deafness (which implies sensorineural impairment)
   - The auditory threshold is very low in one ear and severe in the other
   - The onset of the deafness was prelingual
2) What other factors impact on the ability to communicate with this patient?
   - Does not tolerate her hearing aids (often removes them)
   - Additional visual deficit which will impact on her ability to:

A Practical Approach to Special Care in Dentistry, First Edition. Edited by Pedro Diz Dios and Navdeep Kumar.

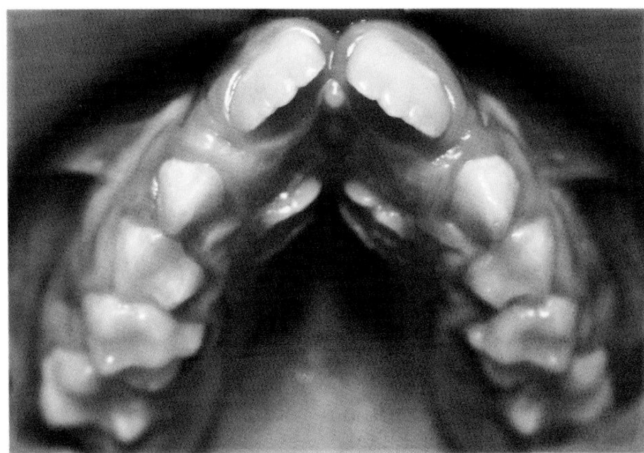

Figure 3.2.1 Bimaxillary compression resulting in a narrow, pointed/ogival arched palate.

- Engage with other communication management techniques such as pictograms and 'tell–show–do' (Figure 3.2.2)
- Ability to lip read or use sign language effectively

- No prior dental experience so unable to relate to surroundings, including the feel and smells associated with a dental office
- Learning disability
- Behavioural issues which may be worsened by heightened anxiety

3) What factors are considered important in assessing the risk of managing this patient?
   - Social
     - Lack of spoken language
     - Limited co-operation
     - Potentially aggressive behaviour
   - Medical
     - Auditory deficit
     - Visual deficit
     - Intellectual deficit
   - Dental
     - No previous experience of dental visits and hence limited co-operation; will require acclimatisation
     - Certain behavioural control techniques are not applicable (e.g. tone of voice)
     - Delayed dental development, malocclusion, tooth agenesis and high arched palate in relation to the foetal alcohol syndrome
4) The foster parent explains that the child is being bullied at school because she looks different. What would you do?
   - Discuss that improving the appearance of the child's teeth may not stop the bullying as the child

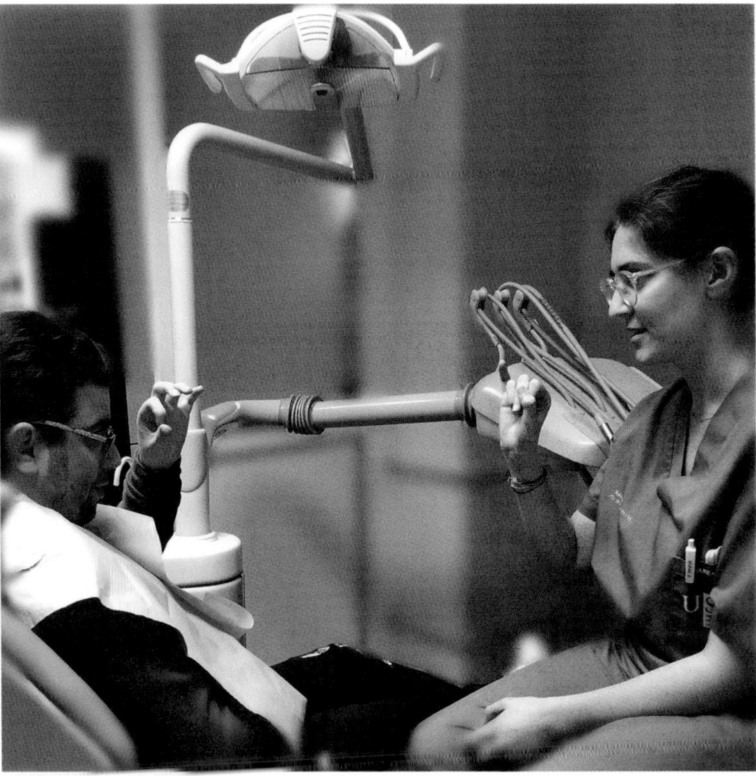

Figure 3.2.2 Sign language can be used to enhance communication.

may have other distinctive facial features of foetal alcohol syndrome which may appear different (small eyes, thin upper lip, short, upturned nose and a smooth skin surface between the nose and upper lip)
- Explain that the child is too young for dental extractions, orthodontics and/or orthognathic surgery to be planned (she is in the mixed dentition stage)
- She also has limited co-operation
- The most important focus is to acclimatise her to visiting the dentist regularly so that her oral health can be maintained and enable more invasive treatment at a later stage
- Encourage the foster parent to discuss the bullying with the school and social services

5) Tooth crowding in anterior sectors has promoted the localised accumulation of dental calculus. What factors would you need to consider when choosing the appropriate technique for removal of these deposits?
   - Manual instruments (curettes) may be preferable to minimise the background noise
   - Ultrasonic instrumentation can cause interference with hearing aids
6) The patient is not co-operative for calculus removal. What factors are important to assess prior to the adjunctive use of inhalational sedation?
   - The nasal hood may not be tolerated or may have a further negative impact on communication
   - Sedation itself may further impede communication
   - The patient has developmental delay – it is important to consider her weight and height before deciding on the appropriate concentration
   - Risperidone and nitrous oxide both have CNS depressant effects

General Dental Considerations

Oral Findings

- The prevalence of caries and the decayed, missing and filled teeth (DMFT) index in children with deafness are determined by their age, socio-economic level and educational level of their parents
- Children and adolescents with and without auditory deficit, whose oral health is supervised, have a similar prevalence of caries
- An increased rate of dental trauma has been reported, especially among males with deafness

Dental Management

- It is important to determine the best method for communicating with the patient that ensures that they understand when explaining oral hygiene techniques, dental procedures and treatment plans (Table 3.2.1; Figure 3.2.3)

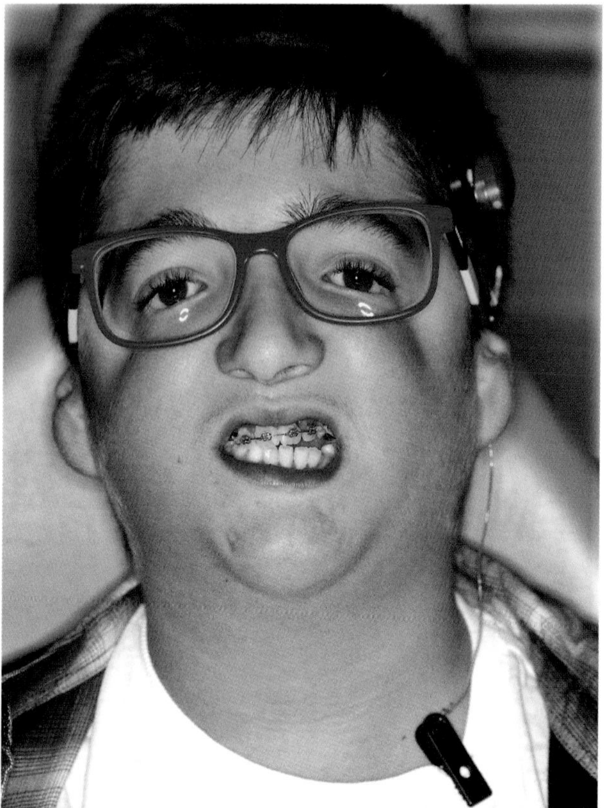

Figure 3.2.3 Orthodontic treatment for a patient with craniofacial dysostosis and associated hearing loss (Treacher Collins syndrome).

Section II: Background Information and Guidelines

Definition

Deafness is the difficulty or inability to use the sense of hearing due to a partial (hearing loss) or total (cophosis) unilateral or bilateral loss of auditory capacity. It is estimated that 7% of the population has an incapacitating hearing loss. Deafness affects men and women equally, and its prevalence increases with age. The condition is classified according to the anatomical area where the injury is located, the degree of hearing loss and the age at onset (Table 3.2.2).

Aetiopathogenesis

- The most common causes for conductive auditory deficit are congenital craniofacial disorders, infections and trauma (Table 3.2.3)

Table 3.2.1 Considerations for dental management.

Risk assessment	• Depending on the onset, degree of hearing loss, type and aetiology, (may impact on intellectual development) and/or the capacity for expression and speech • Cochlear implants are susceptible to electromagnetic interference and can be damaged by excessive electricity, including monopolar diathermy in the head and neck region or bipolar diathermy within 2 cm of the implant • Coexistence of other diseases which have led to the hearing loss
Criteria for referral	• Referral to a specialised clinic or hospital centre is rarely required and will be determined by the presence of comorbidities (e.g. polymalformative syndromes)
Access/position	• Distrust of dentists and anxiety are common • Some patients with auditory deficits can experience positional vertigo (e.g. Ménière syndrome)
Communication	• Patients with mild deficits, those who wear hearing aids/cochlear implants and those who can lip read: – Stand/sit at an appropriate distance from the patient – Position yourself where the patient can clearly see your face/lips – Talk with the face uncovered or use a transparent facemask – Keep the head fixed and talk slowly without raising the tone of voice – Speech should be adapted to the patient's sociocultural level and age – If possible, avoid intermediaries in the conversation • Patients with severe auditory deficit (untreatable): – Use other senses (vision and feel) to facilitate communication – Use mirrors, models, drawings and written language – Use sign language if you are able to (although it is not universal) or mime – Use a sign language interpreter if appropriate
Consent/capacity	• In order to confirm that the patient understands all the information that appears in the consent form and can ask any questions they have, select the most appropriate communication system to be employed (use a sign language interpreter if necessary) • For those who also have a visual deficit, it is essential additional adaptations are in place (e.g. consent form printed in sufficiently large type or a Braille version available) • If the patient cannot read, a close family member/friend acting as a witness can read it for them if hearing is sufficient • If it is not possible for the patient to communicate their decision using alternative adjuncts/methods, a best interest decision may be required
Anaesthesia/sedation	• Local anaesthesia – There are no specific considerations • Sedation – There may be difficulties monitoring the level of consciousness when performing conscious sedation • General anaesthesia – Ensure that the chosen method of communication is effective and communicated to all the theatre and recovery staff
Dental treatment	• Before – Background noise should be reduced as much as possible – Ensure lighting is adequate to allow the face to be clearly seen – Consider the use of signs and pictures to communicate – Transparent facemasks and face shields help lip reading • During – The 'tell–show–feel' (physical contact) technique may be applied – Rotary and ultrasonic instrumentation can cause interference with hearing aids – Electrocautery should not be employed in patients with cochlear implants

(*Continued*)

Table 3.2.1 (Continued)

Drug prescription	• Aminoglycoside antibiotics and macrolides are ototoxic and should be avoided • A number of drugs such as metronidazole, clindamycin and indomethacin can cause reversible hearing disorders (e.g. tinnitus)
Education/prevention	• Oral hygiene is frequently poor, and oral hygiene habits are often inadequate • Effective communication is a key factor in oral health education plans • In view of this, some countries have proposed requiring sign language in their dental curriculum • Dietary counselling is essential (high consumption of sugar and carbonated drinks has been described among patients with deafness)

Table 3.2.2 Auditory deficit classification.

Category	Classification
Lesion location	• Conductive or transmissive hearing loss (external ear, middle ear and labyrinth) • Sensorineural or perceptive hearing loss (internal ear, auditory nerve and temporal lobe) • Mixed
Degree of hearing loss	• Mild (detects sounds between 25 and 29 dB) • Moderate (detects sounds between 40 and 69 dB) • Severe (detects sounds between 70 and 89 dB) • Profound (detects sounds above 90 dB)
Age at onset	• Prelingual (before the development of speech) • Postlingual (after the development of speech)

Table 3.2.3 Auditory deficit aetiology.

Age	Classification
Prenatal	• Infections (rubella, syphilis, toxoplasmosis, HIV) • Hypothyroidism • Hypertension • Ototoxicity • Genetic (craniofacial dysostoses, family history) • Polymalformative syndromes
Perinatal/neonatal	• Prematurity • Low birthweight • Trauma • Infections (herpes simplex, cytomegalovirus) • Jaundice (kernicterus) • Hypoxia
Childhood	• Infections (otitis media, mumps, measles, malaria, meningitis)
Adolescence	• Ototoxicity • Foreign bodies • Exposure to noise • Trauma • Ménière syndrome
Adulthood	• Presbycusis • Ototoxicity • Otosclerosis • Infections (otitis media, encephalitis, meningitis)

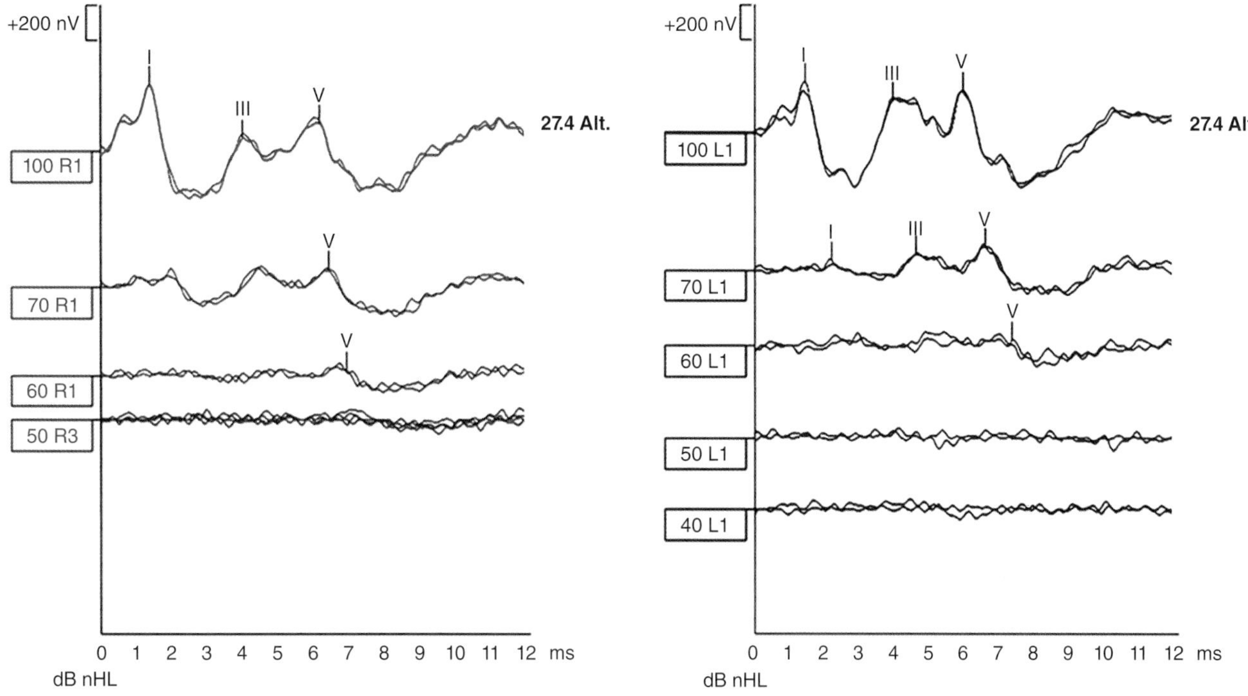

Figure 3.2.4 An audiogram shows the quietest sounds a patient can just hear.

- Sensorineural deafness is commonly associated with genetic disorders, trauma, prematurity, infections, tumours, drug ototoxicity, otosclerosis and presbycusis, among others

Clinical Presentation

- The symptoms of auditory deficit depend on the cause and level of hearing loss
- The presence of comorbidities is in general more common when the auditory deficiency occurs during the prenatal or perinatal stage
- Children younger than 4 months do not turn face to noises; at 12 months, they are unable to articulate a single word and only respond when they can see the speaker or when certain sounds are produced
- Older children talk in a high voice, continuously interrogate the speaker, and their pronunciation is unclear
- Sudden loss of hearing can be a symptom of another disease, such as stroke

Diagnosis

- Initial examination with tuning fork and otoscope

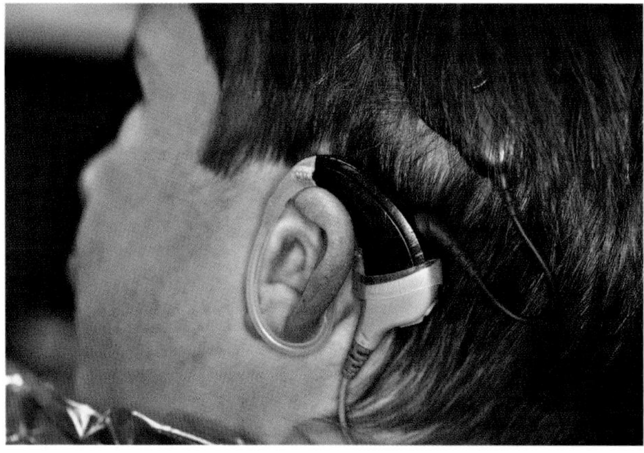

Figure 3.2.5 Cochlear implants in a child with congenital deafness.

- Audiometry (auditory capacity curve that combines intensity and frequency) (Figure 3.2.4)
- Impedance (audiometry of electrical response or otoacoustic emissions)
- Tympanometry and measurement of the stapedial reflex

Management

- Conductive auditory deficits can generally be treated with drugs or surgery (e.g. drainage, tympanoplasty and stapedectomy)
- Sensorineural deafness can be improved with hearing aids and cochlear implants (surgically implanted electrical devices) (Figure 3.2.5)

Prognosis

- The prognosis for deafness depends on its aetiology
- Conductive hearing loss usually has a better prognosis than sensorineural, which in some cases is irreversible
- Deafness in the elderly usually leads to psychological problems and significantly increases the risk of dementia

A World/Transcultural View

- The prevalence of hearing impairment in children and adults is substantially higher in low- to medium-income countries than in high-income countries; the regions with the highest prevalence of hearing impairment are southern Asia, sub-Saharan Africa, Central/Eastern Europe and Central Asia
- A significant percentage of cases of non-syndromic deafness have a genetic origin; a number of mutations (especially in the GJB2 gene) are common in Middle Eastern countries, where carriers belonging to numerous ethnic groups have been identified

Recommended Reading

Alsmark, S.S., García, J., Martínez, M.R., and López, N.E. (2007). How to improve communication with deaf children in the dental clinic. *Med. Oral Patol. Oral Cir. Bucal* 12: E576–E581.

Ávila-Curiel, B.X., Solórzano-Mata, C.J., Avendaño-Martínez, J.A. et al. (2019). Playful educational intervention for improvement of oral health in children with hearing impairment. *Int. J. Clin. Pediatr. Dent.* 12: 491–493.

Bimstein, E., Jerrell, R.G., Weaver, J.P., and Dailey, L. (2014). Oral characteristics of children with visual or auditory impairments. *Pediatr. Dent.* 36: 336–341.

Champion, J. and Holt, R. (2000). Dental care for children and young people who have a hearing impairment. *Br. Dent. J.* 189: 155–159.

Roberts, S., West, L.A., Liewehr, F.R. et al. (2002). Impact of dental devices on cochlear implants. *J. Endod.* 28: 40–43.

Shetty, V., Kumar, J., and Hegde, A. (2014). Breaking the sound barrier: oral health education for children with hearing impairment. *Spec. Care Dentist.* 34: 131–137.

Suhani, R.D., Suhani, M.F., and Badea, M.E. (2016). Dental anxiety and fear among a young population with hearing impairment. *Clujul Med.* 89: 143–149.

Wilson, B.S., Tucci, D.L., Merson, M.H., and O'Donoghue, G.M. (2017). Global hearing health care: new findings and perspectives. *Lancet* 390: 2503–2515.

4

Infectious Diseases

4.1 Tuberculosis

Section I: Clinical Scenario and Dental Considerations

Clinical Scenario

A 43-year-old male presents to the dental clinic complaining of generalised pain in his mouth of several years' duration. He reports that the pain makes eating very difficult and feels that this is linked to his weight loss in the past year. You note that the patient is unable to communicate clearly and appears intoxicated.

Medical History

- Tuberculosis diagnosed at the age of 18 years of age – completed 8 months of drug therapy with pharmacological cure criteria achieved
- Pulmonary mycetoma diagnosed 1 year earlier (pending surgery, which the patient has deferred on several occasions)
- Tuberculous reinfection 4 months earlier (has been undergoing drug therapy since then)
- Post-trauma cataract in the right eye
- Asthma
- Depression/low mood
- Constitutional syndrome (including malaise, fatigue, anorexia, weight loss) with protein-calorie malnutrition

Medications

- Isoniazid and rifampicin
- Tiotropium bromide
- Budesonide/formoterol
- Folic acid
- Lorazepam

Dental History

- Irregular attender as generally feels too tired to go out of the house
- Last visit many years ago
- Reports good co-operation in the past
- Does not brushing his teeth regularly

Social History

- Married but separated and now lives with his mother
- Unemployed/unable to work due to poor general health
- Minimal financial resources
- Tobacco consumption: 20 cigarettes/day since his adolescence
- History of excess alcohol consumption (stopped consuming alcohol 5 years ago)
- Intermittent use of recreational drugs; his wife, whom he sees occasionally, has drug addiction problems

Oral Examination

- Neglected dentition, with numerous caries and severe periodontal disease
- Fixed prosthesis in the aesthetic zone #13–23
- Caries in #16, #24 and #27
- Missing teeth: #11, #12, #14, #15, #21, #22, #36, #37 and #46
- Muscles of mastication tender on palpation

Radiological Examination

- Orthopantomogram undertaken as the patient is unable to tolerate intraoral radiographs (Figure 4.1.1)
- Generalised alveolar bone loss demonstrated
- Caries in #16, #23, #24, #25, #26 and #27

Structured Learning

1) Is it likely that the patient's tuberculosis was active a year ago and led to the development of the pulmonary mycetoma?
   - It is more likely that the patient had latent tuberculosis rather than active tuberculosis disease when the mycetoma was diagnosed
   - A pulmonary mycetoma is a chronic, progressively infectious disease which can occur within a pulmonary

A Practical Approach to Special Care in Dentistry, First Edition. Edited by Pedro Diz Dios and Navdeep Kumar.

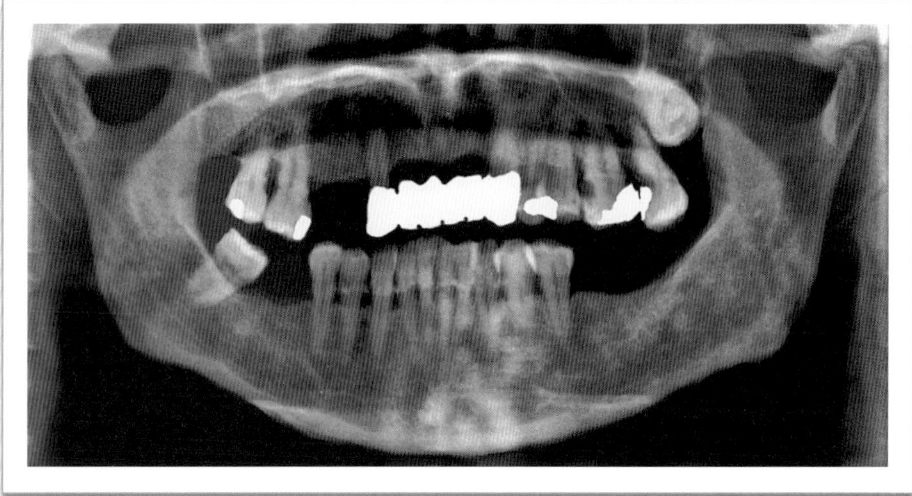

Figure 4.1.1 Orthopantomogram showing multiple caries and alveolar bone loss.

cavity that is usually generated during the previous episode of active tuberculosis
- It consists primarily of fungi, especially of the genus *Aspergillus*

2) What risk factors does this patient have for the development of tuberculosis?
   - The use of recreational drugs is known to increase the risk of contracting tuberculosis, whether or not the individual has HIV
   - This has been linked to the sharing of drug equipment, such as marijuana water pipes
3) What factors could be contributing to the patient's oral symptoms?
   - Poor oral health/recurrent dental infections
   - Temporomandibular dysfunction
   - Depression/atypical facial pain
   - Chronic pain associated with constitutional syndrome
4) The patient requests that all his remaining teeth are removed and dental implants are placed so that he can eat properly and gain weight. What factors should you consider when assessing the risk of managing this patient?
   - Social
     - Unrealistic expectations – the weight loss may be due to other factors, including the constitutional syndrome; orofacial pain may not be related to dental health
     - Impaired capacity due to apparent intoxication – this may be linked to use of recreational drugs; unable to give informed consent, needs to be assessed at each visit
     - Limited commitment to attend the dental clinic/hospital and follow-up
     - Limited financial means
   - Medical
     - Frail, malnourished patient with probable impaired wound healing
     - Recurrent tuberculosis
     - Impaired respiratory function: tuberculosis, mycetoma, asthma
     - Potential side-effects of antituberculosis medication (infection/bleeding risk)
     - Visual impairment due to the cataract and potential blurred vision with tiotropium
   - Dental
     - Neglected mouth/poor commitment to maintaining oral health
     - Active smoking
     - Hyposalivation caused by tiotropium
5) What laboratory tests are recommended before undertaking the dental extractions?
   - Full blood count
     - Rifampicin can cause leucopenia and thrombocytopenia
     - Isoniazid is also associated with a risk of thrombocytopenia, anaemia, aplastic anaemia, haemolytic anaemia
     - Haematological alterations are not uncommon in protein malnutrition
   - Liver function tests
     - Isoniazid can cause toxic hepatitis
   - Coagulation study
     - Coagulation may be impaired due to hepatic dysfunction caused by antituberculosis drugs

  - Rifampicin has also been associated with impaired vitamin K production by oral flora; this reduces the activity of vitamin K-dependent clotting factors

6) You determine that there is acute infection associated with #27. What do you need to consider when prescribing antibiotics and/or analgesics?
   - Do not prescribe medication that is metabolised by the liver
   - Appropriate medications include:
     - Antibiotics such as penicillin V or amoxicillin
     - Analgesics: such as metamizole (unavailable in some countries) or paracetamol at low dosages (<2 g/day)

7) When planning for dental extractions, should you delay due to the diagnosis of tuberculosis?
   - The patient has undergone tuberculosis treatment for more than 3 months following reactivation of the infection
   - Hence treatment can proceed but it is prudent to liaise with the patient's physician given the multiple comorbidities
8) The patient asks whether he can have sedation for dental extractions. What precautions are necessary with this patient?
   - Advise that this cannot be provided if recreational drugs are used
   - Consider the BMI/weight loss of the patient
   - During the active phase of tuberculosis, do not use nitrous oxide as this might contaminate the gas flow system
   - Lorazepam has synergistic action with other benzodiazepines
   - The concomitant use of rifampicin and diazepam should be avoided

General Dental Considerations

Oral Findings

- The most common oral lesion is a chronic ulcer located on the dorsum of the tongue (although it can also appear on the palate, lips, oral mucosa and gums) (Figure 4.1.2)
- Diagnosis is established based on a biopsy of the lesion
- Cervical or submandibular tuberculous lymphadenopathy
  - Often caused by nontuberculous mycobacteria
  - A number of these mycobacteria are multiresistant, particularly among patients with HIV infection
  - Lymphadenopathy can fistulise the skin surface (scrofula)

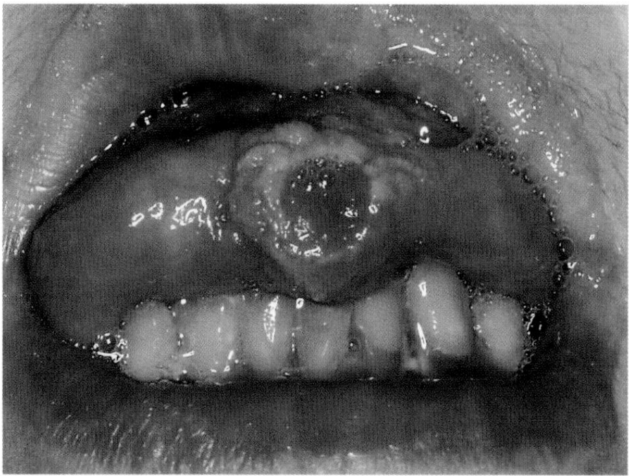

Figure 4.1.2 Primary tuberculosis manifesting as a non-healing, tender ulcer on the tip of the tongue.

  - Diagnosis is established through cultures and/or polymerase chain reaction (PCR) of the nodule biopsy
  - Treatment usually consists of administering clarithromycin and excising the affected nodules
- There have been reported oral findings related to tuberculostatic agents:
  - Rifampicin and rifabutin can stain the saliva red
  - Rifampicin can cause lichenoid hypersensitivity lesions
  - Streptomycin can cause circumoral paraesthesia

Dental Management

- The dental treatment plan will be determined primarily by the disease progression and by the presence of comorbidities (e.g. HIV infection) (Table 4.1.1)

Section II: Background Information and Guidelines

Definition

Tuberculosis is an infectious and transmissible disease caused by *Mycobacterium tuberculosis*, which is characterised by necrotising granulomatous inflammation that mainly affects the lungs (approximately 85% of cases). It is estimated that tuberculosis infects approximately 10 million individuals worldwide each year, 87% of which are concentrated in only 30 countries (predominantly countries with low economic levels). It is a notifiable disease in many parts of the world, with healthcare staff required to inform their health protection teams of a suspected/confirmed case.

Table 4.1.1 Considerations for dental management.

Risk assessment	• Mycobacteria proliferate in the biofilms of dental units • Although the risk of transmission is low, the transmission of tuberculosis in the dental clinic has been reported • Patients who start antituberculosis therapy are considered to not be infectious at 2 weeks, although negative sputum results might not start for up to 2 months • Patients who have completed antituberculosis therapy generally have no risk of disease reactivation • Side-effects of tuberculosis medication: – Especially in those older than 35 years, drug-induced hepatitis can increase the tendency to bleed – Leucopenia, thrombocytopenia and impaired vitamin K production (increasing bleeding risk) have also been described • A number of comorbidities can affect the delivery of dental treatment (alcoholism, drug addiction, hepatitis and HIV infection)
Criteria for referral	• Latent tuberculosis – The patient is not infectious and can be treated in the dental clinic using standard infection control precautions • Active tuberculosis – Standard precautions are insufficient to prevent bacterial transmission – Urgent dental treatment should be undertaken in a hospital setting with access to the appropriate personal protective equipment and ideally a negative pressure room – Non-urgent treatment should be postponed for 3 months • Referral to a specialised clinic or hospital centre is also determined by the patient's general condition (e.g. respiratory distress or concurrent advanced HIV infection)
Access/appointment	• As routine, healthcare staff within the dental clinic should have tests for tuberculosis and evidence of immunity; this is evidenced by tuberculin skin testing or interferon gamma testing within the last 5 years, and/or checking of a BCG (cacillus Calmette–Guérin) scar by an occupational health professional • If the patient has active tuberculosis, schedule the appointment for the last session of the day to minimise the risk of cross-transmission; ensure there is access to filtering face pieces (FFP) – ideally FFP3 as these have the highest level of filtering capacity • Minimise the number of staff in contact
Consent/capacity	• Include any potential risks arising from the drugs used to treat tuberculosis and/or comorbidities
Anaesthesia/sedation	• Local anaesthesia – No specific recommendations; this is the method of choice to enable dental treatment • Sedation – Avoid sedation with nitrous oxide (risk of contamination) – Consider the impact of respiratory depression – The efficacy of diazepam can change in patients who are administered rifampicin – Accelerated metabolism and reduced plasma concentrations of benzodiazepines have been noted • General anaesthesia – General anaesthesia entails a risk of contamination, and some patients also have pulmonary function impairment – Streptomycin increases the activity of neuromuscular blockers (myasthenic syndrome) – Where unavoidable, a plenum-ventilated operating theatre should be used

(Continued)

Table 4.1.1 (Continued)

Dental treatment	• Before – Any patient presenting with symptoms suggestive of active tuberculosis disease should be isolated, instructed to wear a surgical or procedure mask, and referred promptly for medical care – For those patients who require urgent dental treatment/who may be infectious, high-efficiency particulate air (HEPA) filters, ultraviolet germicidal irradiation (UVGI) lamps and appropriate personal protective equipment should be available (FFP3) • During – The use of sprays and the generation of aerosols (ultrasonic scaling equipment and high-speed rotary instruments) should be reduced – Use high-volume suction – Use rubber dams – Use facemasks with eye protection and change them if they get moist • After – Sterilise the instruments with heat (mycobacteria are resistant to disinfectants) – Ventilate the clinic after completing the session (open windows)
Drug prescription	• Avoid paracetamol or recommend low doses (increased hepatic toxicity by rifampicin and isoniazid) • It is prudent to avoid all drugs reliant on hepatic metabolism • Avoid aspirin (increases the risk of ototoxicity by streptomycin, amikacin, kanamycin or capreomycin) • Avoid clarithromycin and azole derivatives (they interact with rifampicin)
Education/prevention	• All staff who provide dental care should undergo a Mantoux test when commencing employment, regardless of the setting's risk classification

Aetiopathogenesis

- The most common infectious agent is *M. tuberculosis*
- The bacilli access the lungs (in the form of aerosol droplets), are phagocytised by macrophages and transferred to regional lymph nodes
- Haematogenous dissemination then occurs
- The granulomatous lesions (tubercles) contain living bacilli and develop by a delayed hypersensitivity mechanism

Clinical Presentation

- Globally, tuberculosis notification data show a male-to-female ratio of 1.7:1 and higher, although the underlying reasons for the male bias remain unclear
- Latent tuberculosis
  - The initial infection is usually asymptomatic
  - Approximately one-quarter of the world's population has latent tuberculosis – at this stage, they cannot transmit the infection
- Active primary tuberculosis disease
  - People infected with tuberculosis bacteria have a 5–15% lifetime risk of progressing to develop tuberculosis disease

    Persons with compromised immune systems, such as those living with HIV, malnutrition or diabetes, or people who use tobacco, have a higher risk of developing the disease
  - Symptoms include fever, night sweats, cough, asthenia, anorexia and lymphadenopathy
  - The symptoms may be mild and persist for many months, leading to delays in seeking care, and in transmission of the bacteria to others
  - Pulmonary impairment may progress, resulting in a productive cough, rales (abnormal rattling sound from the lungs) and, in highly advanced stages, haemoptysis
  - Occasionally, there is extrapulmonary dissemination, which can affect the central nervous system, bones and cardiovascular, genitourinary and gastrointestinal systems
  - Some particularly prevalent conditions such as alcoholism, drug addiction, cancer, diabetes and HIV infection can alter the clinical presentation of tuberculosis
  - Without appropriate treatment, approximately 45% of HIV-negative people with tuberculosis and nearly all HIV-positive people with tuberculosis will die
- Tuberculosis recurrence
  - Latent tuberculosis is associated with 5–10% chance of reactivation, usually within the first 2 years of infection

- Recurrence can be due to either reactivation of the same strain, i.e. relapse, or reinfection with a new strain
- Recurrence due to reinfection is more likely in endemic settings with high rates of HIV coinfection

Diagnosis

- The acquisition of skin reactivity to the tuberculin purified protein derivative or Mantoux test is considered suggestive of tuberculosis (Figure 4.1.3)
- Chest radiography helps establish the suspected diagnosis for patients with symptoms (Figure 4.1.4)
- Sputum smears have poor sensitivity

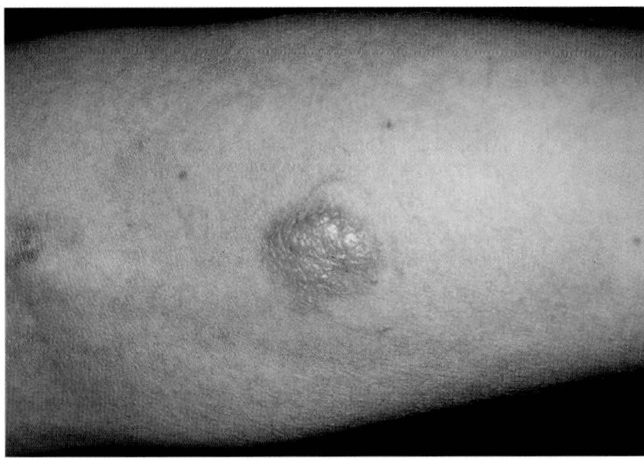

Figure 4.1.3 Positive Mantoux test (also known as tuberculin PPD test for purified protein derivative).

- Sputum cultures provide the definitive diagnosis, but the results are not obtained for up to 4–8 weeks
- PCR provides a rapid and reliable diagnosis
- For extrapulmonary tuberculosis, a histopathological analysis of the infected organs should be conducted . It is characterised by the presence of caseating granulomas formed by epitheloid macrophages surrounging an acelluar necrotic region

Management

- The most widely used regimen is the administration of 4 drugs (isoniazid, rifampicin, pyrazinamide, and ethambutol) for 2 months, followed by 2 drugs (isoniazid and rifampicin) for another 4 months
- Multidrug-resistant tuberculosis is an increasing concern – the disease does not respond to isoniazid and rifampicin, the 2 most powerful medications used to treat the disease
- Alternatives in this situation include diarylquinoline and nitroimidazole
- Treatment regimens can be prolonged, typically lasting 6–12 months
- Treating recurrent tuberculosis that is caused by relapse is challenging as often the bacteria have become resistant to treatment and a different combination of drugs, taken over a longer period of time, is required
- Hence recurrent tuberculosis disease is associated with poor treatment outcomes and higher mortality rates compared to primary tuberculosis infection

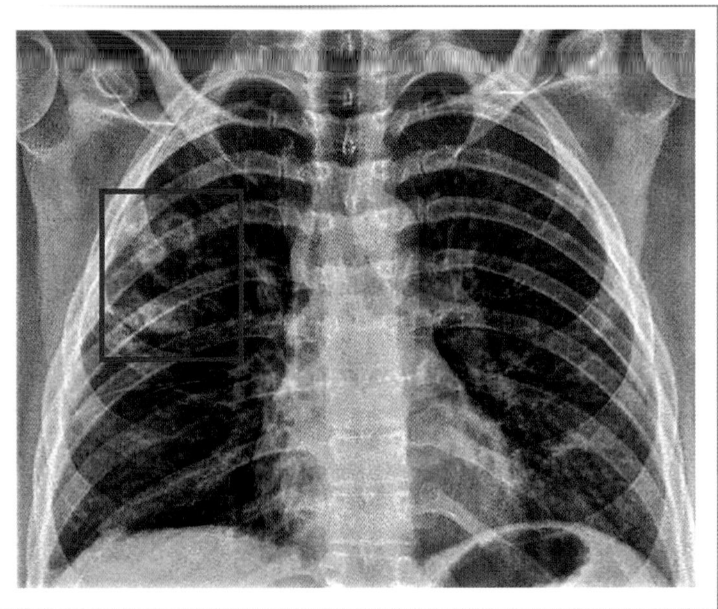

Figure 4.1.4 Chest x-ray showing cavitary lesions typically associated with active pulmonary tuberculosis.

Prognosis

- About 5% of patients infected by *M. tuberculosis* develop active tuberculosis in the first 2 years post exposure
- The incidence of drug-resistant tuberculosis is increasing exponentially
- Although tuberculous mortality has fallen substantially in the past 20 years, it is estimated that 3 million individuals die annually due to complications from this disease
- About 25% of those who die have concurrent HIV infection

A World/Transcultural View

- There is a strong association between the incidence of tuberculosis and a country's gross domestic product per capita
- Marginalised and socially disadvantaged populations, such as indigenous populations, ethnic minorities, immigrants and prisoners, also have a higher incidence of tuberculosis
- Poorer treatment results have been recorded in groups with low socio-economic levels, probably because they have limited access to high-quality care
- Although drug-resistant strains have been previously diagnosed in highly endemic settings, resistance to numerous drugs constitutes a significant problem in the industrialised world

Recommended Reading

Dheda, K., Barry, C.E. 3rd, and Maartens, G. (2016). Tuberculosis. *Lancet* 387: 1211–1226.

Faecher, R.S., Thomas, J.E., and Bender, B.S. (1993). Tuberculosis: a growing concern for dentistry? *J. Am. Dent. Assoc.* 124: 94–104.

Feller, L., Wood, N.H., Chikte, U.M. et al. (2009). Tuberculosis part 4. control of Mycobacterium tuberculosis transmission in dental care facilities. *SADJ* 64: 408–410.

González Mediero, G., Vázquez Gallardo, R., Pérez Del Molino, M.L., and Diz Dios, P. (2015). Evaluation of two commercial nucleic acid amplification kits for detecting Mycobacterium tuberculosis in saliva samples. *Oral Dis.* 21: 451–455.

Jensen, P. A., Lambert, L. A., Iademarco, M. F., Ridzon, R., & CDC (2005). Guidelines for preventing the transmission of Mycobacterium tuberculosis in health-care settings, 2005. MMWR Recomm Rep. 54 (RR-17): 1–141.

Rinaggio, J. (2003). Tuberculosis. *Dent. Clin. North Am.* 47: 449–465.

Sharma, S., Bajpai, J., Pathak, P.K. et al. (2019). Oral tuberculosis – current concepts. *J. Family Med. Prim. Care.* 8: 1308–1312.

4.2 Human Immunodeficiency Virus (HIV) Infection/AIDS

Section I: Clinical Scenario and Dental Considerations

Clinical Scenario

A 45-year-old man is referred by his physician for assessment of extensive but painless oral papillomatous lesions.

Medical History
- Stage 3 human immunodeficiency virus (HIV) infection (HIV infection diagnosed 14 years ago)
- Cryptococcal meningitis (without sequelae)
- Kaposi sarcoma of the skin
- Chronic hepatitis B virus (HBV) infection
- Anal squamous cell carcinoma
- Adjustment disorder and depressed mood

Medications
- Ritonavir (RTV)
- Emtricitabine (FTC) + tenofovir (TDF)
- Citalopram

Dental History
- Irregular dental attender
- Moderate level of co-operation
- Patient brushes his teeth twice a day

Social History
- Lives with his male partner (who is HIV negative)
- Works in a car company as a welder
- Alcohol and tobacco consumption: discontinued 10 years ago

Oral Examination
- Fair oral hygiene
- Numerous exophytic lesions (sessile/flat and pedunculated) that preferentially involve the lips, retrocommissural area and palate; clinically suggestive of warts
- Generalised periodontal disease with numerous pathological periodontal pockets (≥6 mm)
- Caries in #15, #34 and #46
- Lost teeth: #27 and #36

Radiological Examination
- Orthopantomogram undertaken
- No intraoral radiographs due to large number of oral papilloma-type lesions (Figure 4.2.1)
- Restorable caries in #34, #38 and #45
- Extensive, deep and unrestorable caries in #15 and #46
- Periapical osteolytic lesion in #46

Structured Learning

1) What is the cause of the oral lesions?
   - The oral lesions are likely to be due to human papilloma virus (HPV) infection and are benign – oral papilloma/condyloma with focal epithelial hyperplasia
   - HIV and HPV are both infections that can be transmitted sexually

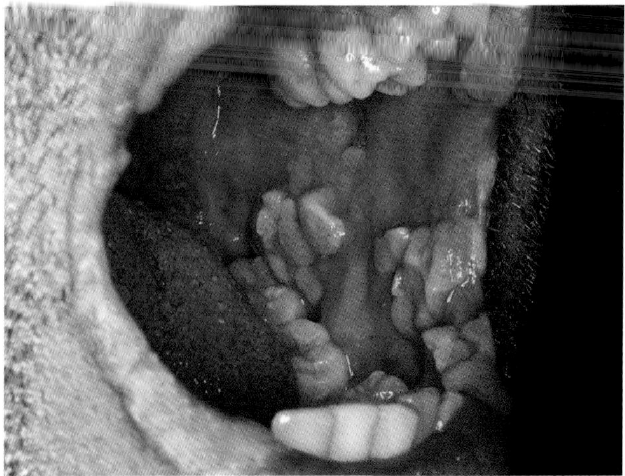

Figure 4.2.1 Oral HPV-associated papillomatosis in AIDS.

A Practical Approach to Special Care in Dentistry, First Edition. Edited by Pedro Diz Dios and Navdeep Kumar.

- Immunosuppression is known to increase the risk of HPV infection
- HPV oral lesions in patients with HIV infection and taking antiretrovirals may be related with the longer life expectancy of individuals with an impaired immune system rather than a direct effect of antiretroviral therapy (ART)

2) The patient's primary concern is removal of the oral lesions as the teeth are asymptomatic. What additional information do you need first regarding his HIV infection?
   - Current viral load: the results are given as the number of copies of HIV per millilitre of blood
   - Current CD4 count: normal CD4 count is from 500 to 1400 cells per microlitre of blood
3) The physician advises you that the last test results are: viral load 13 000 copies/mL and CD4 count of 100 cells/μL. What factors are important to consider when assessing the risk of managing this patient?
   - Social
     - Physical stigma in a work setting that is probably unaware of his HIV infection (i.e. oral warts)
     - Risk of patient not attending appointments due to low mood/depression (see Chapter 15.2)
   - Medical
     - HIV infection in the acquired immune deficiency syndrome (AIDS) stage – CD4 count low leading to an increased risk of infection; viral load high (increased infectivity)
     - Ritonavir may cause thrombocytopenia
     - Chronic HBV infection (see Chapter 4.3) linked to bleeding risk, reduced drug metabolism
     - Anal carcinoma – may be uncomfortable for the patient to sit down if the lesion is symptomatic
   - Dental
     - Oral lesions may impair access to toothbrushing
     - Oral hygiene not optimal – may increase the risk of postoperative infection after removal of the oral papillomas
     - Lesions may recur after removal
     - Dental caries and periodontal disease present
     - Follow-up compromised by the depressive syndrome and previous irregular attendance
4) As the lesions are widespread and some are sessile, vaporisation of the papillomatous lesions using CO_2 laser is planned. What precautions should be in place?
   - Perform the necessary laboratory tests (e.g. complete blood count with differential and coagulation study)
   - Administer antibiotic prophylaxis because the patient has <200 CD4+ T-cells/μL
   - Take a sample with a cold scalpel beforehand to conduct histopathology
   - Maximise protection measures with subsequent use of the CO_2 laser to prevent dissemination of the papillomavirus:
     - Powerful surgical aspirator
     - Facemasks and eye protectors
     - Schedule the appointment for the last hour of the workday and ventilate the dental office after completing the procedure
5) The patient is nervous about the proposed vaporisation of the oral lesions and has been prescribed diazepam to take before he attends. What considerations should be taken into account?
   - Ritonavir can boost the sedative effects of benzodiazepines
   - If the hepatic impairment caused by the HBV is moderate to severe, the use of diazepam should be avoided (liaise with the physician and preferably use lorazepam)
6) The patient returns to you for extraction of the #15 and #46. What laboratory test results should be undertaken before proceeding and why?
   - Full blood count and coagulation study should be undertaken
   - Anaemia, thrombocytopenia and leucopenia/neutropenia may be present
   - Thrombocytopenia can occur in people with HIV due to multiple factors, including HIV infiltration of the bone marrow, as a side-effect of drugs used to treat HIV (e.g. ritonavir), or due to the development of autoimmune (idiopathic) thrombocytopenic purpura
   - Neutropenia is observed in 10% of patients with early asymptomatic HIV infections and in 50% of patients with AIDS (again related to bone marrow infiltration and as a side-effect of some medications)
   - HBV infection can impair the hepatic synthesis of coagulation factors

General Dental Considerations

Oral Findings

Oral lesions in patients with HIV infection are mainly related to the state of immunosuppression and the adverse effects of the antiretroviral drugs (Tables 4.2.1 and 4.2.2; Figures 4.2.2 and 4.2.3)

Table 4.2.1 Potential consequences of HIV disease.

Category	Associated conditions
GROUP 1 Lesions closely associated with HIV infection	• Candidiasis • Hairy leucoplakia • Kaposi sarcoma • Non-Hodgkin lymphoma • Periodontal disease • Linear gingival erythema • Necrotising gingivitis • Necrotising periodontitis
GROUP 2 Lesions less commonly associated with HIV infection	• Bacterial infections: *Mycobacterium avium-intracellulare*, *M. tuberculosis* • Melanin hyperpigmentation • Necrotising stomatitis • Salivary gland enlargement • Thrombocytopenic purpura • Ulcer not otherwise specified (NOS) • Viral infections: *Herpex simplex*, *Papillomavirus*, *Varicela-zoster virus*
GROUP 3 Lesions reported in HIV infection	• Bacterial infections: *Actinomyces israelii*, *Escherichia coli*, *Klebsiella pneumoniae*, Cat scratch disease (*Bartonella henselae*) • Viral infections: *Cytomegalovirus*, *Molluscum contagiosum* • Drug reactions • Fungal infections other than candidiasis • Neurological disorders

Dental Management

- The dental treatment plan will be determined mainly by the patient's general condition, prognosis and prior oral health (Figure 4.2.4)
- Each procedure should take into account the patient's immunosuppression level, potential complications (e.g. tendency to bleed) and presence of comorbidities (e.g. chronic viral hepatitis) (Table 4.2.2)

Section II: Background Information and Guidelines

Definition

The HIV is a retrovirus of the lentivirus group. When transmitted to a patient, HIV mainly targets T helper cells (CD4+ cells), which are essential for the immune response. The initial infection is followed by a long period of gradual deterioration of the immune system, which leads to the AIDS phase. It is estimated that more than 37 million individuals worldwide have HIV/AIDS and that its current rate is 1.7 million new cases per year.

Aetiopathogenesis

- At this time, the main groups exposed to HIV infection are men who have sex with men, individuals who engage in risky heterosexual contact and parenteral drug users (the risk of perinatal transmission has declined dramatically in recent years)
- Two types of HIV, which share the same mechanism of action, have been identified: HIV-1, which has a worldwide distribution, and HIV-2, which is more common among African populations
- HIV infects cells with CD4+ receptors, mainly T-cells, monocytes, tissue macrophages and dendritic cells. Within the cell, HIV replicates using the reverse transcriptase enzyme. The resulting DNA is imported into the cell nucleus and integrated. The infected cells release new virus particles by gemmation and the cells are ultimately destroyed

Clinical Presentation (CDC Classification)

- Stage 1: Initial infection
  - Can be asymptomatic
  - Within 2–4 weeks after infection, may also present as viral symptoms similar to influenza (fever, headache, lymphadenopathy, myalgia and exanthema)
  - High viral load and infectivity

Table 4.2.2 Main antiretroviral drugs with adverse orofacial effects.

Drug class	Adverse orofacial effects							
Generic name	Erythema multif.	Ulcers	Dry mouth	Dysgeusia	Exfoliative cheilitis	Mucosal pigm.	Cushingoid appear.	Lipodys.
Nucleoside/nucleotide reverse transcriptase inhibitors								
• Zidovudine (AZT)	+	+		+				+
• Didanosine (DDI)	+		+					
• Zalcitabine (ddC)	+	+						
• Stavudine (d4T)								+
• Lamivudine (3TC)			+					+
• Abacavir (ABC)	+	+				+		
• Adefovir (ADF)								
• Tenofovir (TDF)								+
• Emtricitabine (FTC)						+		+
Non-nucleoside reverse transcriptase inhibitors								
• Etravirine (ETR)	+	+	+				+	
• Delavirdine (DLV)	+	+					+	
• Efavirenz (EFV)	+		+	+				
• Nevirapine (NVP)	+	+						
Protease inhibitors								
• Saquinavir (SQV)	+	+	+		+		+	+
• Ritonavir (RTV)			+	+	+	+	+	+
• Indinavir (IDV)			+	+	+			+
• Nelfinavir (NFV)			+					+
• Amprenavir (APV)							+	+
• Tipranavir (TPV)	+	+					+	+
• Fosamprenavir (FPV)	+						+	+
• Atazanavir (ATV)	+		+				+	
• Darunavir (DRV)	+					+	+	
Fusion inhibitors								
• Enfuvirtide (ENF)	+		+	+				
Entry inhibitors								
• Maraviroc (MVC)	+			+				
Integrase strand transfer inhibitors								
• Raltegravir (RAL)	+			+				

Erythema multif., Erythema multiforme; Mucosal pigm., Mucosal pigmentation; Cushingoid appear., Cushingoid appearance; Lipodys., Lipodystrophy

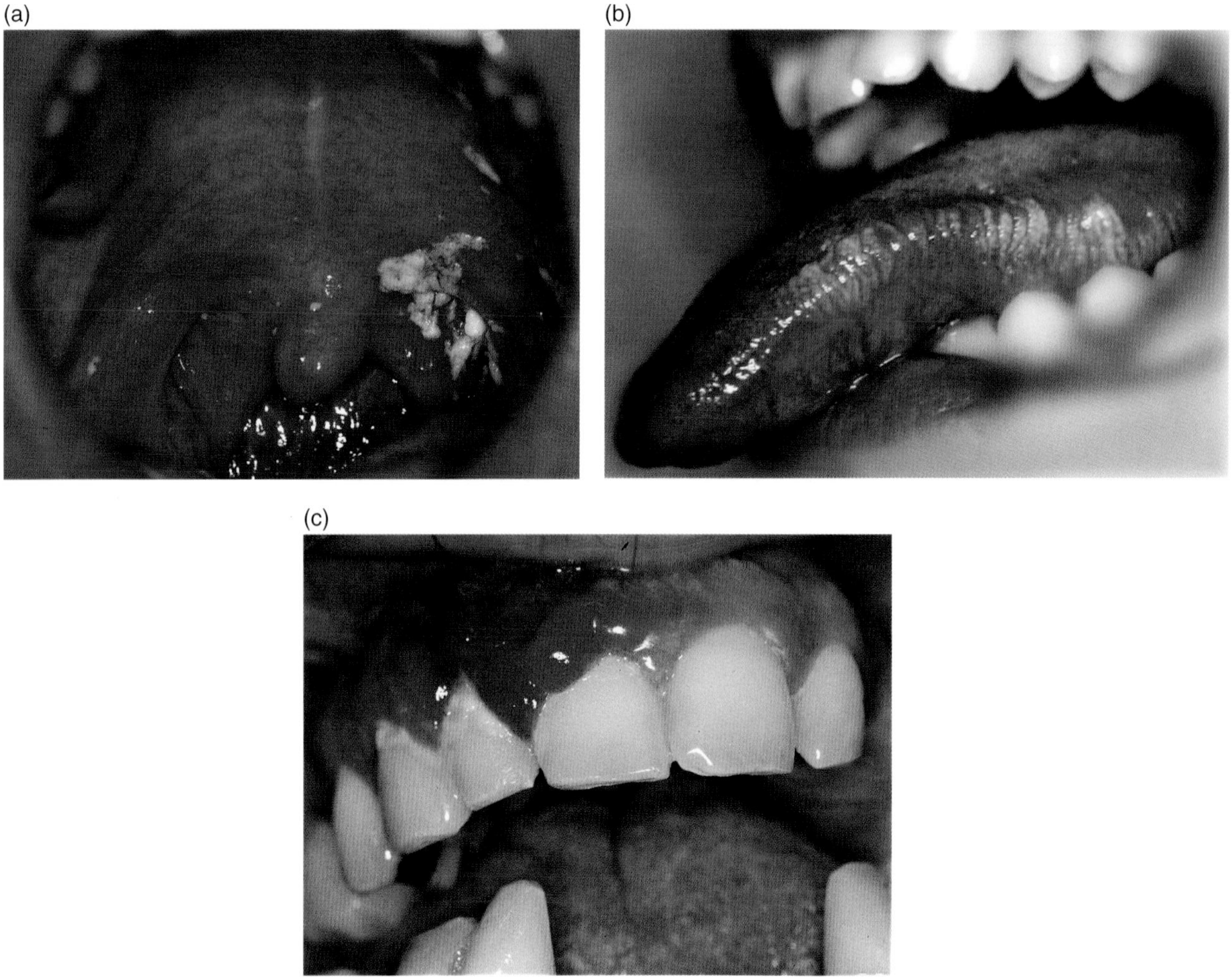

(a)

(b)

(c)

Figure 4.2.2 (a–c) Lesions closely associated with HIV infection: oral candidiasis, oral hairy leucoplakia and Kaposi sarcoma.

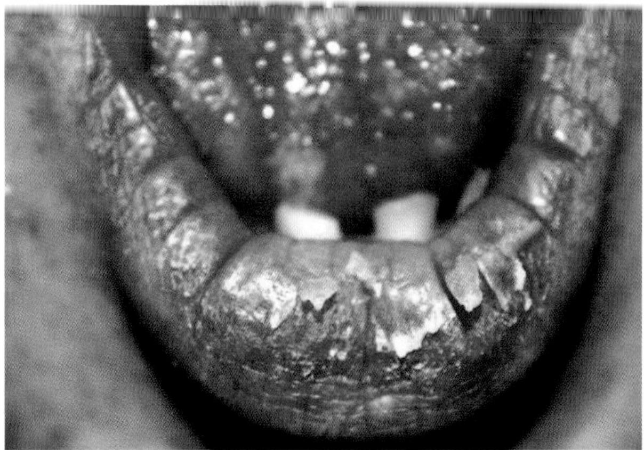

Figure 4.2.3 Exfoliative cheilitis as an adverse oral effect of proteinase inhibitors.

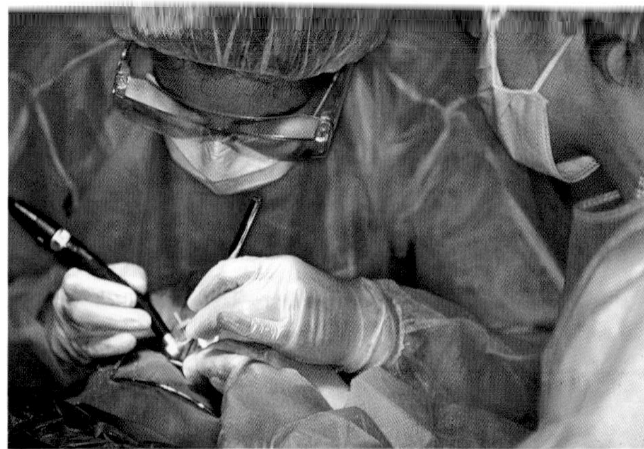

Figure 4.2.4 Infection control in the dental clinic.

Table 4.2.3 Considerations for dental management.

Risk assessment	• There are no absolute contraindications for performing dental treatment on patients with HIV infection • However, due to the HIV-associated immunosuppression, it is important to consider any associated comorbidities (e.g. chronic hepatitis) and side-effects of medication (e.g. thrombocytopenia related to ritonavir, neutropenia related to zidovudine) • The transmission rate is estimated at 0.3% after exposure to contaminated blood by the percutaneous pathway and approximately 0.09% after contact with mucous membranes
Criteria for referral	• Most patients can be treated in a conventional outpatient dental clinic • Referral to a specialised clinic or hospital centre is determined mainly by the patient's general condition, presence of severe immunosuppression, presence of comorbidities and/or increased bleeding risk
Access/appointment	• A number of barriers to treatment have been identified for these patients and include the anxiety caused by the dental setting, reluctance by the dentist to see them, concerns regarding confidentiality, cumbersome administrative processes, long waiting times and psychological problems • If the viral load is high, schedule the patient for the last session of the day to minimise the risk of cross-transmission
Communication	• A significant percentage of patients with HIV infection who receive dental treatment do not report their condition • An HIV diagnostic test and/or the possibility of referring to the family doctor should be offered to patients with suspicious medical histories or oral findings
Consent/capacity	• Patients should be warned of the potential complications resulting from the HIV infection, side-effects of medication and the additional risks associated with existing comorbidities • Neurological involvement in HIV (HIV-associated dementia) is commonly associated with cognitive impairment but is rare in those patients receiving antiretroviral drugs; comorbid conditions can also contribute to impairment
Anaesthesia/ sedation	• Local anaesthesia – Minimise the risk of pricking with contaminated needles after infiltrative anaesthesia (e.g. single-use devices) • Sedation – Minimise the risk of pricking with contaminated needles after percutaneous injection – The activity of benzodiazepines administered for sedation can increase in patients who take protease inhibitors • General anaesthesia – A comprehensive assessment in conjunction with the anaesthetist is essential – The patient's physician should be consulted and investigations undertaken to assess the risk of bleeding, infection and whether there are any concurrent infections which would compromise respiration

(*Continued*)

Table 4.2.3 (Continued)

Dental treatment	• Before – Universal cross-infection control measures should be applied – The treatment plan will be determined by the HIV disease prognosis and the previous oral health condition, among other factors – The dental treatment needs of patients with HIV infection are significantly greater for those with a history of parenteral drug use – Recent blood test results should be available including: ○ CD4+ T-lymphocyte count ○ Viral load ○ Full blood count (risk of anaemia, leucopenia, neutropenia, thrombocytopenia) ○ Coagulation study (in case of liver disease) – If invasive dental procedures are planned, it is advisable to administer antibiotic prophylaxis to patients with <200 CD4+ T-cells/μL and/or those who with moderate neutropenia (500–1000 cells/μL) – For cases of severe neutropenia (<500 cells/μL), antibiotic prophylaxis is mandatory • During – Apply conventional measures for infection control – In the event of accidental exposure in the dental clinic, the contaminated area should be washed with soap and water, and the reference physician should be immediately informed so that they can evaluate the risk of exposure and the advisability of diagnostic tests and prophylactic administration of antiretroviral agents • After – The prevalence and severity of complications after an extraction are similar to those observed in healthy controls – The success rates of osseointegrated implants, sinus lifts and bone regeneration surgery are similar for patients with well-controlled HIV infection and the HIV-negative population – Basic periodontal treatment procedures and periodontal surgery have been successfully performed in this context – The rate of postoperative complications and the elimination of periapical lesions following a root canal are similar to those detected in the general population
Drug prescription	• There is an increased risk of hypersensitivity to some drugs such as beta-lactams • Metronidazole can cause a disulfiram-like reaction in patients who take ritonavir • The risk of haematological toxicity and bleeding in patients who take zidovudine can increase if non-steroidal anti-inflammatory agents are administered concomitantly
Education/prevention	• If a patient is aware of their HIV-positive condition and potential impact on the oral cavity this can promote the need to maintain a healthy mouth and result in an improvement in their oral hygiene habits • Patients should be counselled regarding oral hygiene, xerostomia treatment, smoking cessation and reducing sugar in their diet • Maintaining good oral health can prevent the onset of rapidly progressive periodontal disease • Emphasis should be placed on cleaning the dental prosthesis and disinfecting toothbrushes (with antiseptic solutions such as chlorhexidine) • Patients with peripheral neuropathy might have limited manual dexterity for performing proper oral hygiene

- Stage 2: Latency period/chronic infection
  - Generally characterised by persistent generalised lymphadenopathy
  - Can also be asymptomatic until the first opportunistic infections appear, such as oral candidiasis
  - Very low viral load; if taking antiretroviral therapy, viral load may be undetectable with effectively no risk of viral transmission
- Stage 3: AIDS
  - Characterised by the onset of conditions that have been called 'AIDS-defining'
  - These include oesophageal candidiasis, systemic mycosis (histoplasmosis, coccidioidomycosis, cryptococcosis), cerebral toxoplasmosis, pneumonia by *Pneumocystis carinii* (Figure 4.2.5), retinitis by *Cytomegalovirus*, encephalitis by HIV, tuberculosis and extrapulmonary infections by non-tuberculosis *Mycobacterium*, cervical cancer, Kaposi sarcoma, lymphoma, progressive multifocal leucoencephalopathy and HIV wasting syndrome

Diagnosis

- The initial diagnostic test is the enzyme-linked immunosorbent assay (ELISA), which detects the viral protein p24, an HIV-1 antigen; there can be a window of up to 6 months from exposure to the virus to when it becomes detectable
- If the ELISA is positive, the HIV-1/HIV-2 antibody differentiation immunoassay confirmation test is applied (Western Blot, which was used prior to this test, could not differentiate between HIV-1 and HIV-2). If the result is negative or indeterminate, the nucleic acid test (NAT) may be employed to confirm that this is not an acute infection or a false positive
- Rapid HIV antibody detection tests have been marketed and employ samples of oral mucosa exudate
- The immunosuppression level is established based on the concentration of CD4+ T-cells in peripheral blood and is the best predictor available for the onset of opportunistic infections, disease progression and survival (stage 1, ≥500 cells/μL; stage 2, 200–499 cells/μL; stage 3, <200 cells/μL)
- Determining the viral load consists of quantifying the number of copies of HIV ribonucleic acid (HIV-RNA) in peripheral blood, using the real-time polymerase chain reaction (RT-PCR); this test is applied as a predictor of disease progression and to select the antiretroviral regimen
- A patient is considered to be in the AIDS stage when they have <200 CD4+ T-cells/μL, their CD4+ T-cell count is <14% of the total or they have an AIDS-defining condition

Management

- ART (antiretroviral therapy) is the combination of several antiretroviral agents, and should be commenced as soon as possible after diagnosis
- Antiretrovirals seek to reduce the viral load (below 20–50 copies/mL is considered undetectable, depending

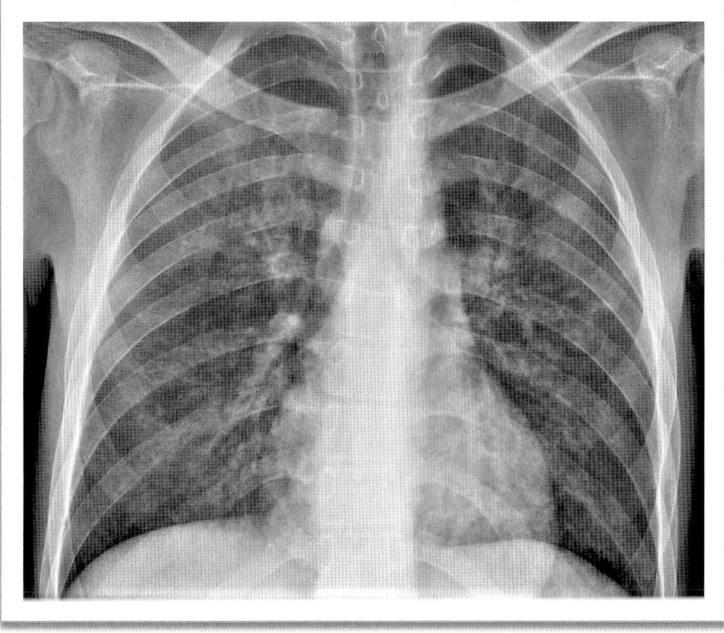

Figure 4.2.5 Pneumonia by *Pneumocystis carinii* as an AIDS-defining condition.

on the test employed), increase the CD4+ T-cell count, prevent opportunistic infections and reduce transmission to others

- The most widely used families of antiretrovirals are:
  - Nucleoside/nucleotide reverse transcriptase inhibitors (NRTI)
  - Non-nucleoside reverse transcriptase inhibitors (NNRTI)
  - Protease inhibitors (PI)
  - Entry or fusion inhibitors
  - Integrase strand transfer inhibitors (INSTIs)
- An initial HIV drug regimen typically includes 3 HIV medications from 2 or more different drug classes:
  - Two NRTIs with an INSTI, NNRTI, or PI
  - Ritonavir (PI) or cobicistat as a booster (cytochrome P450 3A inhibitor)
- The regime varies according to the patient's response and associated side-effects
- ART is associated with adverse effects that are not always predictable and include:
  - Nausea and vomiting, diarrhoea, difficulty sleeping, dry mouth, headache, rash, dizziness, fatigue, and pain
  - Thrombocytopenia caused by ritonavir

Prognosis

- The main markers of disease progression are CD4+ T helper cell counts and the HIV replication rate (viral load)
- The life expectancy of individuals with HIV infection who do not undergo ART is 2–3 years
- About 85% of patients who undergo ART survive for more than 10 years

A World/Transcultural View

- Africa remains the most affected region of the world due to HIV infection/AIDS, especially the sub-Saharan region in which more than 30 million infected individuals live
- The prevalence of HIV-associated oral lesions remains significant in low-income countries. Hairy leucoplakia is more common in Europe and America than in Africa and Asia. Paradoxically, the prevalence of salivary gland disease has decreased in the industrialised world and increased in low-income countries
- Dentists' willingness to provide dental treatment to patients with HIV varies depending on the dentists' origin and country in which they were trained

Recommended Reading

Diz Dios, P. and Scully, C. (2014). Antiretroviral therapy: effects on orofacial health and health care. *Oral Dis.* 20: 136–145.

Gay-Escoda, C., Pérez-Álvarez, D., Camps-Font, O., and Figueiredo, R. (2016). Long-term outcomes of oral rehabilitation with dental implants in HIV-positive patients: a retrospective case series. *Med. Oral Patol. Oral Cir. Bucal* 21: e385–e391.

Ghosn, J., Taiwo, B., Seedat, S. et al. (2018). HIV. *Lancet* 392: 685–697.

Patton, L.L., Shugars, D.A., and Bonito, A.J. (2002). A systematic review of complication risks for HIV-positive patients undergoing invasive dental procedures. *J. Am. Dent. Assoc.* 133: 195–203.

Porter, S.R., Luker, J., Scully, C., and Kumar, N. (1999). Oral lesions in UK patients with or liable to HIV disease-ten years experience. *Med. Oral* 4: 455–469.

Robbins, M.R. (2017). Recent recommendations for management of Human Immunodeficiency Virus-positive patients. *Dent. Clin. North Am.* 61: 365–387.

Santella, A.J. (2020). HIV testing in the dental setting: a global perspective of feasibility and acceptability. *Oral Dis.* 26: S34–S39.

4.3 Viral Hepatitis

Section I: Clinical Scenario and Dental Considerations

Clinical Scenario

A 74-year-old man attends to your clinic for an emergency appointment. He complains of a painful lump in the gum adjacent to the upper left first molar (#26) that presented 24 hours earlier and is getting worse.

Medical History

- Moderate chronic hepatitis C (the patient declined treatment with direct-acting antivirals [DAAs] due to a poor previous experience with interferon)
- Thrombocytopenia (65 000 platelets/μL)
- Arterial hypertension
- Chronic obstructive pulmonary disease (exertional dyspnea)
- Anxiety-depression syndrome
- Road traffic accident in 1988 resulting in a ruptured spleen and a mandibular fracture due to a work accident 40 years earlier – received blood transfusions
- Splenectomy in 1988

Medications

- Telmisartan
- Alprazolam (recently commenced)
- Beclomethasone

Dental History

- It has been 40 years since the patient attended a dental clinic (only went at the time due to his mandibular fracture)
- Admits being afraid of dentists due to a bad experience when he was a child
- Does not brush his teeth regularly

Social History

- Married and lives with his wife (drives his own vehicle)
- Retired
- Ex-smoker (20 cigarettes/day until 4 years ago); alcohol – nil

Oral Examination

- Poor oral hygiene
- Missing teeth: #16, #17, #24 and #25
- Periodontal abscess associated with tooth #26, which extends to the buccal sulcus
- Caries in #26, #36, #47 and #48

Radiological Examination

- Orthopantomogram undertaken (Figure 4.3.1)
- Generalised alveolar bone loss
- Extensive, deep and unrestorable caries in #26
- Restorable caries in #36, #47 and #48

Structured Learning

1) What could have led to this patient having HCV infection?
   - The patient received a blood transfusion in the 1980s
   - This was before the introduction of HCV screening of donated blood in 1991–2
2) The patient requests that the #26 is extracted immediately and does not want any delay. Why is this not advisable?
   - You need further information from his physician regarding the severity/impact of his HCV infection
   - The patient has an increased bleeding risk due to his thrombocytopenia and the likelihood that his HCV infection has also impaired the hepatic synthesis of coagulation factors
   - Antibiotic prophylaxis is mandatory (splenectomised)
3) What could be causing this patient's thrombocytopenia?
   - The pathophysiology of thrombocytopenia in relation to HCV infection is complex

A Practical Approach to Special Care in Dentistry, First Edition. Edited by Pedro Diz Dios and Navdeep Kumar.

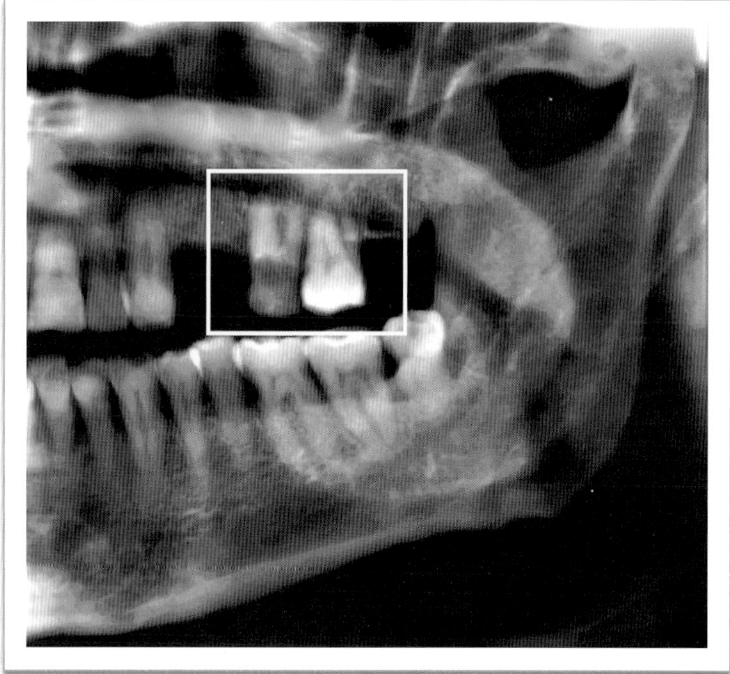

Figure 4.3.1 Orthopantomogram demonstrating unrestorable caries in #26.

- Hypersplenism may contribute to thrombocytopenia but this patient has had a splenectomy
- Hence, in his case, contributory factors include:
  - Bone marrow suppression resulting from HCV itself
  - Aberrations of the immune system resulting in the formation of antiplatelet antibodies and/or immune complexes that bind to platelets and facilitate their premature clearance
  - Thrombopoietin (TPO) deficiency secondary to liver dysfunction

4) What laboratory test results would you need before proceeding with the dental extraction?
   - Full blood count to confirm the platelet count
   - Coagulation study to check the prothrombin time/INR and partial thromboplastin time
5) What factors are considered important in assessing the risk of managing this patient?
   - Social
     - Reduced co-operation due to anxiety-depressive syndrome
     - History of dental anxiety/bad experience of dentistry
     - Alprazolam may impair judgement/cause drowsiness – the patient should not drive and he may not be able to give informed consent
   - Medical
     - Low compliance with medical management with no active antiviral treatment – HCV loads likely to be high
     - Bleeding tendency
     - Increased risk of infection due to the splenectomy
     - Compromised respiratory capacity
     - Risk of a hypertensive crisis (exacerbated by dental anxiety)
     - Drug selection and interactions
   - Dental
     - Poor oral health
     - Acute infection of #26 may prevent effective anaesthesia
     - Lack of regular brushing/mouth cleaning (increases the risk of postoperative infection)
     - Dry mouth as a result of alprazolam
     - Follow-up jeopardised by patient's dental history and depressive symptoms

6) The patient requests sedation due to his dental anxiety. What should you consider?
   - In moderate hepatic impairment, benzodiazepines should not be administered (except for lorazepam in liaison with the physician)
   - Benzodiazepines should also be avoided for patients with chronic obstructive pulmonary disease

- The patient is already taking alprazolam (a benzodiazepine)
- The use of nitrous oxide may be a better option

7) You are unable to achieve effective anaesthesia to enable extraction of the #26. How would you proceed?
   - Prescribe antibiotics: amoxicillin (full dosage) and metronidazole (reduced dosage) may be prescribed but clavulanic acid and azithromycin should be avoided
   - Incision and drainage should be considered
8) What analgesic would you recommend after extracting the tooth root remains?
   - In moderate hepatic impairment, the recommendation is to use metamizole or paracetamol at reduced dosages (<2 g/24 hours)
   - Non-steroidal anti-inflammatory drugs with antiplatelet action should be avoided for this patient due to his tendency to bleed
   - Peripheral thrombocytopenia is an adverse effect of metamizole (unavailable in some countries), which is therefore not recommended when there is baseline thrombocytopenia

General Dental Considerations

Oral Findings

- Pallor of the soft palate and floor of the mouth can appear in patients with jaundice
- In severe cases (with coagulation factor deficiency), petechiae/ecchymosis can present in the oral mucosa, as well as spontaneous bleeding of the gums
- HCV can be associated with Sjögren syndrome, non-Hodgkin lymphoma and lichen planus (especially the erosive type) (Figure 4.3.2)

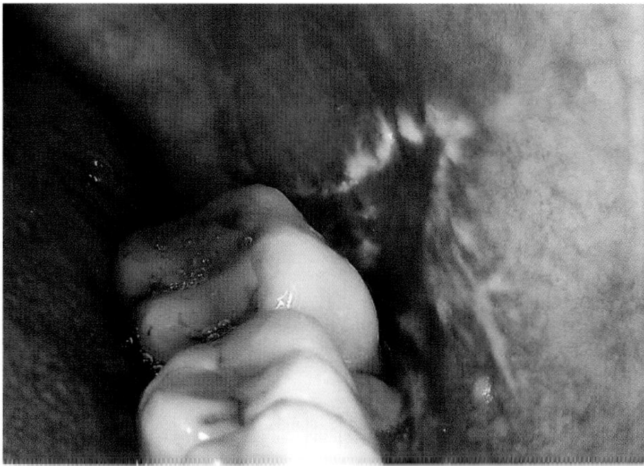

Figure 4.3.2 Erosive lichen planus in an HCV-infected patient.

Dental Management

- Dental management considerations include prevention of transmission of the viral infection in the dental clinic, preventing and treating associated increased bleeding risk during invasive procedures, and avoiding the prescription of drugs metabolised by the liver (Tables 4.3.1 and 4.3.2)

Section II: Background Information and Guidelines

Definition

Hepatitis is an inflammatory process of the liver that is generally caused by viruses, toxins (typically alcohol and drugs) or autoimmune disorders. Viral hepatitis is caused by the action of viruses of the hepatitis virus family (HAV, HBV, HCV, HDV, HEV, HGV, SEN, TTV *[Torque teno virus]), Herpes virus (Cytomegalovirus, Epstein–Barr virus, Herpes simplex) and others (Coxsackie B)* (Table 4.3.3).

HBV and HCV infections are of special interest in dentistry because they can become chronic, causing hepatic dysfunction. Furthermore, these viruses can be transmitted by contaminated blood or other bodily fluids (including saliva). It is currently estimated that more than 240 million individuals are chronic carriers of HBV and more than 70 million are carriers of HCV.

Aetiopathogenesis

- HBV and HCV are non-cytopathic viruses
- The liver damage they cause is therefore considered to be a consequence of an immunopathological process
- Chronic hepatitis is characterised by an ineffective response by T-cells, which are unable to complete the viral clearance and therefore result in continuous cycles of low-level cell destruction

Clinical Presentation

- Hepatitis viruses result in both acute and chronic disease
- Acute phase
  - Can be asymptomatic or subclinical
  - Non-specific symptoms of asthenia (weakness), anorexia and mild fever can sometimes occur
  - Hepatic damage impedes bilirubin conjugation; when bilirubin accumulates above 40 μmol/L, it expresses clinically as jaundice, pruritus, choluria and acholia (Figure 4.3.3)
- Chronic phase
  - Following the initial infection, approximately 80% of individuals do not exhibit any symptoms

Table 4.3.1 Considerations for dental management.

Risk assessment	• Bleeding risk (thrombocytopenia, impaired production of clotting factors) • Impaired drug metabolism • The transmission rate by the percutaneous pathway: – HBV risk varies depending on e-antigen (HBeAg) status of source person; if HBeAg positive, the risk is up to 30%, if HBeAg negative, risk is 1–6% – HCV risk is 1.8%
Criteria for referral	• During the acute phase of the infection, emergency dental treatment should only be performed in the hospital setting • Most patients with chronic hepatitis can be treated in a conventional dental clinic
Access/position	• A number of barriers to treatment have been identified for these patients, including the anxiety caused by the dental setting • Schedule the appointment for the last session of the day to minimise the risk of cross-transmission
Communication	• Some patients with chronic viral hepatitis who undergo dental treatment do not report their condition, for fear of discriminatory attitudes by health professionals
Consent/capacity	• Patients need to be warned of the potential complications resulting from viral hepatic infection, which may require adaptation such as: – Implementation of bleeding prevention protocols – Prescription of drugs that are not metabolised by the liver
Anaesthesia/sedation	• Local anaesthesia – Minimise the risk of pricking with contaminated needles after infiltrative anaesthesia (e.g. single-use devices) – Caution is advised when using lidocaine and mepivacaine (prilocaine and articaine may be preferable) • Sedation – Drug sedation with benzodiazepines in patients with mild hepatic failure may be performed by reducing the dosage – For patients with moderate–severe hepatic failure, benzodiazepines should be avoided • General anaesthesia – A comprehensive assessment in conjunction with the anaesthetist is essential – The patient's physician should be consulted and investigations undertaken to assess the risk of bleeding and infection, and whether there are any concurrent infections which would compromise the procedure
Dental treatment	• Before Universal cross infection control measures should be applied – Recent blood tests results should be available including: ○ Full blood count (risk of thrombocytopenia) ○ Coagulation study (hepatitis/cirrhosis can reduce clotting factors) • During – Invasive procedures can cause prolonged bleeding, which typically is controlled with local haemostasis measures • After – If the bleeding does not stop, the administration of vitamin K may be considered – Avoid drugs that are metabolised in the liver (Table 4.3.2)
Drug prescription	• In general, drugs may be prescribed during short periods at normal dosages, except in cases of moderate–severe hepatic dysfunction (Table 4.3.2)

(Continued)

Table 4.3.1 (Continued)

Education/prevention	• HBV – The vaccine against hepatitis B offers 98–100% protection and is mandatory for dentists – Practitioners infected by HBV who are HBeAg positive or have more than 1000 HBV-RNA copies/mL of blood should not perform procedures with a potential risk of exposure to the virus – In the event of accidental exposure to HBV of an unvaccinated individual, the administration of immunoglobulin (HBIg) and/or starting the vaccination within 24 hours should be assessed • HCV – There is no effective vaccine against hepatitis C – Practitioners infected by HCV should not perform procedures with a potential risk of exposure to the virus – In the event of accidental exposure to HCV, the prophylactic administration of antivirals is not recommended – However, early treatment of the acute infection can prevent chronicity – The dental clinic can also be used as a primary screening centre with the new rapid detection tests for HCV antibodies in saliva

Table 4.3.2 Prescription of drugs for patients with moderate to severe hepatic failure.

	Type of drug	Recommendation
Antibiotics	• Penicillin V	No dosage adjustment required
	• Amoxicillin	No dosage adjustment required
	• Amoxicillin/clavulanic acid	Contraindicated
	• Clindamycin	Reduce dosage (150 mg/8 h)
	• Metronidazole	Reduce dosage (250 mg/8 h)
	• Azithromycin	Contraindicated
	• Clarithromycin	Reduce dosage (250 mg/8 h)
Analgesics	• Paracetamol	Reduce dosage (<2 g/24 h)
	• Metamizole	No dosage adjustment required (under review)
	• Ibuprofen	Contraindicated
	• Diclofenac	Contraindicated
	• Naproxen	Contraindicated
	• Codeine	Contraindicated
	• Tramadol	Contraindicated
Corticosteroids		
Sedatives	• Hydroxyzine	Contraindicated
	• Diphenhydramine	Contraindicated
	• Diazepam	Contraindicated
	• Midazolam	Contraindicated
	• Lorazepam	No dosage adjustment required
	• Alprazolam	Contraindicated

Table 4.3.3 Characteristics of the most common types of viral hepatitis.

	Hepatitis A virus (HAV)	Hepatitis B virus (HBV)	Hepatitis C virus (HCV)
Type of virus	Picornaviridae (RNA)	Hepadnaviridae (DNA)	Flaviviridae (RNA)
Prevalence range*	50-90%	0.7-6.2%	0.6-6.7%
Main transmission pathway	Fecal-oral and sexual	Parenteral and sexual	Parenteral
Transmission in the dental clinic	–	Yes	Yes
Chronicity rate	–	5%	70%
Vaccine available	Yes	Yes	–
	Hepatitis D virus (HDV)	**Hepatitis E virus (HEV)**	**Hepatitis G virus (HGV)**
Type of virus	Delta virus (RNA)	Calicivirus (RNA)	Flaviviridae (RNA)
Prevalence range*	1-40%	0-25%	1-4%
Main transmission pathway	Parenteral and sexual	Fecal-oral	Parenteral
Transmission in the dental clinic	Yes	–	–
Chronicity rate	5-95%[†]	–	–
Vaccine available	Yes (anti-HBV)	–	-

*The wide ranges represent the difference between areas of very low prevalence and endemic areas.
[†] 5% in previously negative HBV (co-infection) and 95% in previously positive HBV (superinfection).

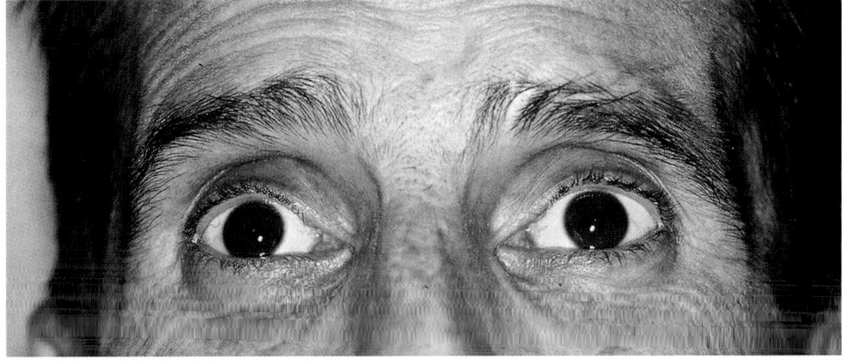

Figure 4.3.3 Jaundice related to liver dysfunction.

- When the bile salts do not reach the intestine, malabsorption, nausea, vomiting, pain and abdominal distension can occur
- Coagulation factor synthesis deficiency and exacerbated fibrinolysis increase the tendency to bleed
- Approximately 1% of persons living with HBV infection are also infected with HIV and hence have additional signs and symptoms related to this coinfection
- HDV infections occur only in those who are infected with HBV, resulting in a more serious disease and poorer prognosis
- Hepatic cirrhosis and liver cancer can develop as a consequence of chronic HBV and HCV infection

Diagnosis

- HBV
  - The laboratory diagnosis of hepatitis B is based on detecting hepatitis B surface antigen (HBsAg) in a peripheral blood sample
  - In the acute phase of the infection, immunoglobulin M (IgM) against the hepatitis core antigen (HBcAg) is also detected
  - The presence of hepatitis antigen 'e' (HBeAg) is indicative of high levels of viral replication and therefore high infection potential
  - Chronic hepatitis by HBV is characterised by the persistence of HBsAg for more than 6 months
- HCV
  - In patients who have been infected by HCV, anti-HCV antibodies are detected in serological tests
  - To confirm the chronic infection in patients who are anti-HCV positive, a nucleic acid test for detecting HCV-RNA is required
  - When the HCV infection becomes chronic, biopsy and other less invasive tests are employed to quantify the hepatic damage

Management

- HBV
  - Only 10–40% of patients with chronic hepatitis B require drug treatment, with tenofovir and entecavir the most widely used antiviral agents
  - In most patients, the treatment suppresses viral replication but does not cure the hepatitis

    HBV can be prevented by vaccines that are safe, widely available and effective; these also provide protection from HDV infection.
- HCV
  - More than 95% of patients with chronic hepatitis from HCV are cured with the administration of pangenotypic direct-acting antivirals (DAAs)
  - These are drug combinations that mainly include sofosbuvir, velpatasvir, voxilaprevir, glecaprevir and pibrentasvir
  - This has reduced deaths due to liver cirrhosis and hepatocellular carcinoma
  - There is currently no effective vaccine

Prognosis

- HBV
  - Causes 650 000 deaths annually as a result of the hepatic damage caused by viral hepatitis
  - HBV infection becomes chronic in only 5% of infected adults
  - However, 20–30% of these develop cirrhosis or liver cancer
- HCV
  - Causes an estimated 400 000 deaths annually
  - HCV infection becomes chronic in 70% of cases
  - The risk of cirrhosis and/or hepatocellular carcinoma within 20 years is estimated at 15–30%

A World/Transcultural View

- Chronic viral hepatitis is especially frequent in low-income countries, where transmission is typically mother to foetus or child to child (e.g. hepatitis B virus in Southeast Asia and sub-Saharan Africa) or through contaminated blood (e.g. hepatitis C virus in Egypt, Pakistan and North Africa)
- A significant number of countries, particularly African, still do not universally administer hepatitis B virus vaccine to infants
- The success of a viral hepatitis detection programme depends on identifying target groups, whose beliefs and health perspectives can affect their acceptance
- Although new treatment strategies for hepatitis C have demonstrated high rates of healing, they have created new inequalities in accessing treatment in low- to medium-income countries

Recommended Reading

Averbukh, L.D. and Wu, G.Y. (2019). Highlights for dental care as a hepatitis C risk factor: a review of literature. *J. Clin. Transl. Hepatol.* 7: 346–351.

Castro Ferreiro, M., Diz Dios, P., and Scully, C. (2005). Transmission of hepatitis C virus by saliva? *Oral Dis.* 11: 230–235.

Carrozzo, M. (2014). Hepatitis C virus: a silent killer relevant to dentistry. *Oral Dis.* 20: 425–429.

Golla, K., Epstein, J.B., and Cabay, R.J. (2004). Liver disease: current perspectives on medical and dental management. *Oral Surg. Oral Med. Oral Pathol. Oral Radiol. Endod.* 98: 516–521.

Jefferies, M., Rauff, B., Rashid, H. et al. (2018). Update on global epidemiology of viral hepatitis and preventive strategies. *World J. Clin. Cases* 6: 589–599.

Klevens, R.M. and Moorman, A.C. (2013). Hepatitis C virus: an overview for dental health care providers. *J. Am. Dent. Assoc.* 144: 1340–1347.

Mahboobi, N., Porter, S.R., Karayiannis, P., and Alavian, S.M. (2013). Dental treatment as a risk factor for hepatitis B and C viral infection. A review of the recent literature. *J. Gastrointestin. Liver Dis.* 22: 79–86.

5

Endocrine Diseases

5.1 Diabetes Mellitus

Section I: Clinical Scenario and Dental Considerations

Clinical Scenario

An 11-year-old girl is referred by her paediatric endocrinologist for urgent management of dental pain. The pain commenced several days ago but has substantially worsened in the last 24 hours. It is localised to #54 which was treated by her family dentist 1 year ago

Medical History

- Type 1 diabetes mellitus, diagnosed at the age of 5 years old
- Two episodes of severe hypoglycaemia in the last 12 months that required hospitalisation
- Currently reviewed by her paediatric endocrinologist every 8 weeks
- Coeliac disease diagnosed 6 months ago
- Generalised anxiety (worsening)

Medications

- Fast-acting insulin
- Long-acting insulin (insulin glargine)
- Strict diet control, including gluten-free foods only for the last 6 months (supervised by her mother)

Dental History

- Regular dental attender (biannual dental check-ups since the age of 6 years)
- Limited cooperation – sedation required when a filling was undertaken a year ago
- Patient brushes her teeth with an electric toothbrush 3 times daily, usually supervised by her mother
- Sporadically uses dental floss
- Rinses with a fluoride mouthwash each night

Social History

- Lives with her mother (divorced) during the weekdays and her father on the weekends
- Her father is not as disciplined as her mother in relation to healthcare (e.g. diet control or tooth brushing)
- Poor relationship between her parents contributing to increasing generalised anxiety for the patient

Oral Examination

- Good oral hygiene
- Buccal fistula adjacent to the carious #54 (disto-occlusal filling in situ) – draining pus
- Hypomineralisation of tooth #73
- Two mouth ulcers on the right buccal mucosa (1 mm diameter)

Radiological Examination

- Orthopantomogram undertaken (Figure 5.1.1)
- Delayed tooth eruption, with persistence of teeth #64, #74 and #84
- Premature loss of tooth #83, due to eruption of #42

Structured Learning

1) Is there any connection with this patient's diagnosis of type 1 diabetes mellitus and coeliac disease?
   - Type 1 diabetes mellitus is often associated with other autoimmune diseases
   - Although the most common coexisting organ-specific autoimmune disease is autoimmune thyroid disease, coeliac disease may also be present
   - Approximately 8% of people with type 1 diabetes will also have coeliac disease
   - Coeliac disease increases the risk of hypoglycaemia if a strict gluten-free diet is not followed

A Practical Approach to Special Care in Dentistry, First Edition. Edited by Pedro Diz Dios and Navdeep Kumar.

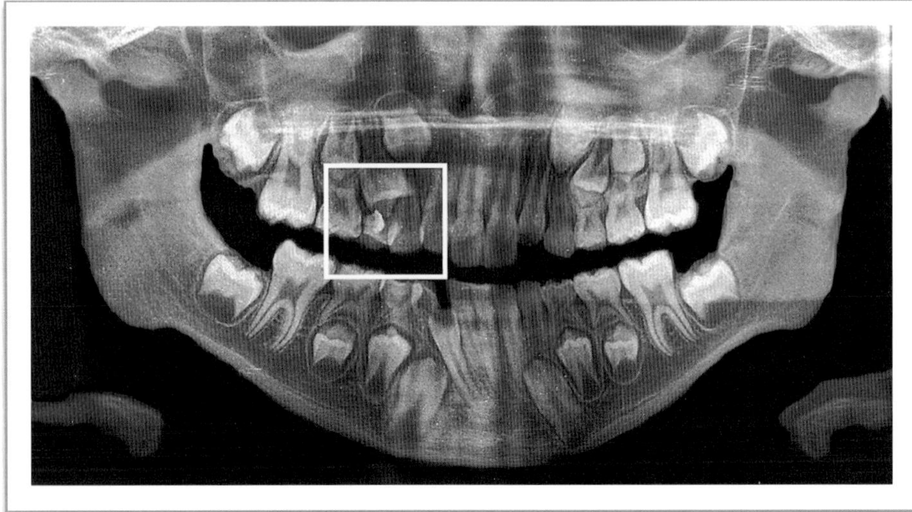

Figure 5.1.1 Panoramic radiography showing caries and a prior filling in tooth #54.

2) Why is a dental abscess of particular concern for this patient?
   - Diabetes mellitus is known to be associated with increased risk of infection and impaired wound healing due to the chronic effects of hyperglycaemia:
     - Neutrophil function (adherence, chemotaxis and phagocytosis) may be downregulated; neutrophils also produce fewer free oxygen radicals, thereby reducing their ability to make toxic metabolites for release against microbes
     - Monocyte, macrophage and fibroblast functions are impaired, resulting in impaired tissue turnover and wound repair
   - Oral infection, pain and stress can result in alteration of blood glucose levels and lead to poor diabetic control
     - The stress response elicited results in the release of hormones such as cortisol and adrenaline which work against the action of insulin
     - As a result, the body's production of glucose increases, which results in high blood sugar levels
     - An insulin adjustment may be required
3) You decide it would be better to control the acute infection in #54 and extract the tooth at a later date. What should you consider when prescribing antibiotics?
   - Administration of antibiotics can alter the blood glucose level and require an insulin dose adjustment
   - Coeliac disease may affect the absorption of antibiotics; antibiotics known to be associated with an increased risk of gastrointestinal toxicity should be avoided
   - Avoid azithromycin and metronidazole because they boost the action of hypoglycaemic agents
4) What factors are considered important in assessing the risk of managing this patient?
   - Social
     - Consent: the parents are divorced and do not have a good relationship; their opinion regarding the proposed extraction of the #54 may differ (although there can be legal differences in the law from one country to another)
     - Anxiety may be heightened due to the above social factors
     - Limited co-operation
   - Medical
     - Hypoglycaemia risk: unable to eat properly due to the dental pain; fasting after dental procedures can also trigger a hypoglycaemic episode
     - Hyperglycaemia risk: emotional and surgical stress can result in increased glucose levels
     - Reduced co-operation may be misinterpreted as related to generalised anxiety instead of abnormal glucose levels
     - Efficacy of oral medication may be impacted by poor absorption secondary to coeliac disease
   - Dental
     - Increased susceptibility to infection
     - Likelihood of delayed healing after dental extraction
     - Increased caries risk (xerostomia; father does not assist with toothbrushing)
     - Coeliac disease can cause enamel defects and mouth ulcers (as observed for this patient)

    - Delayed dental development (coeliac disease and diabetes)

5) The patient injects a daily dose of fast-acting insulin at 8 a.m. and a dose of long-acting insulin at 10 p.m. At what time should you schedule the dental extraction?
    - Fast-acting insulin will have its peak effect between 9 a.m. and noon
    - Long-acting insulin will have its peak effect around 10 a.m.
    - Ideally, the treatment should be performed in the morning, because the risk of hypoglycaemia is lower when the concentration of endogenous corticosteroids increases. This should be as soon as possible after breakfast (also avoids interfering with the next meal)

6) What laboratory tests are recommended before the tooth extraction?
    - Serum glucose concentration before starting the procedure
    - Recent HbA_{1c} reading to determine the degree of metabolic control; postpone treatment if HbA_{1c} > [illegible]

General Dental Considerations

Oral Findings

- Occasionally, oral findings can represent an initial manifestation of undiagnosed diabetes
- Periodontal disease is the most common oral finding (Figure 5.1.2). Its pathogenesis involves vascular changes (microangiopathy), neutrophil dysfunction and collagen metabolism deficiencies. The presence of periodontitis impedes glycaemic control and contributes to the onset of other extraoral complications
- Susceptibility to bacterial (including odontogenic abscesses) and fungal infections (such as oral candidiasis and mucormycosis in the sinuses)
- Xerostomia, which can favour the onset of caries (Figure 5.1.3). Chronic bilateral and asymptomatic inflammation of the parotid glands (sialosis) can develop as a compensatory mechanism
- Burning mouth syndrome (probably related to peripheral neuropathy)
- Circumoral paraesthesia (associated with peripheral neuropathy)
- Glossitis, loss of the filiform papillae and dysgeusia

(a)

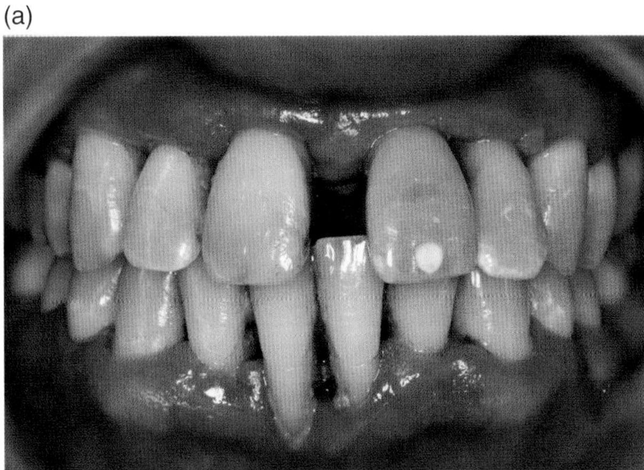

(b)

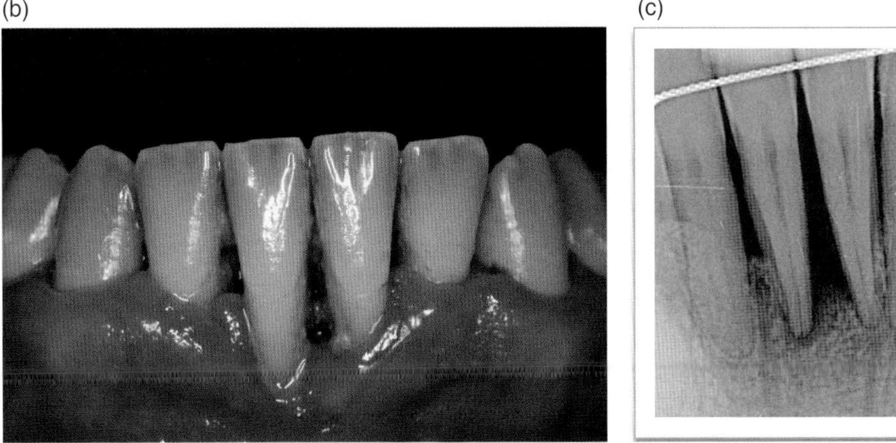

(c)

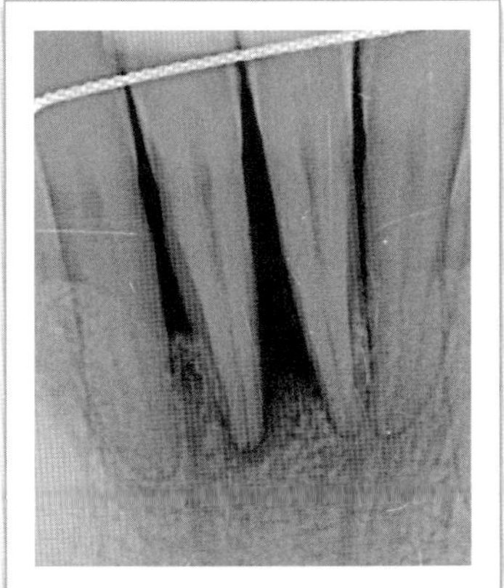

Figure 5.1.2 (a–c) Severe periodontal disease in a 37-year-old male with diabetes mellitus.

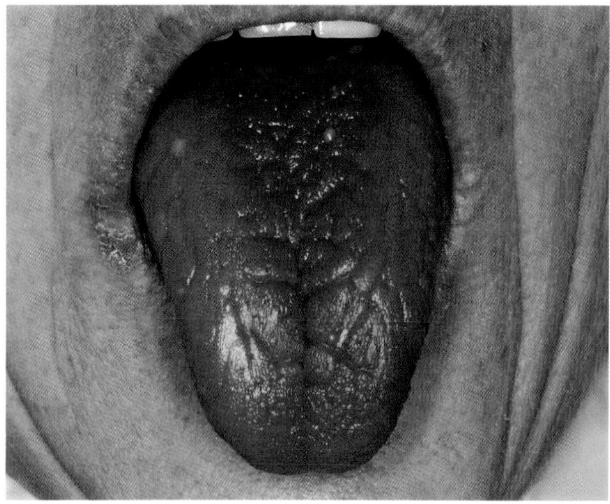

Figure 5.1.3 Xerostomia – depapillated, smooth dry dorsum of the tongue.

- High prevalence of oral lichen planus
- Mucosal lichenoid reactions and facial flushing (secondary effects of antidiabetic drugs)
- Delayed tooth eruption

Dental Management

- The dental treatment plan will be determined mainly by the patient's previous oral health and degree of metabolic control (Table 5.1.1)
- The dental team should be aware of how to manage hypoglycaemic events in the dental clinic (Table 5.1.2)

Section II: Background Information and Guidelines

Definition

Diabetes mellitus is a chronic metabolic disorder characterised by a relative or absolute absence of insulin. Although various types of diabetes have been described (type 1, type 2 and gestational), all are characterised by high blood glucose levels. Worldwide, there are more than 420 million individuals with diabetes (approximately 9% of the worldwide adult population), although it has been estimated that more than 40% of cases are still undiagnosed.

Aetiopathogenesis

- Type 1 diabetes: ~8% (previously known as insulin-dependent or juvenile-onset)
  - The beta cells in the pancreas produce little or no insulin
  - Exogenous insulin must therefore be administered throughout the patient's life
  - Most cases have an autoimmune aetiology, although some are idiopathic
- Type 2 diabetes: ~90% (previously known as non-insulin-dependent or adult-onset)
  - The insulin receptors in the target tissues show reduced sensitivity to the action of insulin (insulin resistance), although insulin production can be normal
  - As the disease progresses, a lack of insulin may also develop
  - Generally associated with a genetic predisposition, obesity or metabolic syndrome (combination of diabetes, hypertension and obesity)
- Gestational diabetes
  - Triggered by an increase in insulin resistance that causes impaired glucose tolerance during pregnancy
- Secondary diabetes can be caused by endocrinopathies (e.g. acromegaly, Cushing disease), drugs (e.g. corticosteroids) or pancreatic disease (surgery, tumour or inflammation)

Clinical Presentation

- Type 1: usually presents before the age of 40 years
- Type 2: average age of onset is 45 years old
- Classic symptoms, especially those of undiagnosed type 1 diabetes
  - Polyuria (frequent voiding), polydipsia (excessive thirst) and polyphagia (excessive hunger)
  - Fatigue, infections, slow wound healing, blurred vision, weight loss
- Hypoglycaemia (onset can be rapid; more frequent; life-threatening)
  - Early signs/symptoms: shakiness, dizziness, sweating, hunger, piloerection, tachycardia, inability to concentrate, confusion, irritability or moodiness, anxiety (due to increased epinephrine activity) or nervousness, headache
  - Later signs/symptoms: clumsiness or jerky movements, inability to eat or drink, muscle weakness, difficulty speaking or slurred speech, blurry or double vision, drowsiness, confusion, convulsions or seizures, unconsciousness, death
- Hyperglycaemia (slower onset, more protracted course)
  - Early signs/symptoms: frequent urination, increased thirst, blurred vision, fatigue, headache
  - Later signs/symptoms: fruity-smelling breath, nausea and vomiting, shortness of breath, dry mouth, weakness, confusion, abdominal pain, coma

Table 5.1.1 Considerations for dental management.

Risk assessment	• Hypoglycaemia is the main risk and must be managed urgently (see Table 5.1.2) • Hyperglycaemia • Fatigue/reduced tolerance for long treatment • Increased risk of infection • Poor wound healing • Increased risk of periodontal disease • Complications related to comorbidities/secondary vascular complications
Criteria for referral	• If HbA1c levels are <7%, any type of dental treatment can generally be performed within the dental clinic • For patients with poorly controlled diabetes (HbA1c >9%), only emergency treatments should be conducted and surgical procedures should preferably be undertaken in a hospital setting • With HbA1c readings >12%, all procedures should be postponed until the glycaemic control has improved
Access/position	• The sessions should preferably be scheduled for the morning (higher endogenous cortisol levels increase blood glucose and decrease the risk of hypoglycaemia) • Avoid scheduling an appointment time that coincides with the maximum insulin activity peak or when it may lead to a meal being missed
Communication	• A significant percentage of individuals with diabetes are unaware of their condition • Patients with signs/symptoms or oral findings suggestive of diabetes should be referred to their doctor for investigation • Communication may be impaired if blood glucose levels are not controlled (slurred speech, confusion)
Consent/capacity	• Patients should be informed that the dental treatment plan and its success will be determined by the degree of diabetic control (e.g. success rates for dental implants are lower for patients with suboptimal diabetes control) • Patients should be warned of the potential for local and systemic complications resulting from diabetes (increased infection risk, delayed healing) • If diabetic control is poor, the patient may be confused, anxious and/or agitated – this will reduce their capacity to give consent
Anaesthesia/sedation	• Local anaesthesia – Any local anaesthetic may be employed by following the routine precautions • Sedation – Controlling the patient's stress is important – For patients with poor metabolic control and comorbidities, sedation should be performed in a hospital setting • General anaesthesia – The use of general anaesthesia is determined by the severity of the comorbidities

(Continued)

Table 5.1.1 (Continued)

Dental treatment	• Before – Confirm that the patient has eaten normally and has taken the scheduled medication – The presence of an oral infection and the administration of antibiotics can change the insulin requirements and might require adjustment by a physician – The physician should also be consulted if the planned procedure is expected to change the normal eating habits – For an oral surgical or periodontal procedure, anticipate the postintervention fasting/changes in diet – Assess the need for antibiotic prophylaxis (not supported by scientific evidence) – Performing a new rapid HbA_{1c} test may be considered • During – Dental implants can be placed successfully in patients with well-controlled diabetes – The main complication during dental treatment is hypoglycaemia • After – Slow healing of the surgical wound is common – Due to the increased risk of infection, consider the need for postoperative antibiotics, if an invasive procedure is undertaken (especially for patients with poor disease control) – Once the session has finished, slowly sit the patient up from the supine position (postural hypotension due to autonomic neuropathy) – Periodontal treatment has been shown to produce a modest improvement in glycaemic control – It has been suggested that the success rate of endodontic treatment is lower than that for the general population, especially for patients with poorly controlled diabetes (as has been reported for dental implants)
Drug prescription	• The antibiotic of choice is amoxicillin • Avoid using metronidazole and azithromycin because they can boost oral hypoglycaemic agents • Avoid ciprofloxacin because it can compete with insulin • The analgesic of choice is paracetamol • Avoid using aspirin, ibuprofen, diclofenac and naproxen because they can boost oral hypoglycaemic agents • Avoid corticosteroids because they can decrease the efficacy of oral hypoglycaemic agents
Education/prevention	• Patients with diabetes usually recognise the signs and symptoms of hypoglycaemia. In any case, dentists should know how to identify and manage urgent episodes, especially hypoglycaemia (see Table 5.1.2) • Maintaining optimal oral hygiene and regular reviews, with a specific focus on periodontal disease, should be routine for patients with diabetes • Removing any removable prosthesis at night and renewing them periodically are essential for preventing denture-induced stomatitis

Table 5.1.2 Managing hypoglycaemia in the dental clinic[a].

Alert/responsive patient	• Check blood glucose level • If <3.0 mmol/L (54 mg/dL), give glucose/sugary drink or pure glucose (2 tablets) • Recheck blood glucose level after 10–15 minutes • Give the patient a complex carbohydrate (biscuits, sandwiches, etc.) to ensure that a sustained release of glucose is maintained
Confused patient	• Check blood glucose level • If <3.0 mmol/L (54 mg/dL), give sublingual dextrose gel (repeated at 10–15 minutes) • Recheck blood glucose level after 10–15 minutes • As the level increases, give the patient a complex carbohydrate (biscuits, sandwiches, etc.) to ensure that a sustained release of glucose is maintained
Unconscious patient (blood glucose <2.8 mmol/L or 50 mg/dL)	• Call for medical assistance • Intramuscular glucagon 1 mg (adults/children over the age of 8 years); 0.5 mg for children under the age of 8 years; not as effective if a patient has liver disease or is anorexic • Monitor airway, breathing and circulation throughout

[a] UK Resuscitation Council.

- Long-term complications cause significant morbidity and mortality
  - Overproduction of reactive oxygen species as a result of metabolic disturbance results in endothelial dysfunction and inflammation; this provokes diabetic vascular changes
  - Macrovascular changes include:
    - Angina pectoris, myocardial infarction, cerebral infarction and claudication
  - Microvascular changes include:
    - Diabetic retinopathy (neovascularisation, vitreous haemorrhaging, retinal detachment and blindness)
    - Diabetic nephropathy, which is the main cause of dialysis and kidney transplantation in high-income countries
    - Peripheral sensory polyneuropathy and autonomic neuropathy
    - Recurrent infections
    - Delayed healing
    - Increased risk of developing dementia

Diagnosis

- When symptoms of diabetes are present, 2 or more repeat tests are undertaken to confirm the diagnosis, as summarised in Table 5.1.3
- Elevated HbA_{1c} is a risk factor for the development of coronary heart disease and stroke
- In conditions associated with increased red blood cell turnover, such as sickle cell disease, pregnancy (second and third trimesters), haemodialysis, recent blood loss or transfusion, or erythropoietin therapy, only plasma blood glucose criteria should be used to diagnose diabetes
- Haemoglobin variants can also interfere with the measurement of HbA_{1c} (e.g. sickle cell trait).
- Serum fructosamine levels may be considered as an appropriate laboratory measurement when monitoring long-term glycaemic control in patients with underlying haemoglobinopathies

Management

- Diet and regular physical exercise

Table 5.1.3 Criteria for the diagnosis of diabetes (WHO).

	Normal	**Prediabetes**	**Diabetes**
• Fasting plasma glucose (FPG)	≤5.5 mmol/L (<100 mg/dL)	5.6–6.9 mmol/L (100–125 mg/dL)	≥7.0 mmol/L (126 mg/dL)
• Oral glucose tolerance test (OGTT) – 2 hours after 75 g anhydrous glucose dose dissolved in water	≤7.7 mmol/L (<140 mg/dL)	7.8–11.0 mmol/L (140–199 mg/dL)	≥11.1 mmol/L (200 mg/dL)
• Glycated haemoglobin in plasma ($HbA1_c$) glycaemic history for lifespan of an erythrocyte (2–3 months)	≤39 mmol/mol (<5.7%)	(39–47 mmol/mol) (5.7–6.4%)	≥48 mmol/mol (≥6.5%)
• Symptoms of high blood sugar and random plasma glucose test	–	–	≥11.1 mmol/L (200 mg/dL)

- Oral hypoglycaemic agents
  - Sulfonylureas (e.g. glipizide, glyburide, glimepiride and tolazamide)
  - Meglitinides (e.g. repaglinide and nateglinide)
  - DDP-4 inhibitors (e.g. sitagliptin)
  - Biguanides (e.g. metformin)
  - Alpha-glucosidase inhibitors (e.g. acarbose and miglitol)
  - Thiazolidinediones (e.g. pioglitazone and rosiglitazone)
- Insulin
  - Several types of human insulin according to the speed and duration of their effects (Table 5.1.4)
  - Generally, individuals with diabetes are controlled with 2 administrations of subcutaneous fast-acting or intermediate insulin (first hour of the morning and middle of the afternoon)
  - Insulin can also be administered with a continuous release pump (especially indicated for patients with considerable blood glucose variability)
- Classically, glycaemic control has been performed with home (electronic glucometers) and professional monitoring (blood glucose and HbA_{1c} levels)
- Continuous glucose monitoring systems consist of a subcutaneous sensor and a transmitter that sends the signal to a receiver by which the reading can be taken (Figure 5.1.4); this process can even be controlled with a smart phone; these devices are also the basis of the so-called 'artificial pancreas', which injects the required insulin doses in real time
- Other treatments under development include the transplantation of pancreatic islets and pluripotent stem cell-derived insulin-producing cells

Prognosis

- Life expectancy of a person with type 2 diabetes mellitus is likely to be reduced, by up to 10 years
- People with type 1 diabetes mellitus traditionally have a life expectancy reduced by over 20 years, although improvements in diabetes care in recent decades have meant that people are now living significantly longer
- The prognosis is better for patients who respond adequately to drug treatment and appropriate dietary and general health measures
- Multiorgan complications (renal failure, heart disease, stroke, blindness, limb amputation and peripheral neuropathy) can affect life expectancy and quality
- Approximately 3% of all deaths worldwide are attributable to diabetes. This percentage increases to 8.5% if we include deaths caused by the cardiovascular disease and renal failure directly related to diabetes, which represent 5 million adult deaths annually

A World/Transcultural View

- The prevalence of diabetes is related to the community's socio-economic conditions, given that 75% of individuals with diabetes live in low- or middle-income countries
- The adoption by some indigenous communities (e.g. in South Africa and Australia) of a Western diet has resulted in a considerable increase in cases of non-insulin-dependent diabetes mellitus
- Countries as heterogeneous as India, the US and Saudi Arabia have shown that dental clinics can be important centres for detecting previously undiagnosed diabetes and prediabetes

Table 5.1.4 Types of insulin and their action profiles.

Main types of insulin	Injection timing	Start of action	Maximum effect	Duration of effect
• Fast-acting insulin	30 minutes before meals	30 minutes	1–3 hours	6–8 hours
• Ultrafast-acting insulin analogues	10 minutes before meals	10–20 minutes	1–2 hours	3–5 hours
• Intermediate-acting insulin	30 minutes before meals	60–120 minutes	4–6 hours	10–12 hours
• Long-acting insulin analogues	At the same time every day	60–90 minutes	12 hours	17–24 hours

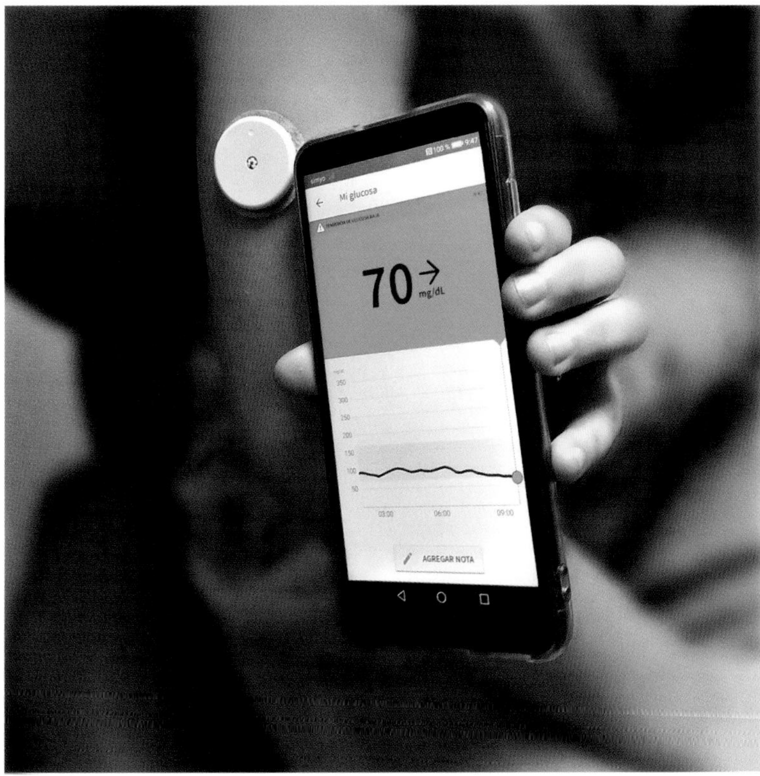

Figure 5.1.4 Continuous glucose monitoring system.

Recommended Reading

Borgnakke, W.S. (2019). IDF diabetes atlas: diabetes and oral health – a two-way relationship of clinical importance. *Diabetes Res. Clin. Pract.* 157: 107839.

Diabetes Canada Clinical Practice Guidelines Expert Committee, Lipscombe, L., Butalia, S. et al. (2020). Pharmacologic glycemic management of type 2 diabetes in adults: 2020 update. *Can. J. Diabetes* 44: 575–591.

Johnson, E., Warren, F., Skolnik, N., and Shubrook, J.H. (2016). Diabetes update: your guide to the latest ADA standards. *J. Fam. Pract.* 65: 310–318.

Lalla, E. and Papapanou, P.N. (2011). Diabetes mellitus and periodontitis: a tale of two common interrelated diseases. *Nat. Rev. Endocrinol.* 7: 738–748.

McKenna, S.J. (2006). Dental management of patients with diabetes. *Dent. Clin. North Am.* 50: 591–606.

Miller, A. and Ouanounou, A. (2020). Diagnosis, management, and dental considerations for the diabetic patient. *J. Can. Dent. Assoc.* 86: k8.

Wilson, M.H., Fitzpatrick, J.J., McArdle, N.S., and Stassen, L.F. (2010). Diabetes mellitus and its relevance to the practice of dentistry. *J. Ir. Dent. Assoc.* 56: 128–133.

Wray, L. (2011). The diabetic patient and dental treatment: an update. *Br. Dent. J.* 211: 209–215.

5.2 Hypothyroidism

Section I: Clinical Scenario and Dental Considerations

Clinical Scenario

A 22-year-old female presents for an emergency dental appointment complaining of unbearable pain in the region of the left angle of the mandible. The patient initially experienced discomfort 3 days ago, but this intensified overnight leading to disturbed sleep and a persistent throbbing ache.

Medical History
- Autoimmune hypothyroidism (Hashimoto' disease) diagnosed 2 years ago
- Autoimmune hepatitis diagnosed 4 years ago
- Poor compliance with the treatment of her autoimmune disease; fails to attend review appointments with her physician, takes medication irregularly
- Obstructive sleep apnoea-hypopnoea syndrome
- Depression/anxiety

Medications (Intermittently taken)
- Azathioprine
- Levothyroxine

Dental History
- Brushes her teeth irregularly
- Irregular dental attender (only attends when in pain)
- Emergency dental treatment last provided in a dental clinic 5 years ago

Social History
- Single; lives with her mother; no contact with father since the age of 5 years
- Has a 4-year-old child (supervised by the grandmother)
- Unstructured social environment (troubled and defiant)
- Unemployed
- Tobacco consumption: 20 cigarettes/day since she was 16 years old
- Alcohol consumption: 30 units weekly

Oral Examination
- Generalised plaque deposits, covering a third of the tooth surfaces
- Gingivitis
- Abundant dental calculus
- Caries: #11, #12, #21, #22, #32 and #38
- Fillings: #16, #17, #26, #27, #37, #46 and #47

Radiological Examination
- Orthopantomogram undertaken (Figure 5.2.1)
- Restorable caries in teeth #11, #12, #21, #22, #32 and #47
- Extensive and unrestorable caries in #16 and #38
- Impacted tooth #48

Structured Learning

1) What factors in this patient's medical history may be linked to the development of obstructive sleep apnoea-hypopnoea?
   - Hypothyroidism is thought to be a risk factor for the development of sleep apnoea
   - The proposed mechanisms include increased mucopolysaccharide and protein deposition in the upper airway, altered regulatory control of pharyngeal dilator muscles from neuropathy, depression of respiratory centres and increased risk of obesity
   - The use of thyroid hormone replacement may reduce the symptoms of sleep apnoea; however, this patient is not compliant with her medical management
2) The patient appears dishevelled and unkempt and her communication is limited. What factors could be contributing to this and what should you be alert for?

A Practical Approach to Special Care in Dentistry, First Edition. Edited by Pedro Diz Dios and Navdeep Kumar.

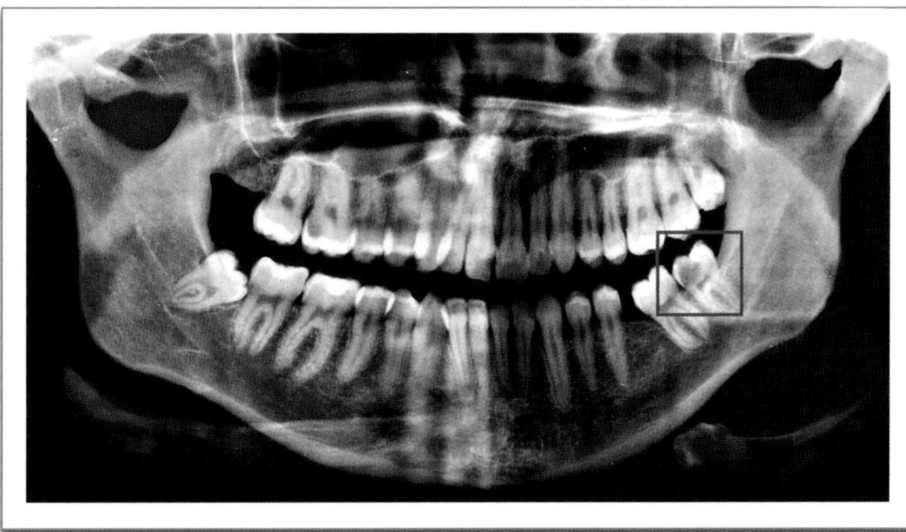

Figure 5.2.1 Orthopantomogram: neglected mouth with unrestorable caries in tooth #38.

- The patient is not compliant with her medical management and hence the psychological and physical dysfunction associated with hypothyroidism is more likely to have an impact on her well-being and quality of life
- Slowing of thought and speech, decreased attentiveness and memory, fatigue and apathy are more commonly observed with hypothyroidism
- Rarely, this can progress to agitation and frank psychosis
- Obstructive sleep apnoea-hypopnoea syndrome (disrupted sleep, leading to fatigue)
- Depression/anxiety
- There are also additional social factors which could have an impact as she is a young, single mother, unemployed, with no contact with her father, and has a high alcohol intake
- Although the patient's 4-year-old daughter is principally looked after by the grandmother, it is important to consider if there are any child safeguarding concerns and raise these

3) The patient has been told that her hypothyroidism is the reason for her hair loss. She believes that the hypothyroidism is also the reason for her teeth 'breaking and falling out'. Is she correct?
   - Hair loss may be related to hypothyroidism, as an adverse effect of azathioprine and/or due to alopecia areata (multifactorial autoimmune aetiology, but in some cases triggered by dental infections)
   - The decline in dental health is more likely to be linked to poor oral care and limited access to dental care – these may be exacerbated by the generalised effects of hypothyroidism, namely fatigue, apathy, depression
   - Hypothyroidism can also be accompanied by salivary gland dysfunction, regardless of the absence of Sjögren syndrome; this may be due to the effect of cytokines in the autoimmune process or because of thyroid hormone dysfunction
   - Additionally, there may be a potential association between hypothyroidism and periodontitis due to the immunological and inflammatory markers found in both (evidence is very limited)
4) You decide that the treatment of choice is to extract tooth #38. What factors are considered important in assessing the risk of managing this patient?
   - Social
     - The social-cultural environment can jeopardise communication with the patient and the interest in any proposed treatment beyond resolving the pain
     - Irregular compliance with medical treatment is a predictor for limited compliance with postdental procedure recommendations
     - Limited compliance with treatment is also more likely due to depression/anxiety
     - A suitable escort may be difficult to find as the grandmother looks after the patient's 4-year-old child
   - Medical
     - Bleeding tendency and drug selection due to liver damage
     - Susceptibility to infections due to azathioprine-induced immunosuppression
     - Untreated hypothyroidism is more likely to be associated with signs and symptoms, including impaired cognition/memory loss (impacts on capacity/consent)

   - Myxoedema coma risk may occur; estimated prevalence around 0.1%, but may be higher as the patient is not compliant with her medical management and is additionally anxious
- Dental
   - Acute pulpitis that requires urgent treatment
   - Dental treatment results compromised by heavy smoking, high alcohol intake and poor oral hygiene
   - Poor patient commitment to complex treatment plan and follow-up visits
   - Increased oral cancer risk due to tobacco and alcohol consumption

5) Given that the patient has uncontrolled hypothyroidism, what should you do prior to extracting the #38?
   - Liaise with the patient's physician
   - Consider referral to a hospital setting if the thyroid function is severely altered
   - Request blood test results
     - Full blood count
       - Haemoglobin; anaemia may be induced by the hypothyroidism and/or by azathioprine
       - White blood cell count; risk of leucopenia secondary to azathioprine
       - Platelet count; risk of thrombocytopenia due to the hepatic dysfunction or secondary to azathioprine
     - Coagulation study
       - Autoimmune hepatitis can cause liver dysfunction
   - Consider pain and infection control in the first instance

6) What sedation technique should be applied to this patient?
   - Nitrous oxide may be employed
   - Benzodiazepines are not recommended due to increased sensitivity; they compromise respiratory capacity and can also trigger a myxoedema coma

7) If there is noteworthy bleeding during the surgical procedure, what could be causing it?
   - Hypothyroidism causes vascular endothelial disorders that increase bleeding tendency (increased subcutaneous mucopolysaccharides, decreasing the ability of small blood vessels to constrict)
   - Von Willebrand disease is associated with hypothyroidism and it potentially may have remained undiagnosed beforehand
   - Thrombocytopenia risk
   - Liver dysfunction

General Dental Considerations

Oral Findings

- In children (cretinism)
  - Thick lips
  - Macroglossia
  - Delayed tooth eruption
  - Enamel hypoplasia
  - Rampant caries
  - Mandibular retrusion
  - Angle class II malocclusion
- In youths and adults
  - Thick lips
  - Macroglossia (Figure 5.2.2)
  - Burning mouth
  - Dysgeusia
  - Xerostomia
  - Lichen planus
  - Susceptibility to caries
  - Periodontal disease

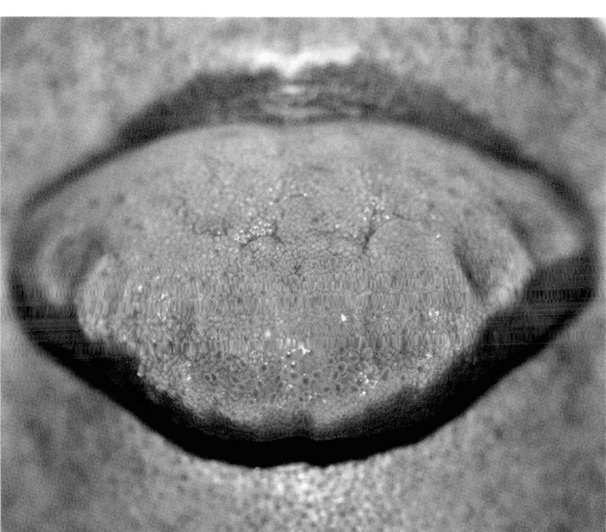

Figure 5.2.2 Macroglossia in a patient with hypothyroidism.

Dental Management

- The dental treatment plan will be determined primarily by the level of hypothyroidism control and the presence of comorbidities (Table 5.2.1)

Table 5.2.1 Considerations for dental management.

Risk assessment	• Myxoedema coma can be triggered under stressful conditions caused by dental treatment • Assess the presence of comorbidities such as hypotension, hypoadrenocorticism, anaemia, cardiac arrythmias, ischaemic heart disease and von Willebrand disease • Potentially increased bleeding risk • Potentially delayed wound healing due to decreased metabolic activity in fibroblasts
Criteria for referral	• Controlled hypothyroidism: dependent on comorbidities, dental care can be provided in the local dental clinic setting • Uncontrolled hypothyroidism: delay elective dental treatment until the hypothyroidism has been controlled; if urgent procedures are required, a hospital setting is preferable
Access/position	• If goitre is present, there may be pressure on the airway; consider a semi-reclined position • If there is a bleeding risk, arrange appointments earlier in the day and week
Communication	• Liaise with endocrinologist/physician if considering urgent dental treatment in a patient with untreated/significant hypothyroidism • Cognitive impairment is a common characteristic of congenital hypothyroidism • Some patients can experience vision loss and/or hearing loss • Bradypsychia-bradylalia has been reported in severe and long-term hypothyroidism
Consent/capacity	• Patients should be warned of the potential local (e.g. bleeding) and systemic complications (e.g. myxoedema coma), which can be triggered by dental treatment • Consider the impact of hypothyroidism on cognition and memory
Anaesthesia/sedation	• Local anaesthesia – Consider risk of increased bleeding at the site of administration • Sedation – Avoid benzodiazepines such as diazepam and midazolam as they can trigger myxoedema coma • General anaesthesia – Procedures under general anaesthesia should be delayed until hormone levels have recovered
Dental treatment	• Before – Ensure that the patient is compliant with their medical management – Determine if there are any additional risks associated with the related comorbidities (e.g. anticoagulants due to arrhythmias) • During – Careful manipulation of soft tissues due to the bleeding and delayed healing risk • After – Reduced bone turnover rate can increase the risk of radicular resorption secondary to orthodontic procedures
Drug prescription	• Increased sensitivity to central nervous system depressants and barbiturates; avoid benzodiazepines and opioid analgesics • Avoid mouthwashes with povidone-iodine (can increase the risk of thyroiditis or hypothyroidism)
Education/prevention	• Due to their susceptibility to caries and periodontal disease, maintaining optimal oral hygiene and periodic professional dental reviews are a priority for these patients

Section II: Background Information and Guidelines

Definition

Hypothyroidism is a common pathological condition characterised by the thyroid gland's inability to produce sufficient thyroid hormone to satisfy the body's metabolic demands. Primary clinical hypothyroidism is defined as the coexistence of thyroid-stimulating hormone (TSH) concentrations above the upper limit of normal and free thyroxine (T_4) concentrations below the reference range. In subclinical hypothyroidism (an early sign of thyroid gland failure), the TSH concentration is also above normal values, while T_4 concentrations are within the reference range. The mean prevalence in countries with adequate iodine intake is estimated at 1–2%. The disease is more common among women, in those older than 65 years and in white individuals.

Aetiopathogenesis

- Primary hypothyroidism (due to thyroid hormone deficiency)
  - May be related to iodine deficiency as iodine is a trace element essential for the synthesis of thyroid hormones, tri-iodothyronine (T_3) and thyroxine (T_4)
  - Iodine (as iodide) is found in the oceans; hence geographical areas that are iodine deficient tend to be inland and mountainous; more cases of congenital hypothyroidism (cretinism) are detected here
  - Autoimmune hypothyroidism (Hashimoto disease) is the most common cause in areas where there is sufficient iodine intake
  - Drugs can interfere with thyroid hormone production (e.g. amiodarone, lithium, some antiepileptic drugs, interferon-alpha, some tyrosine kinase inhibitors)
  - Iatrogenic causes include the administration of radioactive iodine to patients with hyperthyroidism, and those undergoing thyroid surgery or radiation therapy in the neck
  - Infiltrative diseases which involve the thyroid gland may also be responsible (e.g. neoplasia)
- Secondary hypothyroidism
  - Central hypothyroidism: due to thyrotropin-releasing hormone (TRH) deficiency or TSH deficiency and is associated with lesions in the hypothalamus and pituitary gland (mainly hypophysis adenoma), Sheehan syndrome, TRH resistance, radiation therapy to the brain and secondary to drugs such as dopamine, prednisone or opioids

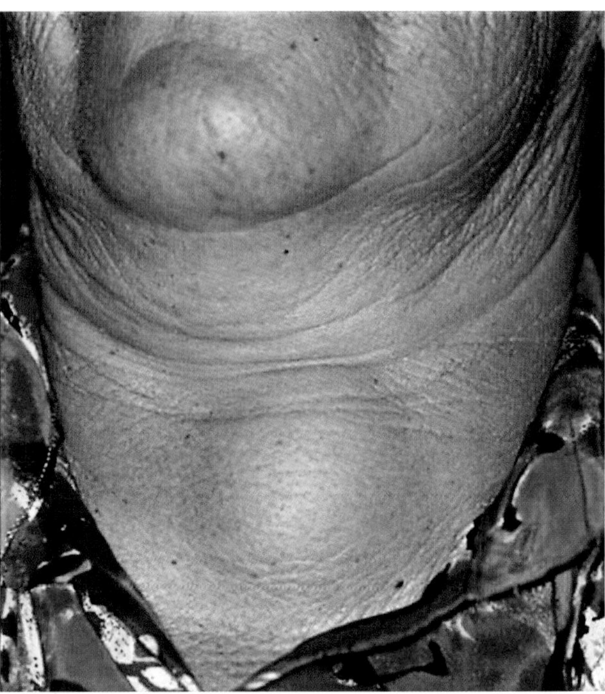

Figure 5.2.3 Goitre (enlarged thyroid gland).

  - Peripheral hypothyroidism: very uncommon and corresponds to an overexpression of deiodinase 3 (an enzyme that inactivates tyrosine) in patients with cancer and those with rare genetic syndromes

Clinical Presentation

- Varies significantly (Table 5.2.2). Enlargement of the thyroid gland (goitre) can occur due to overstimulation in response to low thyroid levels (Figure 5.2.3)
- Determined by age, sex and progression time
- Ranges from asymptomatic forms to myxoedema crisis/coma (encephalopathy, hypothermia, seizures, hyponatraemia, hypoglycaemia, arrhythmias, cardiogenic shock, respiratory failure and fluid retention)
- Cretinism, classically the result of maternal iodine deficiency, is associated with growth retardation, developmental delay, mental retardation and thickened facial features

Diagnosis

- Blood TSH concentration
- If the TSH concentration is high, the test should be repeated and T_4 should be quantified
- The measurement of thyroid peroxidase antibodies can be useful for confirming the diagnosis of primary autoimmune hypothyroidism
- In the presence of additional clinical findings such as an irregular thyroid gland when palpated, ultrasonography is indicated (Figure 5.2.4)

Table 5.2.2 Clinical manifestations of hypothyroidism.

Category	Symptoms	Signs
• General	Fatigue Weight gain Intolerance to cold Drowsiness	Hypothermia Increased body mass index Reduced metabolic activity Myxoedema
• Cardiovascular	Shortness of breath Fatigue with exercise	Hypertension Bradycardia Ischaemic heart disease Pleural effusion
• Haematological	Prone to bleeding	Anaemia Von Willebrand disease
• Musculoskeletal	Joint pain Myalgia	Increased creatine phosphokinase levels
• Gastrointestinal	Intake problems Constipation	Oesophageal motility disorder
• Skin and hair	Dry skin Hair loss	Fine hair Thickened skin Loss of eyebrow tail
• Sensorineural	Husky voice Dysgeusia Vision loss Hearing loss	Neuropathy Cochlear dysfunction
• Endocrinological	Infertility Menstrual disorders Galactorrhoea	Goitre Blood sugar dysregulation Increase in prolactin
• Psychological	Memory loss Depression Dementia	Cognitive impairment

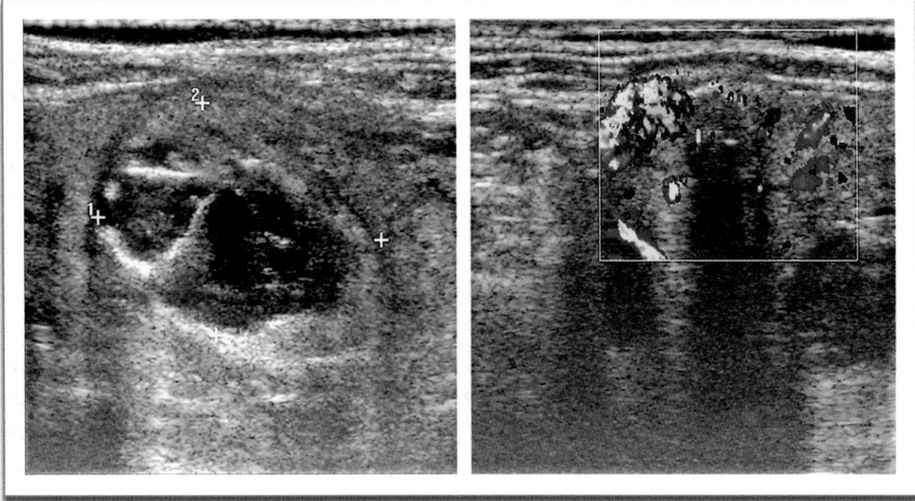

Figure 5.2.4 Grey-scale ultrasound and colour Doppler sonogram showing multiple micronodules in diffuse Hashimoto thyroiditis (right thyroid lobe).

Management

- The treatment of choice is levothyroxine (a synthetic form of T_4), at a dose of 1.5–1.8 μg/kg of body weight daily
- This is reduced in elderly patients or those with atrial fibrillation

Prognosis

- The prognosis of hypothyroidism is dependent on its cause, and whether it is diagnosed and treated in a timely manner
- In the absence of treatment, hypothyroidism may have a risk of high morbidity and mortality, leading eventually to coma or even death
- Congenital hypothyroidism has potentially devastating neurological consequences, with failure to treat resulting in severe intellectual disability
- A leading cause of death in adults is cardiovascular diseases, predominantly heart failure
- Myxoedema coma is uncommon but is a medical emergency with a high mortality rate
- With treatment, most patients have a good prognosis, and the symptoms usually reverse in a few weeks or months

A World/Transcultural View

- Foetal hypothyroidism, which can cause cretinism, has disappeared from the US and Europe thanks to iodine administration campaigns
- However, cretinism still exists in remote rural areas of many countries, and it is estimated that the condition affects 2 million children annually
- The belief that iodine deficiency disorders are hereditary tends to be prevalent in societies where familial goitre is common and where the rate of endogamy is high; this situation makes prophylactic dietary interventions seem useless and wasteful
- Water fluoridation, in regions where it is technically feasible and culturally acceptable, yields proven benefits in terms of public health, including preventing caries; however, it has been suggested that water fluoridation could cause hypothyroidism as fluoride and iodine have an antagonistic relationship

Recommended Reading

Chaker, L., Bianco, A.C., Jonklaas, J., and Peeters, R.P. (2017). Hypothyroidism. *Lancet* 390: 1550–1562.

Chandna, S. and Bathla, M. (2011). Oral manifestations of thyroid disorders and its management. *Indian J. Endocrinol. Metab.* 15: S113–S116.

Huber, M.A. and Terézhalmy, G.T. (2008). Risk stratification and dental management of the patient with thyroid dysfunction. *Quintessence Int.* 39: 139–150.

Little, J.W. (2006). Thyroid disorders. Part II: hypothyroidism and thyroiditis. *Oral Surg. Oral Med. Oral Pathol. Oral Radiol. Endod.* 102: 148–153.

Pinto, A. and Glick, M. (2002). Management of patients with thyroid disease: oral health considerations. *J. Am. Dent. Assoc.* 133: 849–858.

Venkatesh Babu, N.S. and Patel, P.B. (2016). Oral health status of children suffering from thyroid disorders. *J. Indian Soc. Pedod. Prev. Dent.* 34: 139–144.

Wémeau, J.L., Do Cao, C., and Ladsous, M. (2017). Oral and dental expression of thyroid diseases. *Presse Med.* 46: 864–868.

5.3 Hyperthyroidism

Section I: Clinical Scenario and Dental Considerations

Clinical Scenario

A 54-year-old female presents to you for a second opinion. She is unhappy about the appearance of her teeth which she feels look rough and discoloured.

Medical History
- Graves disease/hyperthyroidism diagnosed 4 weeks ago
- Atrial fibrillation – detected at the same time as the hyperthyroidism
- Gastro-oesophageal reflux disease

Medications
- Propylthiouracil
- Dabigatran
- Omeprazole

Dental History
- Irregular attender; only attends if there are dental problems
- Good co-operation; history of multiple fillings and dental extractions
- Brushes twice a day using hard bristle toothbrush to remove the staining
- Highly cariogenic diet, including consumption of tea with 3 spoons of sugar 4–6 times a day
- Likes to chew/suck on citrus fruits
- Also began eating black grapes several times a day since commencing propylthiouracil as she found this helpful with her symptoms of nausea

Social History
- Widowed housewife
- Lives with eldest daughter who works as a secondary school teacher and is responsible for transportation
- No alcohol or tobacco consumption

Oral Examination
- Mild goitre (Figure 5.3.1)
- Generalised pitted hypoplastic enamel and staining present on buccal surfaces of teeth (Figure 5.3.2)

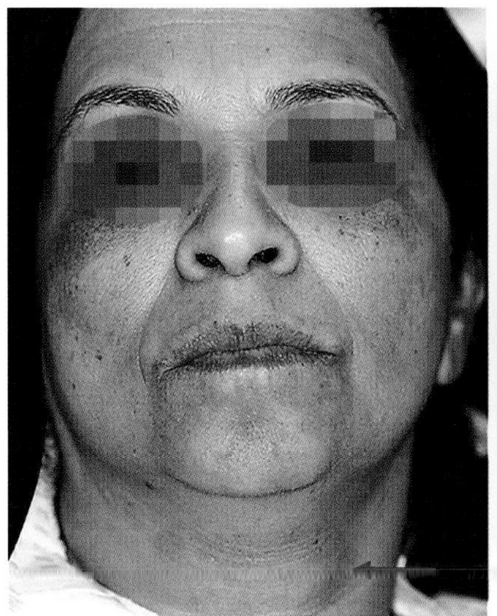
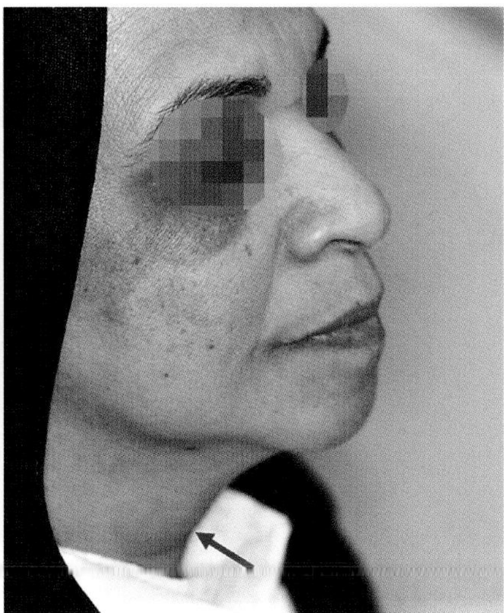

Figure 5.3.1 Mild goitre (anterior and lateral view).

A Practical Approach to Special Care in Dentistry, First Edition. Edited by Pedro Diz Dios and Navdeep Kumar.

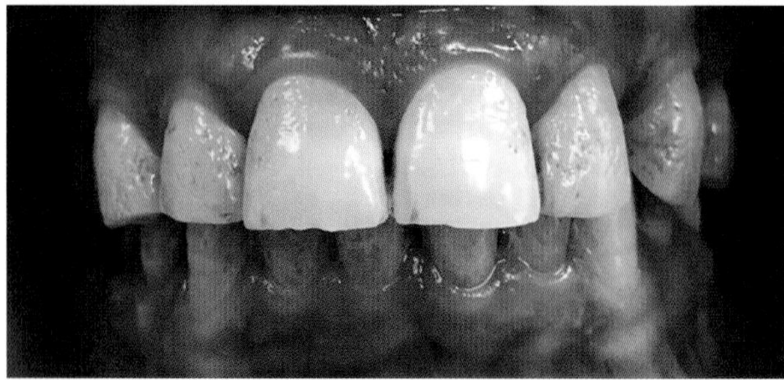

Figure 5.3.2 Pitted hypoplastic enamel and staining present on buccal surfaces of the anterior teeth.

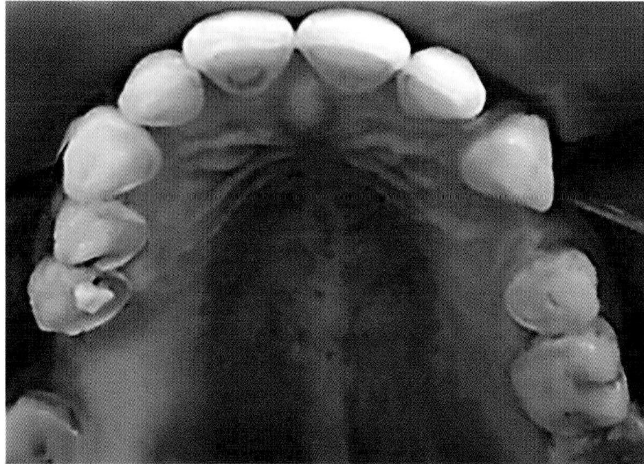

Figure 5.3.3 Generalised moderate to severe tooth surface loss on the palatal and occlusal surfaces of the maxillary dentition.

- Generalised moderate to several tooth surface loss (erosion and attrition) with possible pulpal involvement of #11 (Figure 5.3.3)
- Temporary filling in situ #15
- Caries in teeth #17, #14 and #45
- Supragingival calculus present on the lingual surfaces of the lower incisors
- Generalised gingival recession
- Missing (due to extraction) teeth #16, #24, #36 and #37

Radiological Examination

- Orthopantomogram and long cone periapical radiograph #15 undertaken (Figures 5.3.4 and 5.3.5)
- Generalised bone loss (~60–70%)
- Patchy medullary radiolucency suggestive of osteopenia/osteoporosis
- Periapical radiolucency associated with the apex of tooth #15

Structured Learning

1) What is 'goitre' and how does it affect your dental planning?
   - Goitre is an enlarged thyroid gland which causes a swelling in the front of the neck that moves up and down on swallowing
   - Thyroid function can be normal (euthyroid), which requires regular monitoring, or hyperactive (hyperthyroid)/hypoactive (hypothyroid), which both require active treatment
   - The impact on dental planning is dependent on any associated abnormal thyroid function and complications associated with the enlargement (e.g. respiratory obstruction, cough, voice changes, dyspnoea, tracheal deviation or dysphagia)
2) The patient believes that the appearance of her teeth has worsened due to hyperthyroidism. Is she correct?
   - No – she has enamel pitting; this is a form of enamel hypoplasia which would have been caused at the developmental enamel matrix formation stage of the teeth

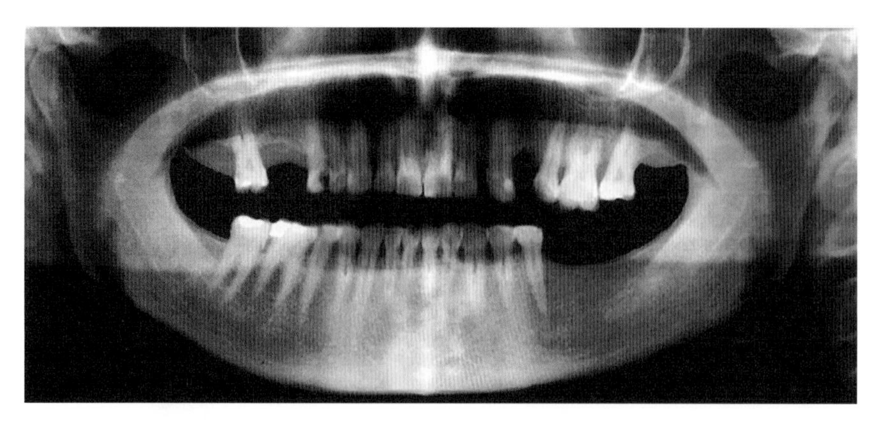

Figure 5.3.4 Orthopantomogram demonstrating patchy medullary radiolucency suggestive of osteopenia/osteoporosis.

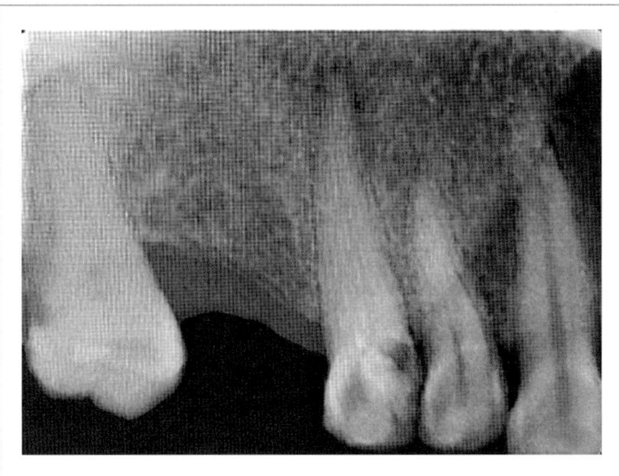

Figure 5.3.5 Long cone periapical radiograph demonstrating periapical radiolucency associated with the apex of tooth #15.

- Defects are divided into 4 categories: pit-form, plane-form, linear-form, and localised enamel hypoplasia
- Causes may include nutritional factors (malnutrition), some diseases (such as undiagnosed and untreated coeliac disease), hypocalcaemia, infection, abnormalities in amelogenesis
- Secondary staining (likely to be linked to increased daily consumption of black grapes) may have made the pitting more noticeable

3) What factors are likely to have contributed to the tooth surface loss?
   - Erosion: gastro-oesophageal reflux disease; dietary – highly acidic/citrus fruits; nausea/vomiting due to propylthiouracil
   - Abrasion: use of a hard toothbrush
   - Attrition: reduced occlusal table due to multiple missing teeth
4) The patient is also concerned about persistent pain from the #15 and wants it extracted at the same appointment. What risk is associated with the propylthiouracil medication?
   - Propylthiouracil has anti-vitamin K activity and can cause hypoprothrombinaemia, leading to an increased risk of bleeding
   - Furthermore, it is a thionamide and hence may cause a rare reaction of agranulocytosis (0.5% of patients) that can result in oral infections and inadequate wound healing
5) What additional risks associated with hyperthyroidism should be considered when planning extraction of the #15?
   - The patient's hyperthyroidism is unlikely to be controlled as the diagnosis/treatment was relatively recent; it is preferable to consider initial pain/infection control using medication until the physician confirms the patient is stable
   - Heightened patient anxiety and irritability likely
   - Elevated blood pressure and heart rate due to the effects of thyroid hormone on sympathetic nervous system activity
   - Patients with high arteriolar pressures may also require increased attention and a longer duration of local pressure to stop bleeding
   - Sympathetic overactivity may lead to fainting
   - A thyroid storm may be provoked during dental treatment by the stress, administration of epinephrine, infection or traumatic surgery
6) What other factors do you need to consider in your risk assessment?
   - Social
     - Reliance on daughter (who works as a school teacher) for transport/to attend appointments
   - Medical
     - Risk of cardiac arrythmias
     - Additional bleeding risk associated with dabigatran (see Chapter 10.4)
     - Gastro-oesophageal reflux disease may be associated with positional limitations
   - Dental
     - Poor oral health and irregular attender
     - Advanced tooth surface loss
     - Partially edentate
     - Osteoporotic changes in the jaw bone secondary to hyperthyroidism
7) The patient requests dental implants to replace the missing teeth. What are the associated risks you should discuss?
   - Poor oral health needs to be stabilised first
   - Compliance and need for regular dental visits and maintenance
   - Bleeding risk
   - Infection risk
   - Osteoporotic changes in the mandible

General Dental Considerations

Oral Findings

- Early tooth eruption and exfoliation of primary teeth
- Alveolar bone osteoporosis
- Increased caries and periodontal disease (due to high sugar intake to satisfy caloric requirement)
- Ectopic thyroid tissue located on the foramen caecum of the tongue is called lingual thyroid, and in some cases may be the only active thyroid tissue present

- Propylthiouracil/carbamizole may cause agranulocytosis, which may result in oral or oropharyngeal ulceration

Dental Management

- Treatment should be modified based on the severity of the condition, the medical management in place and the invasiveness of the proposed dental intervention (Table 5.3.1)

Section II: Background Information and Guidelines

Definition

Hyperthyroidism is characterised by an increase in serum concentrations of the thyroid hormones, thyroxine (T_4) and tri-iodothyronine (T_3). The secretion of T_3 and T_4, which occurs in thyroid gland follicles, is normally controlled by thyroid-stimulating hormone (TSH),

Table 5.3.1 Dental management considerations.

Risk assessment	• These patients may have heightened anxiety and irritability • Sympathetic overactivity may lead to fainting • A thyroid storm may be provoked during dental treatment by the stress, or by epinephrine, infection or traumatic surgery • Bleeding tendency in patients on propylthiouracil • Risk of lymphopenia in patients on propylthiouracil • Carbimazole occasionally leads to agranulocytosis, which may cause oral or oropharyngeal ulceration • Alveolar bone osteoporosis may be present
Criteria for referral	• Controlled hyperthyroidism: depending on the comorbidities, dental care can be provided in the local dental clinic setting • Uncontrolled hyperthyroidism: delay elective dental treatment until the hyperthyroidism has been controlled; if urgent procedures are required, a hospital setting is preferable
Access/position	• If goitre is present, there may be pressure on the airway; consider a semi-reclined position if this is the case • If there is a bleeding/infection risk, arrange appointments earlier in the day and week
Communication	• Liaise with endocrinologist/physician if considering urgent dental treatment in a patient with untreated/significant hyperthyroidism • Speech may be affected if there is goitre or if there is any damage to the laryngeal nerves following surgery
Consent/capacity	• Consider the impact of heightened anxiety on decision making and consent • Patients should be warned of the potential local (e.g. bleeding) and systemic complications (thyroid storm)
Anaesthesia/sedation	• Local anaesthesia – The risks of giving epinephrine-containing local anaesthetics in moderate amounts are more theoretical than real – If there is concern, prilocaine with felypressin can be given, but is not known to be safer • Sedation – Sedation may be considered since anxiety may precipitate a thyroid crisis – Nitrous oxide, which is rapidly controllable, is probably safest for dental sedation – Benzodiazepines may potentiate antithyroid drugs and are thus contraindicated – Antihistamines such as hydroxyzine may also be useful • General anaesthesia – The hyperthyroid patient is especially at risk from general anaesthesia because of the risk of precipitating dangerous arrhythmias – After hyperthyroidism treatment, the patient is at risk from hypothyroidism; this must be borne in mind if a general anaesthesia is required

(Continued)

Table 5.3.1 (Continued)

Dental treatment	• Before – Behavioural control and techniques to control anxiety are essential in patients with untreated hyperthyroidism requiring urgent dental treatment – Definitive dental treatment should be delayed until the patient has been rendered euthyroid – Invasive/surgical treatment will require specialised medical advice • During – The use of topical anaesthesia prior to the local anaesthesia may help pain control and anxiety – Local anaesthesia should be delivered using an aspirating syringe and should include a reduced amount of vasoconstrictor/epinephrine • After – Give patient written postoperative instruction and emergency contact details
Drug prescription	• Benzodiazepines should be avoided • Povidone-iodine and similar compounds are best avoided (iodine is taken up by the thyroid)
Education/prevention	• Reinforce meticulous oral hygiene and regular dental visits to prevent caries, periodontal disease and need for future extractions

a protein secreted from the anterior pituitary gland, which in turn is regulated by thyrotropin-releasing hormone (TRH), produced in the hypothalamus. When serum concentrations of thyroid hormones are elevated, TSH secretion is suppressed by a negative feedback mechanism.

Aetiopathogenesis

- There are multiple causes of hyperthyroidism as summarised in Table 5.3.2
- Graves disease is the most common cause
  - Autoimmune disease that targets the thyroid gland with thyroid-stimulating autoantibodies against TSH receptor antibodies (TRAbs and TMAbs)
  - Predominantly occurs in women (8:1 ratio)
  - Age of presentation 20–40 years old
- General risk factors for hyperthyroidism
  - More common in women
  - Over the age of 60 years old
  - Positive family history
  - Consumption of excess iodine, either from foods or supplements, or from medications containing iodine (such as amiodarone)
  - Pregnancy within the last 6 months
  - Other health problems including pernicious anaemia, type 1 diabetes, primary adrenal insufficiency, myasthenia gravis

Clinical Presentation

- Thyroid hyperactivity mimics epinephrine excess
  - Raised pulse and anxiety
  - Hypertension with tachycardia
  - Eyelid lag/retraction
  - Tremor
  - Dislike of heat
  - Irritability
- Cardiac disturbances are often present, particularly in older patients, and include tachycardia, arrhythmias (especially atrial fibrillation) and cardiac failure
- Additional features:
  - Exophthalmos or proptosis
  - Thyroid swelling/lump (goitre)
  - Warm, moist and erythematous skin
  - Fine brittle hair
  - Change in weight – typically loss of weight although an increased appetite can lead to weight gain
  - Diarrhoea
- Thyrotoxic periodic paralysis (attacks of mild to severe weakness)
- Thyrotoxic crisis/thyroid storm
  - A severe condition that starts with extreme anxiety, nausea, vomiting and abdominal pain
  - Later, it is associated with fever, sweating, tachycardia and pulmonary oedema
  - Finally, stupor, coma and possibly death

Table 5.3.2 Causes of hyperthyroidism.

Category	Causes
Primary	• Increased stimulation secondary to: – Thyroid-stimulating hormone receptor antibodies (TRAb), seen mostly in Graves disease – Excess human chorionic gonadotropin (hCG) secretion in patients with hyperemesis gravidarum – Trophoblastic tumours such as choriocarcinoma or hydatidiform mole – Autonomous thyroid function – Toxic multinodular goitre – Solitary toxic nodule – Familial non-autoimmune hyperthyroidism • Excess release of stored thyroid hormone – Autoimmune (silent or postpartum thyroiditis) – Infective (viral, bacterial, fungal) – Pharmacological (amiodarone, interferon-alpha) • Exposure to excess iodine – Excess iodine intake during radiographic contrast – Consumption of high quantities of iodine-rich foods (e.g. fish, seaweed, egg yolks)/ supplements/medications containing iodine (amiodarone)
Secondary	• Inappropriate thyroid-stimulating hormone (TSH) secretion – TSH-secreting pituitary adenoma – Pituitary resistant to thyroid hormone
Extrathyroid	• Excess intake of thyroid hormone – Iatrogenic/factitious • Ectopic thyroid hormone secretion – Struma ovarii – Functional thyroid metastases

Management

- Symptom control with beta-blockers such as propranolol or nadolol may be used in the first few weeks after diagnosis
- Treatment of hyperthyroidism
  - Antithyroid drugs – carbimazole, propylthiouracil and methimazole; the course of treatment lasts 18 months; 30–50% chance of cure
  - Radioactive iodine – very effective/safe; treatment results in hypothyroidism with the need to take levothyroxine long-term
  - Surgery – considered for younger patients with large goitres and for those in whom antithyroid drugs are not effective; again results in hypothyroidism with the need to take levothyroxine long-term; potential risk to laryngeal nerve

Prognosis

- The severity of hyperthyroidism depends on the amount and duration of hormone excess, age and complications
- Thyrotoxic crisis or thyroid storm may lead to coma and occasionally death

A World/Transcultural View

- Hyperthyroidism is a common condition with potentially life-threatening health consequences that affects all populations worldwide. In advanced economies, the prevalence of undiagnosed thyroid disease is falling owing to widespread thyroid function testing and relatively low thresholds for treatment initiation
- Iodine nutrition remains a key determinant of thyroid function worldwide. More studies are needed in developing countries, especially within Africa, to understand the role of ethnicity and iodine nutrition fluxes in current disease trends

Recommended Reading

Bahn, R.S., Burch, H.B., Cooper, D.S. et al. (2011). American Thyroid Association, American Association of Clinical Endocrinologists. Hyperthyroidism and other causes of thyrotoxicosis: management guidelines of the American Thyroid Association and American Association of Clinical Endocrinologists. *Thyroid* 21: 593–646.

Biron, C.R. (1996). Patients with thyroid dysfunctions require risk management before dental procedures. *RDH* 16: 42–44.

Gortzak, R.A. and Asscheman, H. (1996). Hyperthyroidism and dental treatment. *Ned. Tijdschr. Tandheelkd.* 103: 511–513.

Lee, K.J., Park, W., Pang, N.S. et al. (2016). Management of hyperthyroid patients in dental emergencies: a case report. *J. Dent. Anesth. Pain Med.* 16: 147–150.

Sundaresh, V., Brito, J.P., Wang, Z. et al. (2013). Comparative effectiveness of therapies for Graves' hyperthyroidism: a systematic review and network meta-analysis. *J. Clin. Endocrinol. Metab.* 98: 3671–3677.

Taylor, P., Albrecht, D., Scholz, A. et al. (2018). 2018 global epidemiology of hyperthyroidism and hypothyroidism. *Nat. Rev. Endocrinol.* 14: 301–316.

6

Hepatorenal Diseases

6.1 Hepatic Cirrhosis

Section I: Clinical Scenario and Dental Considerations

Clinical Scenario

A 46-year-old female presents for an assessment appointment, asking you to 'fix her mouth' as she has difficulty chewing because her teeth are so broken down. The medical practitioner has prescribed repeated courses of antibiotics for her due to recurrent episodes of dental infection, but these have not been effective.

Medical History
- Compensated hepatic cirrhosis related to alcohol excess diagnosed 3 years ago (excess alcohol consumption since the age of 24 years)
- Hydropic decompensation (ascites) 1 year ago
- Hypersplenism with thrombocytopenia
- Generalised anxiety with previous anxiety episodes triggered by stress; particularly anxious at the sight of needles
- Chronic insomnia

Medications
- Furosemide
- Spironolactone
- Lorazepam (low dose)

Dental History
- Last visit to a dentist over 20 years ago
- Admits she stopped looking after her mouth when she started consuming excess alcohol
- Now only occasionally brushes her anterior teeth as her molar teeth hurt when she tries to brush them

Social History
- Lives with her husband and their 12-year-old daughter
- Husband works as a lorry driver and is often away from home/working at night
- Family previously unaware of her excess alcohol consumption
- Works part-time for a cleaning company (limited financial resources)
- Smokes 3 cigarettes/day
- Has not consumed alcohol in the past 18 months but previously consumed in excess of 30–40 units a week as a way of coping with her anxiety (secret binge drinker)

Oral Examination
- Neglected mouth
- Very poor oral hygiene
- Advanced tooth surface loss of anterior teeth
- Numerous retained roots and missing teeth
- Caries in teeth #16, #17, #24 and #27

Radiological Examination
- Orthopantomogram undertaken (Figure 6.1.1)
- Restorable caries in #15 and #24
- Extensive, deep and unrestorable caries in #16, #17 and #27
- Retained roots: #22, #25, #26, #44, #45 and #46
- Generalised alveolar bone loss

Structured Learning

1) The patient asks for urgent treatment as her hepatologist has advised her that the poor oral health is linked to the liver disease. Is this correct?
   - Periodontitis may act as a persistent source of oral bacterial translocation, causing inflammation and increasing cirrhosis complications
   - Furthermore, there is some evidence that severe periodontitis is associated with higher mortality in patients who have cirrhosis
2) Other than her very poor oral hygiene, why is this patient at increased risk of repeated oral infections?

A Practical Approach to Special Care in Dentistry, First Edition. Edited by Pedro Diz Dios and Navdeep Kumar.

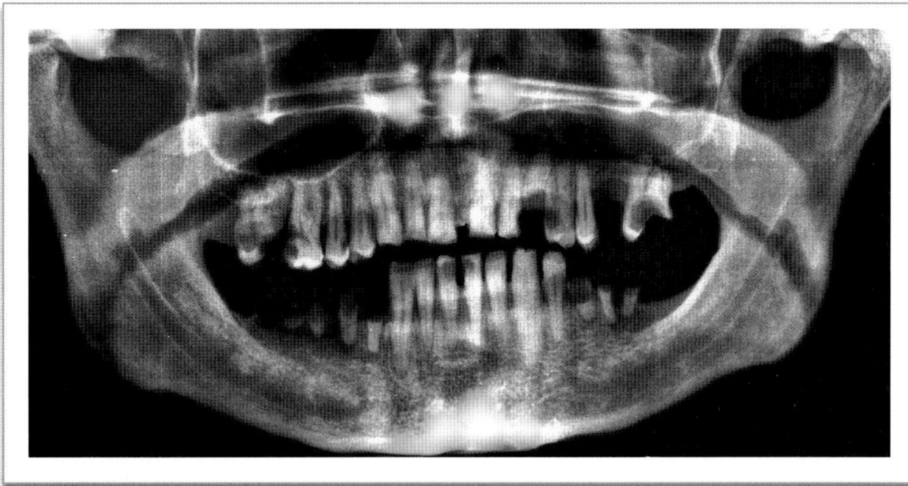

Figure 6.1.1 Orthopantomogram demonstrating a neglected mouth with multiple carious teeth and retained roots.

- Liver cirrhosis impairs the homeostatic role of the liver in the systemic immune response
- Damage to the reticuloendothelial system and the reduction of hepatic synthesis of proteins involved in innate immunity impair the bactericidal ability of phagocytic cells

3) The initial phase of treatment involves removal of the infected retained roots. Why should the patient be referred to a hospital setting for this?
   - Although the cirrhosis is currently compensated, there has been a previous decompensation episode
     - Decompensated cirrhosis is defined as an acute deterioration in liver function in a patient with cirrhosis
     - Typical presenting clinical features include jaundice, ascites, hepatic encephalopathy, hepatorenal syndrome or oesophageal variceal haemorrhage
     - These patients are at high risk of complications/mortality
   - Thrombocytopenia
     - Thrombocytopenia is the most common haematological abnormality in patients with cirrhosis
     - Often attributed to hypersplenism (increased pooling of platelets in a spleen enlarged by congestive splenomegaly secondary to portal hypertension)
     - Pathogenesis also related to decreased platelet production and increased destruction
     - Considered an indicator of advanced liver disease and poor prognosis
4) Apart from the thrombocytopaenia, why would this patient have a tendency to bleed during an oral surgical procedure?
   - Hepatic synthesis of coagulation factors might be impaired
   - Poor absorption and utilisation of vitamin K impairs the synthesis of coagulation factors II, VII, IX and X
   - Bleeding gums due to poor oral hygiene
5) What factors are considered important in assessing the risk of managing this patient?
   - Social
     - Risk of alcoholism relapse
     - Limited financial means
     - Primary carer for her 12-year-old daughter (husband often works away from home)
     - Availability of an adult escort
   - Medical
     - History of alcoholism (see Chapter 15.5); relapses are common in the short term (3 years)
     - Compensated cirrhosis (increased risk of bleeding and infection, avoid drugs metabolised in the liver)
     - Thrombocytopenia (see Chapter 11.4)
     - Anxiety/risk of triggering an acute episode in relation to the planned dental treatment, especially as injections will be required (see Chapter 15.1)
   - Dental
     - Neglected dentition/poor oral hygiene habits
     - High treatment needs
     - Uncertain degree of co-operation in the dental setting
     - Unpredictable commitment to improved oral hygiene measures or to regular follow-up appointments
6) The patient is extremely anxious and requests sedation or general anaesthesia for the planned dental extractions. What should you consider?
   - Sedation and general anaesthetic drugs are potentially dangerous in liver disease mainly due to impaired detoxification; this can result in encephalopathy and potentially coma

- Halothane should be avoided; this risk is higher in obese patients, smokers, middle-aged females and/or if a halothane has been given in the last 3 months
- Newer agents, e.g. enflurane or sevoflurane, are less hepatotoxic
- Relative analgesia with nitrous oxide is preferred to sedation with a benzodiazepine
- A specialist anaesthetist is required even if general anaesthesia is unavoidable
- It should also be noted that this patient is already taking lorazepam

7) Liver function tests, a full blood count and a clotting screen are undertaken prior to the planned dental extractions. The liver function tests and clotting screen are normal. The platelet count is 49×10^9 per litre. What is your approach?
   - Contact the hepatologist/physician for advice
   - Haematological support may include the administration of vitamin K, vasopressin or platelet transfusion. This should preferentially be administered by a specialist
   - Limit the number of extractions undertaken and implement local haemostatic measures (see Chapter 11.4)

8) The patient recalls that the last time she was given penicillin, she developed a mild rash. The hepatologist has advised antibiotic prophylaxis before the procedure as the patient has had a previous episode of bacterial peritonitis. Why are antibiotics indicated and what would you prescribe?
   - Spontaneous bacterial peritonitis is the most frequent bacterial infection in patients with cirrhosis and is associated with a high risk of morbidity
   - Avoid penicillins and also beta-lactam antibiotics due to cross-sensitivity
   - Consider clindamycin, 300 mg 1 hour before the dental treatment session, although a number of authors have proposed a conventional dose of 600 mg
   - A quinolone may be administered without reducing the dose (e.g. ciprofloxacin and norfloxacin)

General Dental Considerations

Oral Findings

- Oral health is frequently poor (especially in alcoholic cirrhosis)
- Jaundiced mucosa
- Some patients can experience chronic, bilateral and asymptomatic inflammation of the parotid glands (sialosis)
- An increase in stimulated parotid salivary flow has been reported, as well as a number of abnormalities in the electrolyte and protein composition of saliva
- Conversely, treatment of liver cirrhosis with diuretics reduces salivary flow (increasing the risk for caries, gingival inflammation and candidiasis)
- Petechiae, ecchymosis and bleeding gums (as an expression of the tendency to bleed due to the deficient synthesis of vitamin K-dependent clotting factors)
- Increased bleeding risk after dental extractions (Figure 6.1.2)
- Periodontal disease is highly prevalent and severe, especially in alcoholic cirrhosis, and has been associated with a state of chronic immunosuppression
- Dental erosion due to gastric regurgitation
- The rate of oral carcinoma is high (in relation to alcohol consumption); lesions representing oral metastases from a hepatocellular carcinoma have also been observed
- Possible delay in wound healing and in the formation of cancellous bone following simple or surgical tooth extractions

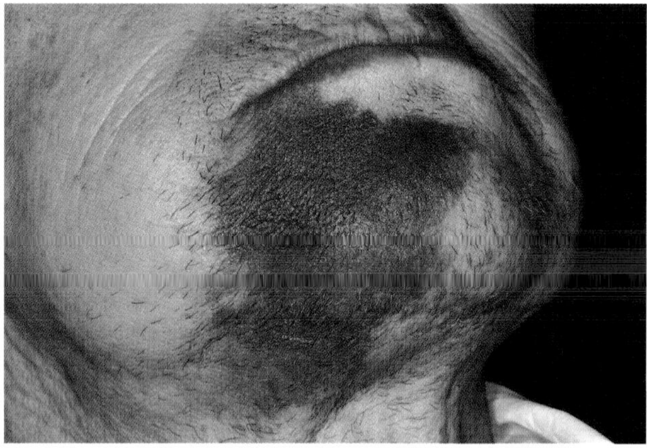

Figure 6.1.2 Postoperative bleeding after dental extraction in liver cirrhosis patient.

Dental Management

- The dental management and treatment plan are contingent on the severity of the hepatic dysfunction, as this determines both the potential complications (e.g. bleeding) and the patient's prognosis (Table 6.1.1)

Table 6.1.1 Considerations for dental management.

Risk assessment	• Increased bleeding tendency • Increased risk of infection • Impaired drug metabolism • Hepatoxicity of drugs • Associated comorbidities (depending on the underlying cause)
Criteria for referral	• The dental treatment should be conducted in a hospital setting in the following circumstances: – Decompensated cirrhosis (Child–Pugh grade B or C) – Compensated cirrhosis with signs of thrombocytopenia or previous episodes of decompensation
Communication	• Potential discrimination by health professionals, due to the erroneous interpretation that the aetiology of cirrhosis is always the excessive consumption of alcohol • Communication can be especially impaired due to fatigue, disturbed sleep patterns, alcohol (see Chapter 15.5)
Consent/capacity	• Patients need to be warned of the potential complications resulting from cirrhosis, which can require: – The implementation of bleeding prevention protocols – The prescription of drugs that are not metabolised by the liver
Anaesthesia/sedation	• Local anaesthesia – Most of the amide local anaesthetics used in dental practice undergo biotransformation in the liver – Avoid lidocaine – Prilocaine or articaine are preferred; articaine is metabolised partly in plasma and prilocaine partly in the lungs – Due to the reduced overall metabolism of all the amides, reduce the overall dose given, depending on the degree of liver cirrhosis • Sedation – Sedatives, hypnotics and opioids can trigger encephalopathy and coma – If a dental treatment with the patient under sedation is planned, nitrous oxide is preferable • General anaesthesia – Avoid halothane and suxamethonium – Isoflurane or sevoflurane are recommended
Dental treatment	• Before – Consult the patient's physician if the liver cirrhosis is significant and/or complex dental procedures are planned – Assess the tendency to bleed – Clotting screen: due to deficient synthesis of vitamin K-dependent clotting factors; determine the prothrombin time, activated partial thromboplastin time and INR – Full blood count: quantitative or functional platelet disorders may be present, especially in alcoholic cirrhosis – Determine whether haematological support is required when invasive dental procedures are planned – Vitamin K parenterally (10 mg/day) 5–7 days prior to the surgery – Desmopressin (IV/SC/intranasal) – Fresh blood, plasma, platelet transfusion – Consider the need for antibiotic prophylaxis (particularly if bacterial peritonitis is a risk) – Consider the presence of concomitant diseases • During – Bleeding can generally be controlled by applying only local haemostatic measures • After – Delay in wound healing and new trabecular bone formation – There is no available evidence on the survival of dental implants in patients with hepatic cirrhosis

(Continued)

Table 6.1.1 (Continued)

Drug prescription	• Avoid drugs that are metabolised in the liver (see Table 4.3.2) • The analgesics of choice are paracetamol and COX-2 inhibitors • The antibiotics of choice are amoxicillin and penicillin V. Clindamycin and metronidazole may be prescribed at reduced doses. Quinolones are a fairly safe option and do not require dose adjustment

Section II: Background Information and Guidelines

Definition

Cirrhosis is the irreversible loss of liver structure due to necrosis and fibrosis. This results in an increased resistance to portal blood flow (responsible for portal hypertension) and impaired hepatic function. A change in terminology to 'advanced liver disease' has recently been suggested because this process is dynamic and has a variable prognosis. The prevalence of cirrhosis is difficult to determine because the disease is asymptomatic in its initial phases. Cirrhosis is estimated to cause more than 1 million deaths worldwide annually. In Europe alone, it is the main indication for performing 5500 liver transplantations every year.

Aetiopathogenesis

- The main causes for the disease in most high-income countries are hepatitis C virus infection, alcohol abuse and, increasingly, non-alcoholic fatty liver disease (linked to fat deposition in the liver; more commonly associated with obesity, insulin resistance, elevated triglycerides)
- In sub-Saharan Africa and most of Asia, the most common cause is hepatitis B virus infection
- The transition of chronic liver disease to cirrhosis involves inflammation, hepatic stellate cell activation with consequent fibrogenesis, angiogenesis and destruction of the parenchyma as the result of vascular occlusion

Clinical Presentation

- There are 2 clinical stages of cirrhosis: compensated and decompensated
- The stages are dynamic and progressive, but there is potential reversibility from the decompensated to the compensated stage
- Most cases are asymptomatic (compensated)
- Clinical decompensation occurs due to an event such as:
  - Ascites
  - Sepsis (spontaneous bacterial peritonitis)
  - Haemorrhagic oesophageal varices
  - Encephalopathy
  - Non-obstructive jaundice
- Other findings include:
  - Leuconychia
  - Palmar erythema
  - Dupuytren contracture
  - Splenomegaly
  - Presence of portosystemic collaterals (e.g. spider veins and caput medusae)
  - Gynaecomastia and testicular atrophy
- General signs/symptoms:
  - Fatigue/exhaustion
  - Loss of appetite
  - Loss of weight
  - Muscle wasting
  - Nausea and vomiting
  - Disturbed sleep patterns

Diagnosis

- In the initial phases of cirrhosis, indirect serum markers may be employed
  - Liver function tests: increased aspartate transaminase (AST) and alanine transaminase (ALT), ALT may also be raised in cardiac or skeletal muscle damage and is therefore not specific for liver disease; gamma-glutamyl transferase (γGT or GGT), when it is raised, usually reflects alcoholic liver disease; alkaline phosphatase levels may be raised in obstructive jaundice but this is not a specific marker
  - Full blood count: platelet count may be abnormal
  - Other serum biomarkers of fibrosis (e.g. FibroTest, Enhanced Liver Fibrosis, FIBROSpect II) and specific imaging modalities (e.g. elastography)
- The diagnosis can be established when an irregular and nodular liver is detected through ultrasound, CT or MRI, along with impaired liver synthesis function
- A liver biopsy is rarely necessary but helps establish the definitive diagnosis and confirm the aetiology (e.g. for compensated cirrhosis where non-invasive parameters may be normal)

Management

- Nutritional supplements
- Diet with low sodium and protein content
- Treatment of the underlying cause to stop disease progression, such as avoiding alcohol consumption and administering immunosuppressants, corticosteroids or direct-acting antivirals
- Prevention and treatment of complications (e.g. surgical treatment of oesophageal varices)
- If the complications are not controlled or the liver stops functioning, liver transplantation may be considered (Figure 6.1.3)

Prognosis

- Cirrhosis is considered a final phase of liver disease (Table 6.1.2)
- Patients with compensated cirrhosis are asymptomatic and overall have median survival times of >12 years
- Patients with decompensated cirrhosis have had at least one complication including ascites, jaundice, variceal haemorrhage or hepatic encephalopathy, and overall they have median survival times of 2 years
- Typically leads to death at 5–10 years if transplantation is not performed
- The disease is associated with a high risk of liver cancer

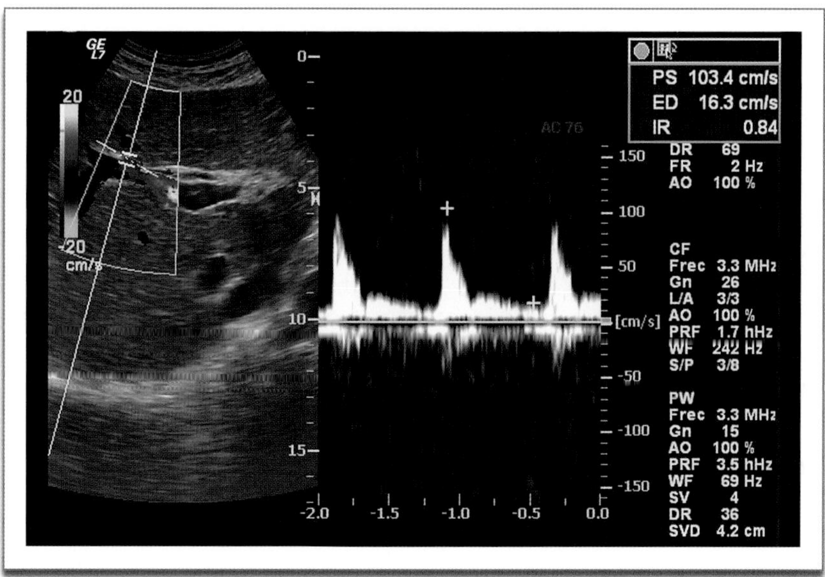

Figure 6.1.3 Grey-scale ultrasound and colour Doppler sonogram showing a liver transplantation in a cirrhotic patient.

Table 6.1.2 Child–Pugh classification of cirrhosis.

		Points		
Factor	**Units**	**1**	**2**	**3**
• Encephalopathy		None	Mild to moderate	Severe
• Ascites		None	Mild to moderate	Severe
• Bilirubin	mg/dL	<2	2–3	>3
• Albumin	g/dL	>3.5	3–3.5	<3
• Prothrombin time	Seconds prolonged	0–4	4–6	>6
	INR	<1.7	1.7–2.3	>2.3

Child–Pugh score (calculated by adding the points of the five factors)

Points	Class	Two-year survival
5–6	Class A (least severe liver disease)	85%
7–9	Class B (moderately severe liver disease)	60%
10–15	Class C (most severe liver disease)	35%

Source: Adapted from Child, C.G. and Turcotte, J.G. (1964). Surgery and portal hypertension. *Major Probl. Clin. Surg.* 1: 1–85; Pugh, R.N., Murray-Lyon, I.M., Dawson, J.L. et al. (1973). Transection of the oesophagus for bleeding oesophageal varices. *Br. J. Surg.* 60: 646–649.

- The most consistent predictor of mortality is the Child–Pugh score and/or its components (albumin, bilirubin, ascites, encephalopathy and prothrombin time)

A World/Transcultural View

- Despite effective interventions for preventing and treating hepatitis B and C, these viruses are still the main cause of cirrhosis worldwide, particularly in low-income countries
- In the near future, non-alcoholic hepatic steatosis is expected to become the main causal factor
- In recent decades, the age-standardised mortality rate decreased or remained constant in all regions, except Western Europe and Central Asia where it increased, mainly due to alcohol consumption
- Sub-Saharan Africa has the highest mortality rate due to cirrhosis (32 deaths/100000 individuals), while high-income regions have the lowest (10 deaths/100000 individuals); the lowest rate is found in Singapore, while the highest is in Egypt

Recommended Reading

Aberg, F., Helenius-Hietala, J., Meurman, J., and Isoniemi, H. (2014). Association between dental infections and the clinical course of chronic liver disease. *Hepatol. Res.* 44: 349–353.

Brigo, S., Mancuso, E., and Pellicano, R. (2019). Dentistry and oral and maxillofacial surgery in the patient with liver disease: key messages for clinical practice. *Minerva Stomatol.* 68: 192–199.

Costa, F.O., Lages, E.J.P., Lages, E.M.B., and Cota, L.O.M. (2019). Periodontitis in individuals with liver cirrhosis: a case-control study. *J. Clin. Periodontol.* 46: 991–998.

Ge, P.S. and Runyon, B.A. (2016). Treatment of patients with cirrhosis. *N. Engl. J. Med.* 375: 767–777.

Medina, J.B., Andrade, N.S., de Paula Eduardo, F. et al. (2018). Bleeding during and after dental extractions in patients with liver cirrhosis. *Int. J. Oral Maxillofac. Surg.* 47: 1543–1549.

Tsochatzis, E.A., Bosch, J., and Burroughs, A.K. (2014). Liver cirrhosis. *Lancet* 383 (9930): 1749–1761.

Zahed, M., Bahador, M., Hosseini Asl, M.K. et al. (2020). Oro-dental health of patients with chronic hepatic failure. *Int. J. Organ Transplant. Med.* 11: 115–121.

6.2 Chronic Kidney Disease (Dialysis)

Section I: Clinical Scenario and Dental Considerations

Clinical Scenario

A 49-year-old male undergoing haemodialysis for end-stage chronic kidney disease (CKD), is referred by his nephrologist for an oral assessment. The request is to eliminate potential oral foci of infection prior to planned kidney transplantation.

Medical History
- End stage CKD (possibly related to workplace exposure to lead)
- Arterial hypertension
- Osteopenia (renal osteodystrophy)
- Iron-deficiency anaemia
- Dyslipidaemia
- Hyperuricaemia

Medications
- Haemodialysis 3 days a week, for 5 years (heparin on days he goes to dialysis)
- Nifedipine
- Irbesartan
- Furosemide
- Calcium acetate
- Vitamin D3
- Iron
- Atorvastatin
- Allopurinol

Dental History
- Last dental visit 15 years ago
- Only attends when he experiences dental pain
- Co-operated with local anaesthesia and dental extractions in the past
- Brushes his teeth 2–3 times a day

Social History
- Single; lives alone, no children or close family/friends
- Not working/on limited disability allowance
- Requires hospital transport for appointments and generally feels too tired to use public transport
- Ex-smoker (20 cigarettes/day until 10 years ago)
- No alcohol consumption

Oral Examination
- Fair oral hygiene
- Caries: #22, #24, #25, #27 and #46
- Missing teeth: #11, #16, #26, #36 and #47
- Generalised alveolar bone loss, extremely advanced in #27

Radiological Examination
- Orthopantomogram undertaken (Figure 6.2.1)
- Tooth root remains in #26, #36 and #47
- Restorable caries in #22, #24 and #46
- Extensive and unrestorable caries in #25 and #27

Structured Learning

1) On oral examination, you note that the patient has marked halitosis, despite brushing his teeth up to 3 times a day. What could be causing this?
   - High salivary urea levels and decomposition of urea into ammonia increases halitosis in people with kidney disease
   - The patient may also be fatigued easily and hence fail to brush his teeth effectively
2) The patient informs you that he also has a metallic taste in his mouth which improves temporarily after a dialysis session. Is there a correlation?
   - Dysgeusia (abnormal taste) is common in those with CKD
   - It may contribute to a poor nutritional intake

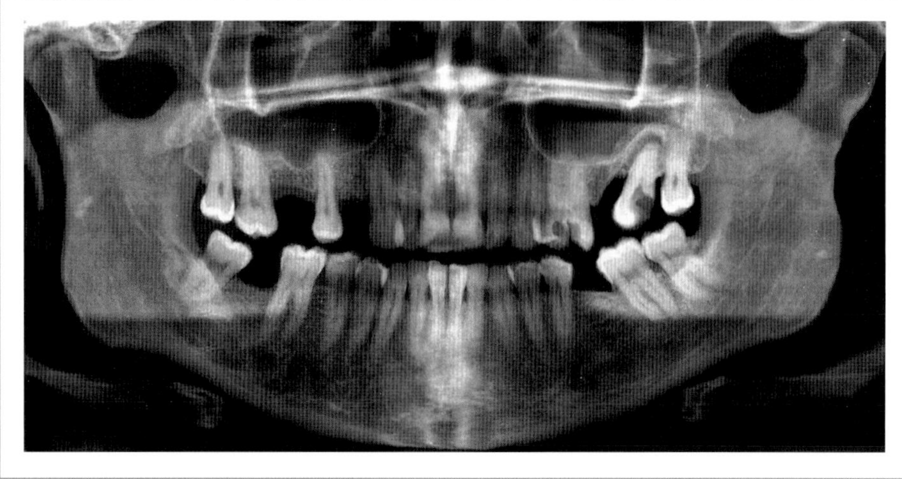

Figure 6.2.1 Orthopantomogram demonstrating multiple carious teeth, missing teeth and generalised alveolar bone loss.

- It has also been related to the urea content in the saliva and its subsequent breakdown to ammonia and carbon dioxide by bacterial urease
- Temporary improvement after dialysis has been reported
- Xerostomia may also contribute to altered taste perception

3) Is this patient's high level of dental decay also related to his CKD?
   - Patients with end-stage renal disease have not been found to have a higher risk of dental decay
   - Elevated salivary urea levels have been suggested as a mechanism that protects the tooth against demineralisation, which render the salivary pH alkaline, even after dialysis
   - This patient's high levels of dental decay are more [illegible] ineffective toothbrushing, fatigue and potentially xerostomia (restricted fluid intake)
4) The patient appears very tired and short of breath. What could be contributing to this?
   - CKD is associated with a reduced red blood cell count and anaemia due to:
     - Lack of erythropoietin, a growth factor predominantly produced in the kidneys that stimulates the production of red blood cells
     - Iron deficiency as a result of nutritional insufficiency or due to increased blood loss
     - Shortened red cell survival due to uraemia
   - CKD also increases the risk of cardiovascular disease due to:
     - Dyslipidaemia which occurs due to downregulation of lipoprotein lipase and the LDL receptor, and increased triglycerides due to delayed catabolism of triglyceride-rich lipoproteins; this can result in increasing arteriosclerosis
     - Diastolic ventricular dysfunction
5) The patient agrees to proceed with dental extractions of the retained roots and the teeth that are unrestorable. He is concerned that his jawbone may break during these, as he has been told by the renal physician that his bone is 'weak due to his renal disease'. What are the risks?
   - Mineral and bone disorder in CKD is common in patients receiving dialysis (e.g. osteoporosis and secondary hyperparathyroidism)
   - Patients have a high rate of vitamin D deficiency, exacerbated by the reduced ability to convert 25-(OH) vitamin D into the active form, 1,25-dihydroxy-vitamin D, by the kidneys
   - Hypocalcaemia arises as a result of phosphate retention and calcium loss in kidneys in chronic renal failure
   - This stimulates parathyroid hormone release and leads to secondary hyperparathyroidism and progressive bone loss, with calcium release from bone by increasing the osteoclastic activity
   - The earliest radiographic indication related to jawbones is the ground-glass appearance that emerges due to the replacement of bone tissue by connective tissue with cortical bone resorption, lamina dura and trabecular bone loss
   - Osteitis fibrosa cystica (brown tumour) may eventually result
   - Caution is advisable when undertaking extractions to avoid the risk of iatrogenic fractures

6) What factors are considered important in assessing the risk of managing this patient?
   - Social
     - Lives alone – no suitable carer/escort
     - Financial limitation
     - Dependent on hospital transport
   - Medical (related directly to CKD)
     - Anaemia and associated fatigue
     - Prone to bleeding
       - Predominantly due to abnormalities in primary haemostasis, particularly platelet function disorder and impairment of the platelet–wall interaction
       - Thrombocytopenia is detected in about 50% of patients undergoing haemodialysis
     - Increased susceptibility to infections due to:
       - Azotaemic state (high levels of nitrogen-rich compounds, such as urea and creatinine in the blood) altering innate immunity
       - Changes in the gastrointestinal microbiota suppress both innate and adaptive immunity
       - Immune responses may also be impaired by poor nutritional status, malnutrition and vitamin D deficiency
     - Arterial hypertension (see Chapter 6.1), a common and often poorly controlled finding, with sodium and volume excess as the prominent mechanism; it may also contribute to increased bleeding risk
     - Osteoporosis (see Chapter 7.1), another prevalent condition in haemodialysis patients due to low bone formation rates, even when bone resorption may be normal
     - Avoid prescription of drugs that are metabolised by the kidneys
   - Dental
     - Prone to oral infections and premature edentulism
     - No commitment to long-term care
     - The procedure should be scheduled the day after the dialysis session (patient often tired and avoids increased bleeding risk due to heparin given at the time of dialysis)

7) Due to the need to raise a flap and remove some bone to extract the remaining tooth roots, you decide to administer an antibiotic postoperatively. What regimen would you recommend without having to adjust the dose?
   - Administer clindamycin (300 mg/8 h) or azithromycin (500 mg/24 h)

8) When prescribing analgesics after surgery, what medications are contraindicated?
   - Ibuprofen and diclofenac are contraindicated for moderate and end-stage renal disease
   - Tramadol is also contraindicated for end-stage renal disease

General Dental Considerations

Oral Findings

- Oral findings in patients with CKD are determined by the severity of the disease and the type of replacement therapy
- In dialysed patients, the lesions are mainly the result of the renal dysfunction (Table 6.2.1; Figure 6.2.2)
- For patients with kidney transplants, the lesions are an expression of the immunosuppression and the secondary effects of the immunosuppressive drugs (see Chapter 12.3)

Dental Management

- These patients' dental treatment is determined by their general condition and overall prognosis (Table 6.2.2)
- The most relevant aspects for the dentist to consider are the tendency to bleed, immune system dysfunction and the selective prescription of drugs (Table 6.2.3)

Section II: Background Information and Guidelines

Definition

CKD is the loss of kidney function for longer than 3 months as a consequence of renal damage, which causes reduced glomerular filtration rates below 60 mL/min/1.73 m^2. If the disease progresses to renal failure or end-stage kidney disease (ESKD), replacement therapy with dialysis or transplantation is required. It is estimated that more than 10% of the adult population has some degree of CKD and that more than 2 million individuals worldwide have ESKD.

Aetiopathogenesis

- Although the aetiology of CKD varies by geographical area, the most common causes include:
  - Diabetes
  - Hypertension
  - Primary glomerulonephritis (immunologically based)
  - Tubulointerstitial nephritis (e.g. drug induced, infection induced and autoimmune)
  - Polycystic kidneys (e.g. hereditary) (Figure 6.2.3)
  - Secondary glomerulonephritis or vasculitis (e.g. drug induced, infection induced and due to systemic diseases)
  - Others (e.g. induced by metabolic disorders or neoplasia)
- The pathogenesis of CKD is characterised by progressive fibrosis and destruction of the renal architecture as a consequence of a sequential process

Table 6.2.1 Oral findings in patients with chronic kidney disease undergoing dialysis.

Gums and oral mucosa	• Pale oral mucosa (anaemia) • Lichenoid reactions (drug induced) • Uraemic stomatitis (grey pseudomembranes that cover painful erythematous macules and/or ulcers) • Petechiae/ecchymosis
Teeth	• Delayed eruption of permanent teeth • Enamel hypoplasia of temporary and permanent teeth (brown discoloration) • Low prevalence of caries • Tartar accumulation • Premature edentulism
Salivary glands	• Swelling of salivary glands • Hyposalivation (due to reduced fluid consumption, drug induced and/or mouth breathing)
Bone disorders due to secondary hyperparathyroidism	• Loss of lamina dura • Loss of cortical bone and trabeculation • Osteolytic lesions • Brown tumours (giant cell focal lesions that arise as a result of abnormal bone metabolism in patients with hyperparathyroidism) • Bone demineralisation (frosted glass appearance) • Bone regeneration jeopardised
Others	• Dysgeusia and/or metallic taste • Halitosis (uraemic fetor) • Paraesthesia of the tongue and lips

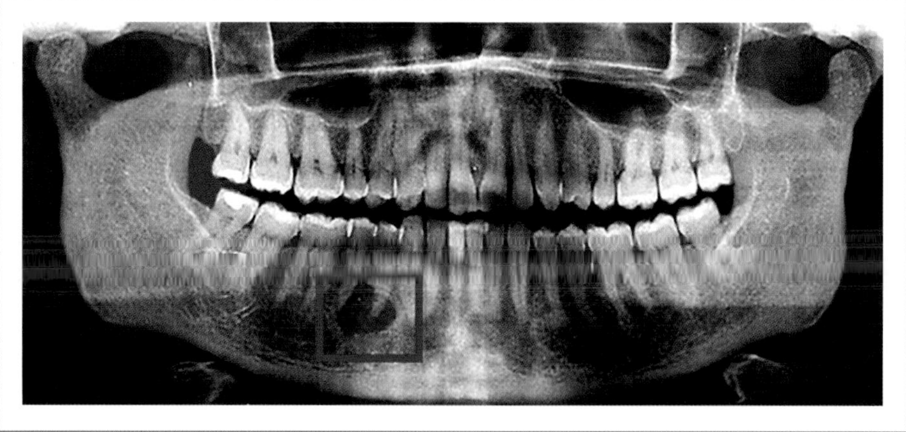

Figure 6.2.2 Brown tumour associated with secondary hyperparathyroidism in a patient with chronic renal failure.

- Infiltration of the diseased kidneys by extrinsic inflammatory cells
- Activation, proliferation and loss (necrosis) of intrinsic renal cells
- Activation and proliferation of extracellular matrix-producing cells (e.g. fibroblasts)
- Replacement of the renal architecture by extracellular matrix deposits

Clinical Presentation

- The clinical manifestations of CKD affect numerous organs and systems but generally do not appear until advanced stages of the disease due to the compensatory activity of the remaining nephrons (Table 6.2.4)
- Common signs/symptoms include fatigue, swollen ankles, feet or hands, shortness of breath, nausea

Table 6.2.2 Considerations for dental management.

Risk assessment	• Tendency to bleed due to thrombocytopenia, platelet dysfunction, increased prostaglandin I levels, factor III deficiency, von Willebrand factor deficiency or anticoagulants (heparin) • Increased risk of arterial hypertension • Increased susceptibility to infections by impaired phagocytic activity, reduced cytokine production and immunosuppressive drugs • Increased risk of demineralisation and bone disorder • Presence of concomitant diseases (mainly diabetes and hypertension) • High prevalence of HCV and HBV infection among patients undergoing haemodialysis in low-income countries
Criteria for referral	• Dental treatment should be conducted in a hospital setting in the following circumstances: • Deteriorated general condition and/or poor vital prognosis (patients who regularly attend dialysis are already classified as ASA III) • Tendency to bleed and/or severe immunosuppression • Significant comorbidities (e.g. pulmonary hypertension)
Access/position	• Determine the regular days when the patient attends for dialysis and preferably schedule dental treatment for the day after (patients are more tired on the day of dialysis; often heparin is administered to prevent clotting during dialysis, increasing bleeding risk) • If an emergency dental treatment needs to be performed on a patient who has taken heparin, protamine sulfate may be administered intravenously (medical consultation should be sought) • Protect the arm with the vascular access (do not use for measuring blood pressure) • Adjust the dental chair's position for patients with continuous ambulatory peritoneal dialysis
Communication	• Patients on haemodialysis frequently experience anxiety and depression; this needs to be taken into consideration during discussions • Direct channels of communication need to be established between the dentist and medical team (e.g. to schedule appointments)
Consent/capacity	• Patients need to be warned of the potential complications resulting from end-stage chronic renal failure, which can require: – Implementation of protocols to prevent bleeding and infection – Prescription of drugs that are not metabolised by the kidneys
Anaesthesia/sedation	• Local anaesthesia – Lidocaine and mepivacaine are preferred – Prilocaine and articaine should be avoided because they are preferentially metabolised in the kidneys – The use of anaesthetics with epinephrine may be determined by the blood pressure levels (arterial hypertension) • Sedation – Nitrous oxide or intravenous midazolam may be used – Do not use the arm with the vascular access for intravenous sedation • General anaesthesia – Contraindicated if the patient has severe anaemia (Hb <10 g/dL) – Avoid the use of halothane (myocardial depression); isoflurane or sevoflurane are preferable

(Continued)

Table 6.2.2 (Continued)

Dental treatment	• Before – Ensure the patient has attended for scheduled dialysis the day before treatment – Verify the bleeding tendency before performing invasive dental procedures/surgery (platelet count, bleeding time, prothrombin time/INR and activated partial thromboplastin time) – In refractory cases, consult the physician to determine what haematological support is required (e.g. transfusions of platelets, cryoprecipitates, conjugated oestrogens) – Desmopressin acetate administered nasally (3 μg/kg) provides haemostasis for 4 hours – Assess the administration of antibiotics before invasive dental procedures (although not supported by scientific evidence, the prophylaxis regimen for bacterial endocarditis may be administered) • During – Apply local haemostasis measures – Narrowing and calcification of the pulp canals can hinder the endodontic treatment – The orthodontics is determined by tooth mobility • After – If surgical procedures are to be performed, bone regeneration can be compromised (alveolar sclerosis following a dental extraction) – The success rate of implants can decrease due to bone demineralisation
Drug prescription	• Patients with chronic kidney disease have abnormal metabolism and elimination of drugs excreted renally (Table 6.2.3)
Education/prevention	• Comprehensive oral hygiene can help reduce dental calculus deposits • Periodic oral health check-ups are recommended to eliminate any focus of infection early • It has been suggested that dental treatment can help protect the vascular access of haemodialysis and improve the prognosis of kidney transplantation • Reinforce healthy attitudes (e.g. regarding nutrition and hydration) in the dental clinic

Diagnosis

- Measurement of the glomerular filtration rate (Table 6.2.5)
- Quantification of the albumin–creatinine ratio
- Imaging tests
  - Ultrasonography
  - Doppler ultrasound
  - Computed tomography
  - Magnetic resonance imaging
  - Angiography
  - Voiding cystourethrography
  - Scintigraphy (e.g. dimercaptosuccinic acid)
  - Kidney biopsy

Management

- General regimens
  - Treat the cause/underlying disease (e.g. can affect recurrence after transplantation)
  - Psychological support (incapacitating disease)
  - Nutritional counselling (protein supply control)
  - Drug treatment (to control hypertension, proteinuria and blood glucose levels in patients with diabetes)
  - Bicarbonate supplementation to treat chronic metabolic acidosis
  - Promote smoking cessation

Table 6.2.3 Prescription of drugs for patients with chronic kidney disease.

	Type of drug	Recommendation for moderate chronic kidney disease (G3, G4)	Recommendation for end-stage kidney disease (G5)
Antibiotics	Penicillin V	Reduce dosage (250–500 mg/8 h)	Reduce dosage (250–500 mg/12 h)
	Amoxicillin	Reduce dosage (500 mg/12 h)	Reduce dosage (500 mg/24 h)
	Amoxicillin/clavulanic acid	Reduce dosage (500 + 125 mg/12 h)	Reduce dosage (500 + 125 mg/24 h)
	Clindamycin	No dosage adjustment required	No dosage adjustment required
	Metronidazole	No dosage adjustment required	Reduce dosage (250 mg/8 h)
	Azithromycin	No dosage adjustment required	No dosage adjustment required
	Clarithromycin	Reduce dosage (250 mg/12 h)	Reduce dosage (250 mg/12 h)
Analgesics	Paracetamol	Reduce dosage (500 mg/8 h)	Reduce dosage (500 mg/12 h)
	Metamizole	No dosage adjustment required	No dosage adjustment required
	Ibuprofen	Contraindicated	Contraindicated
	Diclofenac	Contraindicated	Contraindicated
	Naproxen	No dosage adjustment required	No dosage adjustment required
	Codeine	Reduce dosage (20 mg/6 h)	Reduce dosage (15 mg/6 h)
	Tramadol	Reduce dosage (50–100 mg/12 h)	Contraindicated
Corticosteroids		No dosage adjustment required	No dosage adjustment required
Sedatives	Hydroxyzine	Single dose the night before	Single dose the night before
	Diphenhydramine	Contraindicated	Contraindicated
	Diazepam	Reduce dosage (2.5 mg)[a]	Reduce dosage (2.5 mg)[a]
	Midazolam	Reduce dosage (7.5 mg)[b]	Reduce dosage (7.5 mg)[b]
	Lorazepam	No dosage adjustment required	No dosage adjustment required
	Alprazolam	No dosage adjustment required	No dosage adjustment required

[a] 2 hours before the procedure.
[b] 1 hour before the procedure.

- Haemodialysis
  - Technique in which the patient's blood is taken from a vascular access and fed through an extracorporeal circuit through a filter (dialyser), and once dialysed, reintroduced to the bloodstream using a pump system (Figure 6.2.4)
  - Vascular access is placed on the non-dominant arm through a native arteriovenous fistula, arteriovenous graft or central venous catheter
  - Most patients undergo haemodialysis sessions lasting approximately 4 hours, 2–3 times a week
- Peritoneal dialysis (continuous or intermittent)
  - Technique to filter harmful substances present in the blood through a natural semi-permeable membrane through diffusion (peritoneum), accessed through a catheter; dialysis fluid is poured directly into the abdominal cavity
  - Continuous ambulatory peritoneal dialysis requires 4 cycles of approximately 2 L over the course of the day. In automated peritoneal dialysis, the exchange of dialysis fluid is controlled by an automatic cycler while the patient is asleep (8–10 hours)

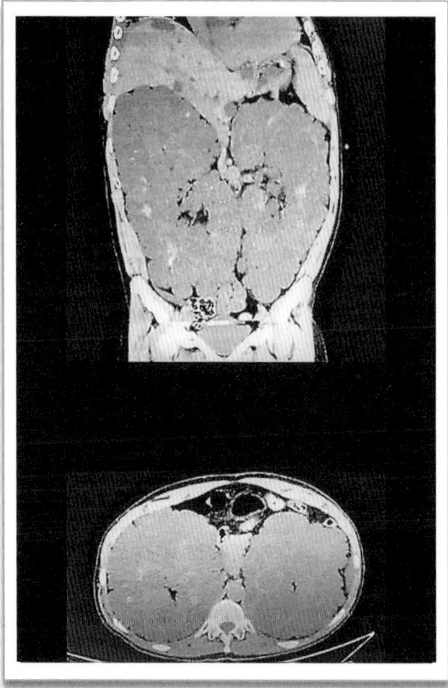

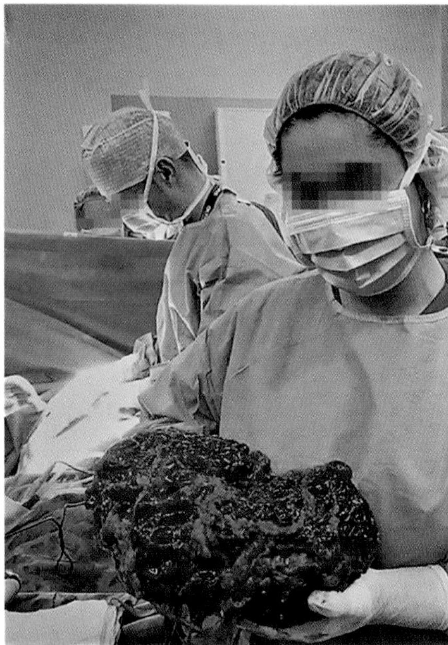

Figure 6.2.3 Autosomal-dominant polycystic kidney disease (ADPKD) may lead to end-stage renal disease usually requiring dialysis and finally removal and renal transplantation.

- Kidney transplantation (living donor or cadaver)
  - The treatment of choice for ESKD, given its superior long-term results (compared with dialysis) for survival and quality of life
  - Estimated graft survival is 90% for the first year and 70% at 5 years
  - Patients who have undergone transplantation require lifelong immunosuppressive therapy to prevent organ rejection (see Chapter 12.3)

Prognosis

- The prognosis is determined by the patient's age, underlying disease severity and onset of complications (e.g. cardiovascular disorders and septicaemia)
- The number of hospitalisations for patients with CKD is threefold higher than for the general population
- The annual mortality rate for patients who undergo haemodialysis is approximately 10%

A World/Transcultural View

- In the US, racial-ethnic minorities have disproportionately high rates of ESKD but are much less likely to undergo kidney transplantation than whites. The identified barriers include a lack of understanding of the benefits of transplantation and concern about the risks that surgery entails
- The survival of patients who undergo haemodialysis is higher in a number of Asian countries, such as Japan, than in any other part of the world. It is also higher in Europe than in the US (these findings have been related to vascular access and the duration and rate of haemodialysis sessions)
- Cultural antecedents can affect the adoption of chronic haemodialysis therapy. The health-related quality of life of patients who undergo haemodialysis varies according to ethnicity

Table 6.2.4 Clinical characteristics of chronic kidney disease.

Skin	Nervous system	Digestive system	Haematological system	Cardio-respiratory system	Osteoarticular system	Endocrine system
Pallor Ecchymosis Haematomas Pruritus Dry skin Waxy colour	Insomnia Tremors Restless legs Paralysis Weakness Headaches Depression Anxiety Cognitive impairment	Anorexia Nausea Vomiting Haemorrhaging Pyrosis Constipation Uraemic fetor Dysgeusia	Anaemia Thrombocytopenia Iron deficiency Vitamin B12 deficiency Dyslipidaemia	Dyspnoea Oedema Arterial hypertension Precordial pain Pericarditis Peripheral arterial ischaemia Arteriosclerosis	Osteodystrophy Calcifications Growth disorders Pathological fractures	Amenorrhoea Sterility Miscarriage Impotence Glucose intolerance Hypoglycaemia

Table 6.2.5 Classification of chronic kidney disease.

Glomerular filtration rate (GFR)	Albumin/creatinine ratio (ACR)
G1: GFR ≥90 mL/min per 1.73 m^2	**A1**: ACR <30 mg/g (<3.4 mg/mmol)
G2: GFR 60–89 mL/min per 1.73 m^2	**A2**: ACR 30–299 mg/g (3.4–34 mg/mmol)
G3a: GFR 45–59 mL/min per 1.73 m^2	**A3**: ACR >300 mg/g (>34 mg/mmol)
G3b: GFR 30–44 mL/min per 1.73 m^2	
G4: GFR 15–29 mL/min per 1.73 m^2	
G5: GFR <15 mL/min per 1.73 m^2 or dialysis	

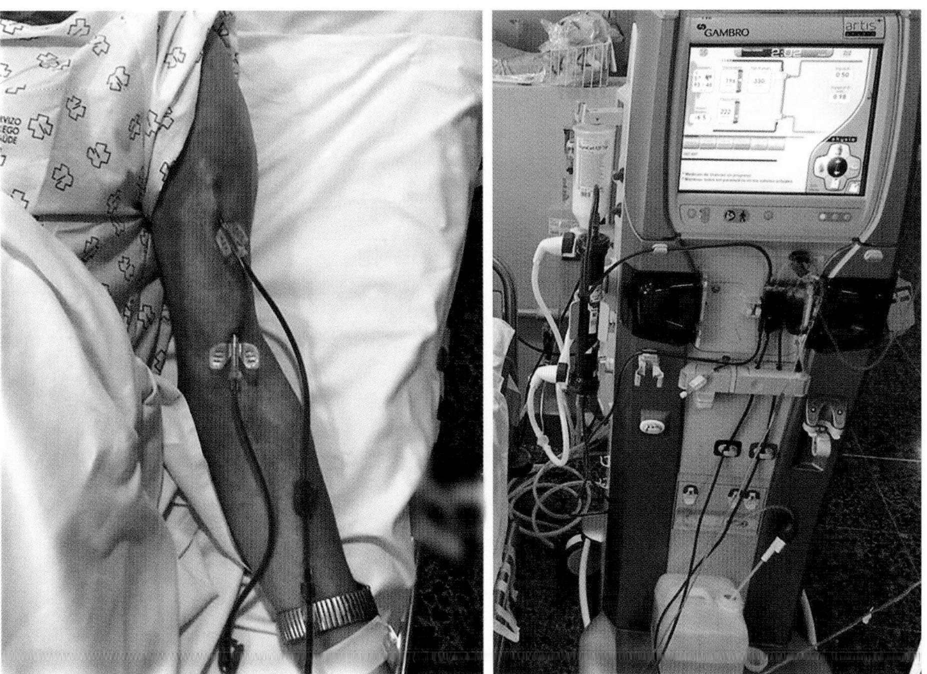

Figure 6.2.4 A haemodialysis system including a blood circuit (with the vascular access), a dialysate circuit and the dialyser.

Recommended Reading

Altamimi, A.G., AlBakr, S.A., Alanazi, T.A. et al. (2018). Prevalence of periodontitis in patients undergoing hemodialysis: a case control study. *Mater. Sociomed.* 30: 58–61.

Brockmann, W. and Badr, M. (2010). Chronic kidney disease: pharmacological considerations for the dentist. *J. Am. Dent. Assoc.* 141: 1330–1339.

King, E. (2013). Dental management of patients in end stage renal failure on dialysis. *J. Mich. Dent. Assoc.* 95: 42–45.

Limeres, J., Garcez, J.F., Marinho, J.S. et al. (2016). Early tooth loss in end-stage renal disease patients on haemodialysis. *Oral Dis.* 22: 530–535.

Proctor, R., Kumar, N., Stein, A. et al. (2005). Oral and dental aspects of chronic renal failure. *J. Dent. Res.* 84: 199–208.

Schmalz, G., Schiffers, N., Schwabe, S. et al. (2017). Dental and periodontal health, and microbiological and salivary conditions in patients with or without diabetes undergoing haemodialysis. *Int. Dent. J.* 67: 186–193.

Sharma, L., Pradhan, D., Srivastava, R. et al. (2020). Assessment of oral health status and inflammatory markers in end stage chronic kidney disease patients: a cross-sectional study. *J. Family Med. Prim. Care* 9: 2264–2268.

Vaidya, S.R. and Aeddula, N.R. (2020). Chronic renal failure. www.statpearls.com/

7

Bone Diseases

7.1 Osteoporosis

Section I: Clinical Scenario and Dental Considerations

Clinical Scenario

A 68-year-old woman presents for an emergency dental appointment complaining of pain and mild swelling in the upper left quadrant. Her symptoms commenced 48 hours earlier and the pain is exacerbated by eating/pressure in the area, but not affected by cold/heat. Sleep is not disturbed.

Medical History
- Osteoporosis, diagnosed 10 years ago
- Well-controlled hypertension
- Dyslipidaemia

Medications
- Risedronate (for the last 6 years)
- Vitamin D
- Calcium
- Chondroitin sulfate
- Enalapril/lercanidipine
- Simvastatin

Dental History
- Good level of co-operation
- However, does not attend for regular dental reviews due to the cost
- In the last 4 years she has only visited the dentist when in pain
- Brushes her teeth irregularly (brushing the molars causes the patient discomfort)

Social History
- Lives with her partner and has good family support
- Can travel independently using public transport
- Retired with limited financial resources
- Nil tobacco consumption; minimal alcohol consumption

Oral Examination
- Poor oral hygiene
- Generalised periodontal disease
- Abscess related to retained roots of #27
- Caries in #34, #44 and #48
- Missing teeth: #15, #16, #24, #25, #26 # and #36

Radiological Examination
- Orthopantomogram undertaken (Figure 7.1.1)
- Generalised alveolar bone loss
- Retained roots of #16, #18 and #27
- Radicular fracture of tooth #28
- Obliteration of the pulpal chambers

Structured Learning

1) What bone changes in this patient's orthopantomogram may be associated with osteoporosis/risedronate treatment?
    - The trabecular bone of the maxilla and mandible has a granular appearance
    - Generalised loss of alveolar bone (periodontal disease also a cause)
    - Paradoxically, the mandibular cortical bone is wider than expected, possibly the result of administering antiresorptive agents
2) You also note that the pulpal chambers appear to be obliterated. Is this likely to be related to the osteoporosis?
    - No, not related directly to the osteoporosis
    - The patient is taking calcium supplements – it has been suggested that pulp obliteration is more common in patients with hypercalcaemia
    - It may be advisable to liaise with the patient's medical practitioner to review her serum calcium level
3) You determine that the retained roots of #27 are the cause of her present discomfort and require extraction. The patient agrees to this but refuses all other treatment as she is worried about the cost. Why is she at particular risk if the rest of the teeth are left untreated?

A Practical Approach to Special Care in Dentistry, First Edition. Edited by Pedro Diz Dios and Navdeep Kumar.

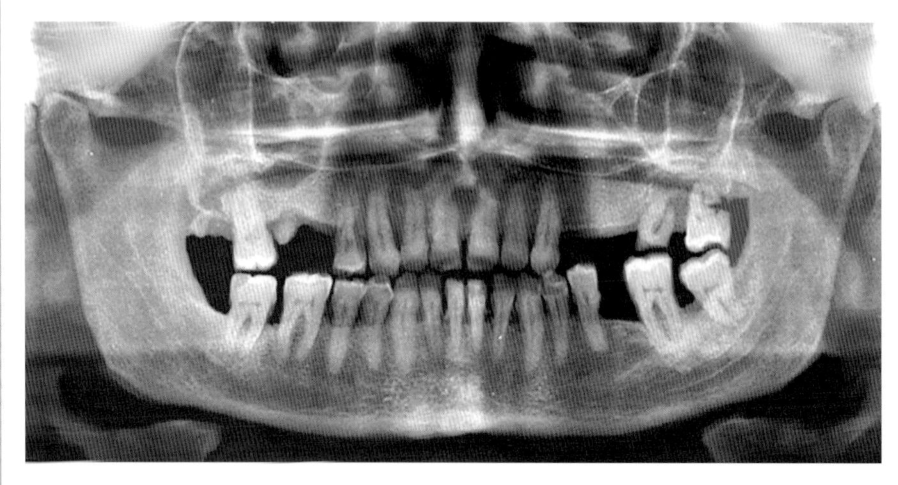

Figure 7.1.1 Orthopantomogram findings suggestive of osteoporosis as well as the effects of risedronate treatment.

- Timely and regular intervention coupled with preventive advice is essential to avoid the risk of further tooth loss and hence reduce the risk of developing medication-related osteonecrosis of the jaw (MRONJ) associated with risedronate
- The #16 and #18 retained roots, as well as #28, may also become symptomatic and require removal
- She has further caries and periodontal disease; left untreated, the prognosis of these teeth will worsen, resulting in further dental extractions

4) What risk factors does this patient have for developing MRONJ? (see Chapter 16.2)
   - Related to the antiresorptive drug: although risedronate is a relatively low-potency antiresorptive drug, the patient has been taking it for an extended time (>4 years)
   - Related to local factors: the patient has an infectious process in relation to #27, periodontal disease and invasive dental procedures need to be performed
5) What factors are considered important in assessing the risk of managing this patient?
   - Social
     - Lack of motivation (only visits the dentist for acute episodes of dental discomfort)
     - Acceptable treatment plan for the patient is determined by her limited financial resources
   - Medical
     - Risk of MRONJ related to the prolonged use of risedronate (see Chapter 16.2)
     - Potential increased bleeding tendency and risk of hypertensive crisis due to high blood pressure (see Chapter 8.1)
     - Drug interactions with antihypertensive drugs and hypolipidaemic agents
   - Dental
     - Poor oral health and motivation to keep the teeth/gums healthy (brushes her teeth irregularly)
     - Requires urgent treatment of dental abscess and the elimination of its cause (#27)
     - Risk of delayed alveolar bone healing
     - Risk of MRONJ
     - Prone to periodontal disease and premature edentulism
     - If a rehabilitation with removable prosthesis is performed (limited financial resources), alveolar ridge resorption may result in an increased risk of movement/trauma from the denture, which in turn increases the risk of MRONJ
6) You decide to prescribe a course of antibiotics and painkillers in view of the acute pain/swelling associated with the roots of #27. What potential drug interactions will determine which drugs you select?
   - Non-steroidal anti-inflammatory drugs, including selective COX-2 inhibitors, attenuate the effect of some antihypertensives such as angiotensin-converting enzyme inhibitors (e.g. enalapril)
   - Macrolide antibiotics interfere with the metabolism of simvastatin, increasing the risk of rhabdomyolysis and hepatotoxicity
7) The patient returns a week later to have #27 removed. She asks if you can remove #16 and #18 at the same visit as she stopped taking risedronate after your explanation regarding the risk of MRONJ. What would you advise her?

- Stopping the drug (drug holidays) does not eliminate the risk of developing MRONJ associated with dental care
- The incidence of MRONJ after tooth extraction is estimated to be ~0.15% in patients being treated for osteoporosis
- The benefits of taking the risedronate to manage the patient's osteoporosis outweigh the small risk of developing MRONJ
- The extractions of the retained roots of #16 and #18 should be planned when healing of the surgical site of #27 has been completed

General Dental Considerations

Oral Findings

- Possible radiographic changes
  - Jawbone may appear thinned and granular (Figure 7.1.2)
  - Thin lamina dura
  - Maxillary sinus may extend between the roots of molars
  - Mandibular cortical bone width may be narrowed/eroded; observed changes on an orthopantomogram have been suggested as useful for the detection/monitoring progression of osteoporosis (Table 7.1.1)
- Potential link between osteoporosis and loss of alveolar bone, increased tooth mobility and tooth loss
- Possible association with periodontal disease (results are inconclusive)

Table 7.1.1 Classification of mandibular cortical bone in assessment of osteoporosis.

Stage	Designation	Radiological findings
C1	Normal cortex	The endosteal cortical margin is even and sharp on both sides
C2	Mild to moderate cortex erosion	The endosteal margin has semi-lunar defects (lacunar resorption) or endosteal cortical residues on one or both sides
C3	Severe cortex erosion	The cortical layer forms heavy endosteal cortical residues and is clearly porous

Source: Modified from Klemetti, E., Kolmakov, S., and Kröger, H. (1994). Pantomography in assessment of the osteoporosis risk group. *Scand. J. Dent. Res.* 102: 68–72.

- Patients may be taking antiresorptive agents and hence have an associated risk of MRONJ (see Chapter 16.2)

Dental Management

- The dental treatment will be determined by the patient's oral health status, the history of antiresorptive or antiangiogenic drugs and the presence of comorbidities (e.g. osteoporosis secondary to chronic liver disease) (Table 7.1.2)

Section II: Background Information and Guidelines

Definition

Osteoporosis is a systemic skeletal disease characterised by reduced mineralised bone mass and microarchitectural

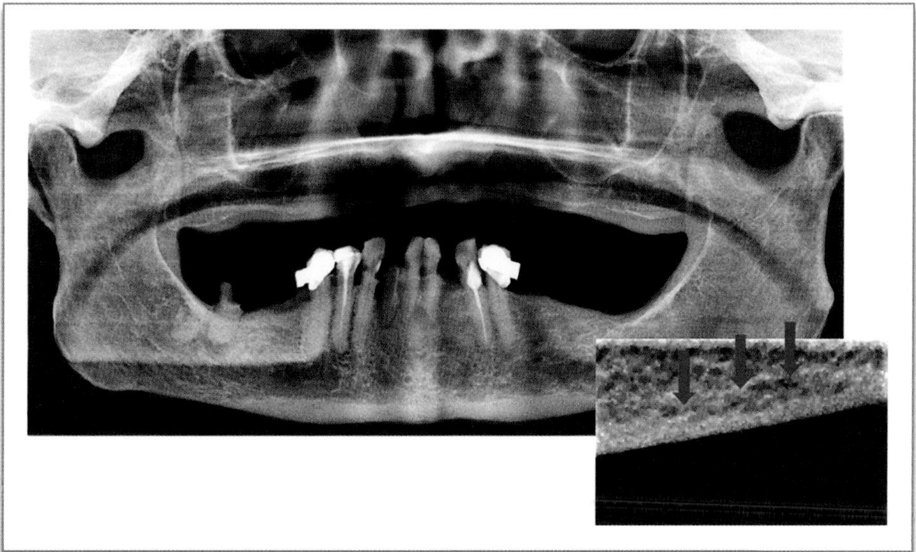

Figure 7.1.2 Granular jawbone and severe cortex erosion in a female patient with osteoporosis.

Table 7.1.2 Considerations for dental management.

Risk assessment	• The dental management of patients taking antiresorptive drugs can trigger medication-related osteonecrosis of the jaw (see Chapter 16.2) • In cases of severe osteoporosis and advanced bone atrophy, a surgical procedure such as insertion of dental implants can cause a mandibular fracture
Criteria for referral	• A medical consultation should be undertaken if the patient has a very high risk of fracture or significant sequelae from previous fractures • If the osteoporosis is secondary to a disease such as diabetes or chronic liver disease, the degree of control over the systemic disease can constitute an indication for dental treatment in a hospital setting
Access/position	• Patients with advanced osteoporosis might have reduced mobility and require assistance/an escort • For patients with a very high risk of fracture or significant sequelae from previous fractures, there can be difficulties positioning the patient in the chair, and fractures can occur during the transfer • Care should be taken to provide adequate neck support
Consent/capacity	• For patients who underwent therapy with antiresorptive agents, the consent form should explicitly reflect the risk of the onset of medication-related osteonecrosis of the jaw (see Chapter 16.2) • Patients should be informed that their osteoporosis can determine the result of certain procedures (e.g. fitting of mucosa-supported dental prosthesis)
Anaesthesia/sedation	• Local anaesthesia – Resorption may result in change in the anatomical landmarks when giving block injections • Sedation – Any sedation technique can be administered • General anaesthesia – General anaesthesia can be associated with increased risk if there is vertebral collapse or chest deformity
Dental treatment	• Before – Specifically ask about the use of antiresorptive and antiangiogenic agents (both current and in the past) – A radiographic evaluation of the remaining bone is always recommended – There is no evidence to suggest that osteoporosis is a contraindication for dental implants – It has been suggested that patients with osteoporosis might not be a suitable risk group for sinus lifts • During – Careful positioning of the patient in the dental chair – Resorption of the alveolar ridge might result in poorly fitting dentures – These patients might require more frequent denture reviews and remakes • After – Delayed alveolar bone healing is not uncommon following tooth extraction – Longer healing times for dental implants may occur
Drug prescription	• Calcium supplements inactivate tetracycline
Education/prevention	• A risk factor analysis (including the use of antiresorptive medication) and patient counselling should be undertaken • Regular dental visits and a healthy lifestyle (e.g. smoking cessation) are necessary to maintain good bone health • Periodontitis and tooth loss after menopause can be useful indicators of bone mineral loss in older women

deterioration of bone tissue, with an increased susceptibility to fractures. It is especially common in older women and is estimated to affect 200 million women worldwide (approximately 10% of women aged 60, 20% of women aged 70, 40% of women aged 80 and 65% of women aged 90).

Aetiopathogenesis

- Metabolic bone disease resulting from an imbalance in osteoblastic and osteoclastic activities
- Primary osteoporosis is caused by androgen-oestrogen deficiency, lack of vitamin D and lack of exercise
- Secondary osteoporosis is caused by corticosteroid use, hyperparathyroidism, diabetes, chronic liver disease, malabsorption or hyperthyroidism
- Key risk factors include genetics, lack of exercise, lack of calcium and vitamin D, personal history of fracture as an adult, cigarette smoking, excessive alcohol consumption, history of rheumatoid arthritis, low body weight and family history of osteoporosis

Clinical Presentation

- No symptoms until bone fractures occur
- Eventually, vertebral crush fractures or femoral neck fractures may occur, resulting in persistent lower back pain, kyphosis and loss of height (Figure 7.1.3)

Diagnosis

- Assessment of bone mineral density (BMD) with dual-energy x-ray absorptiometry (DXA) (Figure 7.1.4)
- Using standard deviation (SD) scores of BMD (related to peak bone mass of healthy young women), osteoporosis is defined as a femoral neck T-score of −2.5 SD or less and osteopenia as a femoral neck T-score between −1 and −2.5 SD
- Additional investigations
  - Blood count, sedimentation rate and C-reactive protein
  - Serum calcium, phosphate, alkaline phosphatase, liver transaminases and creatinine
  - Serum 25-hydroxyvitamin D
  - Thyroid function tests

Management

- Lifestyle measures
  - Proper diet and a programme of weight-bearing exercise
  - Vitamin D and calcium supplements
  - Pharmacological interventions
- Antiresorptive agents to reduce bone resorption leading to an increase in BMD, including oestrogens, selective oestrogen receptor modulators, bisphosphonates and the human monoclonal antibody to receptor activator of NFκB ligand (RANKL)
- Anabolic drugs to promote anabolic skeletal effects through changes in bone remodelling and/or bone modelling; these drugs include the parathyroid hormone receptor agonists teriparatide and abaloparatide

Prognosis

- Almost 3 million hip fractures occur every year worldwide, of which 50% could potentially be preventable if osteoporosis could be prevented

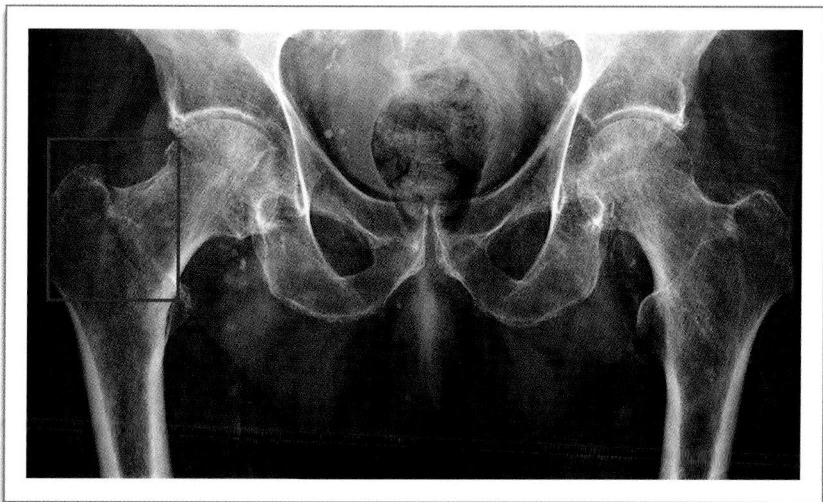

Figure 7.1.3 Right-sided femoral neck fracture (most are due to osteoporosis).

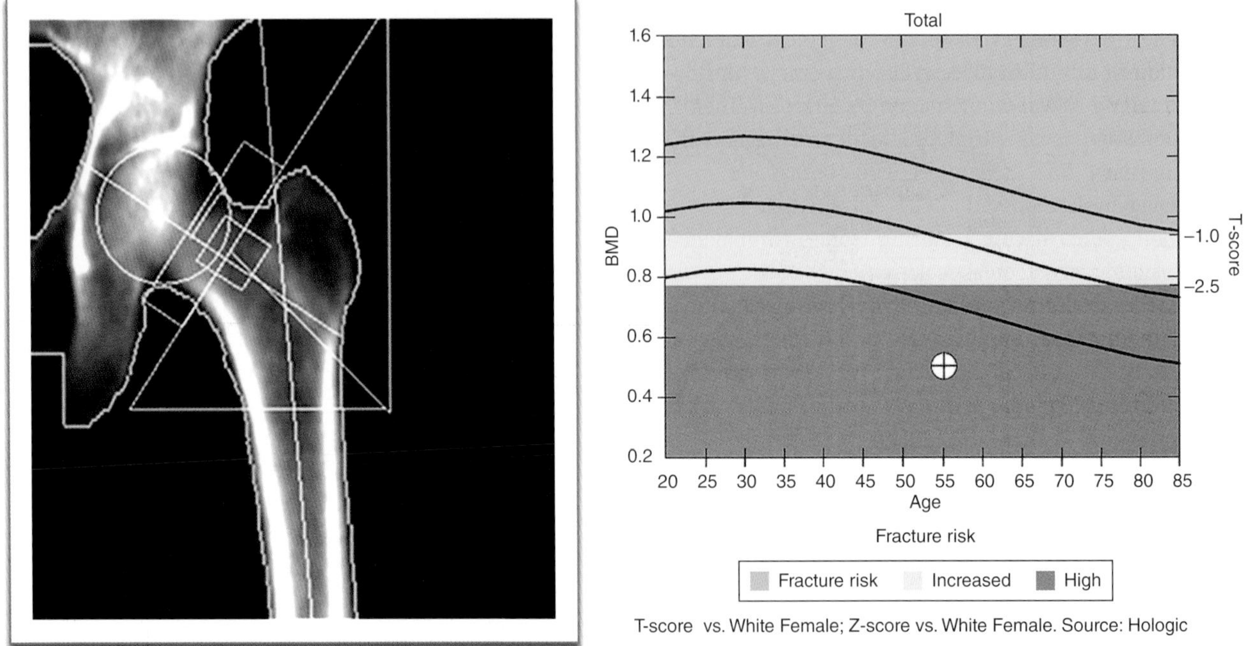

Figure 7.1.4 The gold-standard method to assess bone mineral density (BMD) is dual-energy x-ray absorptiometry (DXA).

- Fractures can cause chronic pain and disability (20–50% of patients with hip fracture require long-term nursing home care)
- Hip fractures are associated with 15–20% increased mortality rate within 1 year (mainly in men) and with a 2.5-fold increased risk of future fractures

A World/Transcultural View

- In the European Union, an osteoporotic fracture is diagnosed on average every 30 seconds; however, BMD measurement is an underused technique in most European countries
- Mortality rates following hip fracture are 2–3-fold higher for populations in the Middle East and Africa than those reported for Western populations
- It is estimated that by 2050, more than 50% of osteoporotic hip fractures worldwide will occur in Asia. Osteoporosis is underdiagnosed and therefore often untreated in Asia, especially in rural areas, where most of the population of countries such as China or India live
- It has been suggested that in Japan, almost all elderly women who visit a dental clinic have osteoporosis

Recommended Reading

Bandela, V., Munagapati, B., Karnati, R.K. et al. (2015). Osteoporosis: its prosthodontic considerations – a review. *J. Clin. Diagn. Res.* 9: ZE01–ZE04.

Black, D.M. and Rosen, C.J. (2016). Postmenopausal osteoporosis. *N. Engl. J. Med.* 374: 2096–2097.

Compston, J.E., McClung, M.R., and Leslie, W.D. (2019). Osteoporosis. *Lancet* 393: 364–376.

Ji, S., Tak, Y.J., Han, D.H. et al. (2016). Low bone mineral density is associated with tooth loss in postmenopausal women: a nationwide representative study in Korea. *J. Womens Health* 25: 1159–1165.

Mattson, J.S., Cerutis, D.R., and Parrish, L.C. (2002). Osteoporosis: a review and its dental implications. *Compend. Contin. Educ. Dent.* 23: 1001–1004.

McCauley, L.K. (2020). Clinical recommendations for prevention of secondary fractures in patients with osteoporosis: implications for dental care. *J. Am. Dent. Assoc.* 151: 311–313.

Mulligan, R. and Sobel, S. (2005). Osteoporosis: diagnostic testing, interpretation, and correlations with oral health – implications for dentistry. *Dent. Clin. North Am.* 49: 463–484.

Otomo-Corgel, J. (2012). Osteoporosis and osteopenia: implications for periodontal and implant therapy. *Periodontol 2000* 59: 111–139.

7.2 Paget Disease

Section I: Clinical Scenario and Dental Considerations

Clinical Scenario

A 60-year-old man is referred to you for an urgent assessment by his medical practitioner. The doctor was examining the patient's throat at the homeless shelter, when he coincidentally noticed a large swelling in the upper left quadrant of the mouth which he is worried may be caused by a cancer. The patient is not aware of the area and has no associated symptoms.

Medical History
- Paget disease of the bone diagnosed 5 years ago; coincidental finding after skull radiographs were taken in hospital after he was hit on the road by a car
- Reports frequent intense headaches have developed over the last 6 months
- Recent hearing loss

Medications
- Initially prescribed alendronate 5 years ago; received a supply for 6 months but has not been able to get repeat prescriptions since then (does not access healthcare due to cost and homelessness)

Dental History
- Does not attend for regular dental reviews due to the cost
- Limited level of co-operation
- Brushes his teeth twice daily with water when he can
- Currently using a toothbrush he was given at the homeless shelter (previous toothbrush 6 months old)

Social History
- Single; lives alone, no children, no close family
- Unemployed and currently residing in a homeless shelter (long-term history of homelessness)
- No financial resources
- Walked to his appointment as could not afford public transport
- Irregular tobacco or alcohol consumption (depending on whether he is given money)

Oral Examination
- Poor oral hygiene with generalised calculus deposits posteriorly
- Largely dentate
- Declines detailed examination of the other areas of his mouth
- Firm/hard expansion of the maxillary bone in the upper left quadrant; warm on palpation (Figure 7.2.1)
- No associated ulceration, induration or mobility of the teeth

Radiological Examination
Declined radiographs as he is worried about the cost

Structured Learning

1) What would you include in your differential diagnosis for the maxillary enlargement in the upper left quadrant?

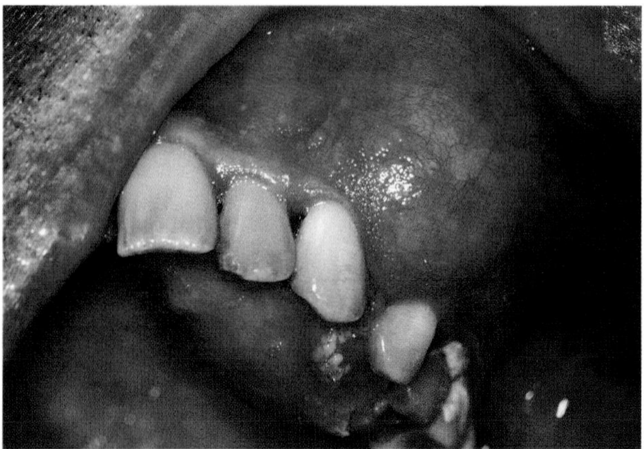

Figure 7.2.1 Enlargement of the left maxillary area.

A Practical Approach to Special Care in Dentistry, First Edition. Edited by Pedro Diz Dios and Navdeep Kumar.

- Paget disease of the bone
- Fibrous dysplasia
- Osteoma
- Osteosarcoma (occurs in less than 1% of patients with Paget disease)

2) There do not appear to be any signs of infection. Why does the area of maxillary enlargement feel warm to the touch?
   - Paget disease is associated with increased vascularity when bone turnover is high
3) How may the patient's recent symptoms of headaches and loss of hearing be related to his Paget disease?
   - Neurological complications occur in the majority of patients over the course of the disease
   - Mechanical compression or reduced blood flow of neural tissue may result in these symptoms
   - This patient has radiologically confirmed skull involvement of Paget disease, and hence neurological symptoms are more likely
   - Cranial involvement is hence likely and may lead to various types of headache, hearing loss or other cranial nerves deficits, hyperaemia of skull and basilar invagination and its consequences
4) You explain to the patient that you need to investigate further and undertake an orthopantomogram. What features on an orthopantomogram would be suggestive of Paget disease?
   - Cotton wool appearance of the bone caused by irregular areas of focal osteosclerosis
   - Loss of lamina dura, hypercementosis, resorption, replacement of tooth roots by bone
5) What factors are considered important in assessing the risk of managing this patient?
   - Social
     - Homeless – no fixed address or contact details
     - Lack of financial resources has led to lack of access to regular healthcare (medical and dental)
     - No family/next of kin/escort
   - Medical
     - Paget disease has been untreated and unmonitored for ~5 years
     - Recent development of headaches/hearing loss
     - Malnutrition may be present due to the lack of financial resources
   - Dental
     - Unable to regularly access facilities and oral healthcare aids which allow him to brush his teeth
     - History of bisphosphonate use associated with the risk of medication-related osteonecrosis of the jaw (MRONJ) (see Chapter 16.2)
6) The patient asks if you can biopsy the area on same day. How would you respond?
   - Oral cancer is not your primary diagnosis
   - Consultation with a physician is required
   - Further bone scans and blood tests are advisable (e.g. serum alkaline phosphatase levels)
   - A bone biopsy may not be required if the investigations confirm that Paget disease is the likely cause of the maxillary enlargement
   - If an incisional biopsy of the region is still considered necessary, it should be undertaken in a hospital setting as there is increased risk due to:
     - Hypervascularity and hence risk of increased bleeding
     - Risk of MRONJ (see Chapter 16.2)
     - Increased susceptibility to postoperative infection, delayed healing and localised osteitis may occur
     - Increased risk of long-term complications of Paget disease as the patient has not had access to regular medical follow-up (e.g. heart failure)
7) The patient decides that if the area in his maxilla may be related to his Paget disease, he does not want any further management as the area does not hurt. What are the risks?
   - The diagnosis is not definitive
   - There is a potential risk of osteosarcoma associated with Paget disease
   - The area may continue to enlarge if it is left untreated
   - The associated irregular bone is prone to pathological fracture
   - The patient needs to access medical help as he is already displaying signs of long-term complications of untreated Paget disease (e.g. headaches and hearing loss)

General Dental Considerations

Oral Findings

- Mandibular/maxillary involvement is present in approximately 17% of patients
- Maxillary involvement is far more common than mandibular involvement
- The alveolar ridges tend to remain symmetrical but become grossly enlarged, causing spacing of the teeth
- Edentulous patients may complain that their dentures no longer fit because of the increased alveolar size
- Hypercementosis and ankylosis may necessitate surgical extraction of teeth (Figure 7.2.2)
- Radiographic changes
  - Early stages associated with decreased radiodensity of the bone and alteration of the trabecular pattern; large

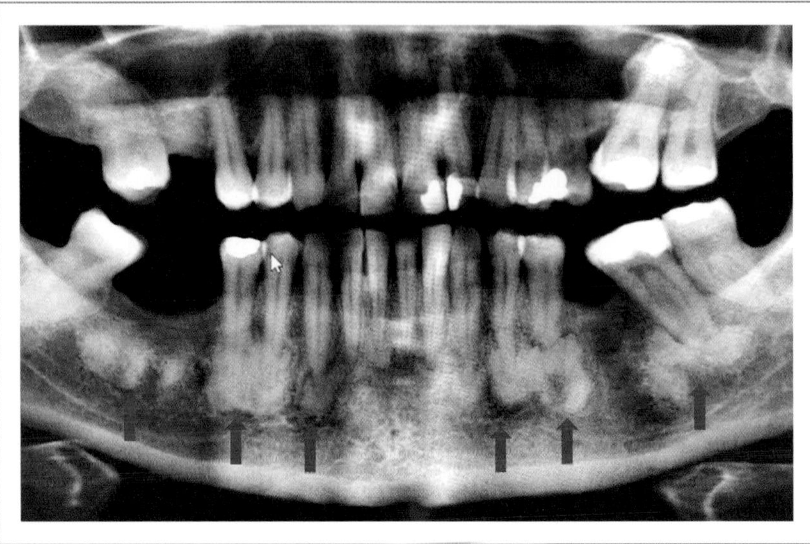

Figure 7.2.2 Hypercementosis associated with Paget disease.

circumscribed areas of radiolucency may be present (osteoporosis circumscripta)
  - Later stages, when there is osteoblastic activity, result in patchy areas of sclerotic bone which tend to become confluent; this is commonly described as a cotton wool appearance

Dental Management

- Dental treatment considerations will be determined by the presence of oral complications of Paget disease (e.g. hypercementosis), the history of antiresorptive or antiangiogenic drugs and the presence of comorbidities (e.g. cardiac failure) (Table 7.2.1)

Section II: Background Information and Guidelines

Definition

Paget disease of the bone is a disorder characterised by excessive bone turnover and is the second most common metabolic bone disease after osteoporosis. It causes remodelling and enlargement of skull, pelvis and long bones. It typically presents in people over the age of 50 years, although there is a less common early-onset variation which presents in teenagers and young adults. Although it occurs worldwide, Paget disease is most common in Europe, Australia and New Zealand. It is estimated to affect 1% of people older than 40 years in the United States.

In addition to Paget disease of the bone, there are several other types of Paget disease, including of the breast/nipple, penis and vulva. These are not discussed within this section.

Aetiopathogenesis

- The aetiology remains unknown, although it is thought that a combination of genetic and environmental risk factors is involved
- Genetic risk factors
  - Recent evidence suggests that mutations in genes that encode components of the RANK [RANK]/NFκB signalling pathway play a vital role in the pathogenesis
  - Variations of *SQSTM1*, *TNFRSF11A*, and *TNFRSF11B* [illegible] involved in remodelling have been identified
  - Studies also suggest that genetic variations in certain regions of chromosomes 2, 5 and 10 are associated with increased risk
  - Familial Paget disease has been described and is associated with more severe disease; the risk of developing Paget disease is seven times higher for those with a close relative with the disease; in 15–40% of cases there is an autosomal inheritance pattern
- Environmental risk factors
- Possible role of viruses (paramyxovirus, measles, canine distemper virus), as the nuclear inclusion bodies in osteoclasts appear to represent viral nucleocapsids

Clinical Presentation

- May be unifocal but more frequently presents as multifocal disease

Table 7.2.1 Considerations for dental management.

Risk assessment	• Hypercementosis may result in the need for surgical extractions • Dental management of patients taking antiresorptive drugs can trigger medication-related osteonecrosis of the jaw (MRONJ) (see Chapter 16.2) • Bleeding from the highly vascular bone • Delayed healing from bone in the later stages of disese due to poor blood supply (increased risk of suppurative osteomyelitis with trauma) • Pathological fractures • In cases of severe Paget disease, there is a higher prevalence of heart disease • Psychosocial problems may be present
Criteria for referral	• A medical consultation should be undertaken if the patient has associated medical complications (e.g. advanced heart failure) • Referral to a specialist in a hospital setting may be required if surgical intervention is planned (e.g. history of bisphosphonates, highly vascular bone or hypercementosis)
Access/position	• Bone deformities (e.g. kyphosis) may require adjustment of the positioning/cushions/support pillows
Communication	• There may be hearing or sight limitations
Consent/capacity	• For patients receiving/having received antiresorptive agents, the consent form should explicitly reflect the risk of the onset of MRONJ (see Chapter 16.2) • Patients should be informed that the bone changes may result in increased bleeding risk/delayed healing/increased risk of infection
Anaesthesia/sedation	• Local anaesthesia – No special considerations • Sedation – Consider the presence of heart failure • General anaesthesia – Consider the presence of heart failure and/or chest deformity
Dental treatment	• Before – Specifically ask about the use of antiresorptive agents (both current and in the past) – A radiographic evaluation of the remaining bone is always recommended – If hypercementosis is severe, a surgical approach with adequate exposure should be planned for dental extractions – The diminished bone quality is a relative contraindication to the use of dental implants, as it may interfere with achievement of osseointegration (limited evidence) • During – Careful positioning of the patient in the dental chair • After – Delayed alveolar bone healing is not uncommon following tooth extraction – Dentures may have to be replaced more frequently as the alveolar ridge enlarges
Drug prescription	• Quinolone and tetracycline antibiotics interact with calcium
Education/prevention	• A risk factor analysis (including the use of antiresorptive medication) and patient counselling should be undertaken • Regular dental visits and a healthy lifestyle (e.g. smoking cessation) are necessary to maintain good bone health

- Predominantly affects the axial skeleton (vertebral column, pelvis, femur, sacrum, skull)
- Usually asymptomatic (up to 90% of cases)
- When symptoms are present, these may include:
  - Bone pain and swelling (the most common symptom)
  - Hypervascularity leading to excessive warmth of the affected area and/or in severe cases, arteriovenous shunting resulting in high output cardiac failure
  - Bony deformity (e.g. bowing deformity of the legs, kyphosis with loss of height, enlarged skull)
  - Secondary osteoarthritis if joints are involved

- Pathological fractures (remodelled bone is weaker and less organised)
- Neurological complications due to nerve compression; may result in headaches, deafness or visual impairment
- Secondary hyperparathyroidism may occur in 10–15% of patients and may be due to inadequate calcium intake in the face of increased demand from extensive bone remodelling
- Impaired quality of life
- Osteosarcoma development (malignant, aggressive), occurs in less than 1% of cases

Diagnosis

- Often a coincidental finding as a result of radiographs/blood tests undertaken for other reasons
- Tests undertaken if there are clinical signs of Paget disease include:
  - Radiography
  - Bone scintigraphy
  - Blood tests
    - Raised bone-specific serum alkaline phosphatase
    - Normal plasma calcium and phosphorus levels
  - Elevated levels of urinary markers, including hydroxyproline, deoxypyridinoline, C-telopeptide and N-telopeptide of type I collagen
  - Computed tomography and magnetic resonance imaging may be useful in assessing the long-term complications of Paget disease

Management

- Analgesia
- Bisphosphonates (e.g. alendronate)
- Calcitonin
- Adequate intake of calcium and vitamin D
- Supportive therapies such as orthotic devices and physiotherapy/rehabilitation
- Surgical management of severe orthopaedic complications and sarcomas

Prognosis

- Generally good, particularly if treatment is given before major changes have occurred in the affected bones
- The decrease in complications is attributed to earlier diagnosis and intervention
- Treatment can reduce symptoms but there is no cure
- Poor prognosis if heart failure or osteosarcoma develops

A World/Transcultural View

- In recent years there has been evidence of a reducing incidence of Paget disease and a reduction of the severity of its potential complications
- This reducing incidence may be due to changes in the ethnic composition of the population because of increased migration; improved public health measures (vaccination programmes and reduced exposure to environmental triggers) may also have contributed to the reduction

Recommended Reading

Alaya R, Alaya Z, Nang M, Bouajina E. Paget's disease of bone: Diagnostic and therapeutic updates. *Rev Med Interne*. 2018;39:185–91.

Hsu E. Paget's disease of bone: updates for clinicians. *Curr Opin Endocrinol Diabetes Obes*. 2019;26:329–34.

Köse TE, Köse OD, Karabas HC, Erdem TL, Ozcan I. Findings of florid cemento-osseous dysplasia: a report of three cases. *J Oral Maxillofac Res*. 2014;4:e4.

Scully C, Langdon J, Evans J. Marathon of eponyms: 16 Paget disease of bone. *Oral Dis*. 2011;17:238–40.

Seehra J, Sloan P, Oliver RJ. Paget's disease of bone and osteonecrosis. *Dent Update*. 2009;36:166–72.

Singer FR. Paget's Disease of Bone. 2020 (Jan 1). In: Feingold KR, Anawalt B, Boyce A, Chrousos G, de Herder WW, Dungan K, Grossman A, Hershman JM, Hofland HJ, Kaltsas G, Koch C, Kopp P, Korbonits M, McLachlan R, Morley JE, New M, Purnell J, Singer F, Stratakis CA, Trence DL, Wilson DP, editors. Endotext [Internet]. South Dartmouth (MA): MDText.com, Inc.; 2000–.

Smith BJ, Eveson JW. Paget's disease of bone with particular reference to dentistry. *J Oral Pathol*. 1981;10:233–47.

7.3 Rheumatoid Arthritis

Section I: Clinical Scenario and Dental Considerations

Clinical Scenario

A 59-year-old woman presents for an urgent consultation because she is unable to open her mouth and has associated pain. She is accompanied to her appointment by her husband who reports that his wife's jaw 'locked open when she was eating lunch'. He reports that this has happened several times in the past but this time the jaw will not go back into place.

Medical History

- Rheumatoid arthritis (RA), diagnosed 14 years ago
- Surgery for herniated disc in the lower back (7 years ago)
- Cataract surgery (4 years ago)
- Macular degeneration
- History of herpes zoster infection (post-therapeutic neuralgia)

Medications

- Methotrexate
- Deflazacort (6 mg); changed 2 months ago from prednisone 10 mg daily for 6 months
- Pregabalin
- Folic acid
- Tramadol/paracetamol
- Omeprazole

Dental History

- Cannot tolerate long dental procedures (fatigue/ pain from jaw)
- Has had 'numerous problems with the teeth and the joint'
- Only visits the dentist when in pain
- Brushes her teeth 2–3 times a day

Social History

- Typically accompanied by her husband
- Impaired mobility – variable; some days she has difficulty walking
- Persistent fatigue
- Significant visual impairment in the past 2 years
- Nil tobacco/alcohol consumption

Oral Examination

- Dislocation of the temporomandibular jaw with protruded mandible and open bite
- Moderate oral hygiene
- Reduced salivary flow
- Generalised periodontal disease
- Generalised dental mobility (grade 3 in #31 and #32)
- Caries in #11, #12, #13, #21 and #22
- Fillings in #11, #12, #13, #27, #31, #32, #36, #45 and #48
- Numerous lost teeth

Radiological Examination

- Orthopantomogram and magnetic resonance imaging undertaken (Figure 7.3.1)
- Bilateral subluxation of the temporomandibular joint
- Deep caries in #21 with probably pulpal involvement (pulp chamber calcified)
- Periapical osteolytic lesion in #22
- Root canal treatment in #31
- Extreme loss of supporting alveolar bone in #31 and #32

Structured Learning

1) Further examination confirms that the patient's mandible is locked in a protruded position and she has an associated anterior open bite. The temporomandibular joint (TMJ) is tender on palpation. What is the most likely cause of these symptoms?
   - TMJ involvement is found ~50% of patients with RA
   - There may be associated pain, swelling, movement impairment and crepitation

A Practical Approach to Special Care in Dentistry, First Edition. Edited by Pedro Diz Dios and Navdeep Kumar.

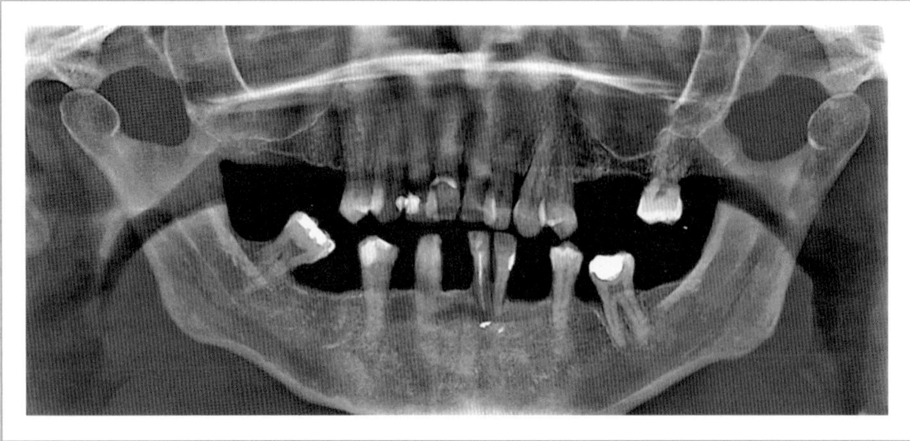

Figure 7.3.1 Orthopantomogram showing conserved structure of the condylar process; MRI is required to confirm subluxation of the temporomandibular joint.

- Dislocation of the TMJ resulting in malocclusion of the teeth and an anterior open bite may occur in advanced stages of RA, such as this patient
- Masticatory effort, particularly with hard, chewy foods, can trigger a TMJ dislocation

2) What are the options to try reposition the patient's TMJ?
   - Intraoral reduction using the wrist pivot method
   - Intraoral Hippocratic method of reduction (Nélaton manoeuvre)
   - Extraoral reduction
   - If the above are unsuccessful, muscle relaxants, analgesics or even general anaesthesia may be required
   - Aftercare includes initial immobilisation, soft food, analgesics and physiotherapy

3) The patient presents for a further appointment a week later, complaining of intense localised pain in the left canine fossa region, which has prevented her from sleeping all night. Clinical and radiographic findings confirm a diagnosis of acute periapical periodontitis of #22. What treatment [illegible] most appropriate: endodontic treatment or dental extraction?
   - Dental extraction of #22 is advisable
   - The reasons for this are:
     - #22: extensive caries and poor restorability; loss of supporting alvelolar bone
     - Mouth opening is limited and painful
     - Endodontic treatment typically requires longer/more frequent appointment (increasing the risk of TMJ pain/dislocation)
     - The patient cannot tolerate long treatment sessions (fatigue)
     - There are numerous lost teeth, with the imminent loss of others; removable prosthetic rehabilitation may be advisable in the long term

4) Before planning the dental extraction, what laboratory test results would you request and why?
   - A recent full blood count with differential would be useful
   - Anaemia of chronic disease is commonly found in patients with RA
   - Neutropenia and thrombocytopenia may be present as adverse effects of synthetic disease-modifying antirheumatic drugs (DMARDs) such as methotrexate

5) What factors are considered important in assessing the risk of managing this patient?
   - Social
     - Lack of motivation as she only visits the dentist for acute episodes
     - Chronic fatigue and joint pain (may result in irregular attendance and reduced tolerance for dental procedures)
   - Medical
     - RA-related positional limitations/discomfort on transfer to the dental chair
     - Adverse effects of methotrexate including nausea/vomiting, hepatotoxicity and severe leucopenia (see Chapter 12.2)
     - Adverse effects of corticosteroids (deflazacort) include adrenal insufficiency risk, delayed wound healing or increased susceptibility to infections (see Chapter 12.1)
     - Visual impairment (due to steroid-induced cataracts and macular degeneration); impaired non-verbal communication; inability to read and sign consent forms
   - Dental
     - Poor oral health, requiring urgent treatment
     - Limited and painful mouth opening

- Previous failed dental treatments
- Prone to periodontal disease
- Hyposalivation
- Impaired oral hygiene

6) Why is this patient at increased risk of infection postoperatively?
   - Drug-induced moderate to severe neutropenia (e.g. methotrexate)
   - If the patient routinely receives corticosteroid doses equivalent to more than 10 mg of prednisone (6 mg deflazacort is equivalent to 5 mg prednisone)

7) What analgesic would you prescribe after the dental extraction?
   - At first, none (only as rescue medication if necessary)
   - The patient already regularly takes tramadol/paracetamol (tramadol is a centrally acting analgesic, included in the second step of the WHO analgesic ladder)
   - The patient is also taking deflazacort, which has an anti-inflammatory effect
   - The risk of methotrexate's adverse haematological effects increases with non-steroidal anti-inflammatory drugs

8) What difficulties may be affecting this patient's ability to maintain her oral hygiene?
   - Limited mouth opening
   - Pain on maximum opening
   - Visual impairment
   - Difficultly holding the toothbrush (RA affecting her hands)
   - Limited manual mobility
   - Hyposalivation

General Dental Considerations

Oral Findings

- Poor oral hygiene, which manifests as a significant accumulation of bacterial plaque (may be related to reduced manual dexterity, fatigue)
- High prevalence of periodontal disease, whose progression is determined by systemic factors such as RA activity and its drug treatment
- Reduced salivary flow (both at rest and stimulated); secondary Sjogren syndrome
- TMJ dysfunction due to joint impairment. Degenerative bone changes may be detectable with imaging tech-

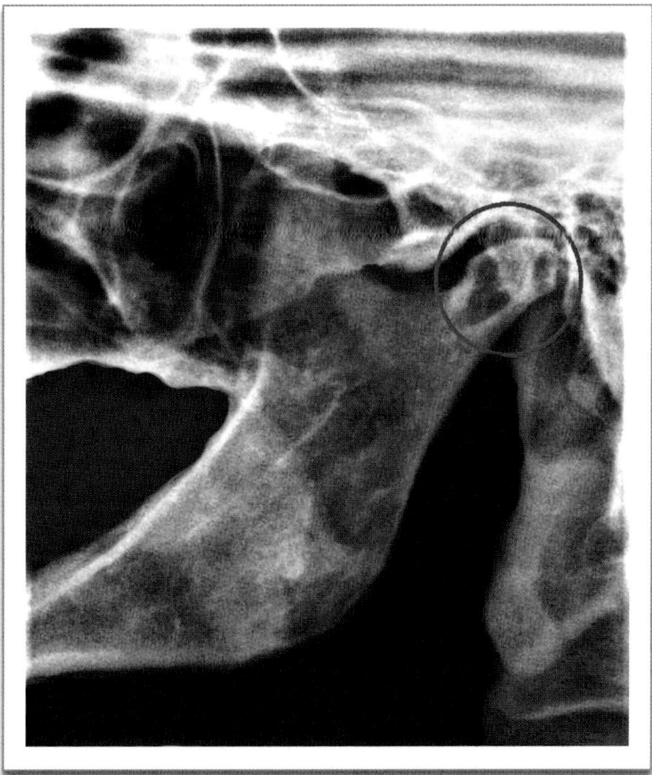

Figure 7.3.2 Condylar process of a rheumatoid arthritis patient showing flattening rough surface and subchondral cysts (Ely cysts).

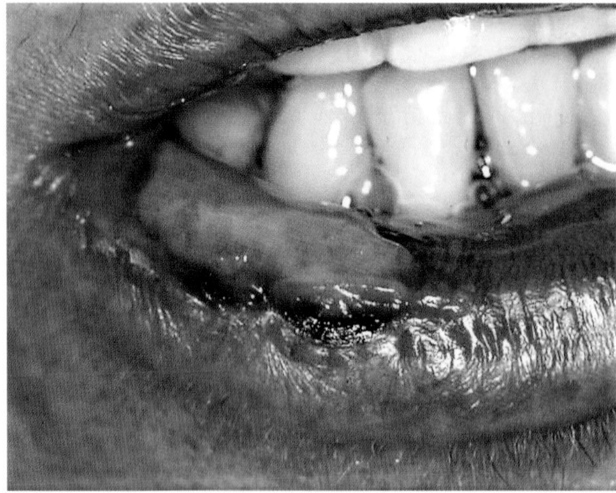

Figure 7.3.3 Methotrexate-induced oral ulcer.

niques in asymptomatic individuals (e.g. erosion and flattening of joint surfaces) (Figure 7.3.2)
- TMJ disease can cause difficulties with swallowing and chewing
- In juvenile RA, the growth pattern and orofacial morphology can be altered, which is characterised by retrognathia, anterior open bite and posterior rotation of the jaw in relation to the cranial base
- Methotrexate can cause stomatitis and mouth ulcers (Figure 7.3.3)
- The administration of biological DMARDs has been related to the onset of mouth ulcers, erythema multiforme, lichenoid reactions and bacterial (e.g. osteomyelitis) and fungal (e.g. candidiasis) infections (Table 7.3.1)
- Biological DMARDs may also be associated with the risk of delayed wound healing (e.g. after dental extractions) and medication-related osteonecrosis of the jaw (MRONJ)

Dental Management

- The dental treatment will be determined mainly by the patient's overall level of impairment, previous oral health, the functional limitations of the TMJ (e.g. mouth opening) and reduced manual dexterity (Table 7.3.2)

Section II: Background Information and Guidelines

Definition

Rheumatoid arthritis is a chronic inflammatory disease that predominantly affects the joints, although it can be associated with extra-articular manifestations such as rheumatoid nodules, pulmonary impairment, vasculitis and other systemic comorbidities. The estimated prevalence of RA among adults is approximately 1% worldwide and it is more common among women than men (2:1 ratio). Although RA can affect patients of all ages, it typically presents between 30 and 50 years of age. RA is more common in Nordic countries than in the southern hemisphere and more common in industrial areas than in rural settings.

Aetiopathogenesis

- RA is considered an autoimmune disease characterised by the production of anticitrullinated peptide antibodies (ACPAs) that cause synovial inflammation and ultimately joint destruction
- The human leucocyte antigen (HLA) system (particularly HLA-DRB1) plays an important role in RA, confirming the role of peptide bonds in the pathogenesis
- A family history of RA multiplies the likelihood of experiencing RA by 3–5 times
- Inheritability is especially relevant in the seropositive forms of the disease (autoantibodies)
- The main environmental risk factor is tobacco

Clinical Presentation

- Joints are painful/inflamed with associated joint stiffness in the morning
- Typically affects the small joints first (hands) and is symmetrical in distribution; may progress to involve the knees, ankles, elbows, hips and shoulders
- The joints most often involved are the wrists, the proximal interphalangeal joints and metacarpophalangeal joints – long-term deformities may occur (e.g. Boutonnière deformity of the thumb, ulnar deviation of the metacarpophalangeal joints, swan neck deformity of the fingers) (Figure 7.3.4)
- Most typically presents as polyarticular disease with a gradual onset
- Less commonly may present with an acute onset, often associated with intermittent or migratory joint involvement, or with monoarticular disease
- Systemic symptoms may also be present in one-third of patients, particularly if the presentation of RA is acute: prominent myalgia, fatigue, low-grade fever, weight loss and depression
- Numerous extra-articular manifestations may occur (Table 7.3.3)

Diagnosis

- There are no clearly defined criteria for the diagnosis of RA
- Diagnosis is established based on both clinical findings and laboratory tests

Table 7.3.1 Orofacial adverse effects of the most common biological disease-modifying antirheumatic drugs (DMARDs).

Target	Monoclonal antibody/fusion protein	Orofacial adverse effects
Anti-TNF agents		
	Adalimumab	• Candidosis • Erythema multiforme • Lichenoid reactions • Carcinoma? • MRONJ?
	Etanercept	• Candidosis • Erythema multiforme • Sarcoid nodules (on face) • Carcinoma?
	Infliximab	• Deep mycoses • Erythema multiforme • Lichen planus • Osteomyelitis • Parotid swelling • Ulcers • MRONJ?
Agents targeting B- or T-lymphocytes		
	Abatacept	• Ulcers
	Rituximab	• Candidosis • Ulcers • MRONJ?

TNF: tumor necrosis factor; ?: suggested but not confirmed; MRONJ: Medication-Related Osteonecrosis of the Jaw

- C-reactive protein levels and erythrocyte sedimentation rates tend to be high in RA
- At diagnosis, 50–70% of patients are seropositive for autoantibodies against ACPAs and IgG (rheumatoid factor)
- The differential diagnosis should be established with other causes of arthritis including reactive arthritis, osteoarthritis, psoriatic arthritis, infectious arthritis and a number of autoimmune conditions such as collagen disease

Management

- Non-steroidal anti-inflammatory drugs reduce the pain and stiffness but do not act on the joint damage or change the disease course
- Glucocorticoids produce rapid symptomatic relief and change the disease progression but have severe long-term adverse effects
- DMARDs reduce synovitis and systemic inflammation and are classified as synthetic (nonbiological) and biological
  - The most common conventional synthetic DMARD is methotrexate; this category also includes leflunomide, hydroxychloroquine and sulfasalazine
  - Biological DMARDs act on specific anti-inflammatory targets; the most widely used of these drugs are the antitumor necrosis factor agents such as adalimumab, certolizumab, etanercept, golimumab and infliximab
  - In recent years, other biological drugs have been administered successfully, such as abatacept, anakinra, rituximab, sarilumab and tocilizumab
  - The first targeted synthetic DMARD (tofacitinib, a pan-janus kinase inhibitor) has also been approved
- When there is advanced joint destruction, orthopaedic surgery may be required (may include joint replacement)

Table 7.3.2 Dental management considerations.

Risk assessment	• Patients can experience movement difficulties and pain when manipulating the joints • Patients with RA undergoing treatment with corticosteroids are at risk of adrenal suppression (see Chapter 12.1) • DMARDs can predispose patients to bleeding, infections, impaired healing and medication-related osteonecrosis of the jaw (MRONJ; see Chapter 16.2) • Methotrexate has a synergistic effect with bisphosphonates and combined with the proinflammatory state of RA, may further increase the risk of MRONJ
Criteria for referral	• Highly limited and/or highly painful oral opening are candidates for treatment in a hospital setting • Significant haematological complications due to DMARDs or at high risk of MRONJ • Significant extra-articular manifestations of RA
Access/position	• Whenever possible, patients who use wheelchairs should be treated in their own chairs • Joint stiffness is more pronounced at the start of the day – hence appointments should preferably be scheduled for the mid-morning or the afternoon • The sessions should be short and should allow for frequent rest and changes of position • Avoid opening the mouth too wide or for an extended time (pain, risk of dislocation) • Some patients are more comfortable in a semi-reclined position • Physical support for the neck and legs might be necessary (e.g. pillows and towels) • In severe RA with impaired cervical spine, there might be difficulties positioning the patient in the chair, and neck hyperextension should be avoided (atlantoaxial instability)
Communication	• It has been suggested that patients with RA are more susceptible to sensorineural hearing loss than the general population (this auditory deficit has also been related to the long-term consumption of analgesics)
Consent/capacity	• Patients may have difficulties due to the hand changes associated with RA • Patients should be informed that the treatment plan will be determined by the potential oral complications of RA
Anaesthesia/sedation	• Local anaesthesia – No special considerations • Sedation – No sedation technique is contraindicated • General anaesthesia – Intubation can be problematic if the oral opening is limited and/or there is cervical ankylosis

(Continued)

Table 7.3.2 (Continued)

Dental treatment	• Before – Check the full blood count and differential blood test results before invasive procedures (in view of the risk of neutropenia and thrombocytopenia) – In general, antibiotic prophylaxis is not recommended for patients with orthopaedic implants before an invasive dental procedure to prevent infection of the prosthetic joint; however, patients with RA treated with biological DMARDs or taking more than 10 mg daily of prednisone are considered immunocompromised; consult the surgeon and consider prophylaxis, applying a regimen similar to that for prevention of bacterial endocarditis (see Chapter 8.5) • During – Limited and/or very painful oral opening may influence the treatment plan and the duration of the sessions – Orthodontic treatment with functional appliances can improve dental malocclusion with minimal skeletal effects – Orthognathic surgery may be considered as few sensorineural sequelae and no severe complications have been observed • After – Non-surgical periodontal treatment improves the clinical and biochemical markers of RA activity – Bleeding in the peri-implantation area and reabsorption of marginal bone are significantly greater in patients with RA who have another concomitant collagen disease than in those who exclusively have RA – There is no direct evidence that RA jeopardises the osseointegration of dental implants, and therefore the success rate is generally similar to the general population
Drug prescription	• The toxicity of methotrexate increases when amoxicillin is administered, and the risk of adverse haematological effects increases when combined with NSAIDs (e.g. ibuprofen, metamizole, indomethacin, diclofenac and naproxen) • Biological DMARDs do not interact with commonly used drugs such as amoxicillin, paracetamol and local anaesthetics
Education/prevention	• Patients with RA have a negative perception of their oral health-related quality of life, based mainly on their physical and functional limitations, which justify the implementation of preventive procedures • Oral hygiene is affected by hyposalivation, reduced manual dexterity and the pain caused by brushing motions • Toothbrushes with custom handles and electric toothbrushes may be helpful • Regular check-ups are recommended to avoid complex dental procedures in the future

RA, rheumatoid arthritis; DMARDs, disease-modifying antirheumatic drugs; NSAIDs, non-steroidal anti inflammatory drugs.

Prognosis

- RA causes progressive impairment in physical functionality and quality of life
- Patients who do not respond satisfactorily to treatment can develop extra-articular manifestations such as vasculitis and interstitial pulmonary disease
- The state of chronic inflammation inherent in RA has been associated with the onset of secondary amyloidosis, lymphoma, cardiovascular disease and increased mortality risk (especially among patients with certain HLA genotypes and those with positive serology for ACPA and rheumatoid factor)

A World/Transcultural View

- The prevalence of RA is particularly high in certain indigenous populations such as Native Americans, native women of Alaska, the First Nations of Canada, the Australian aborigines and the Maori of New Zealand
- In Japan, more than 20% of patients with RA take bisphosphonates

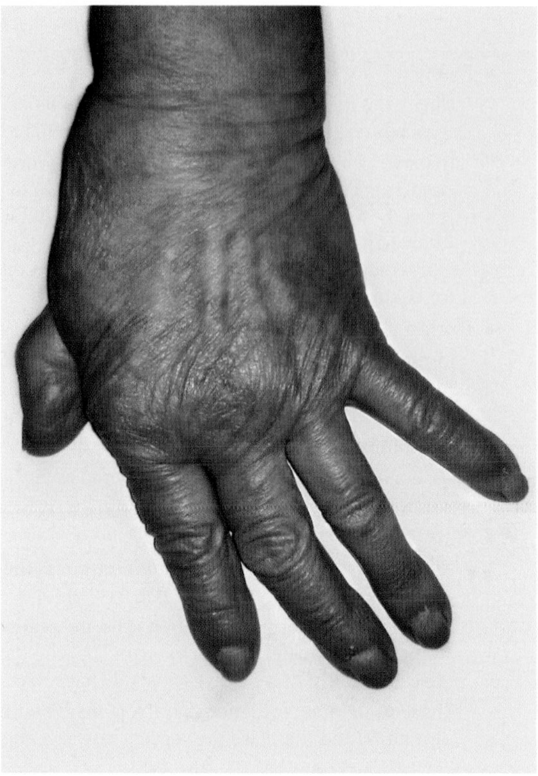

Figure 7.3.4 Stiff fingers and swollen joints in rheumatoid arthritis.

Table 7.3.3 Extra-articular manifestations of rheumatoid arthritis (excluding oral).

Tissue/system affected	Non-severe manifestations	Severe manifestations
Skin	Nodule Raynaud phenomena	Petechiae Purpura Ulcers Gangrene
Cardiovascular	Atherosclerosis Arrhythmias Valvular heart disease	Myocardial infarction Pericarditis
Pulmonary	Bronchiolitis obliterans Organising pneumonia	Pleuritis Interstitial lung disease
Nervous system		Entrapment neuropathy Mono/polyneuritis multiplex Cervical subluxation
Eyes	Secondary Sjogren syndrome	Episcleritis/scleritis
Haematological	Anaemia	Thrombocytosis Eosinophilia Felty syndrome
Renal		Glomerulonephritis Interstitial nephritis
Musculoskeletal	Muscle wasting	Osteoporotic changes Tendon/ligament rupture

Recommended Reading

Bartold, P.M. and Lopez-Oliva, I. (2020). Periodontitis and rheumatoid arthritis: an update 2012–2017. *Periodontol 2000* 83: 189–212.

González-Chávez, S.A., Pacheco-Tena, C., de Jesús Caraveo-Frescas, T. et al. (2020). Oral health and orofacial function in patients with rheumatoid arthritis. *Rheumatol. Int.* 40: 445–453.

Kaur, S., Bright, R., Proudman, S.M., and Bartold, P.M. (2014). Does periodontal treatment influence clinical and biochemical measures for rheumatoid arthritis? A systematic review and meta-analysis. *Semin. Arthritis Rheum.* 44: 113–122.

Krennmair, G., Seemann, R., and Piehslinger, E. (2010). Dental implants in patients with rheumatoid arthritis: clinical outcome and peri-implant findings. *J. Clin. Periodontol.* 37: 928–936.

Schmalz, G., Patschan, S., Patschan, D., and Ziebolz, D. (2020). Oral-health-related quality of life in adult patients with rheumatic diseases – a systematic review. *J. Clin. Med.* 9: 1172.

Silvestre-Rangil, J., Bagán, L., Silvestre, F.J., and Bagán, J.V. (2016). Oral manifestations of rheumatoid arthritis. A cross-sectional study of 73 patients. *Clin. Oral Investig.* 20: 2575–2580.

de Souza, S., Bansal, R.K., and Galloway, J. (2016). Rheumatoid arthritis – an update for general dental practitioners. *Br. Dent. J.* 221: 667–673.

Wasserman, A. (2018). Rheumatoid arthritis: common questions about diagnosis and management. *Am. Fam. Physician* 97: 455–462.

8

Cardiovascular Diseases

8.1 Arterial Hypertension

Section I: Clinical Scenario and Dental Considerations

Clinical Scenario

A 77-year-old woman presents to your dental clinic complaining of mobility problems and discomfort associated with the lower left wisdom tooth. Her symptoms commenced 2 days ago and are especially pronounced when chewing. The painful tooth (#38) serves as an anchor for a removable lower denture that she has been unable to wear since the discomfort started.

Medical History

- Arterial hypertension (AHT) (subclinical secondary target organ impairment)
- Type 2 diabetes
- Osteoarthritis
- Anxiety and sleep disorders

Medications

- Amlodipine
- Metformin
- Dexketoprofen
- Lorazepam
- Omeprazole

Dental History

- Removable upper and lower dentures (~15 years old)
- 10 years since the patient last visited a dental clinic (did not feel the need; feels the denture is adequate and no previous dental pain)
- Good level of co-operation
- Brushes her prosthesis and remaining teeth twice a day

Social History

- Widowed; lives alone and rarely leaves her home
- One of her 2 children escorts her to her appointments if required
- Emotional lability (highly affected by the recent death of her sister)
- Nil tobacco and alcohol consumption

Oral Examination

- Poorly fitting partial upper and lower dental prostheses
- Partially edentate
- Fair oral hygiene
- Loss of periodontal attachment for all remaining teeth
- Grade 2 mobility and pain on percussion of molar #38
- Significant hyposalivation
- Lacy white lesion 1.5 cm in diameter on the left buccal mucosa; asymptomatic; no associated induration/lymph node enlargement

Radiological Examination

- Orthopantomogram undertaken (Figure 8.1.1)
- Generalised horizontal alveolar bone loss
- Severe vertical bone loss in mesial of #38

Structured Learning

1) The patient is concerned about the lesion you have detected in the left buccal mucosa. She did not know it was there and is very worried that it is cancer, particularly as her sister died due to mouth cancer. What is an appropriate response?
   - Reassure the patient and explain that this is unlikely
   - Include the information below in your discussion
     - The lesion does not have the classic signs of cancer (i.e. speckling, ulceration, induration)
     - There are no additional risk factors (no alcohol/tobacco consumption)
     - It is more likely that the lesion is due to a lichenoid reaction
     - A number of medications can cause this type of lesion
     - Although antihypertensive medications are included in these, the patient is taking a calcium

A Practical Approach to Special Care in Dentistry, First Edition. Edited by Pedro Diz Dios and Navdeep Kumar.

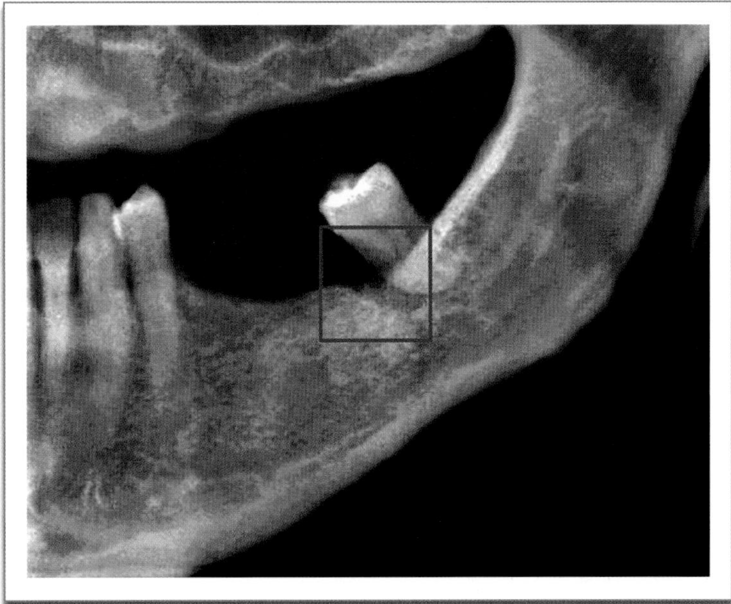

Figure 8.1.1 Orthopantomogram demonstrating severe vertical bone loss in mesial of #38 and multiple missing teeth.

channel blocker (amlodipine), which is not normally associated with this reaction
   - Hence, the lesion is most likely to be related to the hypoglycaemic agent (metformin)
   - A biopsy can help confirm the diagnosis but is not urgent as the lesion does not look suspicious

2) The patient also complains that her mouth has become increasingly dry over the last 5 years. What could be causing this?
   - Anxiety
   - Secondary to diabetes
   - Secondary to medication: lorazepam (benzodiazepine), amlodipine (calcium channel blocker)

3) Following a discussion, the patient agrees to proceed with dental extraction of #38. What factors are considered important in assessing the risk of managing this patient?
   - Social
     - Emotional lability may reduce compliance and ability to cope with dental intervention
     - Emotional distress has also been related to paroxysmal hypertension
   - Medical
     - Hypertension and type 2 diabetes mellitus are both aspects of metabolic syndrome and hence may have shared common aetiological and risk factors; they may also contribute to a worsening of each other's symptoms
     - Increased risk of hypertensive crisis, orthostatic hypotension and potential increased bleeding tendency
     - Diabetes mellitus is known to be associated with increased risk of infection, impaired wound healing and risk of hypoglycaemia/hyperglycaemia in the dental setting (see Chapter 5.1); it may also result in 'silent' heart attacks due to autonomic nerve damage
     - Stress from the dental environment can trigger an anxiety crisis (see Chapter 15.1)
     - Consider the sedative effects of lorazepam
   - Dental
     - Requires an urgent dental extraction (i.e. patient cannot chew)
     - Need for replacement dentures needs to be discussed, taking into account the following factors:
       - Fit of the current dentures is poor
       - Further jeopardised by the loss of a supporting tooth (#38)
       - Previous denture is 10 years old – patient may have difficulty adapting to a new denture
       - Poor prognosis for the remaining teeth
       - Xerostomia can reduce retention and tolerance to a replacement denture
     - Irregular attendance and anxiety may reduce compliance, engagement in improving oral health and engagement in long-term follow-up

4) Before commencing the dental procedure, you check the patient's blood pressure – it is 165/105 mmHg. What is your approach?
   - Do not proceed with treatment
   - Confirm that the patient has taken their antihypertensive medication

- Repeat the blood pressure measurement after a 5-minute interval
- If at 5 minutes the readings are the same or worsen, consult the patient's physician
- Be aware that hypertensive urgency (absence of other symptoms)/emergency (symptoms of target organ involvement) occurs when the blood pressure is 180/120 mmHg or greater – this requires immediate medical review/intervention

5) The physician informs you that the patient's blood pressure is usually well controlled and she has been seen recently for a review. What could have led to the raised readings and what would you do?
   - The patient may not be compliant with her antihypertensive medication, particularly as she is distressed by the recent death of her sister
   - Lifestyle factors may have had an impact (e.g. lack of exercise)
   - The patient has a history of anxiety
   - This coupled with the discussion regarding the buccal lesion and her concern regarding cancer may have caused the elevated readings at the appointment
   - Discuss these factors with the patient
   - Advise further medical review
   - Prescribe medication to control the pain and infection from #38 and rebook an appointment for the dental extraction
6) What should you consider if prescribing an analgesic?
   - The patient is already routinely taking a non-steroidal anti-inflammatory drug (dexketoprofen), although this is not controlling her oral pain
   - Non-steroidal anti-inflammatory drugs can decrease the activity of antihypertensive drugs (especially angiotensin-converting enzyme inhibitors and angiotensin II receptor blockers), but there is no evidence of drug interactions with calcium channel antagonists
   - If she requires a rescue analgesic, she should start with paracetamol
7) The patient asks if she can have sedation when the dental extraction is undertaken in the future. What should you consider?
   - If the hypertension and diabetes are well controlled, no technique is contraindicated: nitrous oxide or drug sedation may be employed (e.g. benzodiazepines)
   - However, it is important to consider that the patient is already taking lorazepam (benzodiazepine) daily, and she is 77 years old

General Dental Considerations

Oral Findings

- Antihypertensive drugs can cause multiple oral side-effects (Table 8.1.1)
  - Facial swelling/flushing (Figure 8.1.2)
  - Xerostomia
  - Lichenoid reactions
  - Dysgeusia
  - Gingival enlargement (Figure 8.1.3)
  - Swelling and pain in the salivary glands
  - Erythema multiforme
  - Angio-oedema
  - Painful mouth or paraesthesia
- Cases of facial paralysis have been reported for patients with 'malignant hypertension' (significant increase in blood pressure, retinal haemorrhage and typically renal impairment)

Dental Management

- The dental treatment considerations are primarily determined by the blood pressure readings and by the target organ impairment such as the kidneys and heart (Table 8.1.2)

Section II: Background Information and Guidelines

Definition

Arterial hypertension is defined as the permanent increase in systolic blood pressure (>140 mmHg), diastolic blood pressure (90 mmHg) or both (in the United States, ≥130/80 mmHg) (Table 8.1.3). AHT is known as the silent killer, due to the typical lack of signs and symptoms until the advanced stages of the disease. There are an estimated 1.13 billion individuals with AHT worldwide, most in low- to middle-income countries. AHT is responsible for more than 7.5 million deaths annually.

Aetiopathogenesis

- AHT is caused by an increase in cardiac output and/or increased peripheral vascular resistance
- Genetic predisposition: complex polygenic disorder, in which more than 25 rare mutations and 120 single-nucleotide polymorphisms have so far been implicated
- Highest risk in those of African or Caribbean origin; increased risk in south Asian origin (AHT secondary to coronary artery disease)
- Two types: primary and secondary

Table 8.1.1 Examples of oral side-effects of antihypertensive drugs.

Class	Adverse effects
Thiazides	• Xerostomia • Lichenoid reactions
Angiotensin-converting enzyme inhibitors	• Erythema • Angio-oedema • Facial swelling • Oral ulcers • Xerostomia • Dysgeusia • Lichenoid reactions • Painful mouth (burning)
Angiotensin II receptor blockers	• Angio-oedema • Xerostomia • Dysgeusia
Calcium channel blockers (dihydropyridines)	• Gingival hyperplasia • Xerostomia • Dysgeusia
Calcium channel blockers (non-dihydropyridines)	• Gingival hyperplasia • Xerostomia • Dysgeusia
Diuretics	• Xerostomia • Dysgeusia • Lichenoid reactions
Beta-blockers	• Erythema • Xerostomia • Dysgeusia • Lichenoid reactions
Direct renin inhibitors	• Erythema • Angio-oedema
Alpha-1 blockers	• Xerostomia • Dysgeusia
Alpha-2 agonists	• Xerostomia • Dysgeusia • Lichenoid reactions • Painful parotid glands
Direct vasodilators	• Facial flushing • Bleeding gums • Lupus-like lesions • Lymphadenopathy

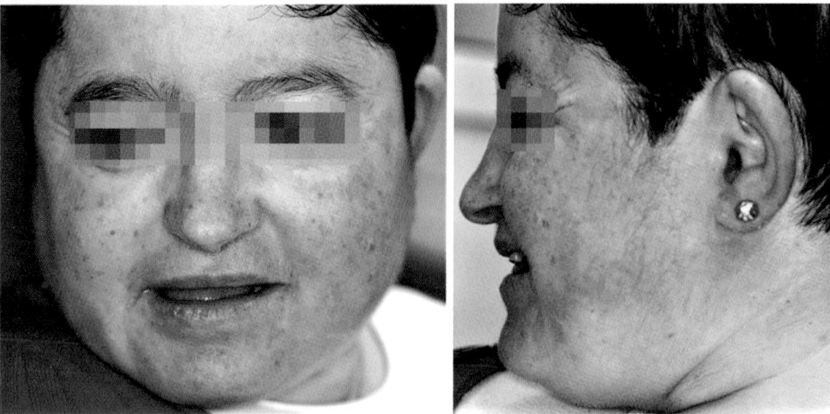

Figure 8.1.2 Angiotensin-converting enzyme inhibitor (enalapril)-induced facial swelling and flushing.

- Primary (or essential) hypertension (~95% of AHT)
  - Specific aetiological factor is not identified
  - Several mechanisms are linked to altered pathways in blood pressure control: genetic factors, diet (especially increased sodium chloride intake), obesity, insulin resistance, endothelial dysfunction, chronic excess alcohol, ageing, stress and sedentary lifestyle

(a)

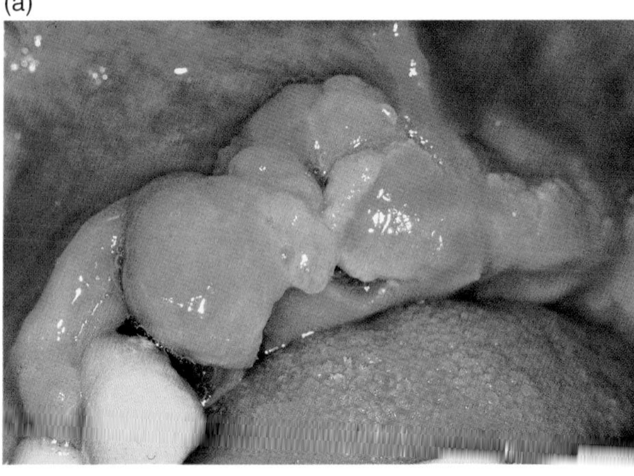

(b)

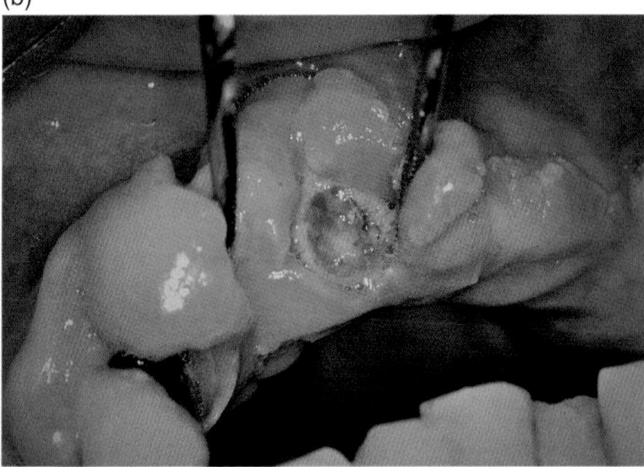

Figure 8.1.3 (a,b) Calcium channel blocker (nifedipine)-induced gingival hyperplasia covering a tooth root remnant.

- Secondary AHT (5–10% of AHT)
  - Related to a known underlying cause
  - Environmental factors
  - Conditions that cause secondary AHT
    - Prescription drugs (e.g. non-steroidal anti-inflammatory drugs)
    - Recreational drugs (e.g. cocaine, amphetamines)
    - Renal disorders (parenchymal and vascular)
    - Endocrine diseases (primary hyperaldosteronism, Cushing syndrome, phaeochromocytoma, hyperthyroidism)
    - Vascular disorders (aortic coarctation)
    - Sleep apnoea syndrome
    - Scleroderma

Clinical Presentation

- Symptoms are frequently non-existent or non-specific (until a target organ is affected) but can include the following:
  - Headaches
  - Blurred vision
  - Tinnitus
  - Fatigue
  - Dizziness
  - Epistaxis
- Hypertensive and atherosclerotic complications can target multiple organs leading to:
  - Retinal damage
  - Left ventricular hypertrophy
  - Heart failure
  - Angina/myocardial infarction
  - Proteinuria and haematuria
  - Renal failure
  - Cognitive impairment (vascular dementia)
  - Stroke

Table 8.1.2 Considerations for dental management.

Risk assessment	• Risk of a hypertensive crisis during dental treatment (systolic blood pressure >180 mmHg and/or diastolic blood pressure >120 mmHg) • Potential increased tendency of bleeding after surgical procedures • Risk of orthostatic hypotension (particularly a risk for older populations – decreased baroreflex and loss of large artery compliance) • The presence of concomitant diseases such as heart and kidney failure needs to be considered (secondary target organ involvement)
Criteria for referral	• With blood pressure readings ≥180/110 mmHg, any type of dental procedure should be postponed (emergency treatments should be performed in a hospital setting) • With blood pressure readings 160–179/100–109 mmHg, dental treatment should not be performed before consulting a physician • Dental treatment can be undertaken without modification if the patient's blood pressure readings are consistently <160/100 mmHg
Access/position	• The appointment should be during the last hour of the morning or the first of the afternoon (endogenous epinephrine levels are higher early in the morning) • Avoid long appointments • Adjust the position of the dental chair slowly to reduce the likelihood of orthostatic hypotension secondary to antihypertensive drugs
Consent/capacity	• Keep in mind that hypertension has become one of the main causes of age-related cognitive impairment • The risk of a hypertensive crisis should be reflected in the informed consent form
Anaesthesia/sedation	• Local anaesthesia – Anaesthetics containing epinephrine should be avoided in patients with severe hypertension – May be used for other hypertensive patients but it is advisable not to exceed a dose of 0.04 mg of epinephrine (approximately 2 cartridges at a concentration of 1:100 000) – Intraligamentary injections with epinephrine concentrations greater than 1:100 000 should not be performed – Caution should be exercised to avoid intravascular injections – The cardiovascular effects of epinephrine are boosted by tricyclic antidepressants (e.g. imipramine), non-selective beta-blockers (e.g. propranolol) and certain anaesthetics (e.g. halothane) • Sedation – Conscious sedation can be achieved with nitrous oxide or benzodiazepines • General anaesthesia – General anaesthesia is not contraindicated, except in cases of severe heart failure, ischaemic heart disease or kidney failure – The antihypertensive therapy should not be interrupted – Diuretics can promote the onset of arrhythmias and increase the sensitivity of muscle relaxants – Avoid administering barbiturates intravenously – Halothane, enflurane and isoflurane can cause hypotension in patients who take beta-blockers

(Continued)

Table 8.1.2 (Continued)

Dental treatment	• Before – Confirm with the patient whether they have taken their prescribed antihypertensive medication – It is advisable to record a blood pressure reading before starting any dental procedure – With blood pressure readings consistently <160/100 mmHg, conventional dental treatment can be performed – If the reading is high, retake after 5 minutes – Consider the impact of anxiety on the reading • During – Bleeding is generally controlled with local haemostatic measures – Avoid the use of retraction cords with epinephrine (its concentration can be up to 12 times greater than that of anaesthetic cartridges) – Prevent episodes of orthostatic hypotension by adjusting the chair position slowly – If there are signs of a hypertensive crisis, stop the procedure, keep the patient recumbent, call for help and follow the protocol for management of medical emergencies in a dental setting • After – Non-surgical periodontal treatment improves blood pressure values and endothelial function (flow-mediated dilation) – Surgery for drug-induced gingival enlargements (e.g. nifedipine) is effective, but discontinuing the drug might sometimes be necessary to completely resolve the symptoms – It has been suggested that the survival of dental implants in patients who take antihypertensive drugs can be even greater than that of dental implants in the general population (antihypertensive drugs promote bone formation and renovation)
Drug prescription	• A number of non-steroidal anti-inflammatory drugs (e.g. ibuprofen, diclofenac and naproxen) can reduce the efficacy of antihypertensive agents such as angiotensin-converting enzyme inhibitors or angiotensin II receptor blockers • Corticosteroids can increase blood pressure
Education/prevention	• Maintenance of good oral hygiene prevents the recurrence of drug-induced gingival enlargement and the onset of periodontitis (there is some evidence of a causal relationship between periodontitis and blood pressure) • Dental visits represent an opportunity for hypertension screening, prevention and education (e.g. promotion of smoking cessation and nutritional counselling)

Table 8.1.3 Blood pressure categorisation in adults.

Category		Systolic blood pressure		Diastolic blood pressure
Normal		<120 mmHg	and	<80 mmHg
High		120–129 mmHg	and	<80 mmHg
Hypertension	Stage 1	130–139 mmHg	or	80–89 mmHg
	Stage 2	≥140 mmHg	or	≥90 mmHg

Diagnosis

- Standard blood pressure determinations using auscultatory measurements calibrated to a mercury column (manual mercury sphygmomanometer) have given way to oscillometers that record variations in pulsatile blood volume (automated oscillometric blood pressure device). The measurement devices need to be validated and should be calibrated periodically
- At least 2 blood pressure measurements (systolic, diastolic or both) on at least 2 different visits need to be recorded for AHT to be diagnosed
- The measurements can be performed in the clinic, at home and through 24-hour outpatient blood pressure monitoring (Figure 8.1.4)

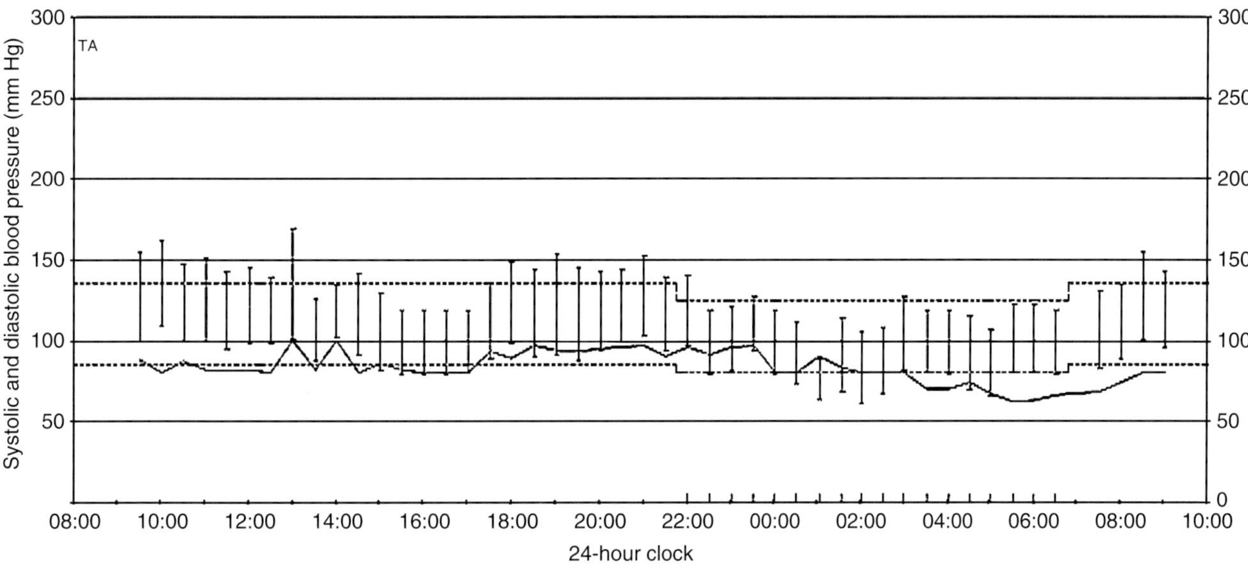

Figure 8.1.4 Ambulatory blood pressure monitoring record over a 24-hour period.

- 'White coat hypertension' is characterised by high blood pressure in the clinic but normal pressure when measured at home or through monitoring
- In 'masked hypertension', the blood pressure readings are normal in the clinic but high when assessed at home or through monitoring
- It has recently been suggested that blood pressure readings recorded at home or through monitoring are more useful than those measured in the clinic for assessing target organ damage and cardiovascular risk
- Criteria for early diagnosis of target organ damage in AHT have also been proposed (Table 8.1.4)

Management

- Non-pharmacological interventions for changing the patient's lifestyle
  - Weight loss
  - Healthy diet (rich in fruits and vegetables)
  - Low-sodium, potassium-enriched diet
  - Physical activity (at least 45 minutes of fast walking daily)
  - Limit alcohol consumption
  - Limit caffeine
  - Stop smoking (to lower the cardiovascular risk)
- Pharmacological interventions (Table 8.1.5)
  - Diuretics

Table 8.1.4 Early diagnosis of target organ damage in hypertensive patients (based on European Society of Hypertension/European Society of Cardiology guidelines).

Test	Cut point
Electrocardiographic (left ventricular hypertrophy)	• Sokolow–Lyon criteria ≥38 mm • Cornell criteria >2440 mm/msec
Echocardiographic (left ventricular hypertrophy)	• Left ventricular mass index (LVMI) ≥125 g/m^2 for men and ≥100 g/m^2 for women
Carotid intima-media thickness	• >0.9 mm or plaque
Carotid-femoral pulse wave velocity	• >12 m/sec
Ankle-brachial pressure index	• <0.9
Serum creatinine	• 1.3–1.5 mg/dL (115–133 μmol/L) for men and 1.2–1.4 mg/dL (107–124 μmol/L) for women
Albumin excretion rate	• Microalbuminuria: 30–300 mg/24 hours • Albumin (mg)/creatinine (g) ratio: ≥22 for men and ≥31 for women
Estimated glomerular filtration rate (GFR)	• GFR <60 mL/min/1.73 m^2 or creatinine clearance <60 mL/min

Table 8.1.5 Main oral antihypertensive drugs.

	Class	Examples
Primary agents	Thiazides	• Chlorthalidone • Hydrochlorothiazide
	Angiotensin-converting enzyme inhibitors	• Captopril • Enalapril • Lisinopril
	Angiotensin II receptor blockers	• Candesartan • Losartan • Valsartan
	Calcium channel blockers (dihydropyridines)	• Amlodipine • Nicardipine • Nifedipine
	Calcium channel blockers (non-dihydropyridines)	• Diltiazem • Verapamil
Secondary agents	Diuretics	• Amiloride • Furosemide • Spironolactone • Triamterene
	Beta-blockers	• Atenolol • Bisoprolol • Carvedilol • Metoprolol • Propranolol
	Direct renin inhibitors	• Aliskiren
	Alpha-1 blockers	• Doxazosin • Prazosin
	Alpha-2 agonists	• Clonidine • Methyldopa
	Direct vasodilators	• Hydralazine • Minoxidil

 - Beta-blockers
 - Calcium channel blockers
 - Angiotensin-converting enzyme inhibitors
 - Angiotensin II receptor blockers

Prognosis

- More than 80% of patients with AHT do not have their blood pressure controlled (they have not been diagnosed, they do not comply with the treatment or do not respond adequately to the treatment)
- AHT is considered the main risk factor for cardiovascular morbidity and mortality, given that approximately half of cases of stroke and episodes of cardiac ischaemia are a direct consequence of AHT
- AHT is the leading cause of premature death and disability worldwide. It is estimated that mean life expectancy of patients with undiagnosed hypertension is 10–20 years shorter than for those with normal blood pressure

A World/Transcultural View

- Hypertension is the leading preventable cause of premature death worldwide
- African Americans have the highest prevalence of hypertension worldwide (41%) and have fewer chances of achieving blood pressure control when prescribed an antihypertensive drug
- Global disparities in AHT, awareness, treatment and control are large and increasing. The prevalence of hypertension is increasing in low- and middle-income countries, while it is steady or decreasing in high-income countries

Recommended Reading

Czesnikiewicz-Guzik, M., Osmenda, G., Siedlinski, M. et al. (2019). Causal association between periodontitis and hypertension: evidence from Mendelian randomization and a randomized controlled trial of non-surgical periodontal therapy. *Eur. Heart J.* 40: 3459–3470.

Hogan, J. and Radhakrishnan, J. (2012). The assessment and importance of hypertension in the dental setting. *Dent. Clin. North Am.* 56: 731–745.

Jordan, J., Kurschat, C., and Reuter, H. (2018). Arterial hypertension – diagnosis and treatment. *Dtsch. Arztebl. Int.* 115: 557–568.

Kaur, B. and Ziccardi, V.B. (2020). Management of the hypertensive patient in dental practice. *Compend. Contin. Educ. Dent.* 41: 458–464; quiz 465.

Southerland, J.H., Gill, D.G., Gangula, P.D. et al. (2016). Dental management in patients with hypertension: challenges and solutions. *Clin. Cosmet. Invest. Dent.* 8: 111–120.

Williams, B., Mancia, G., Spiering, W. et al. (2018). 2018 practice guidelines for the management of arterial hypertension of the European Society of Cardiology and the European Society of Hypertension. *Blood Press.* 27: 314–340.

Wu, X., Al-Abedalla, K., Eimar, H. et al. (2016). Antihypertensive medications and the survival rate of osseointegrated dental implants: a cohort study. *Clin. Implant. Dent. Relat. Res.* 18: 1171–1182.

Yarows, S.A., Vornovitsky, O., Eber, R.M. et al. (2020). Canceling dental procedures due to elevated blood pressure: is it appropriate? *J. Am. Dent. Assoc.* 151: 239–244.

8.2 Angina Pectoris

Section I: Clinical Scenario and Dental Considerations

Clinical Scenario

A 63-year-old man presents to the dental clinic concerned about a lump on the gum in the upper right quadrant which appeared 3 days ago and is causing increasing discomfort. The patient is afraid as he has heard that infections in the mouth can make his heart condition worse.

Medical History
- History of acute myocardial infarction (MI) 3 years earlier
- Stable angina pectoris
- Mild chronic obstructive pulmonary disease (GOLD stage I)
- Dyslipidaemia
- Obese (BMI= 31 kg/m^2)
- Allergy to diclofenac, metamizole and cefuroxime
- Depression syndrome

Medications
- Nitroglycerin (sublingual spray)
- Carvedilol
- Simvastatin
- Acetylsalicylic acid
- Tiotropium bromide
- Amitriptyline
- Lorazepam

Dental History
- Three years since the last visit to a dentist (did not return after his MI)
- Good co-operation
- Brushes his teeth twice a day

Social History
- Married, lives with his wife
- Spends many hours sedentary (truck driver) and several days a week away from home
- Raised BMI related to irregular and unhealthy eating habits while he is working away from home
- Ex-smoker (20 cigarettes/day until 3 years ago)
- Alcohol: nil

Oral Examination
- Fair oral hygiene
- Fixed prosthesis: bridge in the upper right quadrant
- Buccal sinus with draining fistula/purulent discharge adjacent to #15
- Caries in #28 and #37
- Missing teeth #26, #36 and #46

Radiological Examination
- Periapical radiograph undertaken of #14 and #15 (Figure 8.2.1)
- Radiolucent lesion suggestive of periapical cyst, related to #14 and #15 (endodontic treatment 4 years earlier)

Structured Learning

1) Is the patient correct that his dental infection can make his heart condition worse?
   - There is a potential link
   - Dental infection (particularly periodontal disease) is a source of chronic inflammation and is postulated to contribute to the development and progression of atherosclerosis
   - Angina is caused by coronary artery atherosclerosis and can manifest as acute coronary syndrome
   - Acute coronary syndrome is ~3 times more common among people with apical dental infections

A Practical Approach to Special Care in Dentistry, First Edition. Edited by Pedro Diz Dios and Navdeep Kumar.

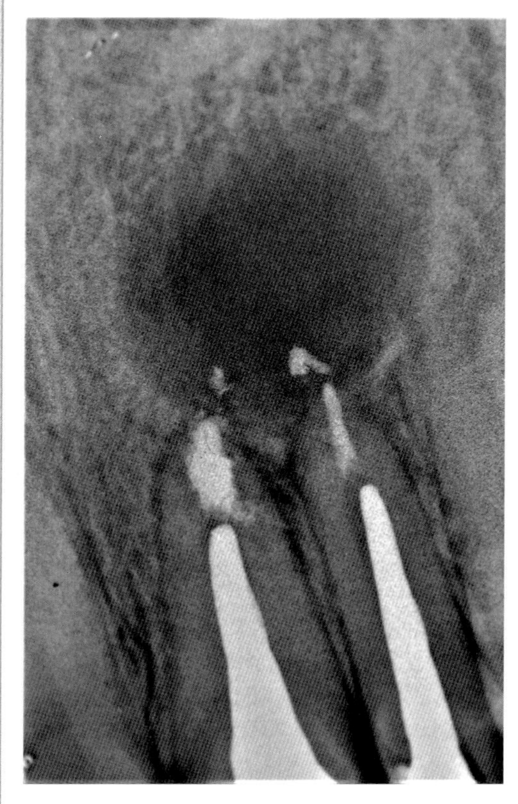

Figure 8.2.1 Periapical dental radiograph showing chronic periapical periodontitis of #14.

- Furthermore, the psychological and physical stress associated with dental pain can trigger an acute angina-related event
- However, it is important to note that dental infection in a patient with angina does not predispose to infective endocarditis, as the latter condition is related to the lining of the heart, not the blood supply to it

2) The patient does not want #14 extracted as it is part of the fixed bridge. He consents to an apicoectomy. What factors are considered important in assessing the risk of managing this patient?
   - Social
     - Limited availability for dental clinic visits (due to his work)
     - Low commitment to following health promotion instructions (e.g. nutrition counselling) as evidenced by his high BMI
   - Medical
     - Risk of an acute presentation of angina-related chest pain in the dental setting
     - Chronic obstructive pulmonary disease may compound hypoxia risk; airflow limitation (e.g. rubber dam use) and drug selection/interactions need to be considered (see Chapter 9.1)
     - Depressive syndrome can result in irregular attendance and lack of commitment to the treatment plan
     - Obesity-related risks (see Chapter 16.4)
     - Tendency to bleed due to the acetylsalicylic acid (minimal risk) (see Chapter 10.5)
     - Drug allergy includes some non-steroidal anti-inflammatory drugs and antibiotics (see Chapter 16.1)
     - Drug interactions
   - Dental
     - Irregular dental attender with suboptimal oral hygiene (this is likely to be related to his job and recent MI)
     - The radiolucent area associated with #14 may require a more extensive surgical approach due to its size (i.e. cystectomy)
     - Orofacial complaints (e.g. dry mouth, chronic facial pain or burning mouth syndrome) are common in depression syndrome (see Chapter 15.2)

3) Avoiding stress during dental treatment is particularly important for this patient. What factors would you consider in relation to the use of pharmacological methods to reduce his anxiety?
   - The patient's chronic obstructive pulmonary disease is mild
   - Nitrous oxide may be used (in addition to relaxing the patient, this also delivers an additional oxygen supply)
   - Benzodiazepines are not contraindicated, although they can present a tolerance problem for this patient (the patient takes lorazepam regularly), and the respiratory disease needs to be considered. It has been suggested that benzodiazepines can worsen the cardiovascular condition
   - Occasionally antihistamines may also be prescribed; however, it is advisable to avoid using hydroxyzine in patients with heart disease
4) What type of local anaesthetic is recommended?
   - Any local anaesthetic may be employed
   - If the decision is made to use an anaesthetic with a vasoconstrictor, ensure a self-aspirating technique is used to avoid intravascular injections
   - Avoid exceeding 2 anaesthetic cartridges with epinephrine
5) What antibiotics should be avoided with this patient?
   - The patient is allergic to cefuroxime, a cephalosporin antibiotic
   - Cross-reaction within the cephalosporin group is rare
   - Cross-reactive allergy between penicillins and cephalosporins is also rare
   - However, as a precaution, do not prescribe cephalosporins or penicillins, if it can be avoided

- Avoid macrolides because they interact with simvastatin, increasing the risk of rhabdomyolysis
- Ampicillin reduces the bioavailability of some beta-blockers such as atenolol, but this interaction has not been confirmed with carvedilol

6) Which should you consider when prescribing postoperative analgesics for this patient?
   - The patient is allergic to 2 non-selective anti-inflammatory cyclooxygenase inhibitors (previously known as selective COX-1 inhibitors) – diclofenac and metamizole
     - Cross-reactivity with other anti-inflammatory agents of this type is therefore possible
     - The probability of cross-reactivity with paracetamol is low
   - Selective anti-inflammatory COX-2 inhibitors are contraindicated for patients with heart problems
   - Additionally, non-steroidal anti-inflammatory drugs can hinder the antihypertensive effect of beta-adrenergic blockers (carvedilol) and can decrease the therapeutic response to nitroglycerin
   - Paracetamol may be administered if no cross-reactivity with this drug has been confirmed; if this information is not available, however, the most advisable course of action is to administer acetylsalicylic acid (which the patient is already taking routinely), despite its disadvantages

7) The patient also reports that he is aware of a bad smell from his mouth but feels that this was present before he developed the gingival swelling. What should you consider if oral/dental factors are ruled out?
   - Undertake an organoleptic assessment (the patient breathes deeply by inspiring the air by nostrils and holds their breath for 5 seconds and then expires by the mouth directly, while the examiner sniffs the odour at a distance of 20 cm – scales of [illegible] commonly [illegible])
   - Approximately 10% of people with halitosis have an extraoral cause of their symptoms, including diet (e.g. garlic, onions, spicy foods), medications (e.g. nitrates and nitrates, disulfiram, amphetamines), respiratory disorders (e.g. tonsillitis, sinusitis), gastrointestinal disease (e.g. gastro-oesophageal reflux disease), hepatic disease, renal failure, haematological or endocrine system disorders and metabolic conditions
   - In this patient, potential contributing factors include:
     - Chronic obstructive pulmonary disease increases mucus production/chronic cough
     - Depression can lead to xerostomia due to related anxiety or as a side-effect of medication (lorazepam); subsequent development of halitosis can worsen the symptoms of depression due to the psychological impact
     - Medication-related halitosis could be due to the nitroglycerin sublingual spray; if dysgeusia is also present, however, the main candidate is the beta-adrenergic blocker with the associated side-effect of a dry mouth (carvedilol)

General Dental Considerations

Oral Findings

- The pain from angina can radiate to the jaw and, less often, to the teeth and oral tissues
- Specific oral lesions have not been reported in angina pectoris
- However, significant accumulations of dental plaque, calculus and a high prevalence of periodontal disease and edentulism have been reported in these patients (possible bidirectional link)
- Oral findings correspond to the adverse effects of anti-angina drugs, such as lichenoid lesions, gingival enlargement and ulcers (Table 8.2.1; Figures 8.2.2 and 8.2.3)

Dental Management

- Dental treatment modifications will be determined by the type of angina (stable or unstable) (Table 8.2.2)

Table 8.2.1 Main oral adverse effects of antianginal drugs.

Class	Adverse effects
Beta-blockers (e.g. propranolol)	• Erythema • [illegible] • Dysgeusia • Lichenoid reactions
Calcium channel blockers (e.g. nifedipine)	• Gingival enlargement • Xerostomia • Dysgeusia
Long-acting nitrates (e.g. dinitrate)	• Halitosis
Selective ion channel inhibitor, which regulates the pacemaker sinoatrial node (e.g. ivabradine)	• Oedema
Potassium channel openers (e.g. nicorandil)	• Oral ulcers
Specific late sodium current inhibitors (e.g. ranolazine)	• Oedema • Xerostomia
Free fatty acid beta-oxidation inhibitors (e.g. trimetazidine)	• Oedema • Erythema

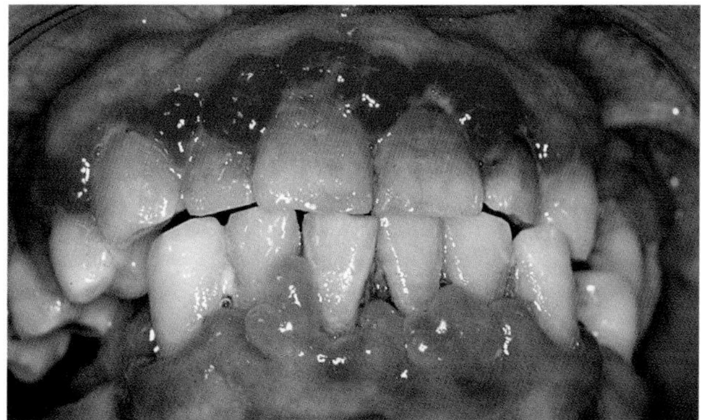

Figure 8.2.2 Gingival hyperplasia caused by nifedipine (a calcium channel blocker).

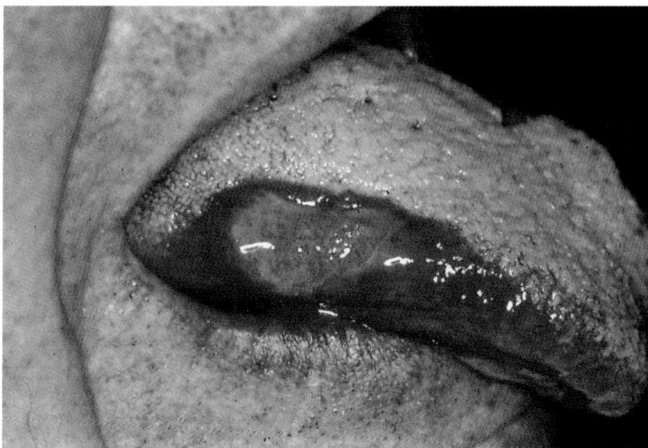

Figure 8.2.3 Nicorandil (a potassium channel opener)-induced oral ulcer.

- It is essential to minimise stress and be prepared to act in the event of a possible acute presentation of angina (Figure 8.2.4; Table 8.2.3)

Section II: Background Information and Guidelines

Definition

Angina pectoris is a clinical condition that occurs due to an imbalance between the supply and demand of oxygen of the myocardium (myocardial ischaemia). The condition is characterised by a feeling of tightness or pain in the front of the chest behind the sternum, generally triggered by physical effort or emotional stress. The pain disappears in less than 10 minutes with rest and the administration of nitrates.

Although its annual incidence rate is low (approximately 1% in individuals younger than 65 years), the importance of angina pectoris lies in the risk of acute coronary events and increased mortality.

Aetiopathogenesis

- A trigger (such as stress, exercise and pain) induces the release of endogenous catecholamines, which cause tachycardia, vasoconstriction and increased blood pressure
- In patients with a narrowing (atherosclerosis), blocking or spasm of one or more coronary arteries, this increased cardiac output translates into a drop in vascular flow and the onset of myocardial ischaemia
- Risk factors include high cholesterol levels, diabetes, obesity, lack of physical activity, age (greater for men over 45 years and women over 55 years), family history of heart disease, hyperthyroidism, stress and anxiety, sleep deprivation; for women, a history of pre-eclampsia and gestational diabetes

Clinical Presentation

- The main symptom is retrosternal pain, which can present as tightness or burning
- The pain can radiate to the throat, jaw, shoulders and arms
- Atypical presentations such as nausea, abdominal pain, extreme fatigue, respiratory distress and mandibular pain are more common in women
- Angina can be classified broadly into stable and unstable variants, although other less common subtypes have been described (Table 8.2.4)
- It is considered chronic and stable when there is no change in the intensity or characteristics of the pain or in the triggers, with the symptoms present for at least 2 months

Diagnosis

- Investigations are triggered based on the medical history and symptoms of possible angina
- Biochemical tests
  - In the acute phase, troponin levels
  - Full blood count, creatinine, lipid profile, glycated haemoglobin and thyroid hormones
- Chest radiography (for atypical presentations or suspected heart failure or pulmonary disease)
- Resting electrocardiogram, stress electrocardiogram and outpatient monitoring (Figure 8.2.5)
- Resting and stress echocardiogram and cardiac magnetic resonance imaging (CMR)
- Coronary computed tomography angiography (CTA)
- Positron emission tomography (PET)
- Single-photon emission computed tomography (SPECT)

Table 8.2.2 Considerations for dental management.

Risk assessment	• The dental setting can cause the onset of an angina attack due to fear, anxiety and/or pain • This can occur in patients with both stable and unstable angina • Without appropriate management, the risk of a serious consequence such as myocardial infarction and/or stroke is significant • Cardiac complications may occur in 10–20% of patients with unstable angina who undergo dental procedures
Criteria for referral	• Patients with unstable angina should be treated in a hospital setting with the following precautions: – The medical team should be consulted and available (specialists in cardiac emergencies) – Appropriate equipment and medication for emergencies should be present – Only urgent dental procedures should be provided – Anxiety control should be considered (e.g. 5 mg diazepam orally, nitrous oxide) – Prophylactic administration with sublingual nitroglycerin or intravenous coronary vasodilators should be considered – Perioperative monitoring of vital signs (oxygen saturation, blood pressure and pulse) is required
Access/position	• The appointment should be during the last hour of the morning or the first of the afternoon (endogenous epinephrine levels are higher early in the morning) • The sessions should be short and relaxed • Consider a semi-recumbent position (some antihypertensive drugs cause orthostatic hypotension)
Communication	• Patients with unstable angina frequently have abnormal moods (anxiety and depression) • Severity of angina is associated with poorer late-life cognitive performance
Consent/capacity	• Cognitive/behavioural changes may impact on capacity/consent • Patients should be advised that the dental treatment may be modified depending on their angina control, and that prophylaxis (e.g. sublingual nitroglycerin) does not exclude the possibility of an acute event
Anaesthesia/sedation	• Local anaesthesia – The use of epinephrine is contraindicated in patients with unstable angina – Do not exceed 2 anaesthetic cartridges with epinephrine at 1:100 000 (0.04 mg) for patients with stable angina – Consider the use of anaesthetics with felypressin as it has been reported to have fewer haemodynamic effects than epinephrine; do not use in high doses as it may cause constriction of the coronary arteries – Ensure that a self-aspirating technique is used to prevent intravascular entry • Sedation – Delay the treatment for at least 3 months from the diagnosis of angina to allow for stabilisation – Diazepam or temazepam may be considered to control anxiety (may be prescribed by the doctor) – A number of authors have suggested that benzodiazepines may worsen the cardiovascular condition and have proposed sedation only with nitrous oxide • General anaesthesia – Delay the treatment for at least 3 months from the diagnosis of angina – Avoid administering barbiturates intravenously

(*Continued*)

Table 8.2.2 (Continued)

Dental treatment	• Before (patients with stable angina) – Medical consultation is recommended to ensure that the angina is well controlled/stable – Anxiety control should be considered (e.g. 5 mg diazepam orally) – Administer prophylaxis with sublingual nitroglycerin (0.3–0.6 mg), 5–10 minutes prior to planned invasive dental treatment; the beneficial effects will last approximately 30–40 minutes; be aware of the adverse effects including postural hypotension, headaches, flushing, reflex tachycardia and occasionally nausea – Monitor vital signs (oxygen saturation, blood pressure and pulse) – The administration of antibiotic prophylaxis for bacterial endocarditis is not indicated • During – Monitor vital signs – Some patients take anticoagulant or antiplatelet drugs and therefore have a tendency to bleed during surgical procedures – Limit the use of epinephrine and avoid using vasoconstrictor-soaked thread retractors • After – Consider drug interactions if medication is to be prescribed – Provide oral and systemic health promotion instructions
Drug prescription	• Some of the non-steroidal anti-inflammatory drugs can reduce the efficacy of antihypertensive agents (e.g. ibuprofen, diclofenac, naproxen) • A number of antibiotics and antifungals can interact with drugs that are typically taken by patients with angina, and should be avoided: – Amoxicillin, metronidazole, azithromycin and clarithromycin interfere with acenocoumarol – Ampicillin reduces serum atenolol levels – Amoxicillin/clavulanic acid, azithromycin and azole derivatives can cause digoxin toxicity – Macrolides and azole derivatives interact with statins and can cause muscle damage (rhabdomyolysis)
Education/prevention	• The dentist, as a healthcare practitioner, should participate in angina pectoris prevention and education (e.g. promotion of smoking cessation and nutrition counselling) • Maintaining good oral hygiene avoids the onset and progression of periodontitis • It has been suggested that periodontal disease is one of the risk factors that determines the course of atherosclerosis in patients with stable angina pectoris

Management

- The goals of treatment are to reduce or eliminate symptoms and prevent long-term complications, such as MI, left ventricular failure and life-threatening arrhythmias
- Change in lifestyle habits and control of risk factors
  - Smoking cessation
  - Healthy diet
  - Moderate physical activity
  - Weight control
  - Evaluation of psychosocial risk factors
- Medications
  - Long-acting nitrates; sublingual nitroglycerin administration used for both acute episodes and for prophylaxis when symptoms are anticipated after exertions; provides symptomatic relief to approximately 75% of patients within 3 minutes
  - Anticoagulants; commonly acetylsalicylic acid
  - Renin-angiotensin-aldosterone system blockers, such as angiotensin converting enzyme inhibitors (ACEI) (e.g. captopril, enalapril)
  - Beta-blockers to reduce heart rate, blood pressure, myocardial contractility, left ventricular afterload (e.g. metoprolol, atenolol, bisoprolol); third-generation selective beta-1 blockers also cause peripheral vasodilation (e.g. carvedilol)
  - Calcium channel blockers to reduce oxygen demand by reducing blood pressure, contractility and afterload (e.g. non-dihydropyridine drugs such as diltiazem and verapamil)
  - Statins have pleiotropic anti-ischaemic effects independent of lipid-lowering activity and can improve endothelial function, enhance ischaemic vasodilatory response and modulate inflammation
  - Additional drug treatments include ivabradine, nicorandil, ranolazine and trimetazidine

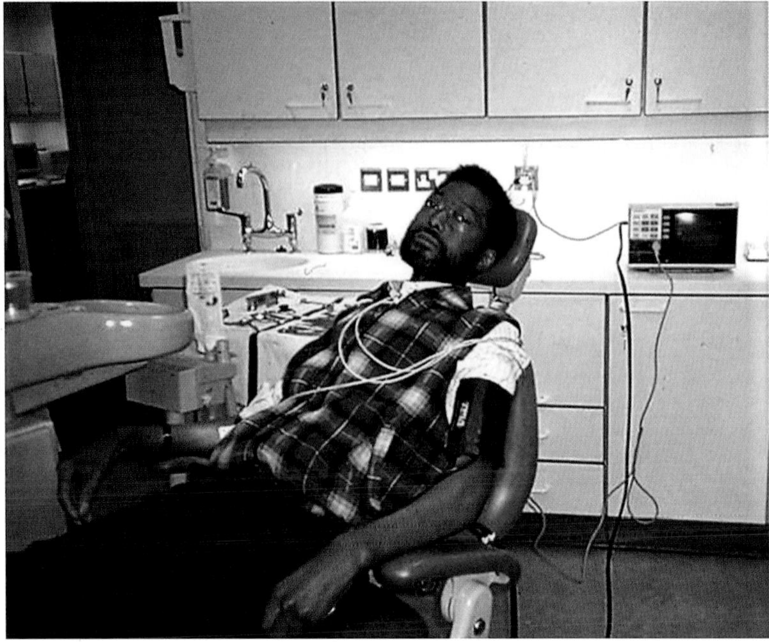

Figure 8.2.4 Patient with unstable angina treated in a hospital setting with perioperative cardiac monitoring.

  - Medication to control underlying conditions such as diabetes or hyperthyroidism
- Myocardial revascularisation
  - Percutaneous coronary intervention
  - Coronary artery bypass grafting

Prognosis

- The prognosis depends on the type of angina, individual risk factors, the therapeutic approach and comorbidities
- Patients with stable angina pectoris often have a poor quality of life and frequently use healthcare services
- Mortality due to angina is estimated at 4% annually, although it depends on the degree of narrowing of the coronary arteries involved

A World/Transcultural View

- Based on data from the US National Health and Nutrition Examination Survey, the prevalence of angina has declined in recent years among white non-Hispanics and among individuals older than 65 years; however, among black individuals, this reduction has not been confirmed
- A number of traditional Chinese medicine techniques, such as moxibustion and acupuncture, have been successfully employed for treating stable angina pectoris

Table 8.2.3 Protocol for the management of an angina pectoris attack (specific recommendations vary globally).

Chest pain during dental treatment in a patient with a history of angina	• Stop the treatment • Administer oxygen at 5 L/min • Sit the patient up • Administer 0.5 mg sublingual nitroglycerin (ensure they do not stand up as their blood pressure is likely to fall) • Monitor vital signs
If the pain disappears in 3–5 minutes	• Consult a physician and arrange a review • Ensure the patient is accompanied home
If there is no pain relief in 3–5 minutes	• Repeat another dose of nitroglycerin (up to 3 doses in 15 minutes, except if the systolic blood pressure is <100 mmHg) • Continue administering oxygen at 5 L/min • Request urgent medical assistance (possible myocardial infarction)
If the pain lasts more than 15 minutes and is accompanied by nausea, vomiting, syncope or hypertension	• Suspect a myocardial infarction • Request urgent medical assistance • Continue administering oxygen at 10–15 L/min • Give the patient 300 mg of aspirin • Morphine sulfate (5–10 mg) and saline solution (0.9%) may be administered intravenously by the medical team

Table 8.2.4 Classification of angina pectoris.

Type of angina	Symptoms	Trigger	Pain progression
Stable angina	Oppressive chest pain that can radiate	Physical exertion/ emotional stress	Relief in 10 minutes with rest or nitroglycerin
Unstable angina	Unpredictable pain	Can appear at rest	Can be prolonged and not respond to nitroglycerin
Other types	*Atypical angina*: without typical chest pain symptoms; characterised by vague discomfort or retrosternal burning, back or neck pain and fatigue *Variant angina (Prinzmetal's angina)*: characterised by nocturnal pain that occurs at rest *Refractory angina*: pain typical of angina that persists for more than 3 months and does not respond to medical treatment, interventions or surgery		

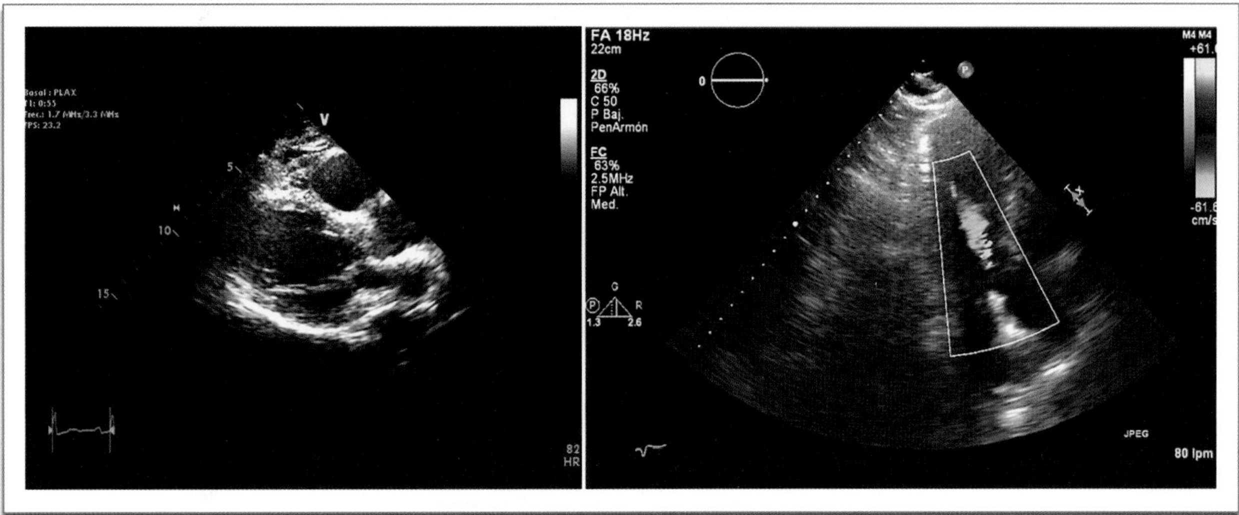

Figure 8.2.5 Stress echocardiography and Doppler echocardiography are established techniques for assessing coronary artery disease.

Recommended Reading

College of Dental Hygienists of Ontario (2017). CDHO Advisory Angina (Angina Pectoris). www.cdho.org/Advisories/CDHO_Advisory_Angina_(Angina_Pectoris).pdf

Herman, W.W. and Konzelman, J.L. (1996). Angina: an update for dentistry. *J. Am. Dent. Assoc.* 127: 98–104.

Hupp, J.R. (2006). Ischemic heart disease: dental management considerations. *Dent. Clin. North Am.* 50: 483–491.

Knuuti, J., Wijns, W., Saraste, A. et al. (2019). ESC guidelines for the diagnosis and management of chronic coronary syndromes. *Eur. Heart J.* 41: 407–477.

Kufta, K., Saraghi, M., and Giannakopoulos, H. (2018). Cardiovascular considerations for the dental practitioner. 2. Management of cardiac emergencies. *Gen. Dent.* 66: 49–53.

Niwa, H., Sato, Y., and Matsuura, H. (2000). Safety of dental treatment in patients with previously diagnosed acute myocardial infarction or unstable angina pectoris. *Oral Surg. Oral Med. Oral Pathol. Oral Radiol. Endod.* 89: 35–41.

Qureshi, W.T., Kakouros, N., Fahed, J., and Rade, J.J. (2020). Comparison of prevalence, presentation, and prognosis of acute coronary syndromes in ≤35 years, 36–54 years, and ≥55 years patients. *Am. J. Cardiol.* 140: 1–6.

8.3 History of Myocardial Infarction

Section I: Clinical Scenario and Dental Considerations

Clinical Scenario

A 63-year-old male presents for an urgent dental appointment complaining of discomfort from his upper right front tooth (#11). This tooth has become increasingly painful since the filling was lost 2 days ago.

Medical History

- Myocardial infarction (MI) 5 years earlier
- Arterial hypertension (without target organ impairment)
- Dyslipidaemia
- Type 2 diabetes (poorly controlled)
- Severe chronic obstructive pulmonary disease (GOLD stage III)
- Obstructive sleep apnoea syndrome (receiving continuous positive airway pressure therapy [CPAP])
- Morbid obesity (BMI= 46 kg/m^2)

Medications

- Acetylsalicylic acid
- Nebivolol
- Amlodipine
- Tiotropium bromide
- Fluticasone
- Metformin
- Simvastatin

Dental History

- Last visit to a dentist ~6 years ago; did not return for regular care as he could not cope when the dental chair was reclined due to difficulty breathing/increasing dental anxiety
- Prior to this, reports visiting the dentist regularly, with several fillings undertaken
- Used to wear a removable lower denture prosthesis but can no longer tolerate it
- Brushes his teeth irregularly

Social History

- Single; no children
- Lives with his 87-year-old mother
- On a minimal disability allowance
- Walks with difficulty
- Came to the dental clinic in taxi
- Frequently cannot leave his home because of fatigue and/or dyspnoea
- Smokes 10 cigarettes/day (although he has tried to quit the habit)
- Alcohol: <7 units a week

Oral Examination

- Poor oral hygiene
- #11 tender on palpation
- Caries in #11, #12 and #33
- Missing teeth #14, #15, #24, #25, #33–37 and #45–47
- Grade 1 mobility of #31 and #41

Radiological Examination

- Orthopantomogram undertaken (Figure 8.3.1)
- Significant alveolar bone loss in the mandibular incisors
- Root canal fillings and intraradicular posts in #13, #27 and #44
- Root canal filling and dentine pin in #32
- Fillings with secondary caries in #21, #22 and #44

Structured Learning

1) You determine that #11 is non-vital. The patient does not want to lose the tooth and requests root canal treatment. What may compromise the success of this treatment option?

A Practical Approach to Special Care in Dentistry, First Edition. Edited by Pedro Diz Dios and Navdeep Kumar.

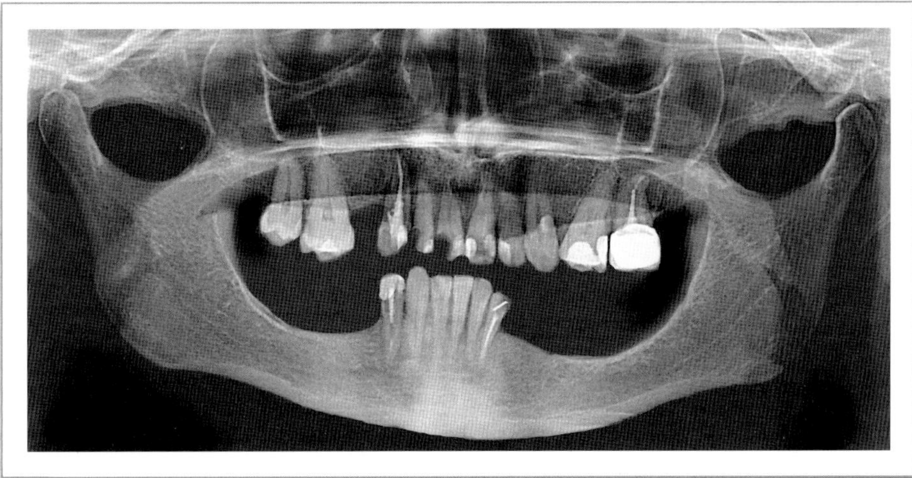

Figure 8.3.1 Orthopantomogram demonstrating loss of multiple teeth and deterioration of dental health.

- Patient may not be able to cope with multiple or longer appointments due to his multiple comorbidities and fatigue
- Access may be compromised (i.e. unable to recline the patient fully due to dyspnoea/chronic obstructive pulmonary disease, further airway compromise in relation to morbid obesity), presence of obesity-related decubitus ulcers
- Adverse effects of the antihypertensive drugs (orthostatic hypotension)
- Co-operation may be limited due to dental anxiety
- May not be able to tolerate rubber dam due to airflow restriction and dental anxiety
- Underlying diabetes may reduce likelihood of success of endodontic treatment (impaired immunity/wound healing)
- Potentially increased bleeding due to medication and underlying hypertension
- Oral hygiene poor and irregular dental attendance
- #11 poor restorability; horizontal bone loss

2) Following a discussion of the factors which may compromise the outcome of endodontic treatment of #11, the patient still wishes to proceed. What additional factors are considered important in assessing the risk of managing this patient?
   - Social
     - Reduced mobility
     - Dependence on adapted taxis
     - Limited financial means
     - No suitable escort
     - Dental anxiety
   - Medical
     - History of MI and higher risk of a repeat episode (multiple risk factors including smoking, raised BMI, hypertension, diabetes)
     - Risk of a hypertensive crisis (see Chapter 8.1)
     - Bleeding tendency due to antithrombotic agents and arterial hypertension
     - Severe limitation of air flow due to advanced chronic obstructive pulmonary disease (see Chapter 9.1)
     - Risk of hypoglycaemia/hyperglycaemia, delayed wound healing and infections due to diabetes mellitus (see Chapter 5.1)
     - Diabetes mellitus also increases the risk of a silent MI (diabetic neuropathy)
     - Morbid obesity and related commodities; may require a bariatric dental chair/facilities as most standard dental chairs have a weight limit of ~20 stone/127 kg (see Chapter 16.4)
     - Drug interactions and adverse effects
   - Dental
     - Multiple missing teeth
     - Unable to wear the previous lower denture
     - Poor prognosis for the remaining teeth (e.g. #43)
     - Poor oral hygiene and irregular toothbrushing
     - Irregular dental attendance

3) Why does dental treatment potentially increase the risk of a further MI?
   - Dental treatment-related pain and stress increase the amount of catecholamine released in blood
   - This results in elevated heart rate and blood pressure; these in turn can reduce the oxygen demand–supply balance in the myocardium and induce myocardial ischaemia
   - In addition, elevated blood catecholamine levels may induce platelet aggregation and coronary spasms, leading to MI

- Conversely, blood pressure reduction due to neurogenic shock or syncope triggered during dental treatment reduces coronary blood flow, increasing the risk of thrombotic occlusion in stenotic sections of the coronary arteries

4) Should this patient be seen for treatment in a hospital or primary care setting?
   - A hospital setting is preferred
   - Although the MI event was 5 years earlier, this patient has multiple comorbidities which increase his risk, including:
     - Severe chronic obstructive pulmonary disease
     - Uncontrolled hypertension
     - Uncontrolled diabetes
     - Morbid obesity
     - Additional risk factor of dental anxiety which may further compromise the existing cardiac and respiratory conditions

5) The patient's care is transferred to a hospital dental service. A medical review is sought prior to scheduling dental treatment as the patient complains of non-specific symptoms of increasing fatigue and dizziness. An ECG confirms that the patient has had a silent MI. What impact does this have on planned dental treatment?
   - Previously it was suggested that only conservative emergency dental treatment procedures should be undertaken during the first 6 months after a MI
   - This advice was based on historical evidence which indicated that for patients with histories of MI within 3 months, the incidence of reinfarction due to general anaesthesia or surgery was as high as 37%; the reinfarction rate decreased to 18% over a 3 month period from 3 to 6 months after MI onset, and to approximately 6% thereafter
   - Management of patients at risk of MI has significantly improved over the last 20 years
   - It has been recognised that although the incidence of reinfarction remains relatively high after major surgical interventions, such as thoracic surgery and vascular surgery, it is considerably lower after minor surgeries under local anaesthesia (e.g. dental extraction and pulpectomy), if the correct support is in place
   - Supportive measures include anxiety management, premedication with nitrates, minimum use of a local anaesthetic with vasoconstrictor, and monitoring of blood pressure, heart rate and ECG in a hospital environment
   - Furthermore, lack of satisfactory dental treatment to eliminate significant dental infection could aggravate myocardial ischaemia, with the pain itself acting as an inducer
   - Severe toothache also interferes with sleep and food intake, causing further physiological and psychological stress
   - Hence the general consensus is that dental treatment should be delayed for 6 weeks
   - However, for this patient, there are additional risk factors in relation to smoking, uncontrolled diabetes and hypertension, in addition to morbid obesity; close liaison with the medical team to address these issues should be in place to reduce the overall risk

6) The symptoms relating to the #11 are controlled with antibiotics and pain relief to allow for his medical status to be stabilised. The patient returns for planned dental care 8 weeks later and sedation is discussed to help reduce his dental anxiety. What should be considered?
   - This patient is considered high risk for conscious sedation due to his severe chronic obstructive pulmonary disease, morbid obesity, obstructive sleep apnoea and cardiac history
   - If sedation is required, it should be given under medical supervision in a hospital setting

7) As a healthcare practitioner, what health promotion advice should you be offering this patient?
   - Smoking cessation
   - Nutrition counselling
   - Prevention and treatment of periodontal disease, given the potential for periodontitis to increase the risk of cardiovascular disease, promote respiratory infections in patients with chronic obstructive pulmonary disease and affect the metabolic control of diabetes

General Dental Considerations

Oral Findings

- The most common oral findings correspond to the adverse effects of drugs administered prophylactically following an MI and include xerostomia, dysgeusia and lichenoid lesions (Table 8.3.1; Figure 8.3.2)
- A significant association has been reported between MI, calcified carotid atheromas (detected in panoramic radiographs) and periodontitis, especially in men
- The extent and severity of the periodontitis are positively related with MI size (evaluated based on serum levels of troponin and myoglobin)

Dental Management

- To minimise the risk of complications, dental clinicians need to consider the time elapsed from the MI episode, the

Table 8.3.1 Main adverse oral effects of drugs administered prophylactically following a myocardial infarction.

Class	Adverse effects
Beta-blockers	• Erythema • Xerostomia • Dysgeusia • Lichenoid reactions
Angiotensin-converting enzyme inhibitors	• Erythema • Angio-oedema • Oral ulcers • Pemphigus-like disease • Xerostomia • Dysgeusia • Lichenoid reactions • Burning mouth
Angiotensin II receptor blockers	• Angio-oedema • Xerostomia • Dysgeusia
Aldosterone antagonists	• Xerostomia • Dysgeusia • Lichenoid reactions

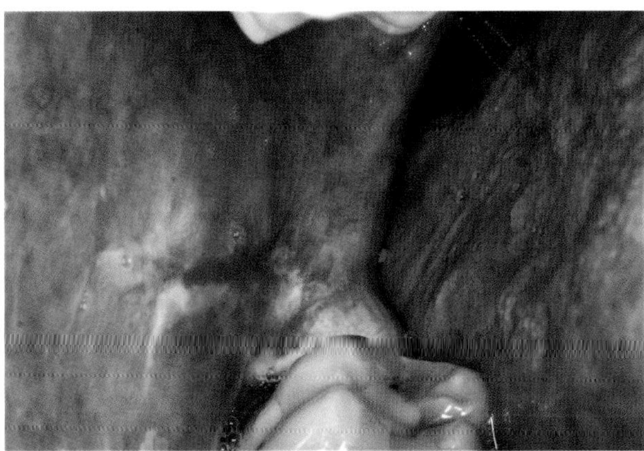

Figure 8.3.2 Oral lichenoid drug reaction triggered by a beta-blocker (nevibolol).

presence of comorbidities, the control of stress and the tendency to bleed (e.g. antithrombotic drugs) (Table 8.3.2)

Section II: Background Information and Guidelines

Definition

Myocardial infarction is the most severe manifestation of coronary artery disease. MI is defined as an acute episode of myocardial ischaemia (with symptoms and/or electrocardiographic criteria of ischaemia), which causes myocyte cell death (detected by specific biomarkers such as cardiac troponin).

Myocardial infarction has a substantial impact on global health, given that it affects more than 7 million individuals worldwide annually. It is defined as one of the acute coronary syndromes, a term which encompasses a range of conditions including unstable angina, ST-segment elevation myocardial infarction (STEMI) and non-ST-segment elevation myocardial infarction (NSTEMI) that are due to a sudden reduction of blood flow to the heart.

Aetiopathogenesis

- STEMI occurs when a coronary artery or one of the smaller branches that supplies blood to the heart becomes suddenly blocked by a blood clot, causing the heart muscle supplied by the artery to die
- In NSTEMI the blood clot causes a reduced blood flow, but not a total blockage so the heart muscle supplied by the affected artery does not die
- MI can be related to a number of causes as summarised in Table 8.3.3
- In most cases, it is due to the disruption of a vulnerable atherosclerotic plaque or the erosion of the coronary artery endothelium (type 1)
- When broken, the plaque releases its thrombogenic content, causing platelet activation, the start of the coagulation cascade, the formation of mural thrombi and the embolisation of atherosclerotic residues
- The end-result is myocyte necrosis, detectable by the increase in cardiac markers in peripheral blood

Clinical Presentation

- The symptoms of ischaemia include various combinations of chest pain (typically intense and lasting longer than 20 minutes), which radiates to the arms, jaw or epigastric area and can appear during exercise or at rest
- MI can sometimes present as an episode of dyspnoea, fatigue, nausea, feeling faint, palpitations and cardiac arrest, and can even be asymptomatic

Diagnosis

- The suspicion of an MI is based on the medical history and symptoms which warrant further investigation
- Changes in the electrocardiogram (ECG) (e.g. ST elevation)
- Increased cardiac troponin levels, particularly of the I and T isoforms (protein found in the cardiac tissue and released in the blood during heart damage)
- Imaging techniques

Table 8.3.2 Considerations for dental management.

Risk assessment	• Risk of recurrent MI • MI may be triggered by a stressful situation such as anxiety, dental phobia or pain • In the past, the recommendation was to delay dental treatment under local anaesthesia for at least 6 months after an MI episode; currently, however, most authors recommend a period of 6 weeks • Six weeks after the infarction, the patient should be treated similar to those with stable angina (see Chapter 8.2)
Criteria for referral	• In the first 6 weeks post infarction, the patient should be treated similarly to those with unstable angina: – Treatment in a hospital setting – The medical team should be consulted and available (specialists in cardiac emergencies) – Appropriate equipment and medication for emergencies should be present – Only urgent dental procedures should be provided – Anxiety control should be considered (e.g. 5 mg diazepam orally, nitrous oxide) – Prophylactic administration with sublingual nitroglycerin or intravenous coronary vasodilators should be considered – Perioperative monitoring of vital signs (oxygen saturation, blood pressure and pulse) is required
Access/position	• The appointment should be during the last hour of the morning or the first of the afternoon (endogenous epinephrine levels are higher early in the morning) • The sessions should be short (30 minutes) and relaxed • Consider a semi-recumbent position (to avoid overloading the pulmonary circulation and causing orthostatic hypotension)
Communication	• The prevalence of depression in patients who have experienced a MI is threefold higher than in the general population and may impact on communication
Consent/capacity	• In certain situations, the treatment should be performed in a hospital setting (e.g. recent infarction and highly anxious patients) • For patients who take antithrombotic agents, the consent form should include the risk of bleeding
Anaesthesia/sedation	• Local anaesthesia – Do not exceed 2 anaesthetic cartridges with epinephrine at 1:100 000 (0.04 mg) – Consider the use of anaesthetics with felypressin as it has been reported to have fewer haemodynamic effects than epinephrine; do not use in high doses as it may cause constriction of the coronary arteries – Ensure that a self-aspirating technique is used to prevent intravascular entry – If an anaesthetic with vasoconstrictor is employed, intraligamentous, intrapulpal and intraosseous techniques are contraindicated • Sedation – Consult the cardiologist – Consider medical support for administration – Diazepam or temazepam may be considered to control anxiety (may be prescribed by the doctor) A number of authors have suggested that benzodiazepines may worsen the cardiovascular condition and have proposed sedation only with nitrous oxide • General anaesthesia – Delay the treatment for at least 3 months after diagnosing the MI

(Continued)

Table 8.3.2 (Continued)

Dental treatment	• Before – Medical consultation recommended – The administration of antibiotic prophylaxis for bacterial endocarditis is not indicated – Anxiety control should be considered – Prophylaxis with sublingual nitroglycerin (0.3–0.6 mg) • During – Monitor vital signs (oxygen saturation, blood pressure and pulse) – Some patients take anticoagulant or antiplatelet drugs and therefore have a tendency to bleed during surgical procedures – Limit the use of epinephrine and avoid using vasoconstrictor-soaked thread retractors • After – Consider drug interactions if medication is to be prescribed – Provide oral and systemic health promotion instructions
Drug prescription	• Non-steroidal anti-inflammatory drugs should be used with caution and limited to 7 days (can increase the risk of another MI) • A number of antibiotics and antifungals can interact with drugs that are typically taken by patients after a MI: – Amoxicillin, metronidazole, azithromycin and clarithromycin interfere with acenocoumarol – Ampicillin reduces the serum atenolol levels – Macrolides and azole derivatives interact with statins and can cause muscle damage (rhabdomyolysis)
Education/prevention	• The dentist, as a healthcare practitioner, should participate in education to prevent a further MI (e.g. promotion of smoking cessation and nutrition counselling) • It has been suggested that there is a relationship between chronic oral infections (periodontal disease and apical periodontitis) and cardiovascular diseases such as MI • Treating the periodontal disease may improve the endothelial function of patients with a history of MI

Table 8.3.3 Clinical classification of myocardial infarction.

	Aetiopathogenesis	Diagnostic criteria
Type 1	Myocardial ischaemia due to an acute disruption of an atherosclerotic plaque (rupture or erosion)	Change in cardiac troponin levels and at least one of the following: • Symptoms of acute myocardial ischaemia • New ischaemic changes in the ECG • Appearance of pathological Q waves • Imaging tests suggestive of ischaemia • Identification of a coronary thrombus by angiography or during autopsy
Type 2	Imbalance between oxygen supply and demand that is not due to an acute disruption of an atherosclerotic plaque	Change in cardiac troponin levels and at least one of the following: • Symptoms of acute myocardial ischaemia • New ischaemic changes in the ECG • Appearance of pathological Q waves • Imaging tests suggestive of ischaemia
Type 3	High suspicion of an acute myocardial ischaemic event, with no evidence of cardiac markers	• Symptoms of myocardial ischaemia • Ischaemic changes in the ECG or ventricular fibrillation • The patient dies before blood samples are collected for cardiac markers or before these increase, or an infarction is detected in the autopsy

(Continued)

Table 8.3.3 (Continued)

	Aetiopathogenesis	Diagnostic criteria
Type 4a	Myocardial infarction caused by a percutaneous coronary intervention	An increase in cardiac troponin levels more than 5 times the 99th percentile of the upper reference limit and at least one of the following: • New ischaemic changes in the ECG • Appearance of pathological Q waves • Imaging tests suggestive of ischaemia • Angiographic findings consistent with a flow-limiting procedural complication
Type 4b	Myocardial infarction related to a stent thrombosis	Identification of a coronary thrombus by angiography or during autopsy and the same criteria for type 1
Type 4c	Myocardial infarction as the result of restenosis	Increase or reduction in cardiac troponin levels and the same criteria as for type 1
Type 5	Myocardial ischaemia during myocardial revascularisation surgery	An increase in cardiac troponin levels more than 10 times the 99th percentile of the upper reference limit and at least one of the following: • Appearance of pathological Q waves • Imaging tests suggestive of ischaemia • Angiographic findings consistent with a new occlusion of the graft or of the native coronary artery

  - Echocardiography
  - Cardiac magnetic resonance imaging (CMR)
  - Myocardial perfusion scintigraphy using positron emission tomography (PET) or single-photon emission computed tomography (SPECT) (Figure 8.3.3)
  - Coronary computed tomography angiography (CTA)

Management

- Drug management of MI in the acute phase
  - Oxygen (15 L/min in an emergency, titrating down to 2–4 L/min as the patient stabilises)
  - Nitroglycerin (0.5 mg sublingual)
  - Aspirin (160–325 mg chewed) or clopidogrel (75 mg orally)
  - Morphine (4–8 mg intramuscularly)
- Coronary flow restoration and myocardial tissue reperfusion
  - Recombinant streptokinase (thrombolytic mechanism of action via the conversion of plasminogen to plasmin; recombinant preferred to streptokinase derived from beta-haemolytic streptococci, as the latter is antigenic and associated with febrile reactions/allergic reactions)
  - Percutaneous coronary intervention (angioplasty and/or stent implantation)
  - Coronary artery bypass grafting
- Secondary drug prevention of cardiovascular events following a MI
  - Beta-blockers
  - Angiotensin-converting enzyme inhibitors
  - Angiotensin receptor blockers
  - Aldosterone antagonists
  - Statins
  - Antiplatelet agents, vitamin K antagonists and new direct oral anticoagulants
- Lifestyle recommendations for patients with a history of MI
  - Smoking cessation
  - Healthy diet
  - Moderate physical activity
  - Evaluation of psychosocial risk factors

Prognosis

- In recent decades, a significant reduction in MI mortality has been confirmed as the result of evidence-based treatment and lifestyle changes
- In the first 5 years post infarction, the relative risk of death and recurrent MI is 30% greater in patients with a history of MI than in the general population
- More than 70% of recurrences occur during the first month after the first MI
- The prognosis is significantly poorer for patients with diabetes, hypertension, peripheral arterial disease, advanced age, reduced renal function and a history of stroke

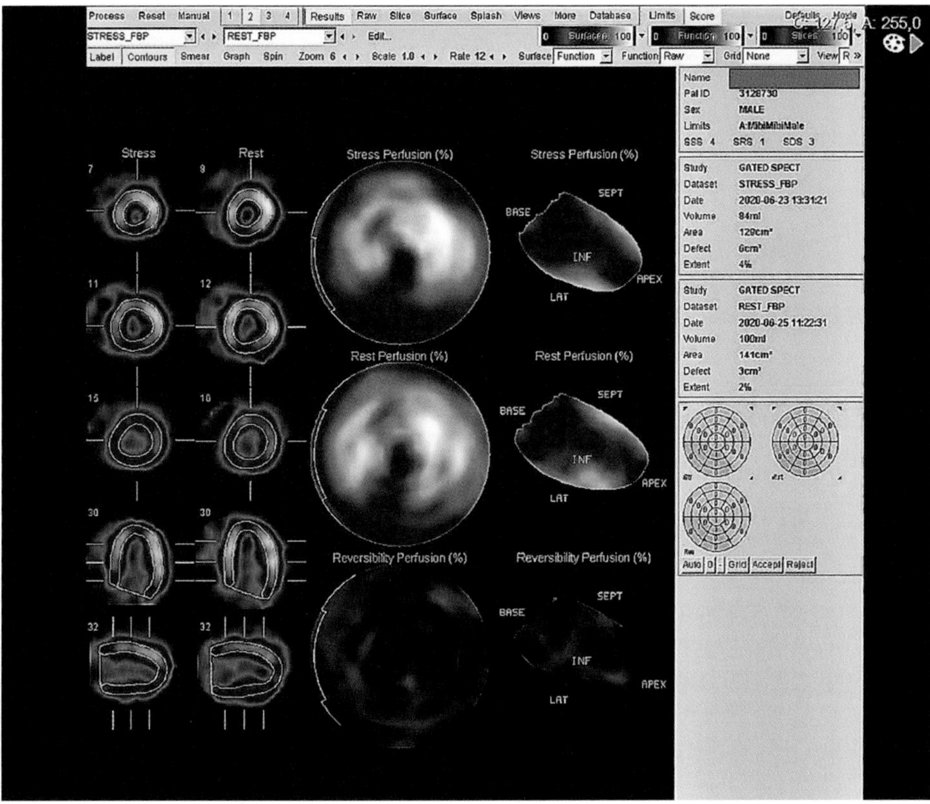

Figure 8.3.3 Myocardial perfusion single-photon emission computed tomography (SPECT) is used to assess the presence and extent of myocardial ischaemia.

A World/Transcultural View

- Acute MI is the main cause of death in developed countries and the third leading cause of death in developing countries, after AIDS and respiratory infections
- Among patients with STEMI, there is a wide regional variation in clinical profiles, hospital care and mortality
- Culturally influenced lay theories about MI have an impact on treatment compliance

Recommended Reading

Gustafsson, N., Ahlqvist, J., Näslund, U. et al. (2020). Associations among periodontitis, calcified carotid artery atheromas, and risk of myocardial infarction. *J. Dent. Res.* 99: 60–68.

Kufta, K., Saraghi, M., and Giannakopoulos, H. (2018). Cardiovascular considerations for the dental practitioner. 2. Management of cardiac emergencies. *Gen. Dent.* 66: 49–53.

Samulak-Zielińska, R., Dembowska, E., and Lizakowski, P. (2019). Dental treatment of post-myocardial infarction patients: a review of the literature. *Dent. Med. Probl.* 56: 291–298.

Singh, S., Gupta, K., Garg, K.N. et al. (2017). Dental management of the cardiovascular compromised patient: a clinical approach. *J. Young Pharm.* 9: 453–456.

Skaar, D., O'Connor, H., Lunos, S. et al. (2012). Dental procedures and risk of experiencing a second vascular event in a Medicare population. *J. Am. Dent. Assoc.* 143: 1190–1198.

Thygesen, K., Alpert, J.S., Jaffe, A.S. et al. (2018). Executive group on behalf of the Joint European Society of Cardiology (ESC)/American College of Cardiology (ACC)/American Heart Association (AHA)/World Heart Federation (WHF) task force for the universal definition of myocardial infarction. Fourth universal definition of myocardial infarction (2018). *J. Am. Coll. Cardiol.* 72: 2231–2264.

8.4 Carrier of Coronary Pacemaker

Section I: Clinical Scenario and Dental Management

Clinical Scenario

An 80-year-old male presents for an assessment appointment at your dental clinic. He is dissatisfied with his full upper denture, as he finds it unstable, particularly on eating. The patient requests implant-supported prosthetic rehabilitation and reports that other dentists have declined to provide this due to his history of heart disease.

Medical History
- Pacemaker carrier (bipolar DDD – dual chamber), implanted 1 year earlier
- Ischaemic heart disease (myocardial infarction 3 years earlier and carrier of coronary stents thereafter)
- Arterial hypertension with target organ damage
- History of prostatectomy/radiation therapy for prostate adenocarcinoma (5 years earlier)
- History of gastrectomy by duodenal ulceration (12 years earlier)

Medications
- Acetylsalicylic acid
- Bisoprolol
- Ramipril
- Furosemide
- Doxazosin
- Atorvastatin
- Pantoprazole

Dental History
- Good level of co-operation
- Irregular dental attender – only attends when he has dental problems/pain; last visit over 10 years ago to construct his current denture
- Poorly fitting removable upper denture
- Brushes the prosthesis and teeth 2–3 times a day

Social History
- Married and lives with his wife
- Both physically active with no impairment of mobility
- Attended the dental clinic with his wife
- Cognitive function unimpaired
- Ex-smoker (20 cigarettes/day until 10 years ago)
- Minimal alcohol intake (2 units a week)

Oral Examination
- Hyposalivation (the patient continuously needs to drink water)
- Significant resorption of the maxillary ridges, with limited support for the denture
- Significant accumulation of calculus on the remaining teeth
- Coronal toothwear due to attrition of #44 and #45
- Caries in #34 and #45

Radiological Examination
- Orthopantomogram undertaken (Figure 8.4.1)
- Severe atrophy of the maxilla
- Radiological signs of osteoporosis

Structured Learning

1) What factors may be contributing to the patient's dissatisfaction with his upper denture?
   - The denture is over 10 years old
   - The residual ridge (denture-bearing mucosa, submucosa and periosteum, and underlying residual alveolar bone) will have resorbed/changed shape significantly over this period, contributing to a deteriorating fit of the denture
   - The patient has a complete upper denture opposing natural teeth – this predisposes to tipping of the denture and generation of lateral forces which can result

A Practical Approach to Special Care in Dentistry, First Edition. Edited by Pedro Diz Dios and Navdeep Kumar.

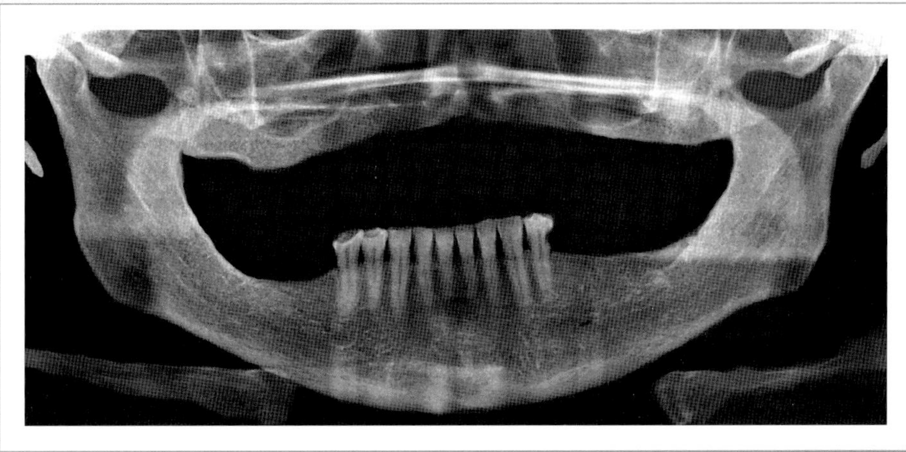

Figure 8.4.1 Orthopantomogram showing severe maxillary atrophy and radiographic features of osteoporosis.

in compression of the periosteum, disruption of vasculature and an accelerated resorptive remodelling response
- With increasing age as is the case for this patient, resorptive processes predominate over new bone formation
- Hyposalivation leading to reduced tolerance and retention of the removable denture because of thin dry atrophic mucosa and lack of a saliva film

2) What is the most likely aetiology of the hyposalivation observed in this patient?
   - Salivary dysfunction in older age is mainly a consequence of systemic diseases and medications although it also reflects reduced functional reserve and reduced fluid consumption
   - For this patient, drug-induced xerostomia is the most likely cause as the patient is taking several medications associated with this side-effect:
     - Beta-blocker (bisoprolol)
     - Angiotensin-converting enzyme inhibitor (ramipril)
     - Diuretic (furosemide)
     - Alpha-1 blocker (doxazosin)
3) Is the patient's heart disease a contraindication for prosthetic rehabilitation with dental implants?
   - Pacemakers do not represent a contraindication for inserting dental implants
   - In carriers of coronary stents, the placement of dental implants is also not contraindicated
   - However, it is advisable to liaise with the cardiologist to ensure that the patient is stable and necessary adaptations are in place prior to proceeding
4) What factors are considered important in assessing the risk of managing this patient?
   - Social
     - Elderly patient with comorbidities – although there is no apparent change in cognition, it is known that coronary heart disease/MI are associated with an increased risk of cognitive impairment or dementia
     - Informed consent must be adapted to specify the possible complications and factors that could affect the prognosis of the implants should the patient's health/cognition decline
   - Medical
     - Risk of pacemaker interference generated by electronic dental devices
     - Risk of hypertensive crisis and orthostatic hypotension episodes (see Chapter 8.1)
     - Tendency to bleed due to the antithrombotic drugs (see Chapters 8.6. and 10.5)
     - Drug selection determined by the prostatic disease and duodenal ulceration
     - Drug interactions
   - Dental
     - Reduced quality/quantity of jaw bone
     - Presence of dental/periodontal disease can contribute to dental implant failure; hence periodontal and conservative treatment is required first to stabilise the patient's oral health (may include endodontic treatment, i.e. #45)
     - History of irregular dental attendance – patient may be lost to follow-up
5) What are the considerations for performing calculus removal on the remaining teeth?
   - The patient carries a modern bipolar pacemaker (DDD)

- This will probably be resistant to the interference generated by electronic devices
- In the event of uncertainty, consult the cardiology team; if no conclusive information is obtained, it is be prudent to use manual instrumentation

6) What antibiotic prophylaxis regimen for bacterial endocarditis would you recommend for this patient?
   - Neither having a pacemaker nor having a coronary stent is considered an indication for endocarditis prophylaxis
7) What are the considerations for prescribing an analgesic to this patient?
   - A number of non-steroidal anti-inflammatory drugs can reduce the antihypertensive effect of beta-blockers (e.g. bisoprolol) and angiotensin-converting enzyme inhibitors (e.g. ramipril)
   - Non-steroidal anti-inflammatory drugs should also be administered with caution to patients with a history of gastroduodenal ulceration; the risk of recurrence and gastrointestinal haemorrhage is greater when these drugs are administered concomitantly with acetylsalicylic acid
   - Metamizole can reduce the antithrombotic effect of acetylsalicylic acid
   - Codeine and other opioid agonists should be avoided in patients with prostatic disease, because they can cause urinary retention and oliguria

General Dental Considerations

Oral Findings

- No oral findings have been reported specifically related to electronic cardiovascular implantable devices
- These patients might have oral lesions due to the adverse effects of the antihypertensive (see Table 8.1.1) or antiarrhythmic medication (Table 8.4.1)

Table 8.4.1 Main oral adverse effects of antiarrhythmic drugs.

Class	Adverse effects
I. Sodium channel blockers (e.g. procainamide)	• White patches and/or ulcers (lupus-like disease) • Xerostomia • Dysgeusia • Lichenoid reactions • Ulcers (agranulocytosis)
II. Beta-blockers (e.g. propranolol)	• Xerostomia • Dysgeusia • Lichenoid reactions • Oedema • Ulcers (agranulocytosis)
III. Potassium channel blockers (e.g. amiodarone)	• Sialorrhoea • Xerostomia • Dysgeusia • Oedema • Grey orofacial/oral mucosal pigmentation (amiodarone)
IV. Calcium channel blockers (e.g. nifedipine)	• Gingival enlargement • Xerostomia • Dysgeusia
V. Others (e.g. digoxin)	• Ptyalism • Xerostomia • Oedema

Dental Management

- Some electronic dental devices can generate interference in pacemakers, although this complication is increasingly rare
- Dental procedures should be performed taking into account the antithrombotic therapy and antiarrhythmic agents (Table 8.4.2)

Section II: Background Information and Guidelines

Definition

An artificial pacemaker is an electronic device designed to generate electrical impulses to stimulate the heart when normal or physiological stimulation fails. Once generated, these impulses require a conductive lead (transvenous

Table 8.4.2 Considerations for dental management.

Risk assessment	• Dental treatment should be delayed by at least 6 months from the implantation of the device to ensure that the cardiac function has stabilised and to avoid the risk of infection around the pacing leads • Antibiotic prophylaxis is not necessary for the prevention of infective endocarditis • The most severe potential complication for patients who carry a pacemaker is the interference generated by electronic dental devices – Classically, the device with the greatest risk has been the electrocautery/thermocoagulator – Ultrasonic scaling equipment, electronic apex locators, electric pulp vitality testers and electronic dental analgesia units have also been considered potentially dangerous • Modern implantable devices are resistant to changes in the electromagnetic field – Although few in vivo studies have been published on the subject, none of these articles have shown that the tested electronic dental instruments interfere with pacemaker function – The risk is lower with bipolar pacemakers – In exceptional cases, the frequency modulation can be deprogrammed during the dental sessions
Criteria for referral	• Dental treatment should be conducted in a hospital environment if the pacemaker activity is irregular and/or the patient's cardiac status is poor • Consulting the cardiologist/doctor is advisable when: – The pacemaker has been implanted for less than 6 months – The device details are unknown in terms of the risk of electromagnetic field generation – Multiple/long sessions of invasive dentistry are planned – The severity and stability of the patient's medical condition are unknown – There are severe comorbidities and/or antecedents (e.g. myocardial infarction)
Access/position	• The appointment should be scheduled for the last hour of the morning or the first of the afternoon (endogenous epinephrine levels are higher early in the morning) • The sessions should be short and relaxed
Communication	• Patients who carry a permanent pacemaker, especially those with a cardioverter-defibrillator, can experience chronic anxiety due to fear that the device will fail • They may have an information card which provides details of the device – this should be brought to the dental appointment in order to help assess the risk generated by electronic dental devices
Consent/capacity	• The consent form should indicate the risk that electronic dental devices can generate interference for pacemakers • Patients who take antithrombotic agents should be advised about the possibility of excessive bleeding
Anaesthesia/sedation	• Local anaesthesia – Do not exceed 2 anaesthetic cartridges with epinephrine at 1:100 000 (0.04 mg) • Sedation – May be helpful to reduce anxiety/cardiac effort (e.g. nitrous oxide) • General anaesthesia – A comprehensive preoperative evaluation should be conducted with the anaesthetist and cardiologist

(Continued)

Table 8.4.2 (Continued)

Dental treatment	• Before – Conventional/digital radiographs and computed tomography (including cone beam computed tomography) do not cause interference – Standard lead protection provides greater shielding for pacemakers – Magnetic resonance is contraindicated except for patients with pacemakers compatible with magnetic resonance imaging (MRI conditional) – Antibiotic prophylaxis has been proposed if an emergency dental procedure needs to be performed within the first 6 months after pacemaker implantation • During – Perioperative monitoring should be considered (heart rate and blood pressure) – If there is no confirmed information on the pacemaker's characteristics, avoid using the electrocautery and other electronic dental devices that could potentially cause interference – Keep electronic dental devices at least 15 cm away from the generator and avoid passing the devices over the area where the generator is inserted – Install the grounding pads as far as possible from pacemakers – Short exposure times are recommended, and repeatedly power cycling of the dental instrumentation should be avoided – Some patients keep a magnet to interrupt the pacemaker activity in case of interference – Patients taking anticoagulant or antiplatelet drugs have a tendency to bleed during surgical procedures – Avoid using vasoconstrictor-soaked thread retractors • After – Consider drug interactions
Drug prescription	• A number of non-steroidal anti-inflammatory drugs can interact with drugs that are typically taken by patients with pacemakers – Ibuprofen, diclofenac and naproxen interfere with acenocoumarol (see Chapter 10.3) – Ibuprofen, diclofenac and naproxen can cause digoxin toxicity • A number of antibiotics can interact with drugs that are typically taken by patients with pacemakers – Amoxicillin, metronidazole, azithromycin and clarithromycin interfere with acenocoumarol (see Chapter 10.3) – Amoxicillin/clavulanic acid and azithromycin can cause digoxin toxicity
Education/prevention	• Electric toothbrushes are considered safe • The recommendation is to keep ultrasonic toothbrushes more than 2.5 cm away from pacemaker generators and more than 15 cm from their battery charger • The dentist, as a healthcare practitioner, should participate in education to prevent further cardiac disease (e.g. smoking cessation) • The important of regular dental visits and good oral hygiene to minimise the need for dental treatment should be emphasised

electrocatheter) that terminates at an electrode attached to the myocardium.

It is currently estimated that more than 4 million individuals worldwide carry a pacemaker or other cardiac rhythm control device.

Mechanism of Action

- Normal cardiac activity commences in the sinus node, whose cells act as a biological pacemaker; the electrical wave passes through the atrium, reaching the atrioventricular node; through the His–Purkinje system, the wave extends rapidly and depolarises the ventricles
- When the intrinsic cardiac automaticity or conduction system fails, a small external electrical stimulus can trigger a group of myocytes, which leads to the depolarisation of the neighbouring myocytes and the subsequent propagation of an electrical wavefront,

which in turn causes almost simultaneous muscle contraction

- Pacemakers can provide this external electrical stimulation

Indications

- Pacemakers were initially designed to prevent catastrophic bradycardia caused by:
  - The sinus node's inability to produce a sufficient number of impulses per minute (sick sinus syndrome)
  - Impulse conduction failure from the atrioventricular node to the myocardium
- The indications for pacemaker placement have since expanded to include the following:
  - Sinus node dysfunction (e.g. sinus bradycardia)
  - Acquired atrioventricular conduction disease (e.g. atrioventricular block)
  - Neurocardiogenic syncope (e.g. carotid sinus hypersensitivity)
  - Neuromuscular disease (e.g. muscular dystrophy)
  - Congestive heart failure (e.g. impaired ventricular function)

Types of Pacemakers

- Based on temporality
  - Temporary pacemakers (transcutaneous or transesophageal)
  - Definitive pacemakers (epicardial or endocavitary)
- Based on the number of cavities the pacemaker stimulates
  - Single-chamber (a single electrode placed in the atrium)
  - Dual-chamber (an electrode placed in the atrium and another in the ventricle)
- Based on the type of electrode
  - Endocardial
  - Epicardial
- In recent years, leadless pacemakers have successfully been developed for clinical use (wireless technology lowers the risk of infection and reduces the recovery time after placement)
- New generations of battery-less pacemakers are currently being tested; some of these pacemakers take advantage of the heart's mechanical movement to generate current while others, known as biological pacemakers, provide automaticity to myocytes through gene therapy techniques
- The particular characteristics of each pacemaker are described using a 5-letter code; the most common combinations are AAI, VVI and DDD (Table 8.4.3; Figure 8.4.2)
- An implantable cardioverter defibrillator (ICD) is a device similar to a pacemaker, but its main function is to send a larger electrical shock to the heart that essentially 'reboots' it to get it pumping again; some devices

Table 8.4.3 Pacemaker coding system. (North American Society of Pacing and Electrophysiology/British Pacing Group)

Position I	Position II	Position III
Heart chamber(s) paced	Heart chamber(s) sensed	Response to sensing
0 - None	0 - None	0 - None
A - Atrium	A - Atrium	T - Triggered
V - Ventricle	V - Ventricle	I - Inhibited
D - Dual (A+V)	D - Dual (A+V)	D - Dual (T+I)

Position IV	Position V
Programmability	Antitachycardia pacing
0 - None	0 - None
P - Programmable	P - Rhythm
M - Multiprogrammable	S - Shock
C - Communicating (telemetry)	D - Dual (P+S)
R - Response rate	

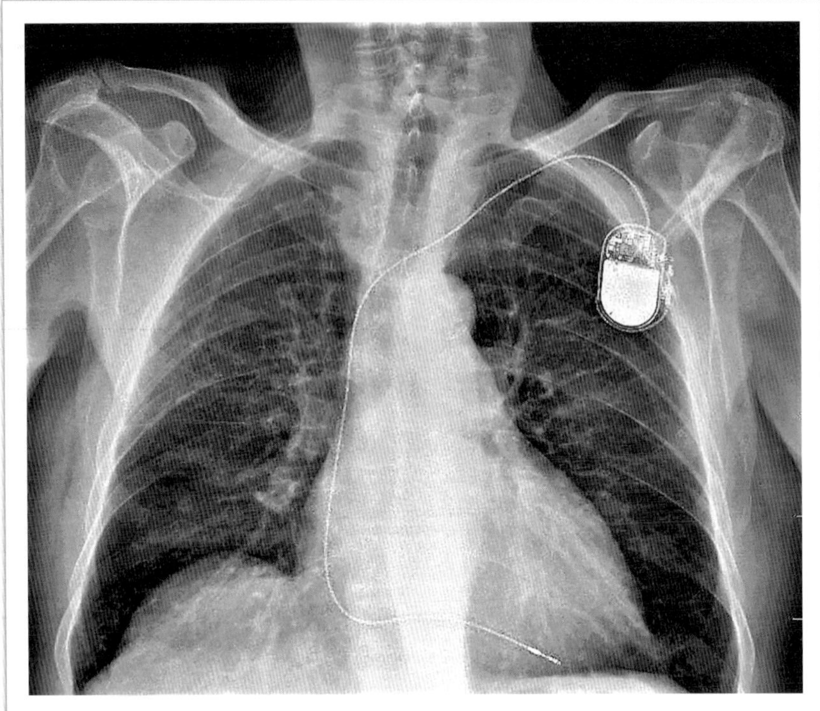

Figure 8.4.2 Heart pacemaker (VVI) on chest x-ray.

contain both a pacemaker and an ICD; conventionally, an ICD has a pacing lead that is implanted along a vein (transvenously), although newer versions have a pacing lead implanted under the skin (subcutaneously) (Figure 8.4.3)

Complications

- The complication rate following placement of a pacemaker is 1–6%, and complications are classified as immediate, intermediate and delayed
- Immediate complications
  - Pneumothorax
  - Haemothorax
  - Haematoma at the device insertion site
  - Cardiac perforation
  - Electrode displacement
- Intermediate complications
  - Device infection
  - Thrombosis or venous stenosis
  - Pain at the device insertion site
  - Mechanical disruption of the tricuspid valve with regurgitation
  - Discomfort with ventricular stimulation
- Delayed complications
  - Electrode fracture
  - Breakage of the insulation that covers the electrocatheter
  - Increase in the stimulation threshold or impedance due to tissue growth or device infection
- Several types of devices and machinery may interfere with ICDs and pacemakers due to electromagnetic interference; the impact depends on the type of device:
  - Microwave diathermy
  - MRI (some ICDs/pacemakers will allow this investigation – check with the physician)
  - Acupuncture with electrical stimulus
  - Cardioversion
  - Electrocautery
  - Electroconvulsive therapy
  - Electrolysis
  - Endoscopic procedures (e.g. colonoscopy or gastroscopy)
  - Hyperbaric therapy
  - Iontophoresis
  - Interferential current therapy

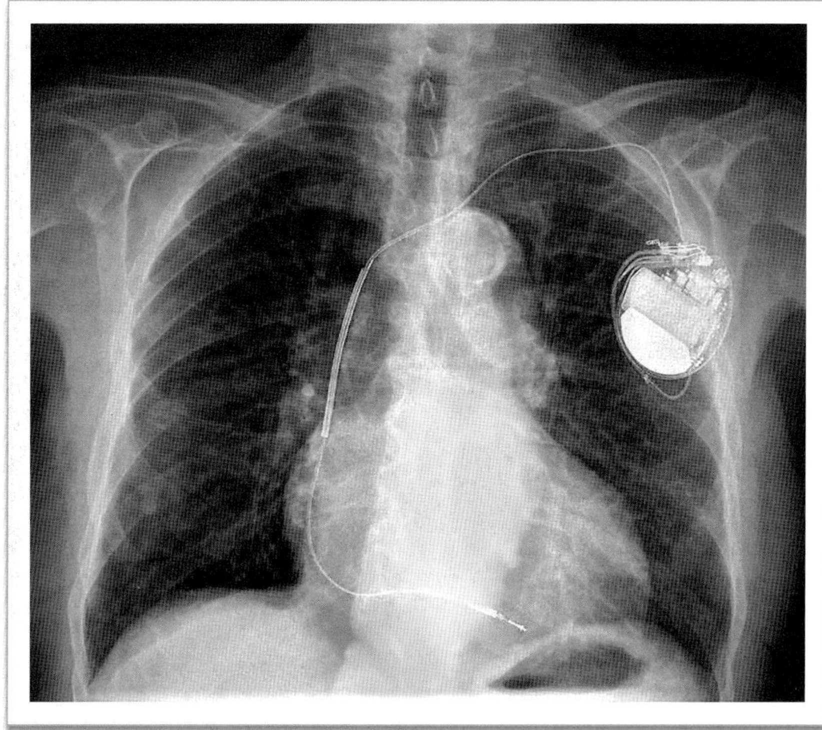

Figure 8.4.3 Implantable cardioverter-defibrillator with 1 lead and 2 shock coils.

- Laser/femtosecond laser in situ keratomileusis (LASIK) for eye surgery
- Lithotripsy
- Radiation therapy
- Radiofrequency ablation
- Therapeutic ultrasound
- Transcutaneous electrical nerve stimulation (TENS)
  Transurethral prostate therapy

Prognosis

- Long-term follow-up is required after pacemaker placement and can be every 3–12 months depending on the type
- Most pacemaker batteries last for 6–10 years; changing the batteries involves replacing the pacemaker box with a new unit; this is usually a simple procedure and may not require an overnight stay in hospital
- The mortality rate for pacemaker carriers is 20% at 3 years and 30% at 5 years
- Among other factors, the prognosis is poorer for elderly patients at the time the device is implanted and for male patients

A World/Transcultural View

- It is estimated that 1–2 million individuals die every year due to lack of access to ICDs or pacemakers
- Despite the medical, legal, cultural and ethical controversies that the postmortem reuse of pacemakers entails, it has been shown that these pacemakers are safe and effective; this option could be worth considering, especially for low-income countries

Recommended Reading

College of Dental Hygienists of Ontario (2016). CDHO Advisory cardiac implantable electronic devices. www.cdho.org/Advisories/CDHO_Factsheet_Cardiac_Implantable_Electronic_Devices.pdf

Conde-Mir, I., Miranda-Rius, J., Trucco, E. et al. (2018). In-vivo compatibility between pacemakers and dental equipment. *Eur. J. Oral Sci.* 126: 307–315.

Mulpuru, S.K., Madhavan, M., McLeod, C.J. et al. (2017). Cardiac pacemakers: function, troubleshooting, and management: part 1 of a 2-part series. *J. Am. Coll. Cardiol.* 69: 189–210.

Puette, J.A., Malek, R., and Ellison, M.B. (2020). Pacemaker. www.statpearls.com/.

Riley, A.D. (2018). Treatment planning and dental technology for patients with implanted cardiac devices. *Gen. Dent.* 66: 56–60.

Tom, J. (2016). Management of patients with cardiovascular implantable electronic devices in dental, oral, and maxillofacial surgery. *Anesth. Prog.* 63: 95–104.

Verma, N. and Knight, B.P. (2019). Update in cardiac pacing. *Arrhythmia Electrophysiol. Rev.* 8: 228–233.

8.5 Carrier of Valvular Prosthesis

Section I: Clinical Scenario and Dental Considerations

Clinical Scenario

An 80-year-old male presents for a dental appointment complaining of a 2-week history of pain from his lower left first molar tooth, which he reports is worse on chewing. The patient had root canal treatment undertaken for this tooth 2 years earlier following similar symptoms.

Medical History

- History of double aortic and mitral lesion (stenosis and insufficiency) of rheumatic fever aetiology
- Mechanical prosthetic valves (aortic and mitral) implanted 5 years earlier
- Chronic atrial fibrillation
- Arterial hypertension with target organ damage
- Dyslipidaemia
- History of bladder cancer (surgical resection 8 years earlier)
- History of cataract surgery

Medications

- Acenocoumarol
- Digoxin
- Bisoprolol
- Furosemide
- Spironolactone
- Rosuvastatin

Dental History

- Good level of co-operation
- Attends the dentist only when there is a problem (the last attendance was 2 years ago)
- Brushes his teeth 3 times a day

Social History

- Widowed; lives with his daughter
- Frail/unable to attend appointments without an escort (usually his daughter)
- Ex-smoker (10 cigarettes/day until 15 years ago); alcohol, nil

Oral Examination

- Good oral hygiene
- Generalised dental attrition
- Missing teeth: #15 and #46
- Periodontal pocket mesial aspect #36 (9 mm), with pain on percussion

Radiological Examination

- Long cone periapical radiograph undertaken of #36 (Figure 8.5.1)
- Root canal treatment in tooth #36; mesial radiolucent lesion suggestive of osteolysis due to radicular fracture (Figure 8.5.2)

Structured Learning

1) The patient reports he has been feeling particularly tired over the last 5 days, and thinks he may have had a raised temperature, although this is not always present. Why is this of particular concern?
   - This patient is at risk of infective endocarditis (IE)
   - There is a confirmed dental infection (#36) which could lead to bacteraemia and the development of IE
   - A low-grade, often intermittent fever is present in up to 90% of patients who develop IE
   - Without treatment, IE may be fatal in approximately 30% of individuals
2) What would you do in response to your concerns?
   - Ensure that you check the patient's temperature
   - Check for other signs of IE
     - Heart murmurs (85%)
     - One or more classic signs (50%)
       - Petechiae – common but nonspecific finding

A Practical Approach to Special Care in Dentistry, First Edition. Edited by Pedro Diz Dios and Navdeep Kumar.

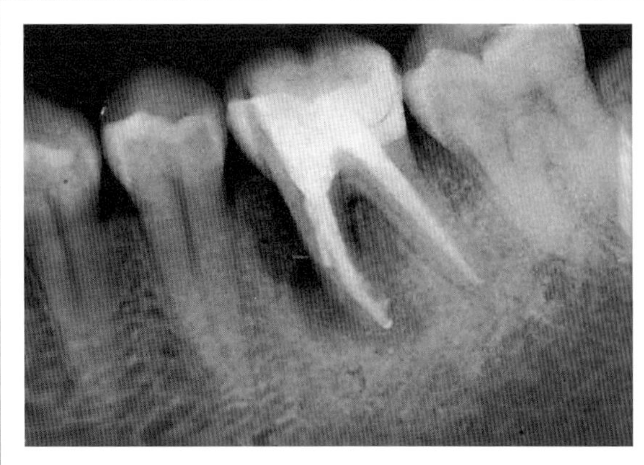

Figure 8.5.1 Periapical radiograph showing radiolucent lesion related to #36.

- Splinter haemorrhages – dark red linear lesions on the nailbeds
- Osler nodes – tender subcutaneous nodules on the distal pads of the digits
- Janeway lesions – non-tender maculae on the palms and soles
- Roth spots – retinal haemorrhages with small, clear centres
- Signs of embolic phenomena
- Haematuria
- Cerebrovascular occlusion

- Signs of congestive heart failure
- Signs of immune complex formation such as vasculitis, arthritis and renal damage

- Contact the cardiologist for urgent review and further investigations (e.g. ECG, echocardiography, blood culture); explain that there is evidence of an infected tooth
- Antibiotics should be prescribed in close liaison with the cardiologist (the patient may receive these from the cardiologist or intravenously if admitted to hospital)

3) The patient is seen by the cardiologist who confirms that the patient does not have any evidence of IE but asks you to remove any source of oral infection urgently. What factors are considered important in assessing the risk of managing this patient?
   - Social
     - Frail – requires an escort who can bring him to the appointment and also look after him on discharge
   - Medical
     - Dental treatment can trigger the onset of prosthetic valves IE
     - Risk of a hypertensive crisis during dental treatment and orthostatic hypotension (see Chapter 8.1)
     - Tendency to bleed due to the acenocoumarol (see Chapter 10.3), arterial hypertension (see Chapter 8.1) and/or digoxin-induced thrombocytopenia
     - Drug interactions mainly with acenocoumarol, digoxin and/or antihypertensive agents
   - Dental
     - The dental treatment proposed is to extract #36 – this is an invasive procedure associated with a higher risk of bacteraemia/bleeding
     - History of irregular dental attendance - the patient may be lost to follow-up

4) Before the appointment for the surgical treatment, you request an INR (international normalised ratio) test as the patient is taking acenocoumarol daily. The test is undertaken the day before the procedure and the result reported as 1.8. What would be your approach?

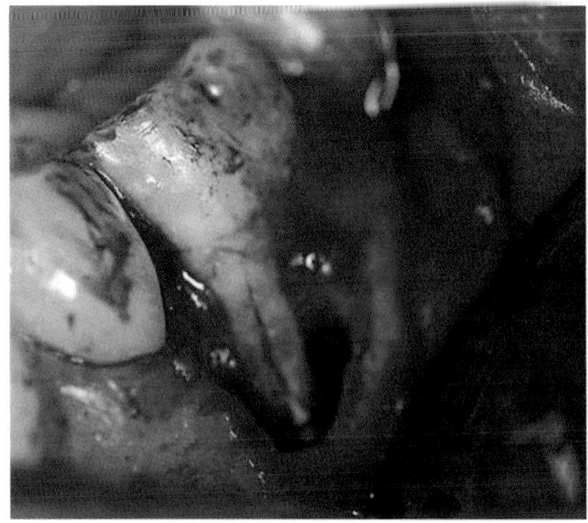
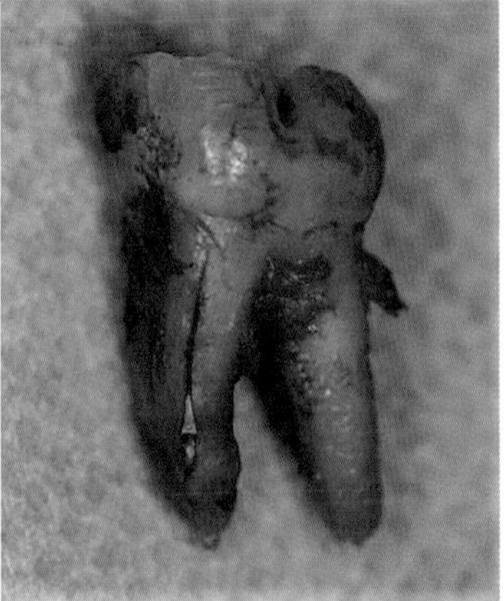

Figure 8.5.2 Exploratory surgery confirmed the radiological suggestion of radicular fracture. As a consequence, dental extraction was undertaken.

- From the dental viewpoint, clinically significant increased bleeding is not expected (see Chapter 10.3) and the surgical procedure can proceed
- However, the patient is considered at high thromboembolic risk, because he has a mechanical mitral prosthesis and an aortic prosthesis, with additional risk due to atrial fibrillation; accordingly, the recommendation is a target INR of 3.0 (range 2.5–3.5)
- The patient should be referred to his anticoagulation clinic/physician for adjustment of the anticoagulant therapy

5) When prescribing antibiotics for bacterial endocarditis prophylaxis, what factors should you consider for this patient?
   - Courses of amoxicillin, azithromycin and clarithromycin increase the bleeding tendency in patients receiving acenocoumarol, although this has not been confirmed following a single antibiotic dose
   - Clarithromycin interacts with digoxin, increasing its concentration
   - Clindamycin does not interact with acenocoumarol or digoxin
   - Although in general no specific modifications in the pharmacotherapy of antibiotics are needed for the healthy geriatric patient, this patient is frail with multiple comorbidities and should be advised to report any side-effects as soon as possible
     - Gastrointestinal symptoms such as pseudomembranous colitis are an important complication of antibiotic therapy in the elderly; although many antibiotics may be implicated, certain drugs such as clindamycin, broad-spectrum penicillins and second- and third-generation cephalosporins are most often reported to trigger symptoms
     - Increased susceptibility to adverse drug reactions and drug interactions associated with antimicrobial therapy (e.g. age-related physiological decline in kidney function, coupled with the severe renal effects associated with congestive heart failure and hypertension, substantially influences the excretion of several antibiotics)

6) The patient copes well with dental extraction of #36 with no signs of anxiety. However, when you raise the dental chair to the upright position the patient starts to faint. What could be the cause and what would you do?
   - The faintness could be linked to an episode of drug-induced orthostatic hypotension – the patient is taking furosemide (diuretic) and bisoprolol (beta-blocker)
   - Appropriate action includes:
     - Laying the patient back in the chair in the supine position until the symptoms subside
     - Determine the blood pressure with the patient lying down
     - Raise the chair up slowly in stages
     - Retake the blood pressure during the first 3 minutes standing; in most cases, there will be a reduction in systolic blood pressure ≥20 mmHg and/or a reduction in diastolic blood pressure ≥10 mmHg
     - If 2 episodes on different weeks are recorded, the recommendation is to consult the physician

7) What can you do to prevent a further episode of orthostatic hypotension during subsequent dental treatment sessions?
   - Avoid scheduling appointments for postprandial periods, especially those after large meals
   - The dental chair's backrest should not be inclined more than 45°
   - Perform changes in position in gradual stages
   - Cross the legs to increase the tolerance to orthostatism (standing up)

8) What should be the first choice for an analgesic for this patient?
   - Paracetamol at dosages that do not exceed 2 g/day is recommended
   - Non-steroidal anti-inflammatory drugs can impair the antihypertensive effect of beta-adrenergic blockers (bisoprolol) and diuretics (furosemide and spironolactone)
   - Some non-steroidal anti-inflammatory drugs increase the risk of bleeding by interacting with acenocoumarol, and some can increase the risk of digoxin poisoning
   - Selective anti-inflammatory cyclo-oxygenase-2 inhibitors (e.g. rofecoxib and celecoxib) can boost the action of acenocoumarol and are contraindicated for patients with heart problems

General Dental Considerations

Oral Findings

- No oral findings have been reported specifically related to prosthetic heart valves
- These patients might have oral lesions due to the adverse effects of antithrombotic drugs (see Chapters 10.3 and 10.5) and other drugs such as antihypertensives (see Chapter 8.1)

Dental Management

- The main preventable risks of dental treatment of these patients are bleeding as the result of antithrombotic drugs and the onset of IE (Table 8.5.1)

Table 8.5.1 Considerations for dental management.

Risk assessment	• Before valve replacement surgery – It has been suggested that any sources of oral infection should be removed in the preoperative period of cardiovascular surgery, as neglected mouths can result in increased morbidity and mortality – However, the effectiveness of dental treatment in improving cardiovascular outcomes has not been confirmed • After valve replacement surgery – Increased risk of endocarditis (delay dental treatment by 6 months) – Tendency to bleed due to antithrombotic drugs
Criteria for referral	• A prior medical consultation is required if a dental procedure needs to be performed within the first 6 months after placement of a valvular prosthesis • For urgent treatments (e.g. dental trauma) in anticoagulated patients with INR >4.0, it is preferable to refer them to a hospital setting
Access/position	• Anticoagulated patients should be treated in the morning, at the start of the working week, in case they have copious bleeding/complications that require emergency care • If the patient is taking antihypertensive drugs, keep the chair semi-reclined to prevent orthostatic hypotension
Consent/capacity	• Patients should be informed of the advantages and disadvantages of antibiotic prophylaxis for infective endocarditis and the decision should be well documented • For patients who take antithrombotic agents, the consent form should include the risk of bleeding
Anaesthesia/sedation	• Local anaesthesia – It is advisable not to exceed a dose of 0.04 mg of epinephrine (approximately 2 cartridges at a concentration of 1:100 000) – Intraligamentary injections should not be performed (increased risk of bacteraemia) • Sedation – Liaise with the cardiologist to ensure cardiac function is stable – Nitrous oxide or diazepam may be employed – The use of hydroxyzine is not recommended • General anaesthesia – Consult the cardiologist – Risk of infective endocarditis and bleeding (e.g. due to endotracheal intubation manoeuvres)
Dental treatment	• Before – The consensus recommendation is to administer antibiotic prophylaxis against infective endocarditis for high-risk dental procedures (those that require manipulating the gingival or periapical region of the teeth or perforating the oral mucosa) in patients with prosthetic valves (including transcatheter valves), with valve repairs using prosthetic material or with prior episodes of endocarditis – The effectiveness of antimicrobial rinses has not been definitively proven (although it may be recommended in terms of risk/benefit) • During – Cardiac monitoring (pulse and blood pressure) – Tendency to bleed during a surgical procedure due to anticoagulants or antiplatelet drugs • After – Monitor postoperatively – Ensure that the patient is alert to any signs/symptoms of infective endocarditis and is able to contact the dental team/doctor urgently if these arise – Consider drug interactions

(Continued)

Table 8.5.1 (Continued)

Drug prescription	• Avoid drugs that interfere with the antithrombotic drugs (see Chapters 10.3 and 10.5)
Education/prevention	• Patients should be educated about the importance of oral hygiene to reduce not only the incidence of bacteraemia from daily activities, but also the need for dental treatment and related risk of complications secondary to dental intervention • The importance of regular dental care and reviews should be emphasised

- IE is a rare but dangerous infection of the endocardial surface of the heart:
  - Platelets and fibrin deposits accumulate at endothelial sites where there is turbulent blood flow (non-bacterial thrombotic endocarditis) to produce sterile 'vegetations'
  - If there is a subsequent bacteraemia, these sterile 'vegetations' can readily be infected
  - Causative organisms include oral pathogens such as viridans group streptococci (~10–30%)
- Antibiotic prophylaxis (AP) (Table 8.5.2)
  - For over 50 years AP was given to patients at risk of IE undergoing dental procedures
  - However, between 2007 and 2009, the European Society for Cardiology (ESC), American Heart Association/American College of Cardiology (AHA/ACC) and the National Institute for Health and Care Excellence (NICE) recommended restriction of AP to varying degrees
  - The rationale for relative or total AP restriction was based on the lack of evidence regarding the efficacy of AP for prevention of IE, an acknowledgement that dental procedures as a cause of IE remained in doubt when bacteraemia levels were compared to those generated by events such as toothbrushing, and the concern that overuse of antibiotics could lead to resistance and/or anaphylaxis
  - In Europe and the US, there was relative AP restriction to those at highest risk (e.g. patients with previous

Table 8.5.2 Antimicrobial prophylaxis for preventing infective endocarditis before dental procedures (see original guidelines for other alternative regimens).

2007 - updated 2021 American Heart Association Guidelines	2015 European Society of Cardiology Guidelines	2008 – revised 2016 National Institute of Clinical Excellence (NICE) UK Implementation advice from the Scottish Dental Clinical Effectiveness Programme (SDCEP) 2018 endorsed by NICE (CG64)
	Patients who require antimicrobial prophylaxis	
• Prosthetic cardiac valve or prosthetic material used for valve repair • Previous endocarditis • Congenital heart disease – Unrepaired cyanotic congenital heart disease, including palliative shunts and conduits – Completely repaired congenital heart defects with prosthetic material or device whether placed by surgery or catheter intervention during the first 6 months after the procedure – Repaired congenital heart disease with residual defects at the site or adjacent to the site of a prosthetic patch or prosthetic device • Cardiac transplantation recipients who develop cardiac valvulopathy	• Any prosthetic valve, including transcatheter valve, or those in whom any prosthetic material was used for cardiac valve repair • Previous endocarditis • Congenital heart disease – Any type of cyanotic congenital heart disease – Any type of congenital heart disease repaired with a prosthetic material, whether placed surgically or by percutaneous techniques, up to 6 months after the procedure or lifelong if residual shunt or valvular regurgitation remains after the procedure	• Antibiotic prophylaxis against infective endocarditis is not recommended *routinely* for people undergoing dental procedures • 'Routinely' was added to NICE guideline in 2016 to add emphasis on NICE's standard advice on healthcare professionals' responsibilities; doctors and dentists should offer the most appropriate treatment options, in consultation with the patient and/or their carer or guardian • SDCEP: patients who should be given 'special consideration' are those who require antimicrobial prophylaxis according to the 2015 European Society of Cardiology Guidelines (see left column)

(Continued)

Table 8.5.2 (Continued)

2007 - updated 2021 American Heart Association Guidelines	2015 European Society of Cardiology Guidelines	2008 – revised 2016 National Institute of Clinical Excellence (NICE) UK Implementation advice from the Scottish Dental Clinical Effectiveness Programme (SDCEP) 2018 endorsed by NICE (CG64)
Recommended antibiotic prophylaxis regimen for those not allergic to penicillin		
• Amoxicillin 2 g orally[a] 30–60 mins before the procedure • Amoxicillin dose for children, 50 mg/kg orally	• Amoxicillin 2 g orally[a] 30–60 mins before the procedure • Amoxicillin dose for children, 50 mg/kg orally	• Amoxicillin 3 g orally[c] (1 sachet) 60 minutes before procedure (3 g prophylactic dose) • Amoxicillin dose for children 6 months – 17 years, 50 mg/kg orally; maximum dose 3 g (prophylactic dose)
Recommended antibiotic prophylaxis regimen for those allergic to penicillin		
• Clindamycin 600 mg orally[b] 30–60 mins before the procedure • Clindamycin dose for children, 20 mg/kg orally • Azithromycin 500 mg orally 30–60 mins before the procedure • Clarithromycin 500 mg orally 30–60 mins before the procedure • Azithromycin and Clarithromycin dose for children, 15 mg/kg orally • Doxycycline 100 mg orally • Doxycycline dose for children, 4.4 mg/kg orally	• Clindamycin 600 mg orally[b] 30–60 mins before the procedure • Clindamycin dose for children, 20 mg/kg orally	• Clindamycin 600 mg orally[c] 60 mins before the procedure • Clindamycin dose for children 6 months–17 years, 20 mg/kg; maximum dose 600 mg (prophylactic dose) • In patients who are allergic to penicillin and unable to swallow capsules, an appropriate oral regimen is azithromycin 500 mg oral suspension 60 mins before the procedure (500 mg prophylactic dose) • Azithromycin dose for children 6 months–11 years, 12 mg/kg; maximum dose 500 mg • Azithromycin dose for children 12–17 years, 500 mg (prophylactic dose)

[a] Unable to take oral medication: ampicillin 2 g intravenous or intramuscular.
[b] Unable to take oral medication: clindamycin 600 mg intravenous or intramuscular.
[c] Unable to take oral medication: amoxicillin 1 g intravenous just before the procedure; dose for children 6 months–17 years, 50 mg/kg (maximum dose 1 g). If allergic to penicillin, clindamycin 300 mg intravenous just before the procedure; dose for children 6 months–17 years, 20 mg/kg (maximum dose 300 mg).

IE, congenital heart disease and rheumatic heart disease, and selected heart transplant recipients) undergoing high-risk dental procedures
  - In the UK, NICE advised against use of AP entirely but updated this advice in July 2016 to state that antibiotics should not routinely be recommended as prophylaxis for dental procedures
- Good oral hygiene and regular dental care remain essential in patients at risk of IE

Section II: Background Information and Guidelines

Definition

The force generated by myocardial contraction propels the blood flow towards the systemic and pulmonary circulation. Myocardial relaxation causes a reduction in pressure that promotes retrograde blood flow. The presence of heart valves that open and close due to these pressure changes prevents the generation of retrograde flow. If a cardiac valve becomes diseased or damaged, resulting in stenosis (incomplete opening of the valve orifice) or regurgitation (incomplete closure of the valve orifice), a replacement valve can be used to correct the haemodynamic impairment and improve quality of life. It is estimated that more than 300 000 prosthetic cardiac valves are implanted annually worldwide.

Aetiology of Valvular Disease

- Rheumatic fever
  - Most common cause in low-income countries
  - An acute systemic inflammatory condition characterised by fever and arthritis 2–4 weeks after pharyngitis caused by certain strains of beta-haemolytic streptococci

- Some patients develop antibodies to the streptococcal cell wall which cause vasculitis and inflammatory lesions of the joints, skin and nervous system, and sometimes the heart (rheumatic carditis)
- Major features of rheumatic disease include polyarthritis, carditis (commonly the mitral valve is affected), skin-subcutaneous nodules or erythema marginatum, Sydenham chorea (St. Vitus dance/involuntary movements)
- Minor features include fever and arthralgia

- Congenital valve defects
- Age-related degenerative lesions

Mechanism of Action of Cardiac Valvular Prostheses

- Mitral and tricuspid valves prevent retrograde flow towards the atrium during systole
- Aortic and pulmonary valves (semilunar) prevent retrograde flow from the great arteries towards the ventricles during diastole
- It is important to note that the placement of a cardiac valve replacement never completely recovers the natural haemodynamics of the native heart valve

Types of Valvular Prosthesis

- Mechanical valves (Figure 8.5.3)
  - Long-lasting but require the lifelong administration of anticoagulants
  - There are 3 basic models:
    - Two semicircular leaflets that pivot in a support ring. These are the most widely used at present; most of these valves are manufactured with pyrolytic carbon covering a titanium and/or graphite core
    - A metal or silicone ball that floats inside a cage-like structure
    - A metal disc that oscillates to allow or impede the blood flow
- Biological valves (Figure 8.5.4)
  - Limited durability – in many cases, they need to be replaced within 10–15 years
  - Main advantage is that in patients without established risk factors, they do not require antithrombotic drugs after the first 3 months
  - These valves can have a nonhuman or human origin:
    - Bioprosthesis of nonhuman origin (xenograft), created from an aortic valve or porcine or bovine pericardial tissue; can be mounted on a metal or polymer support or have no support and attach directly to the native valve ring

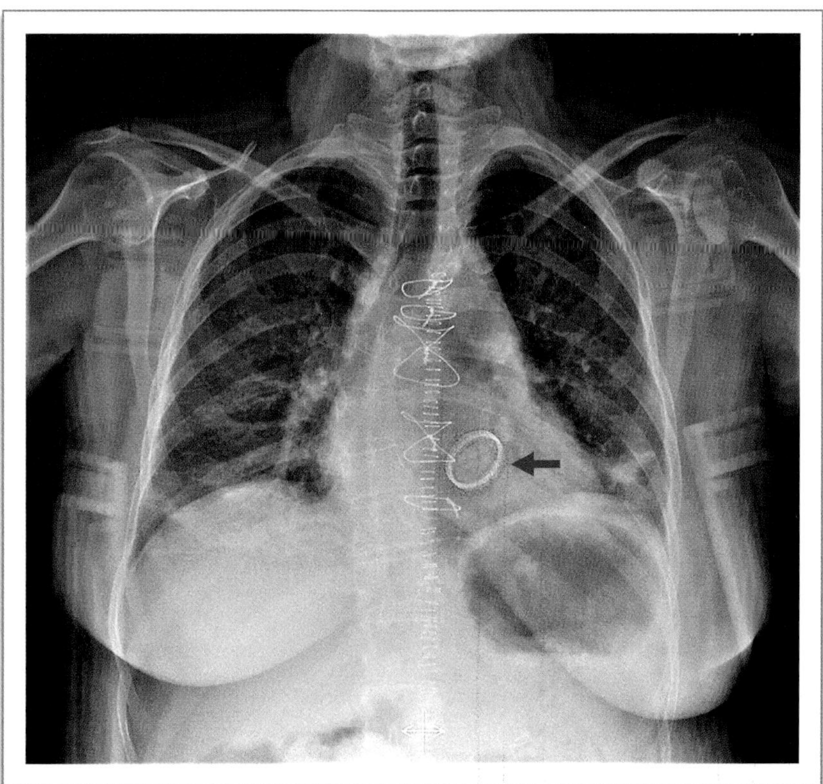

Figure 8.5.3 Mechanical mitral valve prostheses.

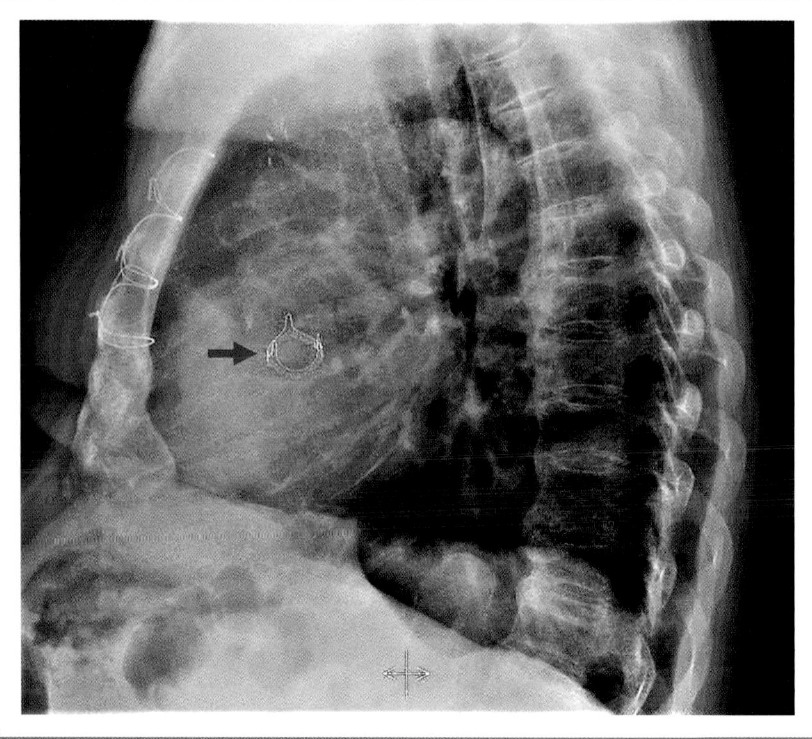

Figure 8.5.4 Biological aortic valve prostheses.

    - Bioprosthesis of human origin, obtained from cadaveric donors (homograft) or transplanted from one location to another in the same individual (autograft); last longer than xenografts, resist infections better and are employed in young individuals, particularly in the presence of endocarditis
- Transcatheter valves
  - Consist of biological tissue mounted within an expandable stent
  - Employed when conventional surgery is high risk or contraindicated
  - Although the surgical procedure is less invasive, the intravascular manipulation and positioning can be difficult

Complications

- Primary failure (deterioration without secondary infection or other identifiable cause)
- Thrombosis/thromboembolism
- Mechanical obstruction due to pannus (endothelial overgrowth)
- Dehiscence
- Haemolysis
- Haemorrhage
- Endocarditis

Prognosis

- Heart valve replacement does not currently provide patients with a definitive cure
- The prosthesis' prognosis is determined by its haemodynamics, durability and thrombogenicity
- The risk of endocarditis increases up to 50-fold for patients with a valvular prosthesis, and morbidity and mortality are significantly increased for carriers of prosthetic valves compared with those with native valves
- Regenerative valves or tissue-engineered valves are being developed
  - Novel approach based on various tissue engineering technologies that provide an alternative crimpable valve replacement device as a definitive solution
  - A tissue-engineered valve would be a living organ, capable of responding and growing like the native valve, ideal for paediatric patients
  - This technology aims to become the most advanced means to improve valve durability but is currently in the preclinical stage

A World/Transcultural View

- In industrialised countries, there is an expected increase in the demand from patients with age-related degenerative valvular heart disease, while in low-income countries, there is an expected increase in the number of young individuals with rheumatic fever who require a valvular prosthesis

- The prophylactic antibiotic regimens to prevent infective endocarditis in each country are variable; their efficacy is determined by geographical factors such as regional variations in antimicrobial susceptibility
- The Australian guidelines on prophylaxis still consider Australian aborigines with rheumatic heart disease a high-risk population
- It seems reasonable to adopt the recommendations proposed by the expert committees of each country or one of the main international guidelines (e.g. US and European guidelines)
- In some countries, the decision to take AP against infective endocarditis is made by the patient, and in others the physician or dentist makes the decision directly

Recommended Reading

Ansell, J., Hirsh, J., and Hylek, E. (2008). Pharmacology and management of the vitamin K antagonists: American College of Chest Physicians Evidence-Based Clinical Practice Guidelines (8th Edition). *Chest* 133: 160S–198S.

Diz Dios, P. (2014). Infective endocarditis prophylaxis. *Oral Dis.* 20: 325–328.

Goff, D.A., Mangino, J.E., Glassman, A.H. et al. (2020). Review of guidelines for dental antibiotic prophylaxis for prevention of endocarditis and prosthetic joint infections and need for dental stewardship. *Clin. Infect. Dis.* 71: 455–462.

Limeres Posse, J., Álvarez Fernández, M., Fernández Feijoo, J. et al. (2016). Intravenous amoxicillin/clavulanate for the prevention of bacteraemia following dental procedures: a randomized clinical trial. *J. Antimicrob. Chemother.* 71: 2022–2030.

Lung, B. and Sjögren, J. (2018). Prosthetic valves. In: *ESC Textbook of Cardiovascular Medicine*, 3e (eds. A.J. Camm, T.F. Luscher, G. Maurer and P.W. Serruys). Oxford University Press.

Millot, S., Lesclous, P., Colombier, M.L. et al. (2017). Position paper for the evaluation and management of oral status in patients with valvular disease: Groupe de Travail Valvulopathies de la Société Française de Cardiologie, Société Française de Chirurgie Orale, Société Française de Parodontologie et d'Implantologie Orale, Société Française d'Endodontie et Société de Pathologie Infectieuse de Langue Française. *Arch. Cardiovasc. Dis.* 110: 482–494.

Pibarot, P. and Dumesnil, J.G. (2009). Prosthetic heart valves: selection of the optimal prosthesis and long-term management. *Circulation* 119: 1034–1048.

Thornhill, M.H., Dayer, M., Lockhart, P.B., and Prendergast, B. (2017). Antibiotic prophylaxis of infective endocarditis. *Curr. Infect. Dis. Rep.* 19: 9.

Tubiana, S., Blotière, P.O., Hoen, B. et al. (2017). Dental procedures, antibiotic prophylaxis, and endocarditis among people with prosthetic heart valves: nationwide population-based cohort and a case crossover study. *BMJ* 358: j3776.

Wilson WR, Gewitz M, Lockhart PB, Bolger AF, DeSimone DC, Kazi DS, Couper DJ, Beaton A, Kilmartin C, Miro JM, Sable C, Jackson MA and Baddour LM (2021); American Heart Association Young Hearts Rheumatic Fever, Endocarditis and Kawasaki Disease Committee of the Council on Lifelong Congenital Heart Disease and Heart Health in the Young; Council on Cardiovascular and Stroke Nursing; and the Council on Quality of Care and Outcomes Research. Prevention of Viridans Group Streptococcal Infective Endocarditis: A Scientific Statement From the American Heart Association. *Circulation*. 143: e963–e978.

8.6 Carrier of Coronary Stent

Section I: Clinical Scenario and Dental Considerations

Clinical Scenario

A 76-year-old male presents to you complaining that he is unable to eat with his removable lower denture and only wears it for aesthetic reasons when leaving the house. The patient reports that he has been unwell due to heart problems and hence has not been to see a dentist in the last 5 years. He now feels able to tolerate dental treatment.

Medical History
- Ischaemic heart disease (angioplasty and coronary stents 6 years earlier)
- Transient ischaemic attack (TIA) due to occlusion of the left internal carotid artery (carotid stent implanted 5 years earlier)
- Arterial hypertension with target organ damage
- Diet-controlled mild type 2 diabetes
- Dyslipidaemia
- Bradyphrenia

Medications
- Nitroglycerin (sublingual spray)
- Acetylsalicylic acid
- Clopidogrel
- Bisoprolol
- Amlodipine
- Ramipril
- Atorvastatin
- Pantoprazole

Dental History
- Six years since the patient last visited a dentist
- Poorly fitting removable dental prosthesis (brought to the dental appointment in a box)
- Brushes his teeth twice a day

Social History
- Married and lives with his family
- Does not drive and relies on his son to drive him to his appointments
- Well presented

Oral Examination
- Fair oral hygiene
- Fillings in #12, #13 and #21
- Metal crowns in #33, #35, #36 and #48
- Caries in #11, #13, #22 and #23
- Missing teeth: #14–17, #24–27, #31, #32, #34, #41, #42 and #44–47

Radiological Examination
- Orthopantomogram undertaken (Figure 8.6.1)
- Caries in #48
- Root canals treatment in #35 and #36
- Radiolucent lesion suggestive of chronic periapical periodontitis related to #36 (with furcation involvement)
- Carotid stent

Structured Learning

1) The patient informs you that his previous dentist alerted his doctor and cardiologist regarding the possibility of a potential problem with the left carotid artery. What could have made the dentist suspect this?
   - In patients undergoing orthopantomogram examination for dental diagnostic purposes, approximately 10% will have evidence of carotid artery calcification
   - It is estimated that 1 in 7 patients with carotid calcification on an orthopantomogram is likely to have a carotid stenosis ≥50%, compared with 1 in 20 patients without carotid artery calcification visible on an orthopantomogram
   - Carotid artery calcification is confirmed by an experienced dental radiologist who should advise the den-

A Practical Approach to Special Care in Dentistry, First Edition. Edited by Pedro Diz Dios and Navdeep Kumar.

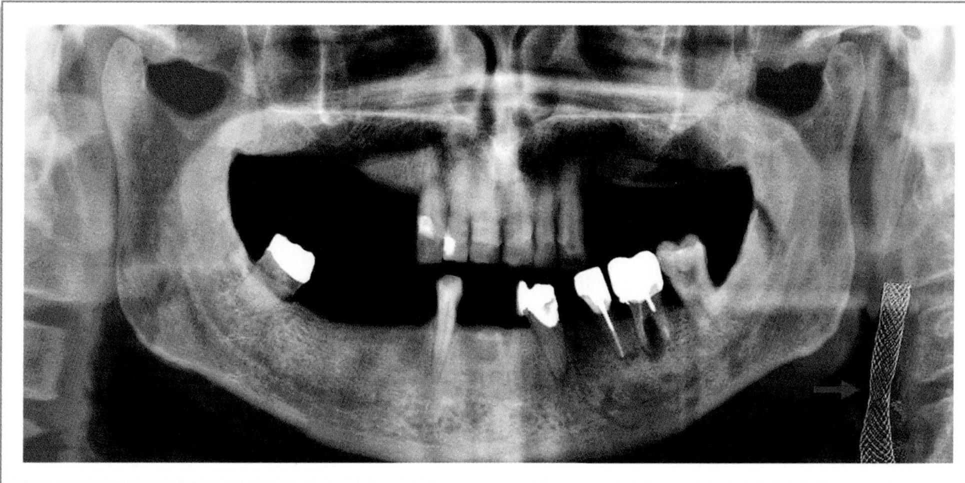

Figure 8.6.1 Orthopantomogram showing carotid stent.

tist that further evaluation is required, especially if there are any symptoms suggestive of cerebral ischaemia
- This patient had a TIA; the dentist may have linked the symptoms to the orthopantomogram findings and referred the patient for urgent medical review, leading to a stent being placed

2) The patient asks about the feasibility of prosthetic rehabilitation with osseointegrated dental implants and whether they would be less successful given his medical problems. What would you discuss?
   - In carriers of coronary stents, the placement of implants is not contraindicated, and there is no evidence that their long-term prognosis is jeopardised
   - Potential complications may occur during the dental procedure and include prolonged bleeding and the onset of a cardiac ischaemia episode
   - A number of antihypertensive drugs may even promote new bone growth (e.g. beta-blockers have been shown to improve bone mineral density in some studies and this patient is taking bisoprolol)
   - The level of diabetes control can determine the success of the implants
3) What could be contributing to the patient's bradyphrenia (slowness of thought)?
   - Health comorbidities, particularly cardiovascular risk factors, are well known to pose risks for cognitive decline in older adults
   - Hypertension has been suggested as a risk factor for subtle executive and memory deficits, above and beyond that conferred by diseases such as Parkinson's
   - Although by definition, symptoms of a TIA subside completely within 24 hours, it is known that there can be more prolonged impairment of cognitive function
4) What factors are considered important in assessing the risk of managing this patient?
   - Social
     - Limited availability for dental clinic visits (requires a companion)
     - Bradyphrenia may make it difficult for the patient to process the information on risks and benefits of any proposed procedure and to obtain informed consent (the presence of his son may be necessary at this stage)
   - Medical
     - Risk of a recurrent ischaemic heart episode triggered by a stressful situation in the dental setting (see Chapter 8.3)
     - Increased risk of a hypertensive crisis and bleeding tendency due to arterial hypertension (see Chapter 8.1)
     - Hypoglycaemia, hyperglycaemia, increased risk of infection and delayed wound healing related to diabetes (see Chapter 5.1)
     - Tendency to bleed due to the antithrombotic drugs (see Chapter 10.5)
     - Drug interactions
   - Dental
     - There is evidence of oral disease elsewhere in the mouth which must be stabilised prior to dental implant planning
     - Placement of dental implants will require commitment to a complex treatment plan with multiple appointments and long-term review
5) The patient agrees to have #36 extracted and the area curettaged. Would you consider a preoperative antibiotic prophylaxis regimen for prevention of infective endocarditis?

- Coronary stents are not considered an indication for endocarditis prophylaxis
- Furthermore, 5 years have elapsed since the placement of the patient's last stent

6) Following successful dental extraction of #36, you decide to prescribe postoperative antibiotics in view of the extensive purulent discharge from the socket. Which antibiotics should you avoid?
   - In this patient, it is preferable to avoid macrolides (erythromycin, azithromycin, clarithromycin) because they increase plasma amlodipine concentrations and interact with atorvastatin (risk of rhabdomyolysis)

7) Which would be the safest analgesic to recommend for this patient postoperatively?
   - Paracetamol is indicated and would be the safest choice
   - Non-steroidal anti-inflammatory drugs increase the risk of ulceration and gastrointestinal haemorrhage in patients who take acetylsalicylic acid
   - A number of non-steroidal anti-inflammatory drugs (e.g. ibuprofen, diclofenac and naproxen) can reduce the antihypertensive efficacy of beta-blockers (e.g. bisoprolol) and angiotensin-converting enzyme inhibitors (e.g. ramipril)
   - Metamizole can reduce the antiplatelet effect of acetylsalicylic acid

General Dental Considerations

Oral Findings

- No oral findings have been reported specifically related to coronary stents
- These patients might have oral lesions due to the adverse effects of antithrombotic drugs (see Chapters 10.3 and 10.5) and other drugs such as antihypertensives (see Chapter 8.1)

Dental Management

Dental treatment should be planned with particular consideration in relation to the control of stress, the presence of comorbidities and the antithrombotic therapy (Table 8.6.1)

Section II: Background Information and Guidelines

Definition

Angioplasty (balloon angioplasty or percutaneous transluminal angioplasty) is an endovascular procedure that consists of dilating a stenotic or occluded artery or vein, generally due to an atherosclerotic lesion, with the aim of restoring blood flow. Coronary stents are designed to prevent the most common complications after balloon dilation (artery retraction and restenosis). A stent is a vascular endoprosthesis consisting of a generally metallic tubular mesh implanted using a catheter into a stenotic or obstructed coronary artery to widen and facilitate blood flow. It is estimated that more than 3 million coronary stents are implanted annually worldwide.

Mechanism of Action

- A coronary angiography is performed through a peripheral vascular access, and a catheter is inserted into the narrowed area of the artery. A deflated 'balloon' is then inserted, which is subsequently inflated to dilate the artery. To prevent the artery from reclosing, a stent is placed, which adapts to the artery walls and keeps them open (Figure 8.6.2)
- The angioplasty and the stent itself cause immediate iatrogenic damage
- The body's response is the elastic retraction of the vascular wall, followed by the formation of mural thrombi and activation of the inflammatory cascade, which promotes neointimal (vascular smooth muscle cells) proliferation and ultimately restenosis

Indications

- Myocardial infarction without ST-segment elevation or acute coronary syndrome
- Myocardial infarction with acute ST-segment elevation
- Stable treatment-refractory angina
- Anginal equivalent symptoms, including dyspnoea, arrhythmia, dizziness and syncope
- Symptomatic patients, with evidence from noninvasive tests of moderate to severe ischaemia in a medium to large area

Types of Coronary Stents

- The selection of the stent type depends on the patient's clinical characteristics (e.g. diabetes, diseases associated with risk of bleeding) and the type of lesions of the coronary arteries (i.e. diameter of the artery to be treated, length of the coronary lesion)
- Metal stents
  - Slotted or coiled-shape structures made of stainless steel or cobalt chromium
  - Disadvantage of easily reclogging or causing restenosis
- Drug-eluting stents
  - Same metallic structural support as conventional stents but are coated with a polymer that elutes

Table 8.6.1 Considerations for dental management.

Risk assessment	• Increased bleeding tendency due to antithrombotic drugs – Dual antithrombotic therapy should not be interrupted during the 12 months after the placement of a drug-eluting coronary stent following acute coronary syndrome or during the 6 months following revascularisation (in the case of stable ischaemic heart disease) – If the antithrombotic therapy is tolerated without haemorrhagic events, it is preferable to extend the therapy (including making it lifelong) • Stent infection – Antibiotic prophylaxis is not indicated, although a number of authors have defended its administration in the first weeks after stent implantation
Criteria for referral	• The recommendation is to perform urgent dental treatment in a hospital setting in the first 6 weeks following the placement of a metallic stent, and in the first 6 months if the stent is drug eluting
Access/position	• The appointment should be scheduled for the last hour of the morning or the first of the afternoon (endogenous epinephrine levels are higher early in the morning) • The sessions should be short and relaxed
Communication	• Anxiety and depression are common in these patients, in which case they may be less receptive to health promotion recommendations provided by health professionals, including dentists
Consent/capacity	• For patients who take antithrombotic agents, the consent form should include the increased risk of bleeding
Anaesthesia/sedation	• Local anaesthesia – It is prudent not to exceed 2 anaesthetic cartridges with epinephrine at 1:100 000 (0.04 mg) • Sedation – Control of anxiety with nitrous oxide or benzodiazepines may be considered – Some antihistamines such as hydroxyzine should be avoided in patients with heart conditions • General anaesthesia – A comprehensive preoperative evaluation should be conducted
Dental treatment	• Before – Elective dental treatment should be postponed for at least 1 year (a number of authors have limited this period to 6 weeks following the placement of a metal stent and 6 months for drug-eluting stents) – The recommendation is to maintain the dual antiplatelet therapy when performing any dental procedure (see Chapter 10.5) – For patients anticoagulated with heparin, acenocoumarol or warfarin, the international normalised ratio (INR) should be assessed before any invasive dental procedure (see Chapter 10.3) • During – Local haemostasis measures should be sufficient to counter the risk of bleeding – It is prudent to avoid using vasoconstrictor-soaked thread retractors • After – Consider drug interactions
Drug prescription	• A number of non-steroidal anti-inflammatory drugs and some antibiotics can interact with the antithrombotic drugs that are typically taken by patients with stents (see Chapters 10.3 and 10.5)
Education/prevention	• Oral healthcare providers should educate patients on strategies for atherosclerotic coronary disease prevention (e.g. smoking cessation, regular exercise and nutrition counselling) • Patients should be advised to take their antithrombotic medication regularly unless advised by the physician to adjust/amend the dose • Regular long-term follow-up to maintain oral health is essential to reduce the need for invasive dental procedures

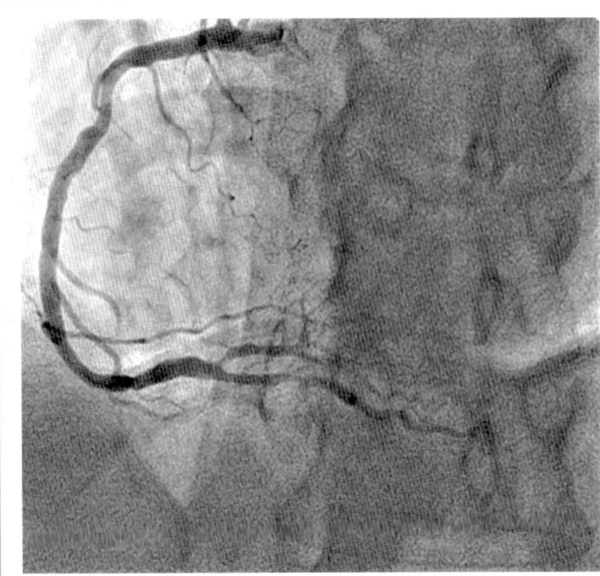
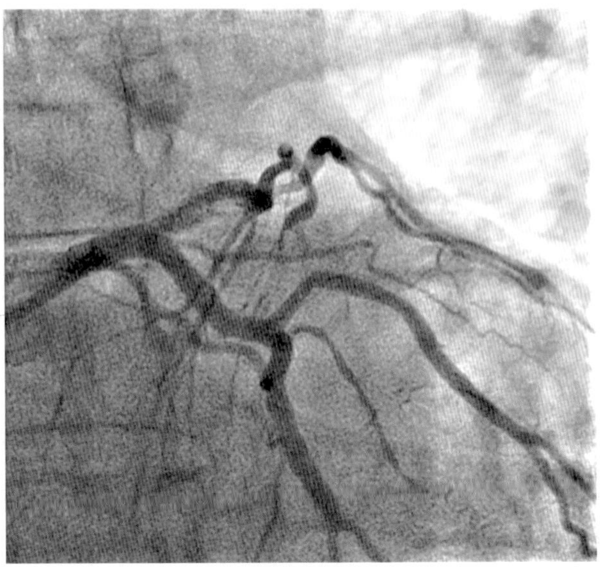

Figure 8.6.2 Invasive coronary angiography remains the standard for the detection of coronary artery diseases.

antiproliferative therapeutic and/or anti-inflammatory agents to minimise the risk of reclogging
  - First-generation drug-eluting stents release sirolimus or paclitaxel
  - Second-generation drug-eluting stents have an improved design, biocompatibility and performance, and dispense paclitaxel, zotarolimus or everolimus
  - Third-generation drug-eluting stents are more flexible, enabling access to more complex coronary anatomies, and release zotarolimus or everolimus (mTOR inhibitors)
- Bioresorbable vascular scaffolds
  - Similar to the above, but the stent structure is formed by a material that is reabsorbed and disappears completely from the coronary artery wall, enabling complete restoration of all vascular wall functions and preventing late mechanical problems

Complications

- Thrombosis: this is an uncommon complication (<1% annually) but leads to acute coronary syndrome with ST-segment elevation, with a mortality rate that can reach 20–40%
- Restenosis: neointimal hyperplasia causes intrastent restenosis in up to 30% of patients with conventional metal stents. With drug-eluting stents, the prevalence of clinical and angiographic intrastent restenosis has been reduced to 5% and 10%, respectively
- Haemorrhagic complications: mainly occurs in vascular access, digestive system and intracranial system, related to antithrombotic drugs

Prognosis

- Percutaneous transluminal angioplasty with stents significantly improves the quality of life of patients who undergo this procedure
- The mortality rate for carriers of coronary stents is 10% at 5 years (although half of the deaths are due to non-cardiovascular causes)

A World/Transcultural View

- The prevalence of atherosclerotic coronary disease is determined mainly by environmental factors
- In the United States, the rate of this disease is similar among ethnic immigrants and the white population
- In Europe, the prevalence of atherosclerotic coronary disease in Norwegian countries is ostensibly greater than that of countries with Mediterranean diets
- In Asia, approximately 300 000 drug-eluting stents are implanted annually, with results similar to those of Western countries
- The limited number of interventional cardiology services in sub-Saharan Africa has resulted in significantly lower rates of percutaneous coronary interventions than in medium- to high-income countries. However, recent evidence points to a rapid increase in the number of patients with atherosclerotic coronary disease as a consequence of the urbanisation and westernisation of rural Africa

Recommended Reading

Brancati, M.F., Burzotta, F., Trani, C. et al. (2017). Coronary stents and vascular response to implantation: literature review. *Pragmat. Obs. Res.* 8: 137–148.

Byrne, R.A., Stone, G.W., Ormiston, J., and Kastrati, A. (2017). Coronary balloon angioplasty, stents, and scaffolds. *Lancet.* 390: 781–792.

Douketis, J.D., Spyropoulos, A.C., Spencer, F.A. et al. (2012). Perioperative management of antithrombotic therapy: antithrombotic therapy and prevention of thrombosis, 9th ed: American College of Chest Physicians evidence-based clinical practice guidelines. *Chest* 141: e326S–e350S.

Grines, C.L., Bonow, R.O., Casey, D.E. Jr. et al. (2007). Prevention of premature discontinuation of dual antiplatelet therapy in patients with coronary artery stents: a science advisory from the American Heart Association, American College of Cardiology, Society for Cardiovascular Angiography and Interventions, American College of Surgeons, and American Dental Association, with representation from the American College of Physicians. *J Am Dent Assoc.* 138: 652–655.

Park, M.W., Her, S.H., Kwon, J.B. et al. (2012). Safety of dental extractions in coronary drug-eluting stenting patients without stopping multiple antiplatelet agents. *Clin. Cardiol.* 35: 225–230.

Roberts, H.W. and Redding, S.W. (2000). Coronary artery stents: review and patient-management recommendations. *J. Am. Dent. Assoc.* 131: 797–801.

9

Respiratory Disease

9.1 Chronic Obstructive Pulmonary Disease (COPD)

Section I: Clinical Scenario and Dental Considerations

Clinical Scenario

A 67-year-old male presents to your dental clinic complaining of 'weak' and 'crumbling' teeth. He feels that his teeth have been progressively breaking down over the last 5 years.

Medical History
- Chronic obstructive pulmonary disease (COPD) – irregular medical reviews
- Asthma
- Hyperlipidaemia
- Recent diagnosis of hypertension
- Low body mass index (BMI= 16.5 kg/m^2)

Medications
- Prednisolone
- Salbutamol (inhaler)
- Ipratropium bromide and albuterol sulfate (combination inhaler)
- Simvastatin
- Enalapril (commenced 2 days ago)

Dental History
- Good level of co-operation
- Irregular dental attender (states he cannot afford dental care)
- Brushes once a day in the morning with a manual toothbrush and water
- No toothpaste used due to the additional cost

Social History
- Married, lives with his wife; has 2 married children who visit infrequently
- Hokkien-speaking (a type of Mandarin dialect)
- Worker at the local hawker food centre for almost 50 years, exposure to long-term inhalation of smoke
- Limited financial means (receives financial support from the government)
- Tobacco consumption: 30 cigarettes daily for the last 50 years
- Diet – eats only at work due to limited income (predominantly fried food, no fresh fruit/vegetables)

Oral Examination
- Very poor oral hygiene
- Smoker's keratosis of the palate
- Numerous dental caries
  - #25, #26 and #27 – gross caries
  - #17 – distal root caries
  - #12 – mesial caries extending onto root surface
  - #11 – mesial and distal caries
  - #14, #33 and #34 – buccal root caries
  - #13, #43, #42 and #44 – interproximal caries
- Retained roots: #21, #22, #23, #24 and #45
- Missing teeth: #18, #28, #38, #37, #36, #46 and #48
- Dental erosion
- Generalised calculus and extrinsic staining
- Multiple periodontally involved teeth with significant attachment loss
- Mobility: #47 (grade III), #12, #17, #25, #26 and #27 (grade II–III), #11 (grade I)

Radiological Examination
- Orthopantomogram undertaken (Figure 9.1.1)
- Generalised horizontal alveolar bone loss

Structured Learning

1) What risk factors does this patient have for the development of COPD?
   - Tobacco consumption: 75 pack-years in total; 1 pack-year is calculated as smoking 20 cigarettes, or

A Practical Approach to Special Care in Dentistry, First Edition. Edited by Pedro Diz Dios and Navdeep Kumar.

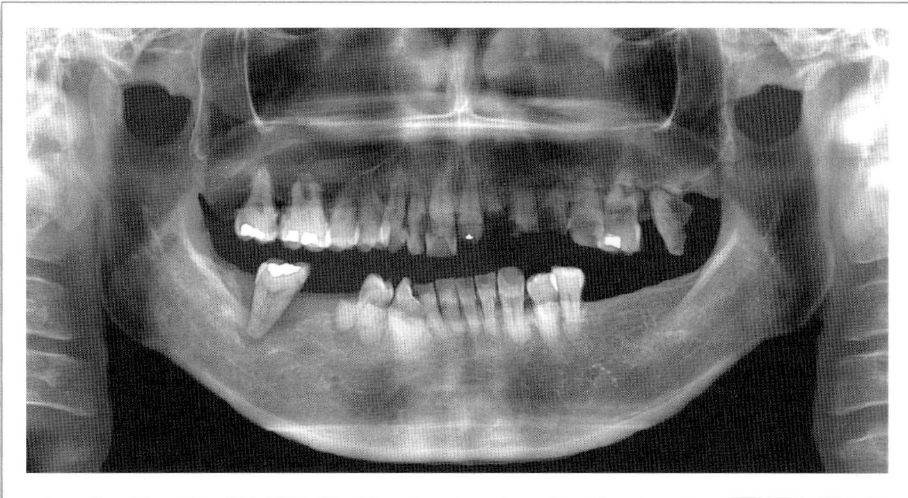

Figure 9.1.1 Orthopantomogram of a patient with chronic obstructive pulmonary disease (COPD) confirming rampant caries and multiple missing teeth.

1 pack, every day for 1 year (or equivalent); a higher pack-year is associated with a higher risk of lung cancer and reduced survival

- Occupation: exposure to cooking fumes from either the use of fossil fuels or liquefied petroleum gas (Figure 9.1.2)
- Low BMI and malnutrition in COPD have been linked with a poor prognosis
- The patient is from a lower socioeconomic group

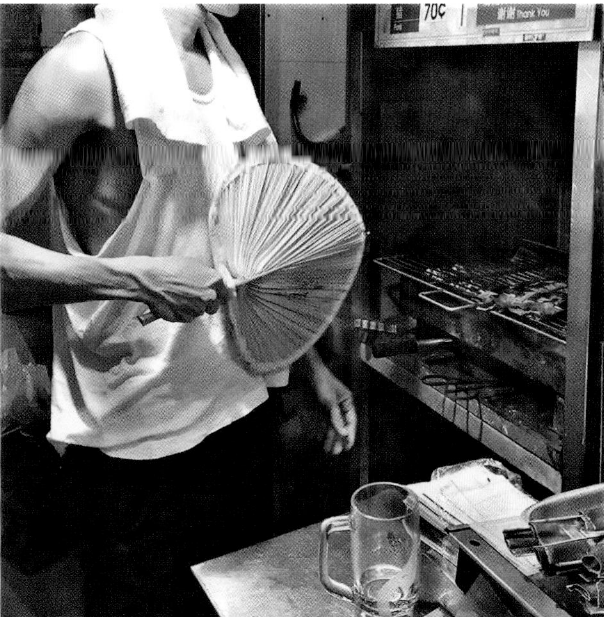

Figure 9.1.2 Inhaling smoke is a chronic work hazard for street hawkers.

2) What factors could be contributing to this patient's high level of dental caries?
   - Poor oral hygiene
   - Not using fluoride toothpaste
   - Irregular dental attender
   - Inhaled drug therapy:
     - Inhaled beta-2-agonists may lead to reduced salivary flow due to the effect of these medications on the receptors in the parotid and other salivary glands
     - This reduction has been associated with a concomitant reduction in pH, increased food retention and increase in cariogenic bacterial load (e.g. *Streptococcus mutans*)
     - Dry powder inhalers also contain fermentable carbohydrates, the most common of which is lactose monohydrate
   - Some studies have found a correlation between tobacco smoking and an increased risk of dental caries
3) Prior to planning the delivery of dental treatment, what additional questions would you ask the patient to assess the severity of his COPD?
   - Is he seen by a specialist in hospital or by his local doctor?
   - How often should he be reviewed (given his limited financial means, this may not be the same as how often he attends)?
   - What triggers a worsening of his symptoms of COPD/breathlessness (e.g. walking, exercise)?
   - Does he take his medications regularly?
   - How often does he need to use his relieving inhalers?
   - How long has he been taking prednisolone and at what dose?

- Have there been any hospital admissions related to his COPD? If so when/how often?

4) The patient has a dry hacking non-productive cough and pitting oedema. You suspect that the patient has significant COPD and contact his respiratory physician for further information and his recent investigation results. These are as follows:
   - Forced expiratory volume in 1 second (FEV1) is 38% of normal
   - Recent chest x-rays showed flattened diaphragm
   - Oxygen saturation (SpO_2) is 90–93% on room air (normal SpO_2 for healthy adults is ~94–99%)
   - Resting heart rate 90–94/minute
   - Respiratory rate is 26 per minute and shallow (normal rate is ~14–20/minute)
5) Given these details, what is your assessment of the severity of his COPD?
   - This patient has severe COPD (low FEV1 and chest x-ray changes due to lung inflation)
   - High resting heart rate is present and associated with poor outcome, including the development of heart failure
   - Reduced cardiac output causes long-term muscle wasting and can contribute to weight loss
   - Rapid compensatory breathing rate
6) Following a discussion regarding the poor prognosis of his teeth, the patient asks for all his remaining teeth to be removed. What factors are considered important in assessing the risk of managing this patient?
   - Social
     - Hokkien-speaking – consider the need for a translator
     - Financial constraints
     - Need for escort/social support
   - Medical
     - Low BMI and malnutrition in COPD are associated with a poor prognosis (a preprocedural full blood count is recommended)
     - The patient has severe COPD which increases the risk of respiratory complications during surgery (hospital-based care preferable)
     - Currently taking systemic prednisolone and may be at risk of adrenal suppression/crisis (see Chapter 12.1)
     - Hypertension recently diagnosed and may not be optimally controlled
     - Drug interactions:
       - Non-steroidal anti-inflammatory drugs can reduce the hypotensive effect of angiotensin-converting enzyme inhibitors (e.g. enalapril)
       - Theophylline is largely (~70%) metabolised by the P450 isoenzyme; inhibitors or inducers of the isoenzyme can interact pharmacokinetically; ciprofloxacin, erythromycin and tramadol are known to significantly increase plasma theophylline levels; theophylline may reduce the anxiolytic and sedative effects of benzodiazepines
       - Azole antifungals, metronidazole and macrolide antibiotics can potentiate the effects of statins in muscle breakdown (e.g. rhabdomyolysis)
   - Dental
     - Multiple dental extractions required
     - Delayed healing likely (COPD, smoking, malnutrition, systemic steroid)
     - Need for replacement dentures needs to be discussed, including the factors below:
       - Xerostomia secondary to medication (e.g. beta-2-agonist) can reduce retention and tolerance to a replacement denture
       - Multiple visits required for denture construction
       - Taking dental impressions may cause respiratory distress if the airway is restricted
       - Irregular attendance/engagement in improving oral health
7) Given the absence of dental pain/acute dental infection, you determine it is advisable to delay treatment until his hypertension is controlled and he has completed his course of prednisolone for the current acute exacerbation of his COPD. When planning his care for the future, should supplemental oxygen be provided to this patient perioperatively?
   - Practices and policies differ widely
   - Hence it is prudent to consult a physician or pulmonologist for patients with moderate to severe COPD as these patients may be dependent on the hypoxic respiratory drive
     - When a patient has long-standing hypercapnia (high levels of CO_2) and resultant acidosis, the body compensates by retaining more plasma bicarbonate; this attenuates the effect of low pH (acidosis) for the central chemoreceptors, and reduces the stimulus for the main carbonic feedback in physiological respiratory drive
     - It is believed that the effect of hypoxia in peripheral chemoreceptors becomes established as a compensation to reduced hypercapnic effect, in generating the respiratory drive – hence the term hypoxic drive
     - Supplemental oxygen raises blood oxygen level, possibly suppressing the hypoxic drive and may contribute to hypoventilation

- In reality, the hypoxic and hypercapnic drive exists with many contributors to respiratory drive, including acidosis/alkalosis balance, metabolic demands, neurological states, physical condition of the patient and drug effects

8) The patient also reports that his throat, tongue, eyes and hands have been feeling slightly swollen over the last 2 days and he also has an itchy rash. What could be the cause?
   - The symptoms are suggestive of angio-oedema
   - When this is acquired, it is typically triggered by an allergic reaction to food or medications
   - The patient commenced enalapril 2 days prior to presentation – this is an angiotensin-converting enzyme inhibitor, a medication known to have angio-oedema as one of its potential side-effects
   - It is important to alert the physician urgently

General Dental Considerations

Oral Findings

- Dry mouth
  - Long-term use of inhaled oxygen (dehydrating)
  - Anticholinergics and beta-2-agonist inhalers
  - Inhaled steroids
  - Mouth breathing is a mechanism to improve aperture for air entry in COPD; it may cause further desiccation of the oral environment
- Taste disturbance
  - Anticholinergics can cause a metallic taste after inhalation
  - Beta-2-agonist inhalers may be associated with an unpleasant taste
- Tobacco stains in smokers
- Increased prevalence of dental caries and periodontal disease has been observed
- Increased risk of dental erosion due to the use of inhaled medications and the development of gastro-oesophageal reflux secondary to the use of beta-2-agonists and methylxanthines (e.g. theophylline)
- Poor wound healing (due to hypoxia)
- Elevated risk of oral mucosal cancers, due to combined tobacco smoking and inhaled corticosteroids
- Oral candidiasis may occur in some patients who use inhaled corticosteroids for long periods of time or at high dose
- Theophylline can rarely produce erythema multiforme; an oral variant of the disease can occur, which presents with ulcerations and targetoid lesions confined within oral mucosa, without the typical skin lesions of the more severe categories

Dental Management

- The dental management considerations are determined by the severity of the COPD, concurrent steroid usage, prolonged tobacco history and risk of comorbidities (Table 9.1.1)

Section II: Background Information and Guidelines

Definition

Chronic obstructive pulmonary disease, or chronic obstructive airways disease, is a common respiratory disease characterised by chronic obstruction of normal lung airflow, with respiratory symptoms. It is progressive, not fully reversible and most frequently diagnosed in people aged 40 years old and above. The more familiar terms 'chronic bronchitis' and 'emphysema' are no longer used but are now included within the COPD diagnosis.

- Chronic bronchitis: long-term cough productive of sputum on most days for 3 months a year, over more than 2 successive years
- Emphysema: enlargement of terminal airspaces

The global prevalence of COPD is estimated at greater than 10%, affecting approximately 380 million people, with 65 million people worldwide diagnosed with moderate to severe COPD. It is predicted to become the third leading cause of death worldwide by 2030.

Aetiopathogenesis

- COPD is caused by factors that trigger inflammation in the lungs
  - Tobacco smoke: 40–50% of lifelong smokers will develop COPD, compared with 10% of people who have never smoked
  - Occupational exposure: 15–20% of COPD cases are associated with exposure to occupational dust, chemicals, vapours or other airborne pollutants in the workplace
  - Pollution: high levels of outdoor air pollution and indoor air pollution (e.g. from biomass fuels for cooking and heating)
  - Early life and environmental factors: lung infections in early life and mothers who smoke
  - Lower educational and income levels (may be related to factors such as nutrition, overcrowding and air pollution)
  - Genetic factors: alpha-1-antitrypsin deficiency

Table 9.1.1 Considerations for dental management.

Risk assessment	• Reduced respiratory function • Diminishing respiratory drive may result in the patient becoming rapidly drowsy or losing consciousness • Patients with COPD have a sensitive upper airway that can be provoked by dental procedures, resulting in frequent coughing that is disruptive to treatment (e.g. moisture control) • Water accumulation, rubber dam placement or the taking of dental impressions may exacerbate respiratory distress • Risk of poor wound healing for extractions and surgical procedures • Comorbid concerns include: – Concurrent steroid usage – Risk of vascular diseases – Pulmonary hypertension – Prolonged tobacco history
Criteria for referral	• Dentists should be able to manage the vast majority of COPD patients • It is good practice to consult a respiratory physician prior to treating moderate–severe patients with COPD for conscious sedation or prolonged surgical procedures • Gold Stage III/IV: referral to a hospital-based dental clinic is appropriate for invasive dental procedures
Access/position	• Consider a semi-upright position (Fowler's position) to optimise breathing rather than reclining the patient to a fully supine position • Postpone elective dental treatment if the patient is experiencing an acute exacerbation of COPD • Exercise intolerance can vary widely – ensure there is ample time for the patient to travel to the dental clinic and whether transport/an escort is required • Consider domiciliary care in selected cases
Consent/capacity	• Mental capacity is not generally affected • In severe COPD/during an acute exacerbation, patients may experience difficulty speaking in complete sentences • Fatigue/exhaustion may impair the ability of the patient to engage in the discussion • Ensure that you discuss the potential for poor wound healing after dental surgical procedures
Anaesthesia/sedation	• Local anaesthesia – It is advisable to limit epinephrine-containing local anaesthesia to 3 cartridges if the patient is taking theophylline (epinephrine-induced hypokalaemia is potentiated by therapeutic concentrations of theophylline) • Sedation – Opioids and benzodiazepines can cause further respiratory depression, particularly in those with severe bronchitis that have a hypoxic respiratory drive – Consult the physician regarding severity of the patient's COPD, suitability of sedation and requirement of supplemental oxygen – Inhalation sedation is generally a safer choice The hypercapnic effect of raising SpO_2 above 94–98% in hypoxic patients is considered insignificant in short-term provision of oxygen in dentistry – Paroxysmal coughing can be disruptive to the sedation • General anaesthesia – Consult the patient's physician – Discuss the need for prior chest physiotherapy and postoperative admission – Postoperative respiratory complications are more frequent

(Continued)

Table 9.1.1 (Continued)

Dental treatment	• Before – Consult a physician prior to the appointment for patients with moderate to severe COPD – Confirm with the patient whether they have any acute symptoms/exacerbations of their COPD symptoms – Ensure that the patient has their bronchodilator inhaler with them at the appointment – Prophylactic use of a bronchodilator (e.g. salbutamol) can be beneficial – Supplemental oxygen can be beneficial for long procedures or during sedation; patients with moderate–severe COPD are ideally given low-flow oxygen and SpO_2 kept in an optimal range of 88–92% to maintain the hypoxic drive (PaO_2 55–60 mmHg) – Evaluate the appropriateness of rubber dam and the potential to restrict respiration (e.g. in mouth-breathers) – Determine the need for steroid cover for surgical procedures – Consider perioperative monitoring depending on the severity of the COPD (e.g. pulse oximetry and blood pressure) – note that a starting SpO_2 of 93% is equivalent to a drop of 40 mmHg in normal arterial blood oxygen • During – Avoid a fully supine position – Monitor for signs of respiratory distress/increased respiratory effort – Ensure effective suction of water/debris – Consider the use of fast-setting impression materials and ensure the impression trays are not overloaded; digital dental impressions technique can be a useful option – Discontinue treatment if paroxysmal coughing occurs • After – Close follow-up after surgery due to the risk of delayed healing – Primary closure of socket may improve healing
Drug prescription	• Ciprofloxacin, tramadol and erythromycin can reduce clearance of theophylline • Theophylline can reduce the effects of benzodiazepines
Education/prevention	• Encourage smoking cessation • High-fluoride regimen is required for patients with high caries risk. This can include 2800 ppm or 5000 ppm sodium fluoride toothpaste, and other fluoride-based dentifrices • Use of specific mouth gels and mouthwashes can help dryness and remineralisation

PaO_2, partial pressure of arterial oxygen; SpO_2, peripheral capillary oxygen saturation.

- Exposure to noxious stimuli stimulates a cascade of inflammatory responses, including activation of polymorphonuclear leucocytes and macrophages, releasing proteases (human leucocyte elastase) that contribute to pulmonary destruction
- Pathological changes occur in the central airways, peripheral bronchioles and lung parenchyma resulting in sputum formation, bullae formation and compression of adjacent parenchymal tissue, limiting blood flow and ventilation
- The main pathological process differs for chronic bronchitis and emphysema

Chronic bronchitis

- Involves damage to endothelium which impairs the mucociliary response that clears bacteria and mucus
- Neutrophilia subsequently develops in the airway lumen's submucosa, causing increased mucous gland activity
- Inflammation and secretions cause the obstructive element of chronic bronchitis
- In contrast to emphysema, the pulmonary capillary bed is relatively undamaged in chronic bronchitis

Emphysema

- Involves destruction of alveoli, usually by inflammation and permanent dilation of airspaces
- This leads to a decline in surface area for gaseous exchange. Secondly, loss of alveoli walls increases scarring (fibrosis) and reduces elastic recoil, which reduces expiratory function
- Loss of alveolar architecture leads to airway collapse, further limiting airflow

Clinical Presentation

- Persistent cough
- Sputum production with phlegm or mucus
- Dyspnoea
- Wheeze

- Respiratory failure or cor pulmonale (right-sided heart failure) – COPD is associated with increased resistance in the pulmonary vasculature, pulmonary hypertension, increased right ventricular workload and in advanced cases right heart failure (cor pulmonale)
- Reduced cardiac output causes long-term muscle wasting, weight loss and other associated medical conditions
- Acute exacerbations of COPD may occur and are defined as 'an acute event characterised by a worsening of the patient's respiratory symptoms that is beyond normal day-to-day variations and leads to a change in medication'
- Up to 30% of patients with COPD have a concomitant diagnosis of asthma and hence additional clinical features
- The type of respiratory failure differs between chronic bronchitis and emphysema (Table 9.1.2)

Chronic bronchitis

- Patients cannot maintain ventilation
- Hypoxia results, leading to central cyanosis and a 'blue bloated' appearance
- Raised jugular veins and ankle oedema are common

Emphysema

- These patients can ventilate
- However, they do not clear CO_2 effectively, giving rise to a 'pink panter' or 'pink puffer' look from the rosy colour from excessive carboxyhaemoglobin

Diagnosis

- Symptoms of chronic cough, dyspnoea and history of respiratory diseases are used to diagnose
- Spirometry (Figure 9.1.3); measures lung function, specifically the amount (volume) and/or speed (flow) of air that can be inhaled and exhaled, and includes the following measurements:
  - Vital capacity (VC) – normal values between 3 and 5 l
  - Forced vital capacity (FVC) – normal 80–120%
  - Forced expiratory volume in 1 second (FEV1) – mild COPD 90%, moderate 50–79%, severe 30–49%, very severe <30%
  - FEV1/FVC – normal value for this ratio is above 0.75–0.85
- Chest x-ray (Figure 9.1.4)
  - Hyperinflation presenting as enlarged spaces in the frontal or sagittal planes, or with flattened diaphragm
  - Lung fields may be hyper-radiolucent
  - Bullae (air pockets) may be observed
- Blood gases analysis – arterial partial pressure of oxygen (PaO_2)
- Staging – The Global Initiative for COPD (abbreviated as GOLD) bases the stage of COPD on several items including symptoms, how many times the COPD has worsened, hospitalisation history and spirometry test results (Table 9.1.3)

Management

- No known cure for COPD
- Control of risk factors (e.g. smoking cessation, avoidance of pollutants)
- Breathing enhancers
  - Bronchodilators
    - Short-acting: beta-2-agonist inhalers (e.g. salbutamol); antimuscarinic inhalers (e.g. ipratropium)

Table 9.1.2 Types of respiratory failure.

Respiratory failure[a]	Description	Gas values	Clinical presentation
Type I Hypoxaemia; 'blue bloater'	Lung damage prevents adequate oxygenation Less lung tissue is required for adequate CO_2 exchange compared to oxygenation	Reduced PaO_2 Normal $PaCO_2$	• Pulmonary oedema • Pneumonia • Acute respiratory distress syndrome • Chronic pulmonary fibrosing alveolitis
Type II Hypercapnic; ventilatory failure; 'pink puffer'	Reduced inability to exchange gases Usually the whole lung is affected	Reduced PaO_2 Raised $PaCO_2$	• COPD • Chest wall deformities • Respiratory muscle defects (Guillain–Barré syndrome) • Central respiratory depression (e.g. oversedation)

[a]Respiratory failure occurs when PaO_2 is 27 kPa (55 mmHg) or lower.
$PaCO_2$, partial pressure of carbon dioxide; PaO_2, partial pressure of arterial oxygen.

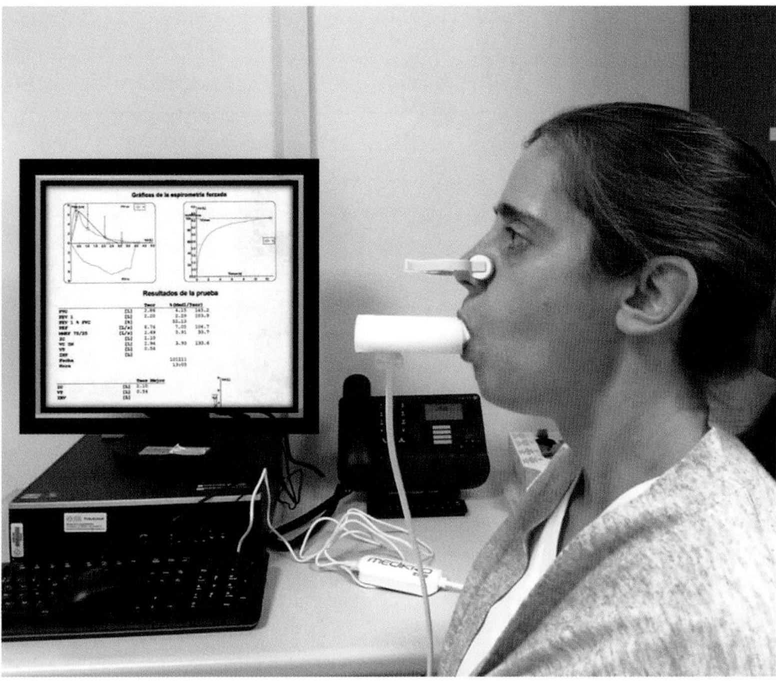

Figure 9.1.3 Spirometry is the standard respiratory function test for case detection of chronic obstructive pulmonary disease (COPD).

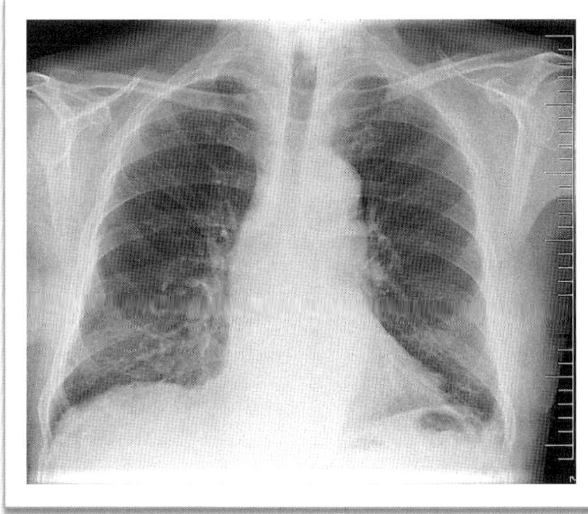

Figure 9.1.4 Chest x-ray of an elderly man with chronic obstructive pulmonary disease (COPD) and bronchiectasis.

    - Long-acting: beta-2-agonist inhalers (e.g. salmeterol, formoterol and indacaterol); antimuscarinic inhalers (e.g. tiotropium, glycopyrronium and aclidinium)
    - Some new inhalers contain a combination of a long-acting beta-2-agonist and antimuscarinic
  - Corticosteroid inhalers
  - Theophylline

- Mucolytics (e.g. carbocisteine)
- Systemic steroid therapy
- Antibiotics as required
- Pulmonary rehabilitation; physical exercise training, education regarding the condition and risk factors, dietary advice, psychological and emotional support
- Roflumilast for severe COPD (phosphodiesterase type-4 inhibitor with anti-inflammatory properties)
- Long-term oxygen therapy – generally not for blue bloaters
- Pulmonary surgery – bullectomy, lung transplantation
- For acute exacerbation of COPD:
  - Non-invasive mechanical ventilation
  - Combination of oral corticosteroids, antibiotic therapy and home-based management
  - Pulmonary rehabilitation after discharge

Prognosis

- 40–70% survival at 5 years
- Frequent COPD exacerbations and requirement for multiple intubation and invasive mechanical ventilation for acute respiratory failure in COPD patients are markers of poor prognosis
- Among different therapeutic modalities in COPD, the only 2 factors that improve survival are smoking cessation and oxygen supplementation

Table 9.1.3 GOLD (Global Initiative for Chronic Obstructive Lung Disease) staging severity.

GOLD stage	COPD severity	FEV1/FVC ratio	FEV1 range[a]
I	Mild	<0.70	>80% of normal
II	Moderate	<0.70	50–79% of normal
III	Severe	<0.70	30–49% of normal
IV	Very severe	<0.70	<30% of normal or <50% of normal with chronic respiratory failure present

COPD, chronic obstructive pulmonary disease; FEV1, forced expiratory volume within 1 sec; FVC, forced vital capacity.
[a]Does not specify pre- or post-bronchodilator.

- It is currently the fourth leading cause of death worldwide, with around 90% of COPD deaths occurring in low- and middle-income countries

A World/Transcultural View

- COPD is a major burden to individuals, societies and healthcare systems across the world
- This is partly due to the continued exposure to risk factors, such as smoking and air pollution, and partly due to an ageing population
- COPD has a variable impact on the quality of life globally, and carries with it a risk of premature mortality
- It is increasingly affecting women, minorities and individuals from lower socio-economic strata
- There are multiple barriers to access health information and medical services for many diverse communities, leading to disparity in COPD treatment outcomes in developing and developed countries
- Tobacco smoking is the biggest risk factor for COPD in middle- to high-income countries; as such, COPD was listed as the fourth leading cause of death in the US for 2018
- Indoor air pollution is the biggest risk factor in low-income countries, where almost 3 billion people worldwide use biomass and coal for household cooking and heating

Recommended Reading

Cunningham, T.J., Eke, P.I., Ford, E.S. et al. (2016). Cigarette smoking: tooth loss, and chronic obstructive pulmonary disease: findings from the behavioral risk factor surveillance system. *J. Periodontol.* 87: 385–394.

Global Initiative for Chronic Obstructive Lung Disease Inc. Pocket Guide to COPD Diagnosis, Management and Prevention – A Guide for Health Care Professionals. (2018). https://goldcopd.org/wp-content/uploads/2018/02/WMS-GOLD-2018-Feb-Final-to-print-v2.pdf

Hupp, W.S. (2006). Dental management of patients with obstructive pulmonary diseases. *Dent. Clin. North Am.* 50: 513–527.

Javaheri, N., Matin, S., Naghizadeh-Baghi, A. et al. (2020). Periodontal status, its treatment needs, and its relationship with airflow limitation and quality of life in COPD patients. *Eur. J. Med.* 52: 259–264.

Lee KC, Wu YT, Chien WC, et al. (2021). Osteoporosis and the risk of temporomandibular disorder in chronic obstructive pulmonary disease. *J. Bone Miner. Metab.* 39: 201–11.

Sapey, E., Yonel, Z., Edgar, R. et al. (2020). The clinical and inflammatory relationships between periodontitis and chronic obstructive pulmonary disease. *J. Clin. Periodontol.* 47: 1040–1052.

Wedzicha, J.A., Miravitlles, M., Hurst, J.R. et al. (2017). Management of COPD exacerbations: a European Respiratory Society/American Thoracic Society guideline. *Eur. Respir. J.* 49: 1600791.

World Health Organization. (2021). Chronic Respiratory Diseases – Chronic Obstructive Pulmonary Disease (COPD). www.who.int/news-room/fact-sheets/detail/chronic-obstructive-pulmonary-disease-(copd)

9.2 Asthma

Section I: Clinical Scenario and Dental Considerations

Clinical Scenario

A 63-year-old male presents for a dental appointment complaining of pain from his upper left wisdom tooth (#28). It affects his eating and sleeping. Due to his dental anxiety, he has not seen a dentist for over 10 years.

Medical History
- Asthma – irregular review with the physician
- Moderate dental anxiety – mainly in relation to the sound of ultrasonic and handpieces
- Rheumatoid arthritis with associated discomfort/swelling of his left knee
- Gastro-oesophageal reflux disease (GORD)
- Low body mass index (BMI)
- History of surgery on the right eye, with some residual visual impairment

Medications
- Salbutamol (inhaler) infrequent use
- Fluticasone with salmeterol (inhaler) infrequent use
- Omeprazole
- *Lignosus rhinocerus*; derived from tiger milk mushrooms, a traditional Chinese tonic with anti-inflammatory and immunomodulating properties used for respiratory ailments (Figure 9.2.1); used regularly instead of prescribed medications

Dental History
- Uses an acrylic partial upper denture fabricated over 10 years ago (overlays retained roots)
- Brushes his teeth once a day and at irregular intervals (due to work shift cycles)
- Diet: mainly rice with mixed vegetables and meat; drinks tea with condensed milk and sugar frequently to keep awake during shifts; irregular mealtimes
- Does not clean/brush denture

Social History
- Divorced, no children
- Lives alone
- Works as a security officer with alternating 8-hour shift cycle of work and rest
- Smoker – currently on 5 cigarettes a day (reduced from 20/day 5 years ago)

Oral Examination
- Poor oral hygiene
- Periodontitis with multiple mobile teeth and pathological tooth migration
- Rampant caries with retained roots, multiple dental caries (Figure 9.2.2)
- Lower anterior crowding
- Creamy white lesions on the hard/soft palate
- Upper denture with dried debris on fitting and smooth surfaces

Radiological Examination
- Orthopantomogram undertaken
- Gross caries in #28 (overerupted)
- Further caries in #36 and #47
- Retained roots: #16, #11, #21, #26, #37, #35, #44 and #45
- Generalised severe bone loss, in particular: #17, #15, #25 and #36 (bone loss 70%) and #47 (bone loss 100%)

Structured Learning

1) What is the most likely cause of the white lesions you have noticed on the patient's palate?
   - Acute pseudomembranous candidiasis, commonly referred to as thrush

A Practical Approach to Special Care in Dentistry, First Edition. Edited by Pedro Diz Dios and Navdeep Kumar.

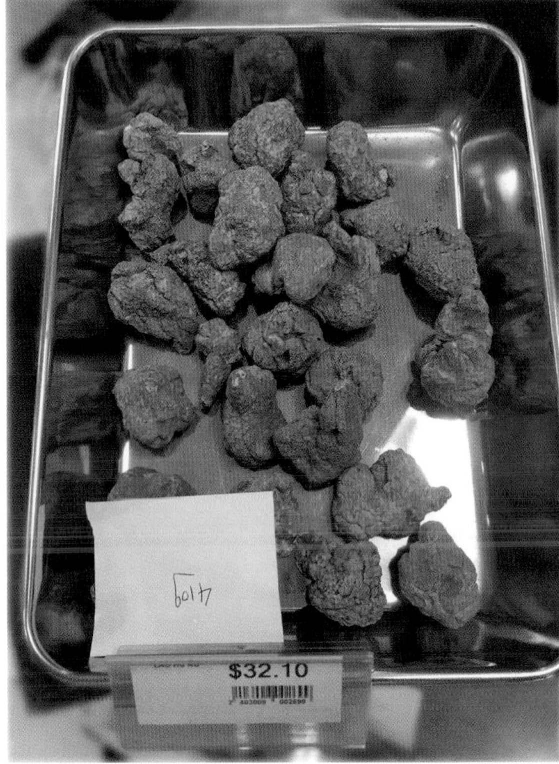

Figure 9.2.1 *Lignosus rhinocerus.*

- This is the most common type of oral candidiasis, accounting for about 35% of cases
- The patient is using a steroid-containing inhaler (fluticasone) which has an immunosuppressant effect and predisposes to the development of these lesions (exacerbated by a poorly cleaned denture)
- It is characterised by a coating of pseudomembranous white slough that can be easily wiped away to reveal an erythematous mucosal base underneath
- The white material is made up of debris, fibrin and desquamated epithelium and infiltrated by candidal hyphae (typically *Candida albicans*) to the depth of the stratum spinosum

2) What advice would you give the patient in relation to the oral lesions?
   - Oral candidal lesions are relatively common (studies vary widely in terms of stated prevalence due to the different diagnostic criteria used)
   - Preventive strategies
     - Review the use of inhaler to ensure that a deep breath is expelled before actuation – this ensures a subsequent deep breath in to draw the medication into the bronchi, rather than allowing it to accumulate in the mouth
     - Rinse the mouth and gargle with water after using an inhaler
     - Consider the use of a spacer to assist in drawing the inhaled medications into the lungs
     - Ensure that the denture is cleaned well, periodically disinfected and not worn at night (it can act as a reservoir for further candidal infection)
   - Therapeutic options
     - Oral candidosis may be persistent in the immunosuppressed patient using steroid inhalers frequently
     - Topical antifungal preparations of nystatin, amphotericin or miconazole are usually effective
     - Occasionally systemic medication, such as fluconazole, is required
3) You notice the patient has a continuous high-pitched whistling sound when breathing. What may be causing this?
   - The sound is likely to be due to a wheeze
   - Wheezes are produced by the oscillation of the airway walls with fluid within the airway

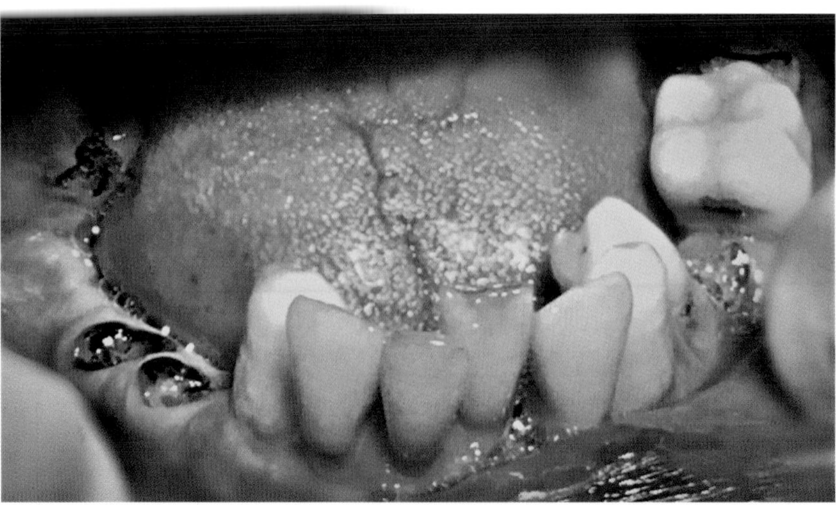

Figure 9.2.2 Mandibular dentition: rampant caries and multiple retained roots.

- It is most often heard on exhalation and is usually a sign of narrowing of the airway
- In this patient it is likely to be caused by his asthma

4) What does the sound tell you about his asthma severity and what other observations may help to clarify this?
   - The patient's asthma is likely to be moderate–severe
   - Other observations that may indicate severe asthma are:
     - Inability to complete sentences
     - Persistently breathless
     - Accessory muscles used to assist breathing (e.g. sternocleidomastoid and scalene neck muscle)
     - Tachypnea (≥25 breaths/min)
     - Tachycardia (heart rate ≥110 beats/min)
     - Pulsus paradoxus (large decrease beyond 10 mmHg in systolic blood pressure during inspiration)
5) The patient requests urgent removal of #28 in your dental clinic. Apart from the patient's wheeze, he has no other signs/symptoms suggestive of severe asthma. You contact the patient's physician who confirms that the patient's asthma is moderately well controlled and you can proceed. What factors are considered important in assessing the risk of managing this patient?
   - Social
     - Lives alone – lack of support/escort
     - Works shifts and hence may not be available during the day or may present for an appointment without having slept overnight
     - Dental anxiety may reduce co-operation and increase the likelihood of an acute exacerbation of his asthma (however, dental extraction of #28 is unlikely to require the use of handpieces due to advanced bone loss)
   - Medical
     - Infrequent attendance for medical review of his asthma may impact on the control of his disease and increase the risk of an acute asthma attack
     - Chinese tonic used regularly instead of prescribed drugs and hence asthma control may not be optimal; although there are as yet no known absolute contraindications to *Lignosus rhinoceros*, it should be used as a complementary medication rather than as an alternative
     - Asthma is associated with an increased risk of other atopic reactions, including drug allergies (e.g. penicillin)
     - Ibuprofen and aspirin are associated with a risk of precipitating asthmatic attacks via hypersensitivity pathways (e.g. Samter's triad syndrome)
     - Reduced mobility in relation to rheumatoid arthritis
     - A low BMI may indicate malnutrition, with an associated increased risk of anaemia and related reduced oxygenation (excessive tea consumption can also cause a deficiency of Fe and folic acid)
     - Visual impairment may impede communication
     - Steroid inhalers (high dose/frequent use) may be associated with adrenal suppression (see Chapter 12.1)
   - Dental
     - Removal of #28 may impact on the retention of his upper overdenture
     - Poor oral hygiene with associated oral health deterioration
     - Frequent cups of sweet tea and irregular mealtimes increase his caries risk
     - Inhaled beta-agonist and steroid increase risk of dry mouth, caries and periodontal inflammation
     - Inhaled steroids may also delay postsurgical wound healing and increase recurrent oral candidiasis risk
     - Oral mucosal malignancy risk is higher in association with long-term smoking and use of steroid inhalers
     - Gastro-oesophageal reflux may cause dental erosion
6) Dental extraction of #28 is uneventful. He requests painkillers postoperatively as the area has been painful and he does not wish to miss more shifts at work. What should you consider?
   - Advise the patient that it is important to rest and allow the area to heal adequately, particularly as healing is likely to be delayed in relation to steroid use
   - Lack of rest may also exacerbate his asthma
   - Advise him of the risk of aspirin-exacerbated respiratory disease, also known as Samter's triad
     - This consists of 3 clinical features: asthma, sinus disease with recurrent nasal polyps, and sensitivity to aspirin and other non-steroidal anti-inflammatory drugs (e.g. ibuprofen) that inhibit the enzyme cyclo-oxygenase-1
     - A single dose of aspirin can provoke an acute asthma exacerbation, accompanied by rhinorrhoea, conjunctival irritation and flushing of the head and neck
     - Approximately 9% of all adults with asthma and 30% of patients with asthma and nasal polyps have Samter's triad
7) The patient feels reassured after his experience of having #28 extracted. He is willing to return for regular care as he does not want to lose all his teeth. What are some effective ways to implement oral health prevention strategies for this patient?

- An oral health prevention programme should take into account the patient's shift patterns
- With the alternating 8-hour work cycle, he is unable to brush his teeth at regular times
- It is important to reinforce that improving oral health can help to avoid further pain, distress and disruption to his work
- Motivational interviewing may be helpful, where the patient is facilitated to establish his own methods in order to elicit the desired behavioural changes, which may include:
  - Rinsing his mouth after each inhaler use, which may not only reduce the risk of oral-mucosal lesions, but can also freshen his breath
  - Mouth rinsing is easier to use during his work shifts, compared to toothbrushing
  - He may consider the option of a fluoride mouthwash to reduce caries risk (0.05% or 225 ppm sodium fluoride) and further reduce halitosis
  - Removing the denture and cleaning it before sleep may reduce smoke stains on the acrylic base and improve halitosis

General Dental Considerations

Oral Findings

- Increased risk of dental caries
  - Saliva flow, composition and pH influenced by asthma medications or the disease itself
  - Decreased saliva secretion rate may be associated with the use of beta-2-agonist inhalers (bronchodilators) and anticholinergics
  - Inhalant medications also decrease salivary pH (reduced buffer capacity and remineralisation)
  - Secretory immunoglobulin A in saliva may be altered
- Increased risk of dental erosion
  - Possibly related to xerostomia and reduced buffering capacity of saliva secondary to medication
  - Gastro-oesophageal reflux symptoms 3 times more prevalent in asthma (bidirectional relationship – acid in the distal oesophagus increases airway reactivity and inhaled asthma medication may be swallowed, causing irritation)
  - Beta-2-agonists and drugs such as theophylline may also cause relaxation of other smooth muscles such as the lower oesophageal sphincter, leading to reflux
- Nasal symptoms, allergic rhinitis and mouth breathing are common in environmental allergy-induced asthma and may be associated with:
  - Higher palatal vault (Figure 9.2.3a)
  - Narrowing of the dental arc
  - Increased overjet (Figure 9.2.3b)
  - Malocclusion, including increased prevalence of posterior cross-bite
- Other medication-associated side-effects:
  - Beta-2-agonist inhalers can be associated with unpleasant taste
  - Inhaled steroids increase the risk of oral candidiasis, gingivitis and/or periodontitis; throat irritation, voice impairment, cough, dry mouth; rarely, angina bullosa haemorrhagica (localised purpura) and tongue enlargement have also been described

Dental Management

- Adaptations to enable the safe delivery of dental treatment are influenced by the severity of the patient's asthma and any related conditions (e.g. atopy resulting in multiple allergies) (Table 9.2.1)
- The features of the patient and management of these can give a broad indication but it is important to consult the patient's physician if moderate–severe asthma is suspected

(a)

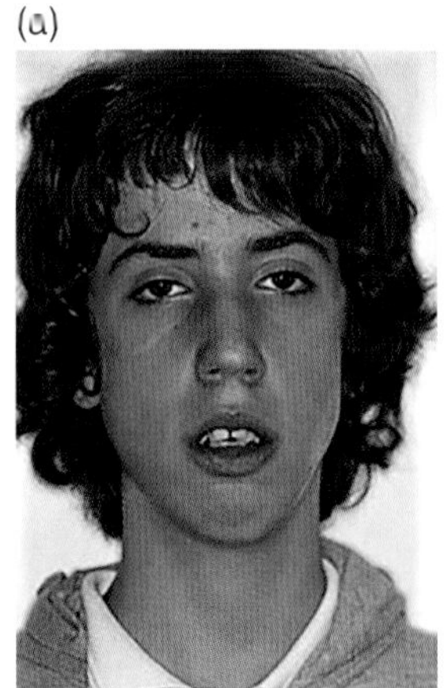

(b)

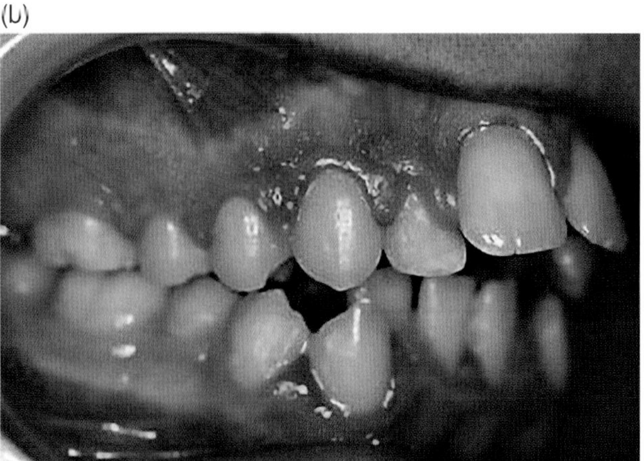

Figure 9.2.3 (a) Characteristic facial features of asthma. (b) Mouth-breathing effects on palate and developing dentition; increased overjet.

Table 9.2.1 Considerations for dental management.

Risk assessment	• Reduced respiratory function and exacerbation of asthma • Patients with asthma may be at risk of exacerbation in winter when it is colder or in spring/summer with seasonal pollen • Others may find attacks more likely in the morning • Risk of poor wound healing for extractions and surgical procedures • Comorbid concerns include: – Concurrent steroid usage – Atopic and concurrent allergy risk, especially allergic rhinitis – Gastro-oesophageal reflux disease – Associated immune dysregulation conditions (e.g. rheumatoid arthritis) – Penicillin allergy – Diabetes mellitus – Depression – Dyslipidaemia
Criteria for referral	• Dentists should be able to manage the vast majority of patients with asthma • It is good practice to consult a respiratory physician prior to treating patients with moderate–severe asthma for conscious sedation or prolonged surgical procedures • Patients with severe asthma, particularly those with severe intrinsic asthma, will require a hospital-based setting for invasive dental procedures
Access/position	• Schedule appointments with consideration of the risk factors which may trigger an exacerbation (e.g. seasonal factors/avoid early morning) • Postpone elective dental treatment for someone with severe asthma until they are stabilised • If breathing is compromised, a 45–60° inclination (Fowler's position) is beneficial compared to a fully supine position • During an acute asthmatic attack, sit the patient upright in the dental chair; patients tend to adopt a tripod position – leaning forward with arms and elbows supported over the knees to maximise lung capacity
Consent/capacity	• Mental capacity is not generally affected • In severe asthma/during an acute exacerbation, patients may experience difficulty speaking in complete sentences • Fatigue/exhaustion may impair the ability of the patient to engage in the discussion • Ensure that you discuss the potential for poor wound healing after dental surgical procedures
Anaesthesia/sedation	• Local anaesthesia – It is advisable to limit epinephrine containing local anaesthetics to 3 cartridges if the patient is taking theophylline (epinephrine-induced hypokalaemia is potentiated by therapeutic concentrations of theophylline) – Sulfite used to preserve vasoconstrictors is a known allergen and should be avoided – Esters-type local anaesthesia is more commonly associated with allergic reactions than amides and should be avoided (e.g. topical tetracaine, benzocaine) • Sedation – Opioids and benzodiazepines can cause further respiratory depression and should be avoided in patients with severe asthma – Oral sedation with antihistamines has an additional anti-allergy effect which may be of benefit; hydroxyzine also has anticholinergic effects which can reduce bronchial secretions – Nitrous oxide is the sedative of choice as it causes minimal depression and maintains oxygenation; however, it may dry the throat and cause irritation • General anaesthesia – Consult the patient's physician – Discuss the need for prior chest physiotherapy and postoperative admission – Postoperative respiratory complications are more frequent

(*Continued*)

Table 9.2.1 (Continued)

Dental treatment	• Before – Consult a physician prior to the appointment for patients with moderate–severe asthma – Confirm with the patient whether they have any acute symptoms/exacerbations – Ensure that the patient has their bronchodilator inhaler with them at the appointment – Prophylactic use of a bronchodilator (e.g. salbutamol) can be beneficial – Supplemental oxygen can be beneficial for long procedures or during sedation: patients with moderat–severe asthma are ideally given low-flow oxygen and SpO_2 is kept in an optimal range of 88–92% to maintain the hypoxic drive (PaO_2 55–60 mmHg) – Evaluate the appropriateness of rubber dam (e.g. in patients with latex allergy) and the potential to restrict respiration (e.g. in mouth breathers) – Determine the need for steroid cover for surgical procedures – Consider perioperative monitoring depending on the severity of the asthma (e.g. pulse oximetry and blood pressure) – note that a starting SpO_2 of 93% is equivalent to a drop of 40 mmHg in normal arterial blood oxygen • During – Avoid a fully supine position – It is reported that in 15% of asthmatics, routine dental treatment can provoke lung function suppression – Monitor for signs of respiratory distress/increased respiratory effort – Ensure effective suction of water/debris but be aware that high-volume suction can exacerbate shortness of breath – Consider the use of fast-setting impression materials and ensure the impression trays are not overloaded; 3D digital impression systems can be useful – Discontinue treatment if acute exacerbation of symptoms occurs • After – Close follow-up after surgery due to the risk of delayed healing – Primary closure of socket may improve healing
Drug prescription	• Ibuprofen and aspirin have a risk of precipitating asthmatic attacks via hypersensitivity pathways (e.g. Samter's triad syndrome) – paracetamol is a safer choice of analgesic • Ciprofloxacin, tramadol and erythromycin can reduce clearance of theophylline • Theophylline can reduce the effects of benzodiazepines
Education/prevention	• Encourage smoking cessation • High-fluoride regimen is required for patients with high caries risk. This can include 2800 ppm or 5000 ppm sodium fluoride toothpaste, and other fluoride-based dentifrices • Use of specific mouth gels and mouthwashes can help dryness and remineralisation • Provide preventive advice in relation to oral candidiasis (e.g. rinse thoroughly after using inhalers, review inhaler technique, consider the use of spacers) • Consider prescription of antifungal therapy if oral candidiasis does not resolve following preventive advice (repeated use of antifungal therapy may cause the emergence of resistant strains)

Section II: Background Information and Guidelines

Definition

Asthma is a common chronic inflammatory disease of the airways characterised by bronchospasm, oedematous swelling of the airway mucosa and hypersecretion of mucus. The major difference between asthma and COPD is that the airflow restriction in asthma is associated with a hyper-responsive component which is largely reversible. Although bronchial inflammation has long been recognised as a major factor, recent evidence suggests that small airways may also play a significant role.

Current evidence suggests that asthma may represent a component of systemic airway disease involving the entire respiratory tract. This is supported by the fact that asthma frequently coexists with other atopic disorders, particularly allergic rhinitis. Worldwide prevalence of asthma is estimated at 339 million people, with approximately 1000 deaths per day attributed to the disease.

Aetiopathogenesis

- Asthma is a type of hyper-reactivity condition which commonly starts from childhood in relation to sensitisation to common inhaled allergens
- It is mediated by stimulation of T helper type 2 (Th2) cell proliferation, resulting in Th2 cytokine and interleukin (IL)-4, IL-5 and IL-13 production and release

- Atopy, or the genetic predisposition to develop specific IgE antibodies directed against common environmental allergens, is the strongest identifiable risk factor for the development of asthma
- Genetic factors
  - Synergistic nature of multiple mutations identified, including polymorphisms in the gene that encodes platelet-activating factor hydrolase
  - It is proposed that a gene-by-environment interaction occurs in which the susceptible host is exposed to environmental factors that are capable of generating IgE, and sensitisation occurs
- Factors that can trigger/contribute to the development of asthma include:
  - Environmental allergens (e.g. house dust mites, animal allergens especially cat and dog, cockroach allergens and fungi)
  - Viral respiratory tract infections
  - Exercise, hyperventilation
  - Gastro-oesophageal reflux disease (GORD)
  - Chronic sinusitis or rhinitis
  - Aspirin or non-steroidal anti-inflammatory drug hypersensitivity, sulfite sensitivity
  - Use of beta-adrenergic receptor blockers (including ophthalmic preparations)
  - Obesity
  - Environmental pollutants
  - Tobacco smoke
  - Occupational exposure (e.g. plants, latex, gums, diisocyanates, anhydrides, wood dust and fluxes)
  - Irritants (e.g. household sprays, paint fumes)
  - Emotional factors or stress
  - Perinatal factors (e.g. prematurity and increased maternal age, maternal smoking and prenatal exposure to tobacco smoke; breastfeeding has not been definitely shown to be protective)

Clinical Presentation

- Classic signs and symptoms of asthma
  - Intermittent dyspnoea
  - Cough
  - Wheezing
- Previously used terms of allergic/extrinsic and idiosyncratic/intrinsic asthma have been replaced by 4 categories which reflect the clinical features and severity of the disease process (Table 9.2.2)
  - Mild intermittent asthma
  - Mild persistent asthma
  - Moderate persistent asthma
  - Severe persistent asthma
- In addition, the likelihood of an exacerbation (asthma attack) in each of the above results in further subclassification as stable or acute asthma
- In acute asthma, there are further subgroups which are related to specific management regimes: moderate acute asthma, acute severe asthma, life-threatening asthma (status asthmaticus) and near-fatal asthma
- Status asthmaticus is a potentially fatal emergency requiring timely management (Table 9.2.3); it is associated with the following clinical features:
  - Does not respond to standard bronchodilators or corticosteroids
  - Inability to complete sentences
  - Expiratory wheeze
  - Use of accessory muscles
  - Respiratory rate elevated to over 25 breaths per minute
  - Reduced oxygen saturation (over 92%)

Table 9.2.2 Asthma severity.

		Persistent		
Components of severity	**Intermittent**	**Mild**	**Moderate**	**Severe**
Symptoms	≤2 days/week	> 2 days/week	Daily	Throughout the day
Night-time awakening	≤2 nights/month	3–4 nights/month	>1 night/week	Often/every night
Short-acting beta-2-agonist used for symptom control	≤2 days/week	>2 days/week but not daily	Daily	Several times per day
Interference with normal activity	None	Minor limitation	Some limitation	Extremely limited
Lung function	Normal FEV1 between exacerbations FEV1 >80% predicted FEV1/FVC >85%	FEV1 >80% FEV1/FVC >80%	FEV1 60–80% FEV1/FVC >75–80%	FEV1 <60% FEV1/FVC <75%

FEV1, forced expiratory volume over 1 second; FVC, forced vital capacity.
Source: Adapted from National Heart, Lung and Blood Institute (NHLBI) Expert Panel Report (EPR3). Guidelines for the Diagnosis and Management of Asthma. www.nhlbi.nih.gov/sites/default/files/media/docs/EPR-3_Asthma_Full_Report_2007.pdf.

Table 9.2.3 Asthma attack severity and emergency management.

	Moderate acute asthma		
Clinical signs and symptoms	• Increasing symptoms of breathlessness, expiratory wheeze, increased pulse rate, use of accessory muscles to optimise ventilation capacity • Peak expiratory flow (PEF) above 50–75% at best (as predicted) • No symptoms of the severe form		
Management of moderate acute asthma	• Stop treatment and sit upright comfortably • Provide supplementary oxygen up to 15 L per minute • Use the patient's own beta-agonist (e.g. salbutamol 100–200 μg/actuation) and repeat as required. Otherwise, this should be within the emergency inventory of the dental clinic • Shake the inhaler well, seal lips around it, exhale, press the puffer and concurrently inhale slowly, hold the breath for at least 4 seconds, and exhale. Repeat until the required actuation is achieved. Children can receive up to 4 actuations from the beta-agonist inhaler and adults 6–8, every 4 minutes • Alternatively, a spacer can be used. The inhaler is inserted onto the spacer and fires 1 puff, taking 4 breaths per puff. Repeat till 4 puffs have been given. In severe or more serious forms of attack, 10 actuations are given via the spacer • A nebuliser contains a small vial of the beta-agonist. Oxygen or compressed air is used to create a small aerosol droplet of the beta-agonist where it is inhaled with the oxygen • Peak expiratory flow and forced expiratory volume are useful and valid measures (see above). In the absence of a suitable test, a predicted percentage can be used as a rough guide • Pulse oximetry can determine the adequacy of supplementary oxygen therapy, where ideally 94–98% saturation is achieved • If response is poor (no relief after 10 minutes or 2 episodes of actuations), start managing as if a severe form, call an ambulance or activate the medical emergency team IMMEDIATELY • If the patient recovers, monitor closely for recurrent attacks. Postpone elective dental treatment. It is good practice to ensure the patient is accompanied home, or to the physician as required		
	Severe acute asthma	**Status asthmaticus (life-threatening asthma)**	**Near-fatal asthma**
Clinical signs and symptoms	Any indication of: • Inability to complete sentences • Increased respiratory rate over 25 breaths/min • Tachycardia (heart rate >110 beats/min) • PEF 33–50% at best (as predicted)	Any indication of: • Reduced respiratory rate under 8 per minute • Bradycardia (heart rate <50 beats/min) • Paleness or cyanosis • Altered mental state • PEF under 33% at best (as predicted)	• Increased $PaCO_2$ with capnography • Person requires mechanical ventilation on increased inflation pressure
Emergency management of asthma attack	• If the acute asthma is at least the severe form, call an ambulance or activate the medical emergency team IMMEDIATELY • A large-volume spacer device can be used with up to 10 salbutamol activations. This can be repeated every 10 minutes until help arrives • Epinephrine (intramuscular or hypodermic injection) can be given to reduce hypersensitivity reaction. In particular if bronchospasm is a feature of an anaphylactic reaction, or if life-threatening signs occur • Someone with status asthmaticus can exhibit a lowered SpO_2 of 92% on room air, but typically not any lower. Monitoring is beneficial while waiting for help to arrive; this helps anticipate deterioration • Corticosteroids have been taken out of the algorithm for acute asthma attacks. However, they may be useful when treating an attack of a different endotype[a] • Continue monitoring of respiratory rate and heart rate. If loss of consciousness ensues, conduct life-support algorithm		

[a] Endotype means a subtype of disease. A disease endotype has a functionally and pathologically distinct molecular mechanism or has distinct treatment responses.

Source: Adapted from British Thoracic Society/Scottish Intercollegiate Guidelines Network (BTS/SIGN). (2019). *SIGN 158 British Guideline on the Management of Asthma*. www.brit-thoracic.org.uk/quality-improvement/guidelines/asthma/.

Diagnosis

- There is no gold standard definition for the diagnosis of asthma
- Diagnosis of asthma is largely based on clinical features
- These include the presence of at least 2 of the following symptoms: wheeze, breathlessness, chest tightness, cough, accompanied by variable airflow obstruction
- More recent descriptions of asthma in children and in adults have included airway hyper-responsiveness and airway inflammation as components of the disease
- Additional investigations which may assist in diagnosis may be used but are dependent on the patient's age in terms of their suitability
  - Spirometry – demonstrates lowered peak expiratory flow rate (PEFR) and forced expiratory volume over 1 second (FEV1) (Figure 9.2.4)
  - Arterial blood gas analysis – measures the acidity (pH) and the levels of oxygen and carbon dioxide
  - Skin prick test (or scratch test)
  - Exercise tolerance test
  - Blood tests: raised total IgE and specific IgE antibody concentrations
  - Chest radiographs are used to exclude other pulmonary disease (e.g. pneumomediastinum, pneumothorax); they are also used in life-threatening asthma, or for those patients who do not respond well to treatment

Management

- Long-term follow-up, functional monitoring and education
- Pharmacological management includes medication which broadly falls into the following categories (Table 9.2.4):
  - Inhalers
    - Relievers (to relieve symptoms)
    - Preventers (to stop symptoms developing)
    - Combination (relieves and prevents)
  - Tablets
    - Leukotriene receptor antagonists (may also come in syrup and powder form)
    - Theophylline
    - Steroid tablets
  - Injections every few weeks
    - Monoclonal antibodies (e.g. benralizumab, omalizumab, mepolizumab, reslizumab)
- Non-pharmacological management
  - Environment control, smoking cessation

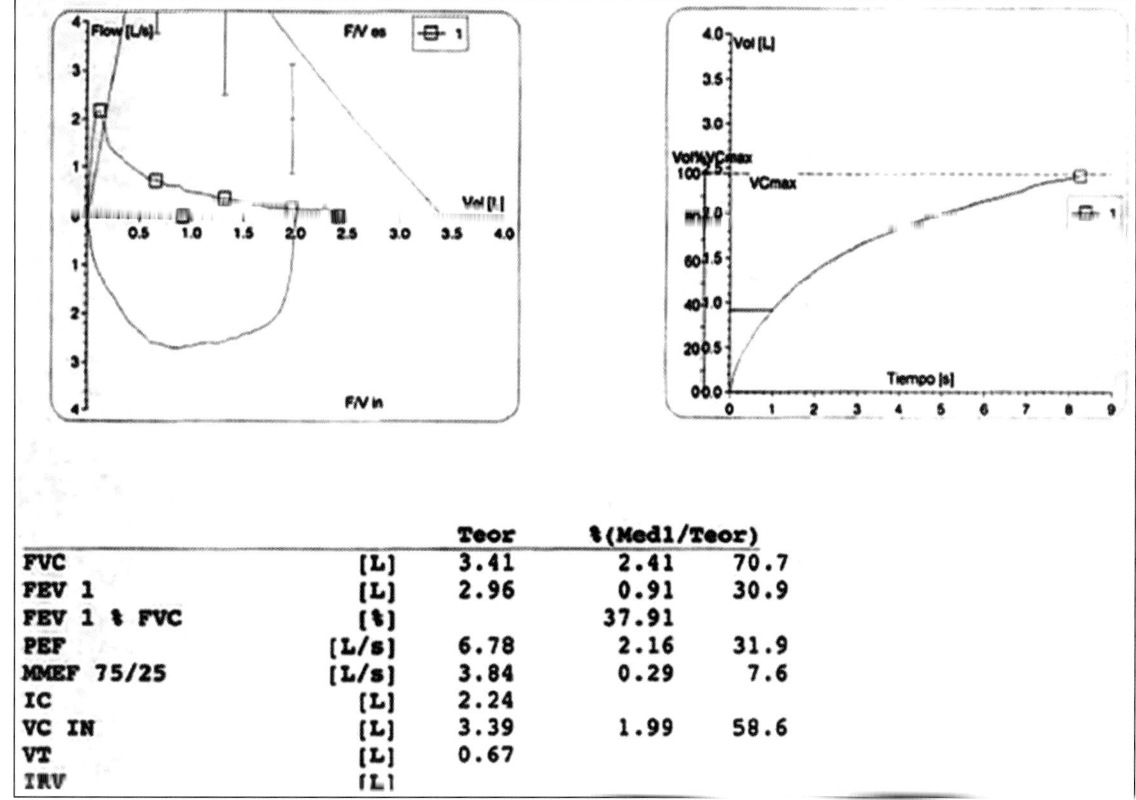

		Teor	%(Med1/Teor)	
FVC	[L]	3.41	2.41	70.7
FEV 1	[L]	2.96	0.91	30.9
FEV 1 % FVC	[%]		37.91	
PEF	[L/s]	6.78	2.16	31.9
MMEF 75/25	[L/s]	3.84	0.29	7.6
IC	[L]	2.24		
VC IN	[L]	3.39	1.99	58.6
VT	[L]	0.67		
IRV	[L]			

Figure 9.2.4 Spirometry is the recommended test to confirm asthma (see also Figure 9.1.3).

Table 9.2.4 Pharmacological management of asthma.

Category of medication	Examples	Details
Beta-2-agonist inhalers (short-acting)	Salbutamol Levalbuterol Fenoterol Terbutaline	Safe and effective bronchodilators with minimal cardiac effects Effect lasts 3–6 hours
Anticholinergic relievers	Ipratropium bromide Tiotropium Oxitropium	Effects lasts up to 8 hours
Beta-2-agonist inhalers (long-acting)	Salmeterol Formoterol Bambuterol	Effect lasts at least 12 hours
Corticosteroid preventers	Beclomethasone Ciclesonide Budesonide Fluticasone	Associated adrenal suppression can occur
Leukotriene receptor antagonists and 5-lipoxygenase inhibitors	Montelukast Zafirlukast Pranlukast Zileuton	May impair liver function
Combination	Fluticasone+salmeterol Budesonide+formoterol	Increased efficacy but also adverse effects
Methylxanthines	Theophylline	For nocturnal asthma High doses may cause cardiac arrhythmias or convulsions Metabolised by cytochrome P450
Mast cell stabilisers	Cromoglicic acid Nedocromil sodium	Prevent release of inflammatory mediators like histamine
Recombinant monoclonal antibodies	Omalizumab (anti-IgE) Mepolizumab (anti-IL5)	For allergic or eosinophilic asthma

  - Lifestyle adjustments such as avoiding aeroallergens with dust mites, pets or food
  - Obese adults and children with asthma should be offered weight loss programmes to reduce other respiratory symptoms and improve control
  - Limiting excessive physical exertion
  - Respiratory rehabilitation including chest physiotherapy is helpful in reducing symptoms and improving quality of life
- Surgery
  - Bronchial thermoplasty, an intervention where controlled thermal energy is applied to the airway via a series of bronchoscopy procedures
- Other therapies
  - Allergen immunotherapy can benefit allergy-induced asthma, where small doses of allergen are regularly infused over 3–5 years
  - Complementary medicine (limited evidence regarding effectiveness): acupuncture, traditional Chinese herbal medicine, homeopathy, dietary supplements

Prognosis

- Prognosis is good, especially when first appearing in childhood
- In adults, asthma may progress to respiratory failure
- Status asthmaticus can persist up to days and is a life-threatening emergency
- Early life atopy such as asthma may be associated with later life proinflammatory disease and immune dysregulation like psoriasis, diabetes, cardiac disease and rheumatoid arthritis

A World/Transcultural View

- Asthma is a common worldwide respiratory condition, prevalent in 1 in 11 children and 1 in 20 adults
- Asthma is common in industrialised nations such as Canada, England, Australia, Germany and New Zealand, where much of the asthma data have been collected
- It has been described that parents of children from ethnic populations do not see asthma as a chronic disease which requires daily use of a preventive medication, but rather as

an acute phenomenon triggered by various factors; this may be missed during medical history collection and has an impact on education and communication

- Traditional Chinese herbal remedies have been used in many parts of the world alongside or in place of conventional therapies

Recommended Reading

Agostini, B.A., Collares, K.F., Costa, F.D.S. et al. (2019). The role of asthma in caries occurence – meta-analysis and meta-regression. *J. Asthma* 56: 841–852.

Bairappan, S., Puranik, M.P., and Sowmya, K.R. (2020). Impact of asthma and its medication on salivary characteristics and oral health in adolescents: a cross-sectional comparative study. *Spec. Care Dentist.* 40: 227–237.

Gani, F., Caminati, M., Bellavia, F. et al. (2020). Oral health in asthmatic patients: a review (Asthma and its therapy may impact on oral health). *Clin. Mol. Allergy* 18: 22.

Moraschini, V., Calasans-Maia, J.A., and Calasans-Maia, M.D. (2018). Association between asthma and periodontal disease: a systematic review and meta-analysis. *J. Periodontol.* 89: 440–455.

Morris, M.J. and Pearson, D.J. (2020). Asthma: Practice Essentials, Background, Anatomy. https://emedicine.medscape.com/article/296301-overview

Baghani, E. and Ouanounou, A. (2021).The dental management of the asthmatic patients. *Spec. Care Dentist.* 41: 309–318.

Shah, P.D., Badner, V.M., Rastogi, D., and Moss, K.L. (2020). Association between asthma and dental caries in US (United States) adult population. *J. Asthma*: 1–8.

10

Bleeding Disorders

10.1 Haemophilia

Section I: Clinical Scenario and Dental Considerations

Clinical Scenario

A 36-year-old male attends for an emergency dental appointment at the end of the day. He complains of persistent dull pain of 2 weeks' duration from the lower right second molar (#47). There is associated buccal swelling. Painkillers have been required daily and he requests dental extraction of this painful tooth.

Medical History

- Haemophilia A with inhibitors to factor VIII (FVIII)
  - Prior to inhibitor development, required recombinant FVIII (rFVIII) on demand only (mild–moderate haemophilia)
  - Inhibitors developed 7 years ago following high-dose FVIII required after an ankle injury, converting patient's phenotype to severe
  - Initially required prophylactic recombinant factor VIIa (rFVIIa) when inhibitor titre was high
  - As inhibitor titre has reduced, rFVIIa now only required on demand
- Left ankle arthrodesis (fusion) 1 year ago due to haemarthrosis
- Chronic hepatitis C infection acquired from blood transfusions as a child

Medications

- Recombinant FVIIa (on demand)
- Paracetamol as required

Dental History

- Irregular dental attender; only presents when he has dental issues
- Dental anxiety due to previous poor experiences with dental extractions
- Three wisdom teeth extracted under general anaesthesia 4 years ago
- Brushes teeth once daily at night only; no interdental cleaning

Social History

- Single, lives alone, no children
- Mixed heritage: Hispanic, Japanese and Anglo-Saxon ethnic origin
- Mother carrier for haemophilia gene (lives overseas)
- Escort: friend as required but needs advance notice due to his job
- Occupation: support worker for adults living with disability; feels haemophilia has limited his employment opportunities (e.g. labour jobs)
- Walks with a limp; unable to walk long distances or run/jog due to previous left ankle injury
- Tobacco consumption nil
- Alcohol: consumes 20 cans of premixed alcohol-containing drinks per week (~30 units)

Oral Examination

- Extensive caries on #36 and #47
- Multiple other smaller dental caries on #15, #21 and #22
- Moderate supra- and subgingival calculus

Radiological Examination

- Orthopantomogram undertaken (Figure 10.1.1)
- Extensive distal caries on #47 with pulpal involvement and periapical radiolucency
- Mesial caries on #36 with likely pulpal involvement
- Missing teeth #18, #28, #38 and #46
- Mild horizontal bone loss ~10%

A Practical Approach to Special Care in Dentistry, First Edition. Edited by Pedro Diz Dios and Navdeep Kumar.

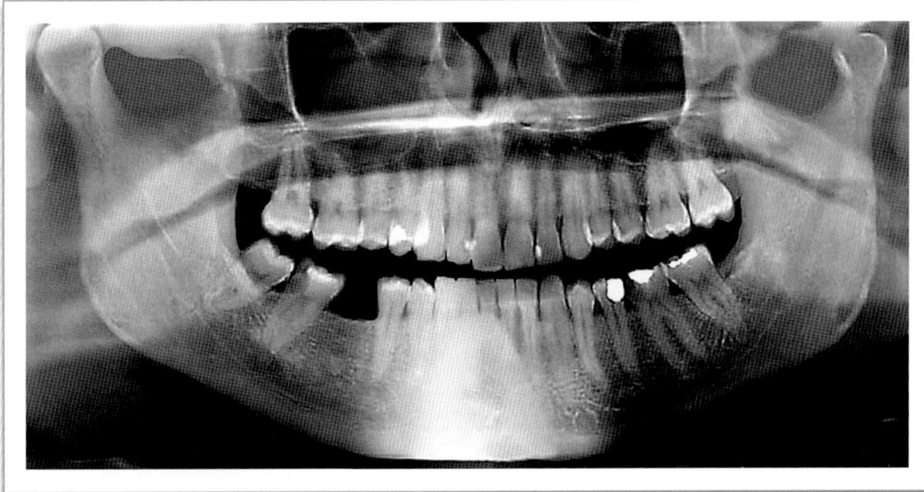

Figure 10.1.1 Orthopantomogram showing extensive caries.

Structured Learning

1) This patient has developed inhibitors to factor replacement therapy for his haemophilia. Why is this?
   - Inhibitors (antibodies) are produced because the body sees the factor concentrates used to treat patients with haemophilia as foreign; this activates an immune response in the patient to destroy the foreign substances
   - Additional risk factors in this patient for the development of inhibitors include:
     - Patients with haemophilia A are more likely to develop inhibitors, i.e. approximately 20–30% of people with haemophilia A develop inhibitors, compared to <6% for patients with haemophilia B
     - This patient received a high dose of factor replacement in relation to the ankle injury which may trigger a strong immune response
     - Patients of Hispanic (or African) heritage have an increased risk of inhibitor formation; the mechanisms that account for these racial/ethnic differences remain unclear
2) The patient reports that his inhibitor level has fallen since first detected. Could he be correct?
   - In approximately two-thirds of cases, the inhibitors disappear on their own or with treatment known as immune tolerance induction
   - Immune tolerance induction with the regular infusion of FVIII in small doses can induce FVIII antigen-specific tolerance
3) What is the significance of the patient's inhibitor development when planning dental care?
   - Although the patient reports that he now has low titres of factor inhibitor, advice of the haematologist must be sought to clarify this
   - Clotting factor replacement may not be effective at preventing excessive bleeding if surgical dental procedures are planned
   - Alternative agents which bypass the need for factor replacement may be required (e.g. recombinant FVIIa or FVIII inhibitor bypassing agent)
   - However, bypassing agents are not as effective in controlling bleeding
   - Furthermore, the cost of treatment is twice that for patients without inhibitors, partly due to the cost of the products required but also related to the need for admission in relation to increased bleeding risk
   - This patient should be managed in a specialised dental unit with appropriate clinical expertise and laboratory support
4) What factors do you need to consider in your risk assessment when planning dental treatment for this patient?
   - Social
     - Lives alone
     - Needs advance notice to arrange an escort if required
     - Reduced mobility
     - High alcohol intake – may impact on his attendance, capacity and also his bleeding risk
   - Medical
     - Haemophilia complicated by development of inhibitors
     - Potential for residual hepatic cirrhosis due to chronic hepatitis C; impact on bleeding, drug metabolism, development of hepatocellular carcinoma
   - Dental
     - Dental anxiety
     - High sugar/acid consumption
     - Poor oral hygiene habits
     - Irregular dental attendance

5) You advise dental extraction of #36 and #47 – the patient wishes to have #47 extracted the same day as his assessment appointment as the tooth is painful. Would you proceed?
   - Do not extract the tooth on the same day – multiple factors need to be considered and appropriate treatment modifications put in place
   - Focus on pain and infection control: review painkillers taken and consider draining any infection through the tooth/antibiotic prescription
   - This patient is at particularly high risk of bleeding due to underlying haemophilia, presence of inhibitors, potential liver cirrhosis secondary to hepatitis C, leading to depletion of clotting factors, and the haematological effects of alcohol excess (see Chapter 15.5)
   - Obtaining further information on liver function status is prudent to identify further potential issues with coagulation and drug metabolism
   - Spontaneous bleeding in patients with haemophilia has also been reported under conditions of emotional stress – this patient has reported dental anxiety in relation to dental extractions
   - Dental anxiety and risk of a failed procedure are high
   - An escort is preferable and is not available on the day
   - The patient has presented at the end of the working day – if he has bleeding issues, he will not be able to return to you/access routine support from the haematology team
   - Close liaison with the haematologist is required; in this case the haematologist advised pre- and postoperative oral tranexamic acid in addition to rFVIIa and DDAVP; observation on the ward for 24 hour postoperatively was also recommended
6) Following completion of dental extractions, the patient returns to you 4 months later and has developed further dental caries. What precautions would you undertake when providing the restorations?
   - Avoid soft tissue trauma
   - Care with matrix bands, wedges and rubber dam clamp positioning
   - Care with high-volume vacuum aspirators and saliva ejectors in the floor of mouth to avoid gingival bleeding/production of haematomas
   - Care with taking mandibular intraoral radiographs
   - Moisten cotton rolls to avoid sticking to mucosa
   - Subgingival restorations performed using retraction cord with haemostatic solution, or local anaesthesia with epinephrine
   - Tranexamic mouthwash may be useful to control bleeding

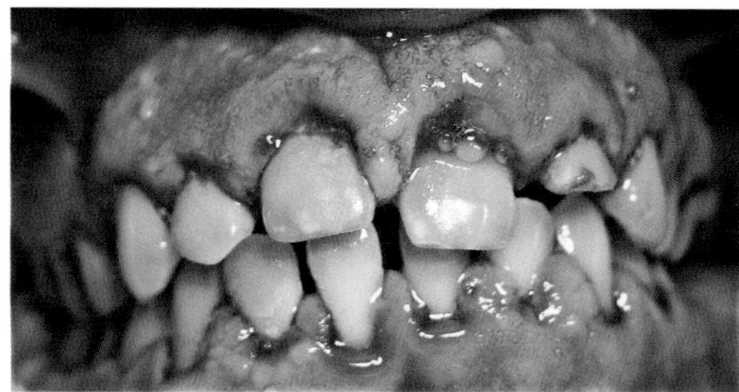

Figure 10.1.2 Spontaneous gingival bleeding.

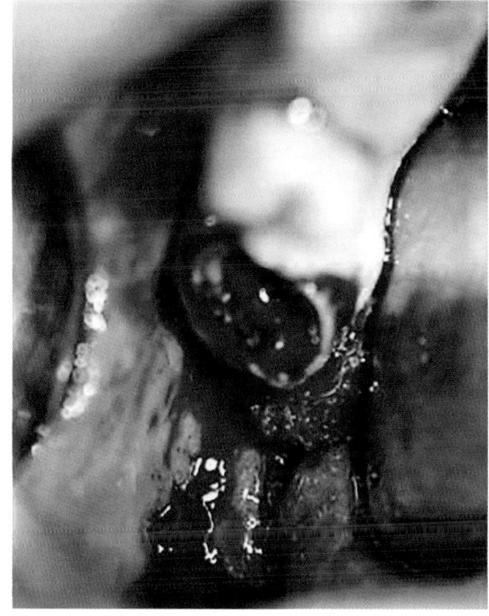

Figure 10.1.3 Persistent bleeding from hyperplastic pulpitis (pulp polyp).

General Dental Considerations

Oral Findings

- Petechiae
- Ecchymoses
- Spontaneous gingival bleeding (Figure 10.1.2)
- Prolonged bleeding after invasive procedures (Figure 10.1.3)

Dental Management

- It is important to determine the severity of the haemophilia and the degree of invasiveness of the proposed dental treatment (Table 10.1.1; Figure 10.1.4)
- This will allow formulation of an appropriate plan in conjunction with the haemophilia team
- The use of topical haemostatic agents should be considered for invasive dental procedures (see Appendix I)

Table 10.1.1 General dental management considerations.

Risk assessment	• Bleeding from surgery and trauma • Mild haemophilia may go undiagnosed until prolonged bleeding results from dental extraction • Impaired mobility and careful positioning (haemarthroses) • Blood-borne viruses in older patients with haemophilia due to unscreened blood transfusions – Hepatitis (increased bleeding, impaired drug metabolism, cross-infection risk) – HIV (infection risks, cross-infection risk) • Analgesic drug tolerance due to chronic pain medications
Criteria for referral	• Most patients with mild haemophilia can receive the majority of their routine dental care in the primary care setting, following the principles below: – Initial liaison with patient's haemophilia centre to confirm disease severity and management – Focus on prevention of dental disease, with regular reviews tailored to the individual's need – Judicious planning of procedures likely to cause bleeding, with close liaison maintained between dentist and haemophilia centre. Prophylactic cover to be arranged by haemophilia unit. Postoperative management with tranexamic acid and local measures – Invasive procedures performed in a specialised/hospital-based dental unit, ideally linked to the haemophilia unit • Dental treatment in patients with moderate/severe haemophilia should be performed in a specialist dental unit where available. The exception is if prior arrangements have been made between the haemophilia centre and primary care dentist • Patients with inhibitors should be managed in specialised dental units with appropriate clinical expertise and laboratory support
Access/position	• Many patients with haemophilia have experienced refusal of treatment by primary care dentists, so may avoid the dentist until in need of extensive treatment • Ensure appropriate setting for invasive dental care • Consider the need for an escort • Timing of treatment: optimally 1 hour after factor replacement therapy, and preferably in the morning and early in the week • Ideally perform treatment in 1 visit or on consecutive days to minimise the number of factor replacement sessions (thus likelihood of antibody development and costs); however, must be weighed up against the need to stage extractions to minimise bleeding risk • Care with patient positioning due to haemarthroses and chronic pain/impaired mobility; consider ground floor surgery
Communication	• Close liaison with the haemophilia team to confirm disease severity and management
Consent/capacity	• Warn patient of the increased risk of intraoral/postoperative bleeding and intra/extraoral bruising • Inform of the measures which will be used to reduce bleeding risk, so as to not discourage patient from attending appointments • Capacity is not impaired unless there is brain haemorrhage/impaired cognition
Anaesthesia/sedation	• Local anaesthesia – No factor replacement is required for buccal infiltrations – Regional block injections, lingual infiltrations or injections into the floor of mouth require factor replacement, due to risk of haemorrhage or life-threatening airway blockage (80% risk of haematomas) – Consider alternative anaesthesia methods: buccal, intraligamentary, intraosseous, papillary or electronic dental infiltrations – Delivered using an aspirating syringe and should include a vasoconstrictor, unless contraindicated – Anaesthetic solution should be delivered slowly to avoid rapid expansion of the soft tissues • Sedation – Oral sedation and nitrous oxide preferred – Intravenous sedation cannulation poses a risk of haematoma formation, though this is rare under factor cover. Dorsum of the hand is preferred to the antecubital fossa • General anaesthesia – Hazards of anaesthesia, especially nasal intubation and intramuscular injections – This must be considered when planning factor replacement – Assessment by the anaesthetist prior to the day of planned surgery; must work in close consultation with haematologist

(Continued)

Table 10.1.1 (Continued)

	– Ensure haematology protocol followed, and that tranexamic acid, DDAVP and factor replacement are available as required – Careful planning prior to surgery to ensure all necessary surgical dental treatment is performed in 1 session. This should include a detailed radiographic survey to identify any other teeth that may also require exodontia – Overnight stay and postoperative follow-up should be considered, especially if the patient has developed inhibitors
Dental treatment	• Before – Liaise closely with the haemophilia team regarding the most recent factor levels and need for factor replacement prior to dental treatment – Non-surgical dental treatment can usually be carried out with minimal problems, with occasional use of antifibrinolytic cover (tranexamic acid mouthwash/tablets) or desmopressin – No current consensus on minimum factor level required for oral surgery; generally minimum 50–75% factor levels recommended for dental extractions and minimum 75% (ideally 100%) for maxillofacial surgery – Confirm haematologist has arranged appropriate cover, and patient has adhered to the haemostatic management plan prior to commencing treatment – Periodontology: placement of non-injectable anaesthetic gels (e.g. 2.5% lidocaine/2.5% prilocaine) using a blunt-ended needle tip into periodontal pockets prior to scaling – Soft vacuum-formed splints may be constructed in advance for patients with inhibitors to aid stabilisation of the clot and protect it from trauma; however, in some circumstances, they may increase the risk of mucosal trauma and ischaemic tissue necrosis and promote sepsis • During – Lubricant/barrier cream used to protect the lips/soft tissue from trauma – Careful manipulation of the cheek and soft tissues – consider the use of gauze when using cheek retractors – Caution with suction to avoid trauma (reduce the volume) and particular care taken to avoid trauma in the floor of mouth – Atraumatic extraction technique preferred – If a mucoperiosteal flap is required, a buccal approach is best since lingual tissue trauma may open up planes into which haemorrhage may track and endanger the airway – Minimal bone removal, teeth sectioned where possible – Local haemostatic measures to control bleeding Bony wound compressed with absorbent gauze – Tranexamic acid 5% mouthwash may be used as an adjunct; this can be soaked in gauze and applied directly over the socket; tranexamic acid 8% gel is also available – Vasoconstrictor local anaesthesia injection locally may assist but haemostasis will not be maintained – Topical haemostatic agents can be used either directly or applied to the area on sterile gauze: minimise use of socket packing agents as they may increase the incidence of dry socket; ensure agent of choice is acceptable to patient as some contain animal based proteins – Suturing: use non-traumatic needles and small number of sutures – Fit soft vacuum-formed splints if these have been constructed – Some patients recognise early symptoms of bleeding, even before physical signs manifest (e.g. 'aura' tingling sensation) – Endodontics: do not instrument beyond the apex (apex locator useful); intracanal anaesthesia with epinephrine may be helpful to reduce bleeding risk; consider factor replacement in patients with severe haemophilia where it is not possible to control bleeding from the canal • After – Extended monitoring. The initial platelet clot may form but can be followed by a slow bleed due to defective clotting factors – Check for haematoma formation with a particular focus on the patient's airways (swelling, dysphagia, hoarseness) – Careful oral cleansing postoperatively – Provide verbal and written postoperative instruction and emergency contact details – Advise the patient to contact the haemophilia unit if bleeding persists – Warn of possibility of postoperative haemorrhage, usually after 7–12 hours (or from 4 to 10 days)

(*Continued*)

Table 10.1.1 (Continued)

	– If a vacuum-formed splint was fitted: ○ Leave in situ for at least 48 hours ○ Advise not to rinse vigorously whilst wearing splint (the patient may eat and drink normally) ○ After 48 hours, remove splint, check socket ○ If clot is stable, splint may be removed and standard mouthcare protocol followed; otherwise, splint may be cleaned and replaced if necessary – Due to inhibitors, consider use of antibiotics to reduce the risk of secondary infection and subsequent fibrinolysis – Arrange close follow-up within 1 week
Drug prescription	• Antiseptics as required (e.g. 0.12–0.2% chlorhexidine rinses every 8 h) • Antibiotics (e.g. amoxicillin, penicillin V, amoxicillin/clavulanic acid or metronidazole at therapeutic doses) • Pain relief (e.g. paracetamol); the patient may already be on chronic pain medication • Avoid aspirin, ibuprofen and diclofenac as these may increase bleeding risk
Education/ prevention	• Patients with moderate/severe haemophilia should have a dental review every 6 months (or as appropriate to dental disease risk) • Patients whose hands/arms have been affected with haemarthroses may benefit from adapting toothbrush and/or toothbrushing technique • Use of fluoride and fissure sealants, oral hygiene education, dietary advice and regular dental visits from an early age (start of tooth eruption) to minimise dental treatment that may cause bleeding complications • Comprehensive orthodontic assessment at 12–13 years old to forestall difficulties resulting from crowding and wisdom teeth

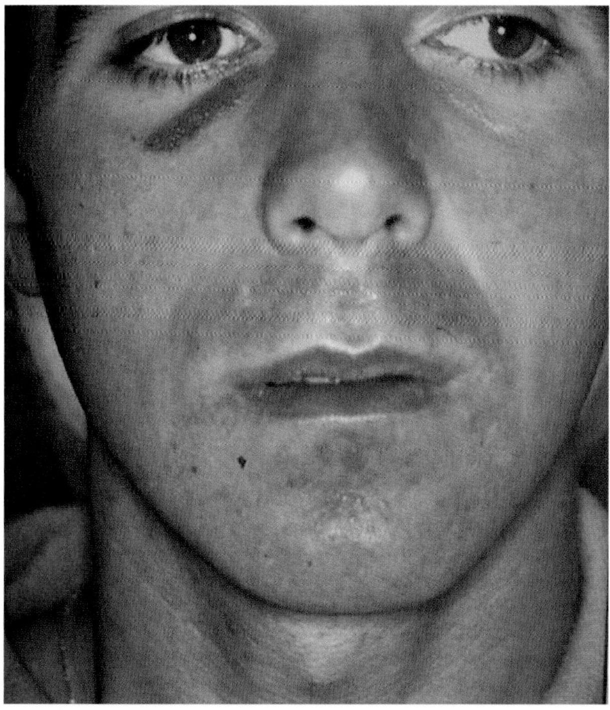

Figure 10.1.4 Infraorbital haematoma following infiltrative local anaesthesia.

Section II: Background Information and Guidelines

Definition

Haemophilia is a predominantly inherited blood coagulation factor defect of which there are multiple variants (Table 10.1.2). Although its prevalence varies among different countries, it affects all ethnic populations and is estimated as occurring in 3–20 cases per 100 000 population.

The most common forms are the congenital X-linked recessive disorders haemophilia A (deficiency of FVIII) and haemophilia B (deficiency of IX). Haemophilia C and other less common inherited autosomal recessive factor deficiencies also exist, as well as acquired haemophilia. The incidence of haemophilia A is 6.6–12.8 per 100 000, and haemophilia B is 1.2–2.7 per 100 000.

Aetiopathogenesis

- Haemophilia A and B
  - X-linked recessive inheritance pattern and hence predominantly affect males on the maternal side

Table 10.1.2 Blood coagulation factor defects in descending order of frequency.

Factor deficient	Inheritance	Prevalence (1 case in)
VIII (haemophilia A)	X-linked recessive	10 000
IX (haemophilia B/ Christmas disease)	X-linked recessive	60 000
VII	Autosomal recessive	500 000
V	Autosomal recessive	1 million
X	Autosomal recessive	1 million
XI (haemophilia C)	Autosomal recessive	1 million
XII	Autosomal recessive	1 million
XIII	Autosomal recessive	1 million
Fibrinogen	Autosomal recessive	1 million
Prothrombin	Autosomal recessive	2 million

  - Approximately 150 different point mutations in the FVIII gene have been characterised in haemophilia A, but a family history can be obtained in only about 65% of cases
  - Women with a spontaneous FVIII or FIX gene mutation may have reduced factor levels, and hence be classified as having haemophilia
  - Some female carriers experience symptoms of haemophilia due to the process of lyonisation (X chromosome inactivation)
  - If a woman has <40% of normal clotting factor, she is classified as having haemophilia
  - A woman with 40–60% of normal clotting factor levels who experiences abnormal bleeding is a symptomatic carrier
- Haemophilia C and the other autosomal recessive inherited factor disorders affect males and females in equal numbers

Clinical Presentation

- Severity of bleeding is correlated with the clotting factor level, and is classified as mild, moderate or severe. Normal plasma contains 1 unit of factor per millilitre, a level defined as 100% (Table 10.1.3)
- Depending on the severity of the deficiency, the first symptoms of haemophilia can arise at various ages

Table 10.1.3 Severity of haemophilia (World Federation of Haemophilia 2012).

Severity	Clotting factor level	Bleeding episodes
Severe	<1 IU/dL (<0.01 IU/mL) or <1% of normal	Spontaneous bleeding into joints or muscles, predominantly in the absence of identifiable haemostatic challenge
Moderate	1–5 IU/dL (0.01–0.05 IU/mL) or 1–5% of normal	Occasional spontaneous bleeding. Prolonged bleeding with minor trauma or surgery
Mild	5–40 IU/dL (0.05–0.40 IU/mL) or 5–<40% of normal	Severe bleeding with major trauma or surgery. Spontaneous bleeding is rare

  - Severe cases of haemophilia usually are diagnosed within the first year of life with excessive bleeding after trauma, and sometimes spontaneously
  - Mild forms may not be apparent until adulthood, with patients first being investigated and diagnosed after they bleed excessively during a surgical procedure
- Typical features
  - Haemorrhage may appear to stop immediately after injury due to normal vascular and haemostatic responses, but after an hour or more reappears as oozing and rapid blood loss
  - Potentially serious, either due to acute blood loss or bleeding into tissues
  - Significant bleeding may occur into the joints (haemarthrosis), muscles or mucous membranes of the mouth, gingiva, nose and genitourinary tract
  - Life-threatening bleeds may be intracranial, gastrointestinal or into the neck/throat
  - Women additionally experience menorrhagia, dysmenorrhoea and increased postpartum bleeding, and have an increased risk of haemorrhagic ovarian cysts and endometriosis

Diagnosis

- Confirmation following clinical suspicion from family history and/or signs and symptoms is via blood tests and measurement of clotting factor levels
- For people with a family history of haemophilia, it is possible to determine during pregnancy if the foetus is affected by haemophilia. This is undertaken via chorionic villus sampling with a small amount of cells taken from the placenta between the 10th to 13th weeks of pregnancy, and a DNA test performed; there is about a 1 in 100 chance of having a miscarriage and if undertaken before

10 weeks of pregnancy, there is a risk of causing birth defects; of note, the FIX level is normally lower than later in life and should be retested at 6–12 months
- In children and adults, a blood test can reveal a clotting factor deficiency
- Screening tests include:
  - Complete blood cell count
  - Activated partial thromboplastin time (APTT) or partial thromboplastin time (PTT) – prolonged
  - Thrombin time (TT) – usually normal
  - Prothrombin time (PT) – usually normal
  - Von Willebrand factor (vWF) antigen test
  - Coagulation factor assays

Management

- The World Federation of Hemophilia (WFH) states that the aims of comprehensive care for patients with haemophilia are:
  - Prevention of bleeding and joint damage
  - Prompt management of bleeding
  - Management of complications
    - Joint and muscle damage and other sequalae of bleeding (e.g. through physiotherapy, rehabilitation, physical activity, joint surgery)
    - Pain from chronic haemophilic arthropathy and inflammation
    - Inhibitor development
    - Viral infection(s) transmitted through blood products
  - Attention to psychosocial health
- Multiple therapeutic approaches have emerged to manage the haemophilia (Table 10.1.4)
- There are 3 main areas of focus to manage bleeding risk and its consequences, namely adjunctive management, factor replacement therapy and joint surgery
- Adjunctive management
  - First aid measures such as protection (splint), rest, ice, compression and elevation (PRICE)
  - Physiotherapy and rehabilitation
  - Antifibrinolytic drugs
  - Pain management of chronic arthropathy and inflammation: paracetamol, COX-2 inhibitors (avoiding other NSAIDs), codeine, tramadol, morphine
- Factor replacement therapy
  - May be given as continuous prophylaxis or episodic ('on demand'), administered when bleeds occur
  - Prophylactic administration reduces the number of bleeds, thereby preserving musculoskeletal function by limiting joint destruction
  - Primary prophylaxis: the WHO and WFH have jointly stated that this is considered to be the optimal form of therapy for a child with severe haemophilia and should be started no later than immediately or shortly after the first recognised joint bleed or clinically significant muscle bleed; benefits and barriers are associated with this approach

Benefits

- ~80% reduction in number of bleeding episodes, ~60% improvement in joint function
- Preserved bone mass density, less clinical and radiological deterioration of joints
- Improved quality of life, fewer days lost from school/work, increased physical activity

Barriers

- Patient factors: activity and lifestyle, adherence, convenience, venous access (especially children), inhibitor formation
- Physician factors: failure rate for review appointments, reduced support to patients
- Clotting factor concentrate factors: access, cost

  - Secondary prophylaxis: regular continuous treatment, started after 2 or more large joint bleeds but before the onset of joint disease
  - Tertiary prophylaxis: regular continuous treatment, started after the onset of joint disease to prevent further damage. Intermittent ('periodic') prophylaxis may also be used as a treatment to prevent bleeding for short periods of time (e.g. during and after surgery)
- Joint surgery
  - Required if extensive damage, pain, deformity or restricted range of motion
- Inhibitors
  - Inhibitors of factors used for replacement therapy are the greatest challenge in the management of haemophilia today
  - The development of inhibitors is related to a number of general and treatment-related risk factors (Table 10.1.5)
  - Inhibitors occur ~20–30% of previously untreated patients with severe to moderately severe haemophilia A, usually within the first 15–20 days of treatment
  - The incidence is lower in patients with haemophilia B (1–6%), although an allergic/anaphylactic reaction to factor replacement is more common
  - Inhibitor development is detected using a Bethesda inhibitor assay, measured in Bethesda units (BU) and whether inhibitor titre increases when a patient is treated with replacement clotting factor:
    - High responding (≥5 Bethesda units); strong immune reaction causing amount of inhibitor to rise quickly to very high levels upon re-exposure to replacement clotting factor (anamnesis)

Table 10.1.4 Therapeutic approaches for patients with haemophilia.

Action	Product	Description
Coagulation factor replacement therapy	Recombinant factor VIII or IX	• Genetically engineered from Chinese hamster ovary cell line • Processed and purified for pharmaceutical use without animal or human proteins in the culture medium or final formulation • Half-life of FVIII is 12 h; FIX is 18–48 h • Currently the treatment of choice
	Extended half-life recombinant factor VIII or IX	• Currently in development • Has potential as the future of recombinant factor in order to reduce frequency of doses and time spent in factor trough levels • Methods: PEGylation, fusion with albumin, fusion of Fc-portion of IgG to a single rFIX molecule • Extends half-life by 1.5–1.8 times for FVIII and 3–5 times for FIX • Currently no major safety issues yet identified, though some theoretical concerns still exist
	Viral inactivated plasma-derived concentrate	• Viral inactivation procedures performed (e.g. heat treatment, solvent/detergent treatment, pasteurisation, nanofiltration) to protect against HAV, HBV, HCV and HIV • Some pathogens are resistant to these processes (e.g. parvovirus B19, prions) • Contains von Willebrand factor • Indications: factor tolerisation, requirement of concentrates containing vWF
	Prothrombin complex concentrates	• Produced by ion-exchange chromatography from cryoprecipitate supernatant of large plasma pools. Different processing techniques to produce either 3-factor (II, IX, X) or 4-factor (II, VII, IX, X) concentrates • Risk of thrombosis or disseminated intravascular coagulation with large doses, since factors II, VII and X may become activated during manufacture • Indicated only when emergency factor replacement required and pure FVIII or FIX concentrate is not available • Originally used to treat haemophilia B, but with development of rFIX, main indication is now congenital or acquired deficiency of vitamin K-dependent clotting factors (e.g. warfarin reversal)
	Cryoprecipitate	• Preparation involves thawing FFP, centrifuging the residues, and collecting the cold-insoluble precipitate which is refrozen • Concerns about safety and quality, since no viral inactivation performed during manufacture. However, may be only available or affordable treatment option in some countries • Contains significant FVIII, vWF, fibrinogen and FXIII (but not FIX or FXI) • Preferable to FFP for treatment of haemophilia A
	Fresh frozen plasma (FFP)	• Concerns about safety and quality, since viral inactivation procedures may impact coagulation factors. However, may be the only available or affordable treatment option in some countries • Contains all the coagulation factors
Release of endogenous factor stores	Desmopressin (1-deamino-8-D-arginine vasopressin, DDAVP)	• Synthetic analogue of vasopressin which induces the release of FVIIIC, vWF and tPA from storage sites in the endothelium • Treatment of haemophilia A only, usually mild or moderate haemophilia • Administration via intranasal, subcutaneous or slow IV infusion routes • Patient response must be tested prior to therapeutic use due to variability of responses • Case reports of thrombosis (including myocardial infarction) in patients with cardiovascular disease

(Continued)

Table 10.1.4 (Continued)

Action	Product	Description
Improving clot stability (antifibrinolytic drugs)	Tranexamic acid	• Derivative of amino acid lysine • Competitively inhibits the activation of plasminogen to plasmin through blockage of the lysine-binding site on the plasminogen molecule • Administration as mouthwash (4.8–5%, 10 mL, 4 times/day), oral tablet (usually 3–4 times/day), intravenous infusion (2–3 times daily) • Peak plasma levels in saliva 30 min after mouthwash, remains at therapeutic levels for 2 h • Undetectable levels in saliva following oral administration • As effective as factor replacement therapy to control gingival haemorrhage • Due to risk of thromboembolism, contraindicated if receiving prothrombin complex concentrates for haemophilia A or B treatment
	Epsilon-aminocaproic acid	• Similar antifibrinolytic activity to tranexamic acid, but less widely used due to shorter plasma half-life, reduced potency and increased toxicity
FIXa and FX bridging	Emicizumab (ACE910)	• Humanised bispecific monoclonal modified IgG4 antibody that binds to and bridges FIXa and FX • Substitutes the activity of missing FVIIIa • No structural relationship or sequence homology to FVIII, so does not induce or enhance the development of inhibitors to FVIII • Indications: haemophilia A only, prophylaxis for patients with or without inhibitors
Gene and stem cell therapy (under development)	Gene therapy	• Introduction of exogenous genetic material (usually DNA) to manipulate a patient's cells to produce a missing protein/coagulation factor • Virus vector-mediated gene transfer is currently being researched • Adeno-associated viruses have been selected as vectors since they infect humans without known symptoms – modified to infect hepatocytes with the genetic material to produce FIX and FVIII • Has been more successful in haemophilia B due to the smaller size of cDNA of FIX (more amenable to insertion into different gene transfer vectors)
	Stem cell therapy	• Infusion or transplantation of intact cells into a patient • Foreign cells may be enclosed in immune-protective devices before implantation to prevent rejection • Research is under way into the utilisation of stem cells to differentiate into hepatocytes and liver sinusoidal endothelial cells, combined with gene therapy
Rebalancing agents	Anti-tissue factor pathway inhibitor (TFPI) monoclonal antibodies	• Currently under development (e.g. concizumab) • 'Rebalance' the equilibrium between bleeding and clotting by decreasing the naturally occurring anticoagulants • Anti-TFPI monoclonal antibodies: monoclonal humanised antibody directed against TFPI; TFPI inhibits the coagulation cascade by blocking the function of FXa and the activity of the tissue factor–FVIIa complex; inhibiting TFPI could thus increase procoagulant activity
	Fitusiran (ALN-AT3SC)	• A synthetic investigational RNA interference (RNAi) therapy that targets antithrombin messenger RNA, to suppress antithrombin III production in the liver • Though a death from severe intracranial blood clot led to the manufacturer halting its production, studies into its use have recommenced

Table 10.1.5 Risk factors for inhibitor development in haemophilia.

General risk factors	Treatment-related risk factors
• Genetic mutations related to factor production • Ethnicity: Afro-Caribbean and Hispanic > Caucasian • Unique individual immunological traits (no consistent pattern yet identified) • Family history of inhibitors • Severity of haemophilia: severe > mild/moderate	• Number of days treated with clotting factor concentrate: typically occurs in first 50 treatment days; risk diminishes after 200 days • Age at first exposure: majority develop during childhood; low rate of new inhibitor development through 6th decade • Intensity of first exposure: early intense therapy related to high inhibitor formation • Type of factor product: recombinant > plasma-derived; particular rFVIII products thought to be higher risk

  - Low responding (<5 Bethesda units); immune response slower and weaker with immune titre remaining low
- The inhibitor titre may increase and decrease over time and without further exposure to the factor, the titre may be transient and become undetectable
- In severe haemophilia, inhibitors do not change the site, frequency or severity of bleeding
- In moderate or mild haemophilia, the inhibitor may neutralise endogenously synthesised FVIII, converting the patient's phenotype to severe; predominance of mucocutaneous, urogenital and gastrointestinal bleeding increases, and hence the risk of severe complications or death
- The primary aim of treatment is permanent eradication of the inhibitor by immune tolerance induction (ITI) therapy to allow effective replacement therapy and prophylaxis
- If this is not possible, other management options are available (Table 10.1.6)
- Efforts to develop therapies that best prevent or eradicate inhibitor formation are continuing and are in various stages of development

Prognosis

- Life expectancy is variable, depending on disease severity and whether patients receive appropriate treatment
- Before factor concentrates were available, life expectancy for those with severe haemophilia was only 11 years
- In the 1980s, the impact of the human immunodeficiency virus (HIV) and hepatitis-associated infections associated with blood transfusions increased mortality rates

Table 10.1.6 General management of patients with inhibitors.

Treatment	Description
Immune tolerance induction (ITI) therapy	• Frequent doses of factor concentrate over several months to years to train the body to recognise the treatment product without reacting • Preferred management in haemophilia A with high-titre inhibitors • Relatively high risk of severe complications (nephrotic syndrome, anaphylaxis) and lower success rate (30%) in haemophilia B with high-titre inhibitors • Improved results for eradication of high-titre inhibitors to FIX when combined with immunosuppressive regimens (e.g. rituximab, dexamethasone, mycophenolate mofetil)
Bypassing agents	• Usually used whilst awaiting inhibitor eradication, and in patients failing ITI – Recombinant FVII (rVII) – Prothrombin complex concentrates (PCCs) ○ 3-factor PCC: factors II, IX, X ○ 4-factor PCC: factors II, VII, IX, X ○ Activated prothrombin complex concentrates (aPCC): factor VIIa, with small variable amounts of activated factors II, IX, X; available as factor VIII inhibitor bypassing agent
Antifibrinolytics	• Tranexamic acid • Epsilon-aminocaproic acid

(Continued)

Table 10.1.6 (Continued)

Treatment	Description
Recombinant porcine factor VIII	• Prepared from the plasma of pigs to treat haemophilia A patients with inhibitors to endogenous FVIII • Theoretical advantage of decreased cross-reactivity of anti-human FVIII antibodies towards porcine FVIII compared to human factor • Reserved for use in haemophilia A when life- or limb-threatening bleeding cannot be controlled with a bypassing agent
Plasmapheresis	• Removes inhibitors from the bloodstream when inhibitor titre needs to be reduced quickly and bypassing therapy is not effective (e.g. limb- or life-threatening bleeding) • Temporary measure, since factor administration will stimulate the body to make large amounts of new antibody within several days
High-dose factor concentrates	• Final option for individuals with bleeding and an inhibitor • May be effective for patients with haemophilia A or B with: [1] low titre <5 BU or a low-responding inhibitor without infusion reactions; [2] high-responding inhibitors currently at a low titre or titre lowered by plasmapheresis
Non-factor therapies	• Emicizumab • Rebalancing agents (e.g. anti-TFPI monoclonal antibodies, fitusiran) • Currently under development • Since non-factor therapies differ completely from factor replacement therapy, holds future promise for improved quality of life for patients with inhibitors • Particularly useful if immune tolerance induction therapy is ineffective against inhibitors • Constantly evolving, must consult most recent literature and guidance for current status

- Prophylaxis and early treatment with factor concentrate that is safe from viral contamination have dramatically improved outcomes
- Currently, with appropriate education and treatment, patients with haemophilia may live full and productive lives
- However, approximately one-quarter of patients with severe haemophilia aged 6–18 years demonstrate below-normal motor skills and academic performance; an increase in emotional and behavioural problems has also been observed

A World/Transcultural View

- Haemophilia A represents 80–85% of the total haemophilia population, though in some Asian populations the frequencies of haemophilia A and B are almost equal
- The costs of haemophilia prophylaxis treatment are significant, at approximately USD $200 000–400 000 per patient per year. As such, 75% of the world's haemophilia population is inadequately treated
- Factor usage (international units) per capita in developed countries is significantly higher than in developing countries, correlating with lower morbidity
- Low-dose/ultra low-dose primary prophylaxis and extended half-life products are being investigated as options in countries with restricted healthcare economies. In such countries, dentists may be seeing undiagnosed individuals with haemophilia, or patients for whom access to appropriate haemophilia care is limited

Recommended Reading

Anderson, J.A., Brewer, A., Creagh, D. et al. (2013). Guidance on the dental management of patients with haemophilia and congenital bleeding disorders. *Br. Dent. J.* 215: 497–504.

Bajkin, B. and Dougall, A. (2020). Current state of play regarding dental extractions in patients with haemophilia: consensus or evidence-based practice? A review of the literature. *Haemophilia* 26: 183–199.

Brewer, A. (2008). *Dental Management of Patients with Inhibitors to Factor VIII or Factor IX*. World Federation of Hemophilia: Quebec www1.wfh.org/publications/files/pdf-1200.pdf.

Brewer, A. and Correa, M.E. (2006). *Guidelines for Dental Treatment of Patients with Inherited Bleeding Disorders*. World Federation of Hemophilia: Quebec www1.wfh.org/publications/files/pdf-1190.pdf.

van Galen, K.P., Engelen, E.T., Mauser-Bunschoten, E.P. et al. (2019). Antifibrinolytic therapy for preventing oral bleeding in patients with haemophilia or Von Willebrand disease undergoing minor oral surgery or dental extractions. *Cochrane Database Syst. Rev.* (4): CD011385.

Halpern, L.R., Adams, D.R., and Clarkson, E. (2020). Treatment of the dental patient with bleeding dyscrasias: etiologies and management options for surgical success in practice. *Dent. Clin. North Am.* 64: 411–434.

Scully, C., Diz Dios, P., and Giangrande, P. (2008). *Oral Care for People with Hemophilia or a Hereditary Bleeding Tendency*. World Federation of Hemophilia: Quebec www1.wfh.org/publications/files/pdf-1164.pdf.

Srivastava, A., Santagostino, E., Dougall, A. et al. (2020). WFH Guidelines for the Management of Hemophilia, 3rd edition. *Haemophilia* 26: S1–S158.

10.2 Treatment with Heparin

Section I: Clinical Scenario and Dental Considerations

Clinical Scenario

A 55-year-old woman presents to you concerned about her deteriorating oral health and 'crumbling teeth'. Most recently, the upper right second premolar (#15) has lost a filling and feels sharp. It is cutting her tongue, causing bleeding. She has not been able to find a dentist who will see her as they have all refused care due to her medical history.

Medical History

- Alport syndrome
  - Chronic renal failure (chronic kidney disease stage 5, patient not suitable for renal transplant and undergoing haemodialysis)
  - Visual impairment (yellow flecks/dots behind the retina)
  - Hyperparathyroidism (parathyroidectomy 1 year ago)
  - Osteoporosis (no plan for bone-altering medications)
  - Secondary hypertension
- Kartagener syndrome
  - Primary ciliary dyskinesia
  - Bronchiectasis
  - Situs inversus totalis and dextrocardia
  - Partial hearing loss
- Chronic obstructive pulmonary disease
- Osteoarthritis
- Chronic pain
- Gastro-oesophageal reflux disease
- Depression
- Anxiety, difficulties sleeping and restless legs syndrome
- Breast carcinoma (diagnosed 2 years ago; surgical treatment only as medical comorbidities posed high risk for chemotherapy; reviewed annually)

Medications

- Dalteparin 5000 IU injection (every second day in own home; native/tissue arteriovenous fistula)
- Folic acid
- Cinacalcet
- Calcium/ vitamin D
- Amlodipine
- Amoxicillin/clavulanic acid
- Azithromycin
- Prednisolone (10 mg daily)
- Fluticasone/salmeterol (inhaler)
- Tiotropium bromide (inhaler)
- Salbutamol (inhaler and nebuliser solution)
- Methadone
- Paracetamol
- Pantoprazole
- Metoclopramide
- Citalopram
- Diazepam
- Temazepam
- Pramipexole

Dental History

- Irregular dental attender
- Stopped attending regularly due to competing medical issues and difficulties with access
- Brushes her teeth twice daily, flosses teeth once weekly. Dexterity still satisfactory
- Consumes lollies to pass the time during haemodialysis, and sips on 5 cups of coffee with sugar during day. Recommended lemonade and sugary/fatty foods by her doctors and dietician in order to maintain energy and weight

Social History

- Independent ability for activities of daily living have rapidly declined over past 2 years. Increased dependence on adult son and ex-husband (good relationship remains)

A Practical Approach to Special Care in Dentistry, First Edition. Edited by Pedro Diz Dios and Navdeep Kumar.

- Lives alone, divorced, frequently visited by son who acts as primary carer
- Driven in private car to appointments by son or ex-husband
- Tobacco consumption: 10 cigarettes/day for the past 30 years
- Alcohol consumption: nil
- Walks slowly with walking stick; wheelchair required for long distances
- Patient does not have a telephone due to her hearing impairment; she provides the telephone numbers of her son and ex-husband in the contact details

Oral Examination

- Primary concerns
  - #27: carious retained roots; tender on buccal palpation
  - #15: lost restoration
  - 0.5 cm diameter superficial traumatic ulcer of the tongue caused by the sharp #15
- Multiple other decayed and defective heavily restored teeth (Figure 10.2.1)
  - #14: large glass-ionomer restoration with fractured margins
  - #17: stabilised with temporary restoration, residual subgingival caries present
  - #26: metal underlay of porcelain-fused-to-metal crown only (no porcelain remaining)
  - #36: distal caries, large amalgam restoration
  - #46: distal caries, large amalgam restoration with fractured margins
  - #47: carious/fractured amalgam restoration
- Soft deposits present in all quadrants
- Generalised mild chronic periodontal disease

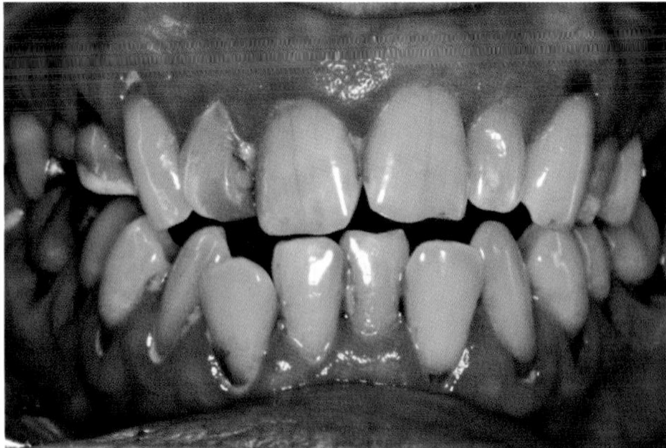

Figure 10.2.1 Multiple other decayed and defective heavily restored teeth.

Radiological Examination

- Orthopantomagram and periapical radiographs undertaken (Figure 10.2.2)
- Lost restoration: #15
- Carious retained root: #27
- Caries: #17 (residual decay underneath restoration), #36 (distal), #46 (distal) and #47 (distal)
- Mild horizontal bone loss ~10%

Structured Learning

1) Why is this patient receiving dalteparin on alternate days?
   - Dalteparin is a low molecular weight heparin (LMWH) and is given as a single-bolus dose with its mechanism of action lasting up to 4 hours
   - In this patient it is indicated for prevention of thrombosis during haemodialysis
   - This ensures that the vascular access (arteriovenous fistula) remains patent
   - In some countries, unfractionated heparin (UFH) is still preferred to enable haemodialysis instead of LMWH (e.g. United States) – it is given as a bolus dose at the start of dialysis and followed by either a continuous or hourly intermittent infusion
2) Why is it important to differentiate whether a patient is on UFH or LMWH?
   - UFH and LMWH have different pharmacological effects and clinical indications
   - Hence their impact on dental treatment differs (Table 10.2.1)
   - For this patient, elective dental treatment should be planned on the day following dialysis so that the effects of heparin administration have declined
3) Why does this patient have renal failure?
   - This patient has Alport syndrome, a genetic condition characterised by kidney disease, hearing loss and eye abnormalities
   - People with Alport syndrome experience progressive loss of kidney function
4) What is the impact of Kartagener syndrome on the dental management of this patient?
   - Kartagener syndrome is an autosomal recessive genetic primary ciliary dyskinesia disorder, comprising the triad of situs inversus (positioning of some or all of the vital organs reversed or mirrored), chronic sinusitis and bronchiectasis
   - The signs and symptoms vary but may include frequent lung, sinus and middle ear infections beginning in early childhood

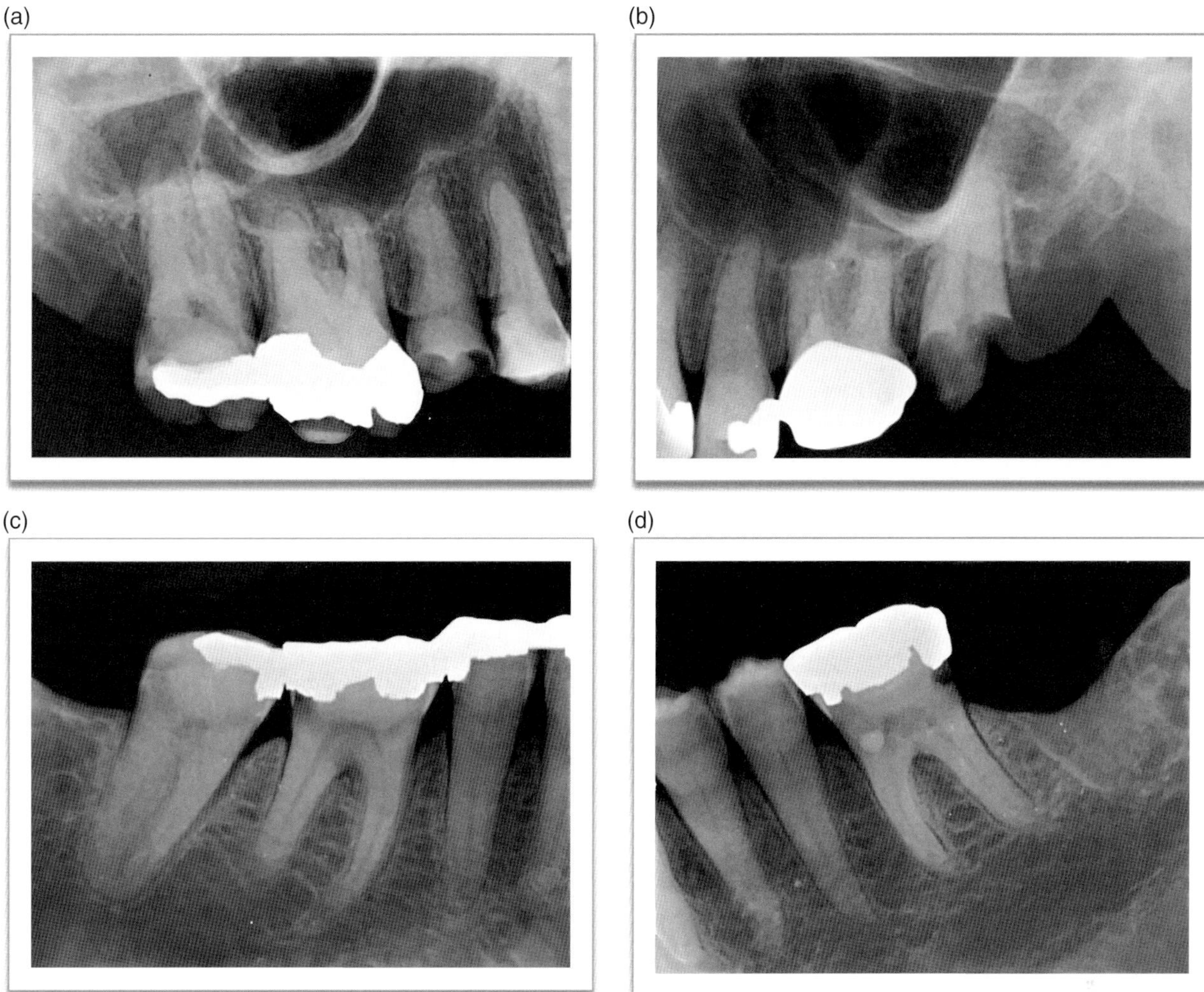

Figure 10.2.2 (a) Periapical radiograph upper right quadrant showing fractured #15. (b) Periapical radiograph upper left quadrant showing retained root #27. (c) Periapical radiography lower right quadrant showing distal caries #47. (d) Periapical radiograph lower left quadrant showing distal caries #36.

- This patient is taking multiple medications to maintain airway patency including high-dose steroids
- Steroid prophylaxis will need to be considered for invasive dental procedures (see Chapter 12.1)

5) You note the superficial traumatic ulcer of the tongue caused by the sharp #15, which is bleeding continuously. The patient reports it has been bleeding all night and she woke in the morning to find her pillow soaked with blood. How would you manage this?
   - Apply pressure and use local haemostatic agents such as tranexamic acid 5% mouthwash applied directly to the tongue
   - Place a temporary dressing/adjust the #15 to avoid further trauma
   - Liaise with the physician to alert them to the persistently bleeding tongue ulcer and obtain their advice
   - Check when the last dose of dalteparin was given and when the next dose is planned – the physician may delay the next dose or if bleeding is significant, and urgently review the patient in a hospital setting
6) Can reversal agents for LMWHs be used by the medical team to reduce the bleeding from the tongue?
   - Protamine sulfate given by slow infusion results in partial reversal of LMWH
   - It is considered if patients are suffering significant haemorrhage following recent (<12 hours) administration of a therapeutic dose of LMWH
7) The patient also complains of discomfort from the retained roots in the upper left second molar (#27) region which has been associated with swelling in the past. She requests antibiotics. What factors should you consider?

Table 10.2.1 Unfractionated heparin and low molecular weight heparin – different approaches when undertaking dental procedures associated with bleeding risk.

Unfractionated heparin (UFH)

- Most patients on UFH are hospitalised and will be placed on warfarin/a direct oral anticoagulant (DOAC) once discharged
- Elective dental treatment should be delayed until heparin treatment has ceased
- Treat dental emergencies as conservatively as possible, in consultation with medical specialist
- If urgent invasive dental treatment cannot be delayed, it should be undertaken at least 6–8 h after injection of UFH or on the following day when its effects have ceased (prior to the next dose of UFH, which may be delayed by the medical team to enable dental treatment)
- Consider the need to confirm the aPTT, anti-Xa factor assay and platelet counts

Low molecular weight heparin (LMWH)

- Patients on LMWH may receive this (or self-administer) in an outpatient setting
- Outpatients taking LMWH may be able to have invasive dental procedures performed without altering their LMWH medication depending on the dose and frequency
- However, if significant bleeding is anticipated, liaise with the physician to either discontinue LMWH (miss 1 dose) and restart following haemostasis, or wait until LMWH therapy is completed if possible
- Patients on renal dialysis having LMWH treatment should have dental surgery on the following day when effects have ceased (renal dialysis is typically given 3 times a week – see Chapter 6.2)
- These patients are not typically monitored with laboratory tests

- The patient is already taking amoxicillin 875 mg/clavulanic acid 125 mg (daily) and azithromycin 250 mg (Monday, Wednesday, Friday)
- Liaison with renal and respiratory specialists is required in view of background of immunosuppression balanced with the underlying renal failure/reduced clearance (see Chapter 6.2)

8) What factors do you need to consider in your risk assessment for managing the oral health of this patient?
   - Social
     - Reduced mobility (wheelchair access), falls risk
     - Impaired hearing
     - Visual impairment
     - Reliance on third party to attend appointments
     - Recent rapid decline in activities of daily living, chronic pain, weakness and fatigue, anxiety, impact on consent due to fatigue/depression/medication
   - Medical
     - Bleeding risk due to heparin and renal failure
     - Drug toxicity and interactions
     - Caution in relation to the arm with the arterio-venous fistula (avoid this arm for intravenous access, blood pressure monitoring, etc.)
     - Susceptibility to infection (prednisolone and renal disease)
     - Adrenal suppression risk
     - Impaired wound healing (prednisolone and smoking)
     - Impaired respiratory exchange
   - Dental
     - Caries risk (highly calorific diet and dental erosion due to gastro-oesophageal reflux disease)
     - Increased susceptibility to oral candidosis (inhalers, immunosuppression)
     - Hyposalivation (polypharmacy)
     - Oral side-effects of tobacco smoking
     - Pain control requirements (already taking methadone)

General Dental Considerations

Oral Findings

- Petechiae
- Ecchymoses
- Spontaneous gingival bleeding
- Prolonged bleeding after invasive procedures

Dental Management

- Heparinised outpatients may still present in the primary care dental setting, with varied conditions and drug regimes, including:
  - Pregnant women with indications for anticoagulation (once to twice daily, at prophylactic or therapeutic doses)
  - Recent joint replacement
  - Treatment of deep venous thrombosis or asymptomatic pulmonary embolism
  - Venous thrombosis with a background of cancer (once to twice daily, at prophylactic or therapeutic doses)
  - Haemodialysis for end-stage renal disease (usually 3 times per week)
  - Patients intolerant to warfarin
  - Prophylaxis for patients with lupus anticoagulant factor
- Clinical evidence regarding the dental management of patients taking heparin is lacking, probably in part due to them being used in limited patient groups (Table 10.2.2)

Table 10.2.2 General dental management considerations.

Risk assessment	• Spontaneous bleeding/bleeding from surgery and trauma • Consider the impact of the underlying condition for which the heparin is being given • Consider the required dental procedure, other medical conditions that may contribute to bleeding risk, and other medications that may contribute to bleeding risk
Criteria for referral	• Dentists can treat the majority of outpatients on heparin in primary care • Need for referral would be based on the acuity, severity and complexity of the underlying medical conditions necessitating the heparin, if there are multiple comorbidities and/or the invasiveness of the proposed dental procedure
Access/position	• Plan treatment for early in the morning /week to allow for monitoring and management of bleeding complications, should they occur • Since the effects of heparin are relatively short-lived, it is often possible to delay dental treatments likely to cause bleeding to the following day • Consider the need to stage invasive treatment to minimise bleeding risk • Consider the need for an escort
Communication	• If procedure is likely to cause bleeding, consult general medical practitioner or specialist • Heparinisation may not be the life-long plan – hence elective dental treatment should be delayed where possible until heparin is ceased • If heparinisation is being discontinued, consult with medical practitioner regarding timing of heparin recommencement (depending on complexity of the extraction and patient's thromboembolic risk)
Consent/capacity	• Warn patient of the increased risk of intraoral/postoperative bleeding and intra/extraoral bruising • Inform patient of the measures to be used to reduce bleeding risk
Anaesthesia/sedation	• Local anaesthesia – Delivered using an aspirating syringe and should include a vasoconstrictor, unless contraindicated – Anaesthetic solution should be delivered slowly to avoid rapid expansion of the soft tissues • Sedation – Intravenous sedation cannulation poses a risk of haematoma formation – Avoid use of arteriovenous fistula arm for cannulation and sphygmomanometer • General anaesthesia – Hazards of anaesthesia, especially nasal intubation and intramuscular injections
Dental treatment	• Before – Consider limiting initial treatment area (e.g. perform a single extraction or debride 3 teeth only initially and assess bleeding before continuing) – For procedures with higher risk of postoperative bleeding, consider carrying out staged treatment • During – Lubricant/barrier cream used to protect the lips/soft tissue from trauma – Careful manipulation of the cheek and soft tissues – consider the use of gauze when using cheek retractors – Caution with suction to avoid trauma (reduce the volume) and particular care taken to avoid trauma in the floor of mouth – Atraumatic extraction technique preferred – If a mucoperiosteal flap required, a buccal approach is best since lingual tissue trauma may open up planes into which haemorrhage may track and endanger the airway – Minimal bone removal, teeth sectioned where possible – Local haemostatic measures to control bleeding – Bony wound compressed with absorbent gauze – Tranexamic acid 5% mouthwash/8% gel may be used as an adjunct; this can be soaked in gauze and applied directly over the socket – Haemostatic packing agents: minimise usage to reduce incidence of dry socket; ensure agent of choice is acceptable to patient as some contain animal-based proteins – Suturing: use non-traumatic needle and small number of sutures • After – Extended monitoring – Careful oral cleansing postoperatively – Provide verbal and written postoperative instructions and emergency contact details

(*Continued*)

Table 10.2.2 (Continued)

Drug prescription	• Antiseptics as required (e.g. 0.12–0.2% chlorhexidine rinses every 8 h) • Antibiotics (e.g. amoxicillin, penicillin V, amoxicillin/clavulanic acid or metronidazole at therapeutic doses) as required • Pain relief (e.g. paracetamol) • Avoid aspirin, ibuprofen and diclofenac as these may increase bleeding risk
Education/ prevention	• Use of fluoride and fissure sealants, oral hygiene education, dietary advice and regular dental visits to minimise dental treatment that may cause bleeding complications

- Consider the invasiveness of the proposed dental procedure, the impact of the underlying medical condition for which the heparin is being taken and determine the dose and frequency of heparin administration

Section II: Background Information and Guidelines

Definition

Heparin is a natural sulfated glycosaminoglycan found in the mast cells that line the vasculature in the lungs, liver and intestines. It is released in low concentration in response to injury. In vivo heparin function is not fully understood – in addition to a mild physiological anticoagulant effect, it may aid in the packaging and storage of histamine and other inflammatory mediators stored in mast cell granules that are released upon IgE-stimulated degranulation.

Pharmaceutical heparin is an injectable anticoagulant predominantly derived from bovine lung and porcine intestinal mucosa. It is given subcutaneously or intravenously. Some heparins are also being used for other effects, such as immunosuppression. Recombinant oral heparin is under development.

Mechanism of Action

- Anticoagulant activity and duration of action of heparins are variable
- Heparin binds to the enzyme inhibitor antithrombin III, causing a conformational change that results in its activation through an increase in the flexibility of its reactive site loop
- This conformational change in antithrombin mediates its inhibition of factor Xa
- It then dissociates and binds to further antithrombin molecules, accelerating the inactivation of factors IIa (activated prothrombin), IXa and Xa
- For thrombin inhibition, however, thrombin must also bind to the heparin polymer at a site proximal to the pentasaccharide, resulting in a tertiary complex – this effect is size dependent and hence not present for all heparins

Classification

- Heterogeneous with respect to molecular size, anticoagulant activity and pharmacokinetic properties
- There are 2 main groups of heparins (Table 10.2.3)
  - Unfractionated heparin (UFH)
    - Immediate effect on coagulation
    - Cleared more rapidly, usually lost within 6 hours of stopping heparin
    - Inactivates several coagulation enzymes, including factors IIa (thrombin), IXa, Xa, XIa and XIIa
    - Requires daily blood monitoring to check the aPTT
    - Long-term use is associated with the risk of developing osteoporosis
  - Low molecular weight heparin (LMWH)
    - LMWHs have gradually replaced UFH for most indications
    - Each LMWH has a specific molecular weight distribution that determines its anticoagulant activity and duration of action – hence one product cannot always be substituted for another (Table 10.2.4)
    - Interact with factor Xa
    - Given once daily because they have a longer duration of action
    - More predictable dose–response, superior efficacy, better bioavailability, longer half-life, fewer non-haemorrhagic side-effects, do not require laboratory monitoring, and can be used in an outpatient setting
- Other injectable anticoagulants
  - Fondaparinux
    - Synthetic anticoagulant based on the pentasaccharide sequence that makes up the minimal antithrombin binding region of heparin
    - Similar to LMWH, it is an indirect inhibitor of factor Xa, but does not inhibit thrombin at all
    - Longer half-life than heparin and does not interact with platelets, both of which may be advantageous in certain circumstances
  - Direct thrombin inhibitors (argatroban, bivalirudin, lepirudin)
    - Bind directly, selectively and reversibly to the active site of thrombin
    - Main alternative therapeutic agents in heparin-induced thrombocytopenia

Table 10.2.3 Comparison of the characteristics of unfractionated heparin and low molecular weight heparin.

	Unfractionated heparin (UFH)	**Low molecular weight heparin (LMWH)**
Composition	Heterogenous mixture of polysaccharide chains, with mean molecular weight of 12 000–16 000 Da	Derived from UFH by depolymerisation, yielding heparin fragments with mean molecular weight of 4000–6000 Da
Onset of action	Instantaneous (intravenous bolus)	20–30 minutes
Peak plasma concentration	2–4 hours	3–5 hours
Half-life	45 minutes–1 hour	3–7 hours
Duration of anticoagulant effect	4–5 hours (dose dependent)	24 hours (dose dependent)
Metabolism	Liver	Liver
Excretion	Renal function irrelevant at therapeutic doses. High doses: renal excretion (50%), reticuloendothelial system excretion clearance (unpredictable)	Renal excretion (10–40%)
Bioavailability	Inconsistent, unpredictable	99%
Mechanism of action	Activation of antithrombin III, resulting in inhibition of thrombin IIa, IXa, Xa, XIa, XIIa, i.e. inhibits FXa and thrombin equally Reduces platelet aggregation by inhibiting thrombin-induced activation	Activation of antithrombin III, resulting in more selective inhibition of Xa, i.e. greater activity against FXa than thrombin Reduces platelet aggregation by inhibiting thrombin-induced activation
Reversal	Protamine sulfate if urgent Discontinuation usually sufficient due to short half-life Under development: ciraparantag	Protamine sulfate (incomplete) if urgent Discontinuation usually sufficient due to short half-life Under development: ciraparantag and andexanet alfa
Laboratory tests	aPTT or anti-Xa assay monitoring required to assess anticoagulation Platelet count monitoring to identify complication of heparin-induced thrombocytopenia	Usually none or anti-Xa assay aPTT is normal since FX inhibited more specifically
Administration	Intravenous (usually in hospital setting) or subcutaneous	Subcutaneous (outpatient setting)
Advantages	Rapid onset and offset (flexibility in dose titration and discontinuation); ideal for surgery Ability to monitor aPTT and anti-factor Xa activity Rapid reversal using protamine sulfate Reduced renal excretion (allows use in renal failure/insufficiency) Extensive clinical experience Preservative-free preparation does not cross placenta Does not accumulate in breast milk	More predictable dose–response (dosage based on body weight), no laboratory monitoring required Longer half-life, allowing administration only 1–2 times/day in the outpatient setting Improved bioavailability and superior efficacy Fewer non-haemorrhagic side-effects Lower risk of heparin-induced thrombocytopenia and osteoporosis than UFH Extensive clinical experience Preservative-free preparation does not cross placenta Does not accumulate in breast milk

(*Continued*)

Table 10.2.3 (Continued)

	Unfractionated heparin (UFH)	Low molecular weight heparin (LMWH)
Disadvantages	Laboratory monitoring of aPTT or anti-factor Xa activity required due to highly variable dose–response relationship Short half-life, usually requiring continuous intravenous administration in hospital setting Achieving and maintaining therapeutic levels often challenging Higher risk of haemorrhagic complications compared with LMWH Side-effects of long-term use: heparin-induced thrombocytopenia (1% risk during days 4–14 of heparinisation), skin reactions, osteoporosis (>6 months)	Slightly delayed onset of action compared to instantaneous action of UFH Longer duration of action (less flexibility with dose titration and discontinuation) Monitoring less widely available, if required (i.e. anti-factor Xa assay with rapid turnaround time) Protamine sulfate less effective for reversal Prolonged half-life in patients with renal failure Higher risk of local skin reactions and skin necrosis than UFH

aPTT, activated partial thromboplastin time.

Table 10.2.4 Low molecular weight heparin (LMWH) medications.

Drug name	Average molecular weight (daltons)	Ratio anti-Xa/anti-IIa activity	Units of anti-factor Xa activity per mg
Enoxaparin	4500	3.9	100
Dalteparin	6000	2.5	156
Tinzaparin	6500	1.6	70–120
Nadroparin	4300–4500	2–4.1	Various formulations
Other LMWH products under development: ardeparin, reviparin, parnaparin, certoparin			

Laboratory Findings

- The prothrombin, activated partial thromboplastin (aPTT) and thrombin times (TT) are prolonged in persons on UFH
- Most patients under UFH are monitored with the aPTT and are maintained at 1.5–2.5 times the control value (the therapeutic range)
- Large doses of heparin can increase the international normalised ratio (INR)
- Platelet counts should also be monitored if heparin is used for more than 5 days, since heparin can cause thrombocytopenia – this risk is reduced for LMWH and fondaparinux
- Autoimmune thrombocytopenia can occur within 3–15 days, or sooner if there has been previous heparin exposure

Indications

- Treatment and prevention of venous thromboembolism (deep venous thrombosis or pulmonary embolism) and acute coronary syndrome (unstable angina and myocardial infarction)
- Deep venous thrombosis prophylaxis in medium- and high-risk groups (hospitalisation procedures; surgical, medical, orthopaedic patients)
- Coronary interventions, cardiopulmonary bypass surgery, maintaining patency of catheters and cannulas
- Treatment of venous thromboembolism in pregnancy
- Treatment of symptomatic venous thromboembolism with a background of solid tumour cancers
- Bridging therapy for warfarin
- Prevention of thrombosis in the extracorporeal circulation during haemodialysis

A World/Transcultural View

- Heparin remains one of the most widely used anticoagulant drugs globally, with an annual market in 2018 estimated at USD 6.4 billion
- It remains an animal-derived product, commercially derived from porcine intestine. A public health contamination crisis occurred in 2007–2008, prompting research into improved methods for synthesising safer products.

- From the 1940s to the 1990s, heparin was commercially produced from both bovine and porcine intestine. Bovine heparin was withdrawn from the market due to the spongiform encephalopathy epidemic, which had implications for Jewish and Muslim patients who follow strict Kosher and Halal regulations, respectively
- There is growing concern about a shortage of heparin. This is due to the number of animals that must be slaughtered to meet current need, and because most of the world's heparin is produced from a single animal in a single country (China) whose pig herds have been afflicted by African swine fever since August 2018. As such, a worldwide reintroduction of bovine heparin manufactured in different countries has been proposed as a way to mitigate against a fragile supply chain

Recommended Reading

Bloomer, C.R. (2004). Excessive hemorrhage after dental extractions using low-molecular-weight heparin (Lovenox) anticoagulation therapy. *J. Oral Maxillofac. Surg.* 62: 101–103.

Erden, İ., Çakcak Erden, E., Aksu, T. et al. (2016). Comparison of uninterrupted warfarin and bridging therapy using low-molecular weight heparin with respect to the severity of bleeding after dental extractions in patients with prosthetic valves. *Anatol. J. Cardiol.* 16: 467–473.

Eziafa, I.O., Robert, J.L., and Susan, T.S. (2016). Heparin: past, present, and future. *Pharmaceuticals* 9: 38.

Jagels, A., Young, J., and Mathers, S. (2016). *Guidelines for Anticoagulation and Prophylaxis Using Low Molecular Weight Heparin (LMWH) in Adult Inpatients*. Brisbane: Department of Health, Queensland Government www.health.qld.gov.au/__data/assets/pdf_file/0023/147533/qh-gdl-951.pdf.

Karslı, E.D., Erdogan, Ö., Esen, E., and Acartürk, E. (2011). Comparison of the effects of warfarin and heparin on bleeding caused by dental extraction: a clinical study. *J. Oral Maxillofac. Surg.* 69: 2500–2507.

Pettinger, T. and Owens, C. (2007). Use of low-molecular-weight heparin during dental extractions in a Medicaid population. *J. Manag. Care Pharm.* 13: 53–58.

Scottish Dental Clinical Effectiveness Programme. (2015). Management of dental patients taking anticoagulants or antiplatelet drugs. Dundee: SDCEP. www.sdcep.org.uk/published-guidance/anticoagulants-and-antiplatelets

Yong, J.W., Yang, L.X., Ohene, B.E. et al. (2017). Periprocedural heparin bridging in patients receiving oral anticoagulation: a systematic review and meta-analysis. *BMC Cardiovasc. Disord.* 17: 295.

10.3 Treatment with Warfarin (Acenocoumarol)

Section I: Clinical Scenario and Dental Considerations

Clinical Scenario

A 56-year-old male presents to you requesting extraction of his upper right first premolar (#14). The tooth is currently painful with a 2-week history of periodic swelling and pus discharge.

Medical History

- Peripheral vascular disease, resulting in left leg below-knee amputation 9 years ago
- Pulmonary embolism 9 years ago
- Chemical sympathectomy 2 years ago (ineffective; phantom leg pain persists)
- Hypercholesterolaemia
- Fatty liver disease
- Hepatitis C – no detectable liver cirrhosis at present
- Osteoarthritis affecting right knee and lower spine
- Surgery for lumbar disc herniation 20 years ago, current lower back pain

Medications

- Warfarin
- Simvastatin
- Pregabalin
- Amitriptyline
- Oxycodone

Dental History

- Regular dental attender for over 20 years
- Long history of generalised chronic periodontal disease – also seen by a periodontal specialist
- Brushes twice daily with electric toothbrush and uses interproximal brushes after each meal
- Previous periodontal surgery for debridement
- Fruit juice once per day, cordial once per day, coffee with sugar once per day

Social History

- Wheelchair user; able to self-transfer to dental chair
- Attends appointments by public transport and driving non modified automatic car
- Lives alone, independent with activities of daily living, has supportive adult children
- Stopped working 10 years ago due to lower back issues
- Stopped smoking tobacco 3 years ago; history of 20–25 cigarettes/day for 25 years prior to this

Oral Examination

- #14 associated with buccal swelling, pus discharge and grade II mobility
- Generally good oral hygiene with minimal plaque deposits present; no gingival inflammation

Radiological Examination

- Periapical radiograph upper right quadrant (Figure 10.3.1)
- #14: perio-endo lesion: extensive bone loss to apex of the tooth; root filled
- #15, #16 and #17: advanced bone loss (>50%)
- Previous orthopantomogram (taken 18 months prior to the appointment) demonstrates:
  - Severe periodontal disease
    Furcation involvement all posterior teeth
  - Advanced vertical and horizontal bone loss, most severe in relation to the lower anterior teeth

Structured Learning

1) Why is this patient taking warfarin?
   - It is used as an anticoagulant for the prevention of thromboembolic events due to the patient's history of pulmonary embolism and peripheral vascular disease
2) What specific questions should you ask the patient in relation to his warfarin medication?
   - Check the therapeutic/target INR
   - How, where and how often is the INR monitored – it may be undertaken at an anticoagulation clinic via a standard

A Practical Approach to Special Care in Dentistry, First Edition. Edited by Pedro Diz Dios and Navdeep Kumar.

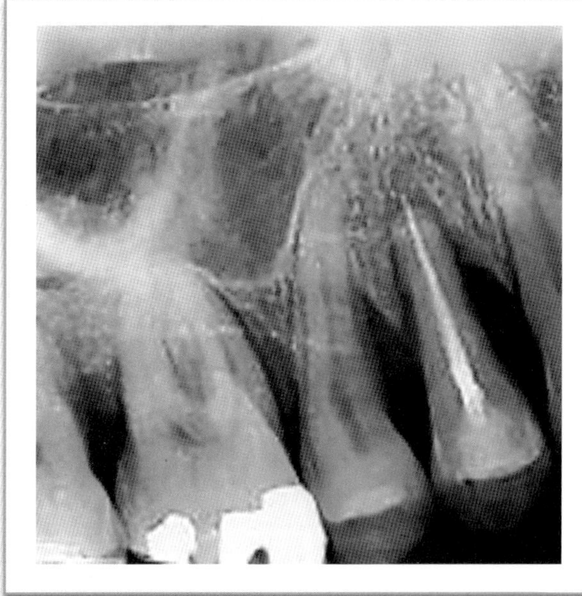

Figure 10.3.1 Periapical radiograph of the #14 demonstrating extensive bone loss.

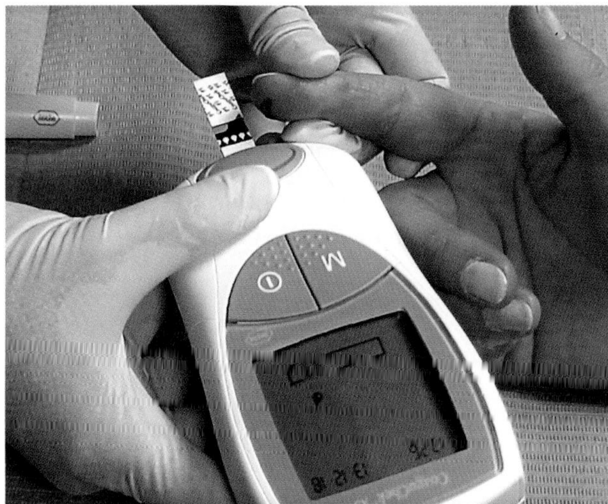

Figure 10.3.2 International normalised ratio (INR) testing in the dental clinic.

blood test/point of care device, or the patient may have his own machine for use at home (Figure 10.3.2)

- Stability of INR results (related to how often the warfarin dose is adjusted/frequency of testing) – this can be determined from the INR record book that most patients have in their possession
- Confirm when the last INR test was undertaken
  - Ideally this should be no more than 24 hours prior to an invasive dental procedure

    If the patient has a stable INR profile, an INR test result no more than 72 hours prior to the procedure may be acceptable depending on local protocols

3) The patient informs you that he last had an INR test undertaken at his local anticoagulation clinic 1 day ago. The result was 4.3. How does this impact on your dental management?
   - As the INR was >4.0, elective dental treatment, namely extraction of the #14, should be delayed (Table 10.3.1)
   - The anticoagulation service already advised the patient to reduce his warfarin dose and arranged to retest the INR in 1 week
   - Liaise with the service to advise them that a dental extraction is planned and arrange a dental appointment within 24 hours of the planned repeat INR
   - Once the INR is <4.0, the patient can receive dental treatment in primary care without needing to stop or adjust warfarin dose
4) The patient asks if you can give him medication to reverse the effect of warfarin to allow extraction of the #14 on the same day. Is this possible?
   - Warfarin is reversible by vitamin K, but this is not commonly used in relation to dental treatment
   - It may be used if there is prolonged bleeding following an invasive procedure
   - Fresh frozen plasma and prothrombin complex concentrate have also been used for life-threatening haemorrhages
5) Tooth #14 is painful and infected. It is not possible to drain the buccal swelling. What do you need to consider if you decide to prescribe antibiotics until you can extract the tooth?
   - Many antibiotics can interact with warfarin
   - They commonly inhibit warfarin metabolism, prolonging its action and raising the INR
   - Antibiotics in the same class have similar effects on INR (Table 10.3.2)
   - The effect is generally more pronounced in older patients and/or those with multiple medical comorbidities, such as this patient
   - Metronidazole should be avoided where possible
   - Consider empirical dose reduction of other antibiotics
   - If antibiotics are prescribed:
     - The patient should be advised of the risk of the INR being affected
     - The anticoagulation clinic should be contacted as more frequent INR testing may be required (INR can be affected within 2-3 days, causing potentially severe bleeding risk)
6) The patient returns to you a week later for dental extraction of #14. He informs you that he decided to omit his warfarin dose the day before his dental appointment so

Table 10.3.1 Management of patients taking warfarin undergoing dental procedures associated with bleeding risk.

Prior to dental procedure

- Check the international normalised ratio (INR), ideally no more than 24 h prior to an invasive dental procedure
- Checking no more than 72 h before is acceptable if the patient has a stable INR (i.e. patient does not require weekly monitoring and has not had any INR measurements above 4.0 in the last 2 months)
- If there is reason to believe a test result obtained 72 h prior to the dental procedure is not reflective of current level, INR should be retested within 24 h before dental procedure
- If extensive maxillofacial surgery is required, an approach of discontinuing warfarin and introducing heparin as a bridging agent may be used, owing to heparin's rapid onset and short half-life
  - Warfarin is ceased and intravenous heparin instituted to allow INR to decrease to a level appropriate for surgery
  - Warfarin is then reinstituted post surgery
  - INR is checked on a daily basis until it is within therapeutic range, and heparin therapy discontinued once this has been achieved
  - As this requires inpatient hospital management, significant social and financial costs, and interdisciplinary co-operation, it is not an appropriate management protocol for less complicated surgery or low-risk patients

If INR is >4.0

- Delay elective dental treatment and inform the patient's general medical practitioner or anticoagulation service if they are not already aware
- Refer to secondary care if urgent treatment is required
- Be aware that prescribing amoxicillin for the dental condition may affect the INR level; ideally the INR should be checked 24 h after starting the antibiotic
- Enquire if there have been any recent health or dietary changes that may have contributed to increased INR

If INR is <4.0

- Treat without interrupting vitamin K antagonists
- Consider limiting initial treatment area (e.g. perform a single extraction or limit subgingival periodontal scaling to 3 teeth, then assess bleeding before continuing)
- For procedures with a higher risk of postoperative bleeding complications, consider staging treatment over separate visits
- Use local haemostatic measures to achieve haemostasis; actively consider suturing and packing, taking into account patient factors
- Consider tranexamic acid 5% mouthwash 10 mL for 2 min, 4 times daily for 2–5 days (utility of tranexamic acid as an additional haemostatic measure in warfarinised patients is controversial)
- Advise patient to take paracetamol, unless contraindicated, for pain relief rather than aspirin or other non-steroidal anti-inflammatory drugs
- Caution with prescription of metronidazole, erythromycin, broad spectrum antibiotics, sulfonamides, tetracycline and azole antifungals
- If prescribing more than a single dose of antibiotic, consider reviewing patients routinely at 2–3 days postoperatively to check INR, remembering that absence of bleeding does not rule out an elevated INR
- Be aware that presurgery fasting and problems eating due to multiple extractions may have an effect on INR

that he would not bleed after the procedure. Why is this not advisable?

- There is strong evidence of increased risk of serious thromboembolic complications, including death, in patients whose anticoagulant therapy is interrupted
- This risk is significantly higher than the risk of bleeding complications in patients whose anticoagulant therapy is continued
- The overwhelming majority of patients taking warfarin before and after extractions whose INR is <4.0 at time of extraction do not have clinically significant bleeding postoperatively that requires more than local haemostatic measures, and any increase in bleeding is manageable at home

7) What other factors do you need to consider in your risk assessment?
   - Social
     - Reduced mobility
     - Wheelchair accessibility to/within dental clinic
   - Medical
     - Bleeding risk due to warfarin and liver disease (in addition to INR, may need coagulation blood test results)
     - Careful positioning due to back pain and osteoarthritis
   - Dental
     - High risk of periodontal disease
     - High sugar consumption in his daily drinks

Table 10.3.2 Major–moderate drug interactions between warfarin and antibiotics.

Direction and severity of effect on INR	Drug	Mechanism
Major increase in INR	• Metronidazole	Inhibits warfarin metabolism via CYP2C9
	• Moxifloxacin	May inhibit warfarin metabolism via CYP1A2+
	• Sulfamethoxazole	Inhibits warfarin metabolism, displaces protein binding
Moderate increase in INR	• Amoxicillin	May be due to decreased intestinal flora production of vitamin K
	• Azithromycin	Possibly decreases warfarin metabolism
	• Ciprofloxacin	May be due to CYP1A2 inhibition
	• Clarithromycin	Inhibits warfarin metabolism via CYP3A4
	• Cloxacillin	Unknown
	• Doxycycline	May inhibit warfarin metabolism via CYP3A4
	• Erythromycin	Inhibits warfarin metabolism via CYP3A4
	• Isoniazid	Inhibits warfarin metabolism via CYP2C9
	• Levofloxacin	May inhibit warfarin metabolism via CYP1A2
	• Tetracycline	Reduces plasma prothrombin activity
Moderate to severe decrease in INR	• Rifampin	Induces hepatic warfarin metabolism
Can increase or decrease INR	• Terbinafine	Unknown

8) Following planned extraction of #14, bleeding from the socket appears to cease after the use of local haemostatic measures, including suturing/placement of a haemostatic pack. However, the patient returns following discharge with persistent bleeding. How would you manage this?
   - Be aware that #14 was very infected and infection may induce fibrinolysis
   - Apply local pressure to the socket for 10–15 minutes
   - Bleeding may initially appear to stop with the formation of a platelet plug
   - Warfarin affects the clotting factors (II, VII, IX and X) and hence the subsequent clot may not form as rapidly
   - Following the application of pressure, observe the socket continually for 10 seconds to check for bleeding around the edges of the socket
   - Consider the use of tranexamic acid (TXA) or epsilon-aminocaproic acid (EACA) mouthwash applied to the socket with a gauze swab and given for use at home if bleeding persists
     - Use of TXA and EACA is not universally recommended and depends on local protocols
     - Although initial studies found TXA mouthwash to be of benefit, later studies found it offered no benefit over resorbable haemostatic agents plus suturing
     - As such, whilst some consensus guidelines recommend the use of TXA mouthwash as an additional haemostatic measure (e.g. British Society for Haematology, British Dental Association, National Patient Safety Agency, Australian Oral & Dental Therapeutic Guidelines, American Dental Association Council on Scientific Affairs, American Heart Association, American College of Cardiology), others conclude that there is insufficient evidence to indicate any additional benefit of TXA mouthwash when used in conjunction with other haemostatic measures for dental procedures (e.g. Scottish Dental Clinical Effectiveness Programme, UK Medicines Information)
   - If the patient continues to bleed, contact the patient's physician and arrange for them to be reviewed by the medical team as they may consider:
     - Reversal of warfarin; best achieved with a prothrombin complex concentrate and fresh frozen plasma
     - Vitamin K (1 mg) is essential for sustaining the reversal achieved by prothrombin complex concentrate and fresh frozen plasma

General Dental Considerations

Oral Findings

- Petechiae
- Ecchymoses
- Spontaneous gingival bleeding

(a)

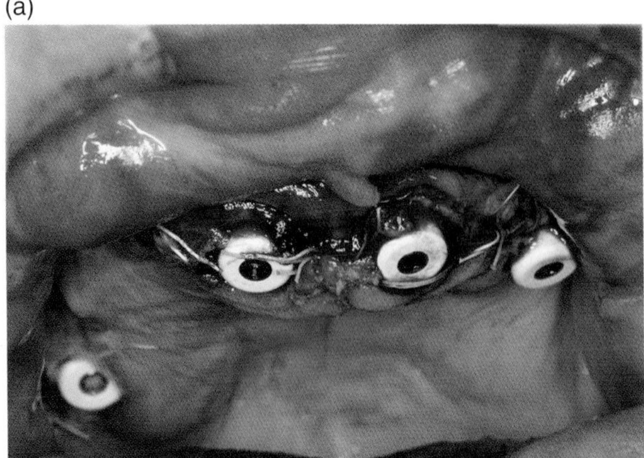

(b)

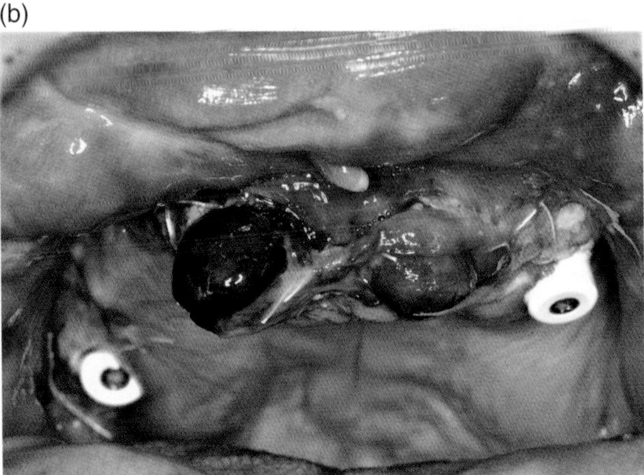

Figure 10.3.3 (a,b) Prolonged bleeding and bruising (haematoma) after dental implant insertion.

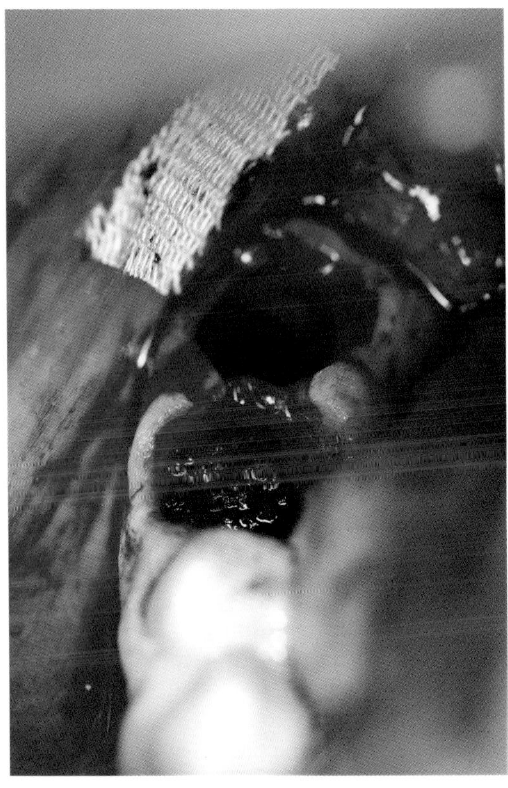

Figure 10.3.4 Prolonged bleeding after dental extractions; haemostatic pack (oxidised cellulose) placed.

- Prolonged bleeding after invasive procedures (Figures 10.3.3 and 10.3.4)

General Dental Management

- Do not withdraw anticoagulation due to the risk of thromboembolic events
- Instead, dental treatment modifications are recommended to minimise the risk of bleeding (Table 10.3.3)

Section II: Background Information and Guidelines

Definition

Vitamin K antagonists (VKAs) are drugs administered to decrease blood coagulability. They were developed around 1940, and until relatively recently were the only available oral anticoagulants.

Mechanism of Action

- VKAs prevent vitamin K conversion to its active form, thereby reducing vitamin K-dependent synthesis of several coagulation factors in the liver (II, VII, IX and X), and proteins C, S and Z (Table 10.3.4)

Classification

- VKAs include warfarin, phenprocoumon and acenocoumarol
- Genetic polymorphisms affect drug metabolism differently according to the type of VKA
- The CYP2C9 isoenzyme may be more important for warfarin clearance than for acenocoumarol or phenprocoumon clearance
- Acenocoumarol is structurally different from warfarin (characterised by a nitro group in the *para* position of the phenyl ring) and may be a more potent anticoagulant compared to warfarin and phenprocoumon

Advantages

- Oral administration
- Low initial costs
- Reliable lab test to measure level of coagulation (INR); availability of point-of-care testing machines (may be

Table 10.3.3 General dental management considerations.

Risk assessment	• Prolonged bleeding from surgery and trauma • Consider the impact of the underlying condition for which the warfarin is being given • Additional systemic conditions that may aggravate the bleeding tendency include any condition or drug that affects the vascular, platelet or coagulation phases of haemostasis
Criteria for referral	• Dentists should be able to treat the vast majority of patients in primary care • Refer to specialist services if the patient has: – Other medical comorbidities that affect haemostasis – Other medications affecting haemostasis – An INR that remains above 4.0, or erratic INR control – Urgent dental care needs when INR is >4.0
Access/position	• Timing of treatment: in the morning and early in week • Consider the need to stage invasive treatment to minimise bleeding risk • Consider the need for an escort
Communication	• If the dental procedure is likely to cause bleeding, consult the general medical practitioner and/or specialist physician • Liaise with the anticoagulation clinic regarding the timing of an INR test in relation to planned invasive dental treatment
Consent/capacity	• Provide information to the patient regarding warfarin and invasive dental treatment at the assessment appointment to allow the patient time to consider the information • Emphasise the importance of not ceasing anticoagulation medication due to the thromboembolic risk outweighing the bleeding risk from dental extractions • Explain the steps that will be undertaken to reduce bleeding, so as to not discourage patients from taking their warfarin medication • Warn patient of the increased risk of intraoral/postoperative bleeding, and intra/extraoral bruising • Inform the patient of the measures which will be used to reduce bleeding risk
Anaesthesia/sedation	• Local anaesthesia Delivered using an aspirating syringe and should include a vasoconstrictor, unless contraindicated – Anaesthetic solution should be delivered slowly to avoid rapid expansion of the soft tissues – Regional block local anaesthetic injections, or those in the floor of the mouth, may be a hazard since bleeding into the fascial spaces of the neck can threaten airway patency – Intraligamentary or intrapapillary injections are preferred • Sedation – Intravenous sedation cannulation poses a risk of haematoma formation • General anaesthesia – Hazards of anaesthesia, especially nasal intubation and intramuscular injections
Dental treatment	• Before – Consider limiting initial treatment area (e.g. perform a single extraction or debride 3 teeth only initially, and assess bleeding before continuing) – For procedures with higher risk of postoperative bleeding, consider carrying out staged treatment – Check INR, ideally no more than 24 h prior, or no more than 72 h if INR is stable – If INR is >4.0, delay elective dental treatment and inform the patient's general medical practitioner or anticoagulation service. Refer to secondary care if urgent treatment is required – If INR is <4.0, treat without interrupting warfarin therapy • During – Lubricant/barrier cream used to protect the lips/soft tissue from trauma – Careful manipulation of the cheek and soft tissues – consider the use of gauze when using cheek retractors – Caution with suction to avoid trauma (reduce the volume) and particular care taken to avoid trauma in the floor of mouth – Atraumatic extraction technique preferred – If a mucoperiosteal flap is required, a buccal approach is best since lingual tissue trauma may open up planes into which haemorrhage may track and endanger the airway – Minimal bone removal, teeth sectioned where possible

(Continued)

Table 10.3.3 (Continued)

	– Local haemostatic measures to control bleeding – Bony wound compressed with absorbent gauze – Tranexamic acid 5% mouthwash may be used as an adjunct; this can be soaked in gauze and applied directly over the socket – Haemostatic packing agents: minimise usage to reduce incidence of dry socket. Ensure agent of choice is acceptable to patient as some contain animal-based proteins – Suturing: use non-traumatic needle and small number of sutures • After – Extended monitoring – Careful oral cleansing postoperatively – The patency of the airway must always be ensured – Care should be taken to watch for haematoma formation which may manifest itself by swelling, dysphagia or hoarseness – Provide verbal and written postoperative instructions and emergency contact details
Drug prescription	• Antiseptics as required (e.g. 0.12–0.2% chlorhexidine rinses every 8 h) • Antibiotics (e.g. amoxicillin, penicillin V, amoxicillin/clavulanic acid at therapeutic doses) as required but consider their potential effect on warfarin metabolism • Pain relief (e.g. paracetamol) • Avoid aspirin, ibuprofen and diclofenac, antifungals (miconazole, fluconazole) and antibiotics (erythromycin, tetracycline, metronidazole, quinolones, sulfonamides, possibly broad-spectrum antibiotics) as these may increase bleeding risk • Carbamazepine may increase thromboembolic risk
Education/prevention	• Use of fluoride and fissure sealants, oral hygiene education, dietary advice and regular dental visits to minimise dental treatment that may cause bleeding complications

Table 10.3.4 Pharmacokinetics and pharmacodynamics of warfarin.

Mechanism of action	Vitamin K antagonist, inhibiting factors II, VII, IX, X and anticoagulant proteins C and S
Peak plasma concentration	2–8 hours
Half-life	25–60 hours
Anticoagulation duration	48–96 hours
Metabolism	Liver via CYP450 system; S-isomer: CYP2C9; R-isomer: CYP1A2, CYP3A4
Excretion	Renal (90%)
Reversal	Vitamin K, fresh frozen plasma, prothrombin complex concentrate
Drug interactions	• Lower INR: antiepileptic drugs (carbamazepine); homoeopathic medications (ginseng, St John's wort) • Increase INR: amiodarone; analgesics (aspirin, other non-steroidal anti-inflammatory drugs); antidiabetic drugs (chlorpropamide); antiepileptic drugs (phenytoin); antifungals (miconazole, fluconazole); antibiotics (erythromycin, tetracycline, metronidazole, quinolones, sulfonamides, possibly broad-spectrum antibiotics); fluorouracil (5FU); homoeopathic medications (garlic, ginger, *Ginkgo biloba*, ginseng); lipid-lowering agents (statins); omeprazole; selective serotonin reuptake inhibitors
Food interactions	• Lower INR: diets high in vitamin K such as avocado, beetroot, broccoli, Brussels sprouts, cabbage, chick peas, green peas, kale, lettuce, spinach, turnips • Increase INR: cranberry juice, grapefruit, pomegranate
Comorbidities affecting dosage	Biliary disease; congestive heart failure; diarrhoea; fever; hypo- and hyperthyroidism; liver disease; malignant disease; malnutrition (undernourishment, malabsorptive disorders, presurgery fasting); vitamin K excess or deficiency

Table 10.3.5 Indications for oral anticoagulation and target INR.

Indication for warfarin	Target INR
• First episode of deep vein thrombosis or pulmonary embolism (including those associated with antiphospholipid syndrome or for recurrence in patients no longer receiving warfarin) • Peripheral vascular disease (acute arterial embolism requiring embolectomy) • Atrial fibrillation • Myocardial infarction • Dilated cardiomyopathy • Bioprosthetic heart valves (treat for 3 months) • Mitral stenosis or regurgitation with atrial fibrillation/history of systemic embolism/left atrial thrombus/ enlarged left atrium • Cardioversion (3 weeks preprocedure, 4 weeks postprocedure)	2.5
• Cardioversion (day of procedure)	3.0
• Mechanical prosthetic heart valves (target dependent on prosthesis thrombogenicity and patient risk factors)	2.5–3.5
• Recurrent deep vein thrombosis or pulmonary embolism in patients currently receiving anticoagulation and with an INR above 2	3.5

Source: Keeling, D., Baglin, T., Tait, C., et al. (2011). British Committee for Standards in Haematology. Guidelines on oral anticoagulation with warfarin – fourth edition. *Br. J. Haematol.* 154 : 311–324.

used in anticoagulation clinics, at home by patients or in the dental clinic)

- Increased compliance due to accountability of regular monitoring tests
- Vitamin K reversal agent available

Disadvantages

- Dose response variability due to:
  - Genetic polymorphisms (CYP450 system) producing variation in patient's sensitivity
  - Non-genetic factors including age, body weight, dietary vitamin K intake, concomitant diseases and medications
- Need for dose titration
- Less predictable pharmacokinetics and pharmacodynamics
- Delayed onset and offset of action (may require bridging therapy)
- Narrow therapeutic window
- Overall higher longer-term costs as regular monitoring is required
- Higher incidence of adverse effects, including:
  - Multiple dietary interactions
    - A diet high in vitamin K (avocado, beet, broccoli, Brussel sprouts, cabbage, chickpeas, green peas, green tea, kale, lettuce, liver, spinach and turnips) can reduce the INR
    - Alcohol ingestion can inhibit warfarin, but can have the converse effect if there is liver disease
  - Multiple drug interactions
    - Warfarin effect may be enhanced by many drugs such as non-steroidal anti-inflammatory agents, antibiotics and azole antifungal agents
    - Aspirin and other non-steroidal anti-inflammatory agents can enhance warfarin by displacing it from plasma proteins; they may also interfere with platelet function and also cause gastric bleeding
    - COX-2 inhibitors such as celecoxib appear not to have a significant effect on platelets or INR (but may be cardiotoxic)
    - Paracetamol (acetoaminophen) in excessive and prolonged administration can enhance the action of warfarin, presumably by inhibiting its metabolism; an intake of less than 6 tablets of 325 mg of paracetamol per week has little or no effect on INR; however, 4 tablets a day for a week significantly affects the INR, with initial effects observed within 18–48 hours of administration
    - Tramadol occasionally interferes with warfarin and raises the INR
    - Where antibiotics are indicated, a single dose of amoxicillin, as required, for example, in endocarditis prophylaxis, does not cause significant alteration in the INR; however, extended doses may cause an impact
  - Disorders/diseases such as diarrhoea, liver disease and malignant disease can increase the INR

Indications/Laboratory Findings

- The World Health Organization introduced the international normalised ratio (INR) as the standard to measure warfarin activity in 1983
- INR is a prothrombin ratio, calculated by dividing prothrombin time by the laboratory control prothrombin time (to correct for the quality of thromboplastin used in the test against an international standard thromboplastin)
- Individuals with normal coagulation have INR around 1.0
- The risk of bleeding increases as INR increases
- Target values (rather than ranges) are now recommended
- The target INR varies with the condition being treated (normally between 2.0 to 4.0) (Table 10.3.5)
- An INR which is within 0.5 units of the target value is generally satisfactory, with larger deviations requiring dosage adjustment
- However, only 50% of INRs in patients taking warfarin are within range at any one time

A World/Transcultural View

- The popularity of VKAs has exhibited a constant decline, particularly since the introduction of the direct oral anticoagulants (DOACs)
- However, the initial cost of warfarin is considerably less than DOAC medications; hence affordability across the world may impact prescription numbers relative to DOACs, especially in countries where patients pay for their own medications
- Of the VKAs, warfarin is the drug of choice for anticoagulation in the UK, North America, Australia and Scandinavia
- In contrast, the VKAs of first choice in many continental European countries are phenprocoumon (e.g. Germany) and acenocoumarol (e.g. Spain)
- Views on the utility of tranexamic acid as an additional haemostatic measure vary

Recommended Reading

NHS National Patient Safety Agency, British Dental Association, Haemostasis and Thrombosis Task Force of the British Committee for Standards in Haematology (2004). *Managing Patients Who Are Taking Warfarin and Undergoing Dental Treatment*. London: NHS National Patient Safety Agency.

Pirmohamed, M. (2018). Warfarin: the end or the end of one size fits all therapy? *J. Pers. Med.* 8: 22.

Quciroz, S.I.M.L., Silvestre, V.D., Soares, R.M. et al. (2018). Tranexamic acid as a local hemostasis method after dental extraction in patients on warfarin: a randomized controlled clinical study. *Clin. Oral Investig.* 22: 2281–2289.

Scottish Dental Clinical Effectiveness Programme (2015). *Management of Dental Patients Taking Anticoagulants or Antiplatelet Drugs*. Dundee: SDCEP www.sdcep.org.uk/published-guidance/anticoagulants-and-antiplatelets.

Shaer FE, Raslan I, Osaimi NA, et al. Documentation of various approaches and outcomes in patients on warfarin undergoing dental procedures: a review article. *Am. J. Cardiovasc. Dis.* 2016; 6: 109–17.

Verhoef, T.I., Redekop, W.K., Daly, A.K. et al. (2014). Pharmacogenctic-guided dosing of coumarin anticoagulants: algorithms for warfarin, acenocoumarol and phenprocoumon. *Br. J. Clin. Pharmacol.* 77: 626–641.

Weltman, N.J., Al-Attar, Y., Cheung, J. et al. (2015). Management of dental extractions in patients taking warfarin as anticoagulant treatment: a systematic review. *J. Can. Dent. Assoc.* 81: f20.

10.4 Treatment with Direct Oral Anticoagulants

Section I: Clinical Scenario and Dental Considerations

Clinical Scenario

A 75-year-old female presents as an emergency to your dental clinic first thing in the morning, accompanied by her husband. She complains of pain from her upper left second molar tooth, which she reports is worse on clenching and chewing. This commenced 2 weeks ago when she was eating and part of the tooth fractured. The tooth is currently asymptomatic.

Medical History

- Deep vein thrombosis (DVT) 2 years ago following hip replacement surgery
- Osteoarthritis
- Stage 2 chronic kidney disease (glomerular filtration rate of 60–89 mL/min)
- Body mass index (BMI): 32 kg/m^2

Medications

- Rivaroxaban
- Paracetamol
- History of 2 corticosteroid injections in the involved joint 4 years ago

Dental History

- Attends the dental practice yearly
- Brushes her teeth twice a day but after her DVT became reliant on her husband to help her; uses a soft toothbrush only once a day as her gums bleed and she is worried that this will not stop because she is taking rivaroxaban
- Clenches her teeth due to pain related to her osteoarthritis
- Previous history of fractured lower molar teeth, including a lower left tooth which was stabilised 1 year ago with a large composite filling

Social History

- South Asian origin
- Lives with her husband
- Attends appointments using their modified private car (husband drives)
- Uses a walking stick
- No tobacco or alcohol

Oral Examination

- #27: probably fractured; likely to require a surgical extraction
- Generalised soft deposits and plaque-induced gingivitis

Radiological Examination

- Long cone periapical radiograph: root canal treatment in tooth #27 (Figure 10.4.1)

Structured Learning

1) How do you assess the bleeding risk of rivaroxaban in relation to dental procedures?
   - Rivaroxaban is the first orally active direct factor Xa inhibitor/anticoagulant (DOAC) developed
   - Unlike warfarin, routine laboratory monitoring of INR (international normalised ratio) is not necessary
   - Although the activated partial thromboplastin time (aPTT) and HepTest (a test developed to assay low molecular weight heparins) are prolonged in a dose-dependent manner, neither test is recommended for the assessment of the pharmacodynamic effects of rivaroxaban
   - Anti-Xa activity and inhibition of anti-Xa activity monitoring is also not recommended despite being influenced by rivaroxaban
   - The patient's previous bleeding history is often more helpful in determining the risk of bleeding
   - The invasiveness of the proposed procedure should also be assessed

A Practical Approach to Special Care in Dentistry, First Edition. Edited by Pedro Diz Dios and Navdeep Kumar.

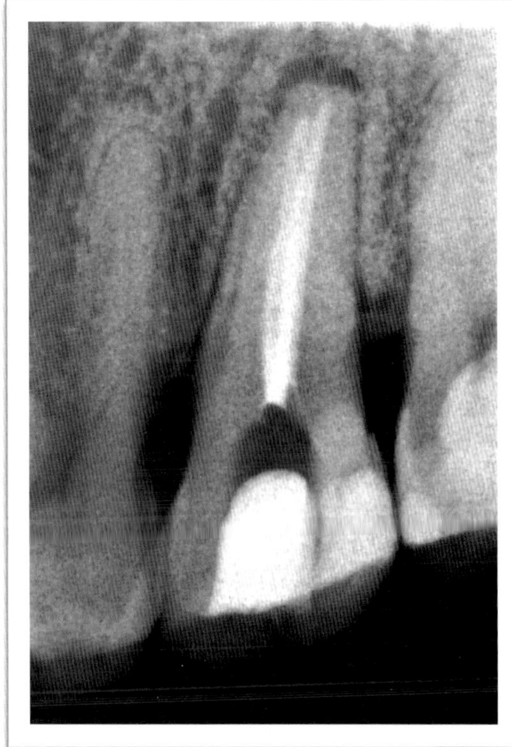

Figure 10.4.1 Periapical radiograph showing root canal treatment in tooth #27 and a small radiolucent periapical lesion.

2) The patient reports that she has taken her rivaroxaban earlier in the morning, before attending her dental appointment. What are the treatment options for managing the fractured tooth in this patient?
   - #27 is likely to require a surgical extraction
   - Plan for surgical dental extraction at a later date as:
     - The patient has already taken her rivaroxaban
     - The tooth is asymptomatic and does not require urgent removal
   - Smooth the rough tooth surface and/or place a temporary dressing to avoid further trauma to the tongue; particularly important as there is an increased bleeding risk; advise the patient to avoid eating on the tooth
3) The patient is upset that you are not going to extract the tooth the same day as she finds travelling to the dental clinic tiring. Can you use reversal agents for rivaroxaban to facilitate invasive dental treatment the same day?
   - Andexanet alpha is a recombinant form of human factor Xa protein which binds specifically to apixaban or rivaroxaban, thereby reversing their anticoagulant effects
   - It is used in life-threatening or uncontrolled bleeding (specialist supervision in hospital)
   - It is not used in relation to dental treatment
4) How would you plan the exploratory surgery of the #27?
   - Exploratory surgery and eventual surgical extraction of the #27 should be considered as a high-risk invasive dental procedure (Figure 10.4.2)
   - Consult with the physician regarding the proposed dental extraction, as the patient is elderly and has chronic kidney disease – both factors may have a negative impact on the clearance of the DOAC and hence increase its duration of action
   - Highlight that the procedure is at high risk of bleeding given that a surgical approach is likely
   - The patient's previous bleeding history may also assist in determining the risk of bleeding
   - Confirm the plan regarding the timing of the extraction in relation to the DOAC medication
   - In most cases advice would be to withhold the morning dose of the rivaroxaban until haemostasis is achieved after the dental extraction
5) What other factors do you need to consider in your risk assessment?
   - Social
     - Reduced mobility
     - Escort required – husband, who will also need to drive the patient to her appointments
   - Medical
     - Bleeding risk due to DOAC
     - Comorbidity related to chronic renal failure (including prescribing considerations), osteoarthritis, obesity and related complications (moving

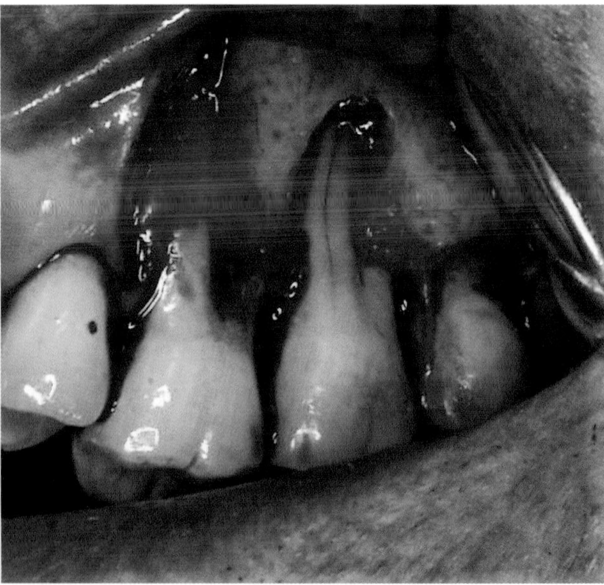

Figure 10.4.2 Exploratory surgery showing radicular fracture. Consequently, dental extraction was performed in the same treatment session.

  - and handling, bariatric complications) (see Chapters 16.2 and 16.4)
- Dental
  - Dental trauma due to clenching, with a history of fractured teeth
  - Reliance on husband to clean her teeth
  - Reduced brushing frequency
  - Use of a soft brush

6) What advice would you give in relation to the patient's bleeding gums?
   - Reassure the patient that it is important to continue to clean her teeth as usual even though she is taking an oral anticoagulant
   - Explain that poor oral hygiene can lead to gingivitis and periodontal disease, where the gums become swollen and bleed more easily – this will have a significantly greater impact than the anticoagulant
   - A soft brush may not be effective and she needs to brush at least twice daily

7) How would you manage the tendency that this patient has to fracture her teeth?
   - Provide advice regarding clenching/bruxism and its relation to chronic pain/illness
   - Explain that it is likely to be the cause of the history of multiple tooth fractures
   - Consider provision of a mouthguard to protect remaining dentition; ensure the gingival health has improved first to avoid a deterioration in relation to higher plaque accumulation inside the guard; the design should avoid excessive contact with the soft tissues (minimise trauma due to anticoagulant medication)
   - Review the remaining dentition and consider the need for full-coverage crowns on heavily restored teeth
   - Consider other underlying diseases (e.g. gastro-oesophageal reflux)

General Dental Considerations

Oral Findings

- Petechiae
- Ecchymoses
- Spontaneous gingival bleeding
- Prolonged bleeding after invasive procedures (Figure 10.4.3)

General Dental Management

- It is important to stratify the risk of bleeding for any proposed dental procedure as this determines the appropriate perioperative management of patients on DOACs (Tables 10.4.1 and 10.4.2; Appendix H)

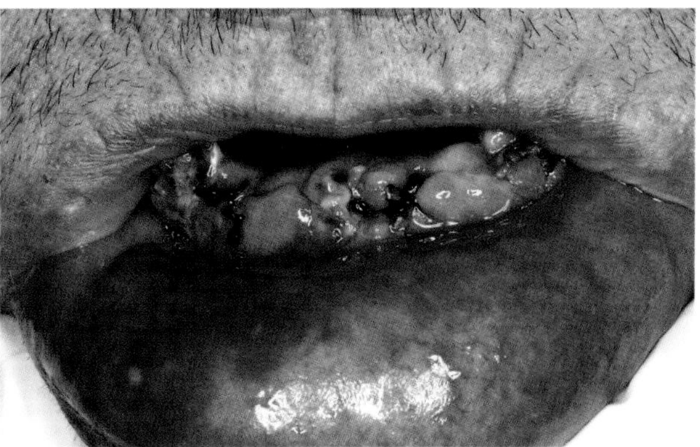

Figure 10.4.3 Bruising (haematoma) following dental extractions.

- There is emerging evidence that DOACs do not need to be omitted for all invasive dental procedures

Section II: Background Information and Guidelines

Definition

Due to the many limitations of traditional anticoagulant medications, a new category of drugs has been developed. Initially known as 'new oral anticoagulants' (NOACs), these drugs have now been renamed as 'direct oral anticoagulants' (DOACs). Clinical use of the DOACs began in 2008 when dabigatran and rivaroxaban were first approved in the European Union for the prevention of venous thromboembolism after elective hip or knee replacement surgery. Since then, several other DOACs have become available for use.

Mechanism of Action (Table 10.4.3)

- Directly inhibit activated factor II/thrombin (dabigatran)
- Directly inhibit activated factor X (rivaroxaban, apixaban, edoxaban, betrixaban)

Advantages (Table 10.4.4)

- Oral administration
- Rapid onset and offset of action (reducing the need for bridging)
- Largely predictable pharmacokinetics
- Fewer drug and dietary interactions
- Overall reduced longer-term cost as regular monitoring not required in the majority of patients (exceptions include acute liver/renal failure, extremes of body weight, suspected pregnancy)

Table 10.4.1 Management of patients taking direct oral anticoagulants (DOACs) undergoing dental procedures associated with bleeding risk.

Dental procedures associated with low bleeding risk

- Do not interrupt DOAC medication (if the patient has another relevant medical condition or is taking other medications that may increase bleeding risk, consult with physician as appropriate)
- If the patient is on a time-limited course of DOAC, delay non-urgent invasive dental procedures where possible until the medication has been discontinued
- Patients with acute deep vein thrombosis or pulmonary embolism may be taking high-dose DOACs (e.g. apixaban or rivaroxaban) for the first 1–3 weeks of treatment – delay until standard dose is reached
- Plan treatment for early in the day/week to allow for monitoring and management of bleeding complications, should they occur
- Perform the procedure as atraumatically as possible
- Use local haemostatic measures (haemostatic packing material/sutures)
- Consider tranexamic acid 5% mouthwash
- If travel time to emergency care is a concern, consider limiting the initial treatment area, staging treatment, haemostatic measures and extended post-treatment monitoring
- Advise the patient to take paracetamol, unless contraindicated, for pain relief rather than non steroidal anti-inflammatory drugs such as aspirin, ibuprofen, diclofenac or naproxen
- Provide the patient with written post-treatment advice and emergency contact details

Dental procedures associated with higher bleeding risk

- Advise the patient to miss (apixaban/dabigatran) or delay (rivaroxaban/edoxaban) their morning dose on the day of their dental treatment
- If the patient usually takes once-a-day rivaroxaban/edoxaban in the evening, there is no need to modify their medication schedule prior to the dental treatment
- If the patient is on a time-limited course of DOAC, delay non-urgent invasive dental procedures where possible until the medication has been discontinued
- Patients with acute deep vein thrombosis or pulmonary embolism may be taking high-dose apixaban or rivaroxaban for the first 1–3 weeks of treatment – delay until standard dose is reached
- Plan treatment for early in the day/week to allow for monitoring and management of bleeding complications, should they occur
- Perform the procedure as atraumatically as possible
- Use local haemostatic measures (haemostatic packing material/sutures)
- Consider tranexamic acid 5% mouthwash
- If travel time to emergency care is a concern, consider limiting the initial treatment area, staging treatment, haemostatic measures and extended post-treatment monitoring
- Advise the patient to take paracetamol, unless contraindicated, for pain relief rather than non-steroidal anti-inflammatory drugs such as aspirin, ibuprofen, diclofenac or naproxen
- Provide the patient with written post-treatment advice and emergency contact details
- Advise the patient when to restart their medication
  - For rivaroxaban/edoxaban (taken once a day), the delayed morning dose may be taken 4 h after haemostasis has been achieved. The next dose should be taken as usual the following morning. If the patient normally takes their rivaroxaban in the evening, they can take this at the usual time on the day of treatment as long as no earlier than 4 h after haemostasis has been achieved
  - For apixaban or dabigatran (taken twice a day), having missed the morning dose, the patient should take their evening dose at the usual time as long as no earlier than 4 h after haemostasis has been achieved
- Advise the patient to contact the practice for advice if rebleeding occurs before or after restarting their DOAC
- The patient should avoid missing subsequent doses of their DOAC, unless absolutely required in an emergency situation to control bleeding

Disadvantages

- Initial cost of the DOAC
- Potential risk of lack of compliance due to no regular monitoring tests
- Limited availability of reversal agents
- Caution in the elderly or renal disease
- Risk of bleeding increased in patients >75 years of age
- Increased gastrointestinal bleeding with high dosing of dabigatran
- Increased dyspepsia with use of dabigatran
- Lack of reliable laboratory tests to measure levels of DOACs
- Selective antidotes are now becoming available but their use is restricted to emergency use (emergency surgery/life-threatening bleeding)
  - Dabigatran: reversible by idarucizamab within 5 minutes
  - Xa DOACs: reversal by andexanet alpha

Table 10.4.2 General dental management considerations.

Risk assessment	• Prolonged bleeding from surgery and trauma • Consider the impact of the underlying condition for which the DOAC is being given • Consider the impact of any additional systemic conditions that may aggravate the bleeding tendency
Access/position	• Plan treatment for early in the day/week to allow for monitoring and management of bleeding complications, should they occur • Consider the need to stage invasive treatment to minimise bleeding risk • Consider the need for an escort
Criteria for referral	• Dentists should be able to treat the vast majority of patients taking DOACs in primary care • Need for referral is based on the severity and complexity of the underlying medical conditions necessitating the use of a DOAC, if there are multiple comorbidities, and/or the invasiveness of the proposed dental procedure
Communication	• If procedure likely to cause bleeding, consult general medical practitioner or specialist • Provide information to the patient regarding DOACs and invasive dental treatment at the assessment appointment to allow the patient time to consider the information
Consent/capacity	• Warn patient of the increased risk of intraoral/postoperative bleeding, and intra/extraoral bruising • Inform the patient of the measures which will be used to reduce bleeding risk
Anaesthesia/sedation	• Local anaesthesia – Delivered using an aspirating syringe and should include a vasoconstrictor, unless contraindicated – Anaesthetic solution should be delivered slowly to avoid rapid expansion of the soft tissues – Regional block local anaesthetic injections, or those in the floor of the mouth, may be a hazard since bleeding into the fascial spaces of the neck can threaten airway patency – Intraligamentary or intrapapillary injections are preferred • Sedation – Intravenous sedation cannulation poses a risk of haematoma formation • General anaesthesia – Hazards of anaesthesia, especially nasal intubation and intramuscular injections
Dental treatment	• Before – Consider limiting initial treatment area (e.g. perform a single extraction or debride 3 teeth only initially, and assess bleeding before continuing) – For procedures with higher risk of postoperative bleeding, consider carrying out staged treatment • During – Lubricant/barrier cream used to protect the lips/soft tissue from trauma – Careful manipulation of the cheek and soft tissues; consider the use of gauze when using cheek retractors – Caution with suction to avoid trauma (reduce the volume) and particular care taken to avoid trauma in the floor of mouth – Atraumatic extraction technique preferred – Minimal bone removal, teeth sectioned where possible – If a mucoperiosteal flap is required, a buccal approach is best since lingual tissue trauma may open up planes into which haemorrhage may track and endanger the airway – Local haemostatic measures to control bleeding – Bony wound compressed with absorbent gauze – Tranexamic acid 5% mouthwash may be used as an adjunct; this can be soaked in gauze and applied directly over the socket – Haemostatic packing agents: minimise usage to reduce incidence of dry socket; ensure agent of choice is acceptable to patient as some contain animal-based proteins – Suturing: use non-traumatic needle and small number of sutures

(Continued)

Table 10.4.2 (Continued)

	• After – Extended monitoring – Careful oral cleansing postoperatively – The patency of the airway must always be ensured; care should be taken to watch for haematoma formation which may manifest itself by swelling, dysphagia or hoarseness – Provide verbal and written postoperative instructions and emergency contact details – If the DOAC dose has been delayed to enable invasive dental treatment, confirm with the physician when it should be taken – in general this is 2–4 h after haemostasis is achieved
Drug prescription	• Antiseptics as required (e.g. chlorhexidine rinses) • Antibiotics (e.g. amoxicillin, penicillin V, amoxicillin/clavulanic acid or metronidazole at therapeutic doses) as required • Pain relief (e.g. paracetamol) • Drug interactions are emerging – avoidance or dose reduction should be considered as appropriate: – Strong P-gp and CYP3A4 inhibitors including itraconazole, ketoconazole, posaconazole, voriconazole, clarithromycin – Aspirin and other non-steroidal anti-inflammatory drugs
Education/ prevention	• Use of fluoride and fissure sealants, oral hygiene education, dietary advice and regular dental visits to minimise dental treatment that may cause bleeding complications

Table 10.4.3 Direct oral anticoagulation medications[a].

Drug name	Mechanism of action	Dose/frequency for long-term use[b]
Dabigatran	Thrombin inhibitor	110–150 mg twice daily
Rivaroxaban	Factor Xa inhibitor	15–20 mg daily
Apixaban	Factor Xa inhibitor	2.5–5.0 mg twice daily
Edoxaban	Factor Xa inhibitor	30–60 mg daily
Betrixaban	Factor Xa inhibitor	80 mg daily

[a] Other factor Xa inhibitors in development include darexaban, otamixaban, letaxaban and eribaxaban.
[b] Reduced dose in relation to age and reduced creatinine clearance (dabigatran contraindicated if <30 mL/min; rivaroxaban, apixaban, edoxaban and betrixaban if <15 mL/min).

Indications

- Prophylaxis of stroke and systemic embolism in those with non-valvular atrial fibrillation, treatment and prevention of recurrent DVT and pulmonary embolism
- Prophylaxis of thromboembolic events in those who have undergone hip or knee replacement surgery (dabigatran, rivaroxaban, apixaban)
- Prevention of atherothrombotic events following acute coronary syndrome (rivaroxaban)

A World/Transcultural View

- The popularity of DOACs is constantly increasing around the world, whereas that of warfarin has exhibited a constant and inexorable decline
- However, the initial cost of DOAC medications is considerably more than warfarin and antiplatelet medication; hence patient affordability across the world may impact on their use in countries where patients pay for their own medications

Table 10.4.4 Comparison of the characteristics of warfarin and direct oral anticoagulants (DOACs).

	Warfarin	DOACs
Reversibility	Warfarin is reversible with vitamin K	D is reversible by idarucizamab within 5 min Xa DOACs are reversible by andexanet alpha antidote
Need for dose titration	Laboratory monitoring required	Laboratory monitoring not required
Laboratory test	International normalised ratio (INR)	Not routinely undertaken; concentration of the drug in plasma can be undertaken D – thrombin time (TT) and activated partial thromboplastin time (aPTT) R – prothrombin time (PT) A/E/B – no reliable test
Therapeutic window	Narrow	Broad
Effectiveness	Dose response variability	Predictable anticoagulation
Adverse effects	Higher incidence	Lower incidence, except gastrointestinal bleeding and dyspepsia with D (>25%)
Interactions	Many food and drug interactions	Few food and drug interactions (especially D)
Half-life	Long: 20-60 h	D: 12–17 h; R: 5–13 h; A: 12 h; E: 10–14 h; B: 20–27 h
Time to peak in plasma	4 h	D: 1 h; R: 2–4 h; A: 3–4 h; E: 1.5 h; B: 3–4 h

D, dabigatran; R, rivaroxaban; A, apixaban; E, edoxaban; B, betrixaban.

Recommended Reading

NICE (National Institute for Health and Care Excellence). Anticoagulants, including direct-acting oral anticoagulants (DOACs). (2016). www.nice.org.uk/advice/ktt16

Wigle, P., Hein, B., and Bernheisel, C.R. (2019). Anticoagulation: updated guidelines for out patient management. *Am. Fam. Physician.* 100: 426–434.

Costantinides, F., Rizzo, R., Pascazio, L., and Maglione, M. (2016). Managing patients taking novel oral anticoagulants (NOAs) in dentistry: a discussion paper on clinical implications. *BMC Oral Health.* 16: 5.

Hassona, Y., Malamos, D., Shaqman, M. et al. (2018). Management of dental patients taking direct oral anticoagulants: Dabigatran. *Oral Dis.* 24: 228–232.

Lupi, S.M. and Rodriguez y Baena, A. (2020). Patients taking Direct Oral Anticoagulants (DOAC) undergoing oral surgery: a review of the literature and a proposal of a peri-operative management protocol. *Healthcare.* 8: E281.

Kaplovitch, E. and Dounaevskaia, V. (2019). Treatment in the dental practice of the patient receiving anticoagulation therapy. *J. Am. Dent. Assoc.* 150: 602–608.

Kwak, E.J., Nam, S., Park, K.M. et al. (2019). Bleeding related to dental treatment in patients taking novel oral anticoagulants (NOACs): a retrospective study. *Clin. Oral Investig.* 23: 477–401.

Manfredi, M., Dave, B., Percudani, D. et al. (2019). World Workshop on Oral Medicine VII: direct anticoagulant agents management for invasive oral procedures: a systematic review and meta-analysis. *Oral Dis.* 25: S157–S173.

10.5 Treatment with Antiplatelets

Section I: Clinical Scenario and Dental Considerations

Clinical Scenario

A 50-year-old male presents at the end of the day complaining of increasing mobility of his lower anterior incisors. The teeth were splinted as a temporary measure during a period of acute illness but have recently become increasingly loose.

Medical History

- Non-ST-elevation myocardial infarctions (NSTEMI) 9 years ago and three years ago. One coronary stent placed after each episode
- Controlled hypertension
- Multicentric Castleman disease – MCD (HHV8 positive): diagnosed one year ago and managed with chemotherapy, recently confirmed in remission
- Human immunodeficiency virus (HIV) positive: diagnosed 9 months ago. Recent CD4 counts 263 cells/μL, viral load undetectable
- Type 2 diabetes mellitus: diagnosed three months ago; recent HbA1c 7.1%
- Depression
- Allergy: sulfamethoxazole/trimethoprim (rashes)

Medications

- Aspirin
- Ticagrelor
- Metformin
- Empagliflozin
- Emtricitabine/tenofovir alafenamide
- Raltegravir
- Terbinafine
- Paroxetine

Dental History

- No history of regular dental attendance
- Currently brushes twice daily, no interproximal cleaning
- Uses a fluoride toothpaste
- Self-care was more difficult during recent period of acute illness and had days without brushing teeth

Social History

- Polish origin
- Unable to work for the past three years due to medical issues
- Rental accommodation with one cotenant
- Socially supported by a friend; family live overseas

Oral Examination

- Lingual composite splinting of #31/#32 and #41/#42/#43; both splints starting to debond
- #31 and #41: grade III mobility; negative response to cold sensibility testing
- #32 and #42: grade II mobility; positive response to cold sensibility testing
- #23 large mesial restoration; positive response to cold sensibility testing; asymptomatic
- #21 and #22: porcelain-fused-to metal crowns; root filled 20 years ago; asymptomatic
- Moderate subgingival calculus accumulation
- Generalised moderate chronic periodontal disease, localised severe disease of lower anterior teeth
- Metal partial upper denture

Radiological Examination

- Orthopantomogram and periapical radiographs (lower anterior teeth) undertaken (Figure 10.5.1)
- Generalised horizontal bone loss ~40–50% (~20–40% lower incisor teeth)
- Multiple prosthetic crowns: #11, #21, #22 and #37

A Practical Approach to Special Care in Dentistry, First Edition. Edited by Pedro Diz Dios and Navdeep Kumar.

(a)

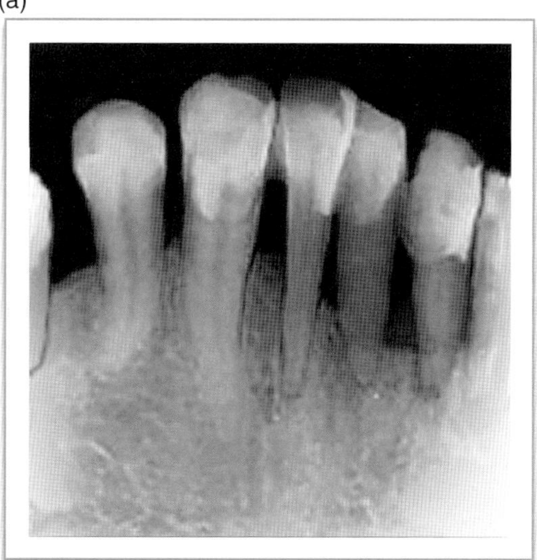

(b)

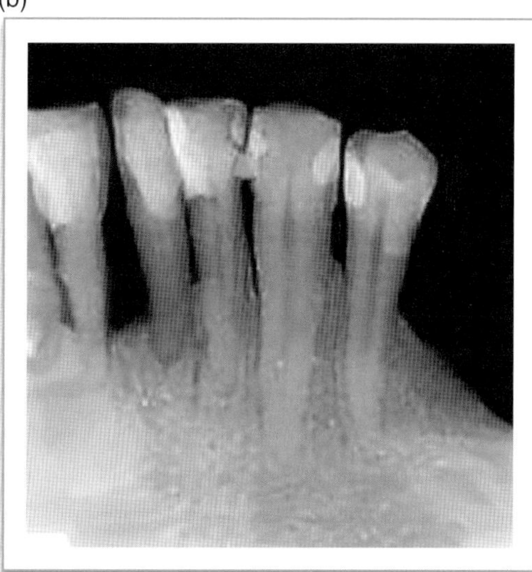

Figure 10.5.1 (a,b) Long cone periapical radiographs of lower anterior teeth showing advanced bone loss #31, #32, #41 and #42.

Structured Learning

1) The patient requests that you resplint his mobile lower teeth as he does not want them extracted. What would you advise?
   - There is generalised advanced bone loss, most advanced in relation to the lower incisors, with evidence of periapical infection of the lower central incisor teeth
   - Retaining these teeth poses a local and focal infection risk
   - Splinting may compromise adjacent teeth and will make cleaning and maintenance more problematic
   - Discuss with the patient his oral health priorities and tolerance for dental treatment given his recent period of ill health
   - If the patient is relatively stable, it is a good opportunity to undertake invasive dental treatment
2) Why is dental infection a particular concern for this patient?
   - Castleman disease: involves multiple regions of enlarged lymph nodes, flu-like symptoms, abnormal blood counts and dysfunction of vital organs due to uncontrolled infection with human herpes virus 8 (HHV-8), leading to excessive production of inflammatory cytokines
   - HIV positive: immunocompromised, i.e. CD4 glycoprotein found on the surface of immune cells, such as T helper cells, monocytes, macrophages and dendritic cells, is lower than normal range (500–1200 cells/µL)
   - Recent chemotherapy
   - Diabetes: poor mobilisation and phagocytosis of granulocytes, leucocyte adherence and bactericidal activity
   - Coronary stent: risk of focal infection of oral origin
3) What is the connection between multicentric Castleman disease (MCD) and HIV?
   - Persons with HIV are at increased risk of developing HHV-8-associated MCD
   - In some cases, MCD diagnosis may have led to HIV testing and subsequent positive diagnosis
4) Why is surveillance for oral cancer of particular importance in this patient?
   - Patients with HHV-8-associated MCD are at increased risk of developing Kaposi sarcoma and non-Hodgkin lymphoma which may present in the mouth
   - The risk is compounded by the associated HIV-positive diagnosis and recent immunosuppression with chemotherapy
5) The patient agrees to dental extraction of #41, #42, #31 and #32 but is concerned about bleeding excessively after the procedure. He reports that he did not stop bleeding for two days after the upper right canine (#13) spontaneously exfoliated one year ago. What could be contributing to his increased bleeding risk?
   - Local infection/inflamed tissue: the patient has active periodontal disease
   - Dual antiplatelet therapy

- Patients taking clopidogrel, dipyridamole, prasugrel or ticagrelor single or dual therapy (in combination with aspirin) may present with prolonged bleeding compared to aspirin monotherapy
- However, this is not clinically significant and can be controlled by local measures

- Medical comorbidities associated with increased bleeding risk
  - Arterial hypertension
  - HIV: immune-mediated thrombocytopenia
  - MCD: multiorgan involvement; possible impaired liver function
  - Chemotherapy: thrombocytopenia due to chemotherapy-induced pancytopenia

6) Would you discontinue the antiplatelet therapy to enable dental extractions?
   - No – do not interrupt antiplatelet therapy prior to dental treatment
   - The invasiveness of the proposed procedure, other medical conditions and the patient's other prescribed or non-prescribed medications should be assessed and the relevant physician consulted if there are additional concerns
   - There are no significant differences in the occurrence or degree of excessive blood loss between patients on single or dual antiplatelet therapy compared with control subjects
   - Discontinuation of antiplatelet therapy can increase the risk of a thromboembolic event if the drug is stopped prior to surgery
   - A thromboembolic event is significantly more consequential (e.g. a stent thrombosis is a catastrophic event) whereas bleeding from the mouth is usually manageable by local haemostatic measures
   - Given the relative ease with which the incidence and severity of oral bleeding can be reduced with local measures during surgery, and the unlikely occurrence of bleeding once an initial clot has formed, there is no indication to interrupt antiplatelet drugs for dental procedures

7) What additional factors do you need to consider in your risk assessment?
   - Social
     - Depression associated with multiple medical comorbidities
     - Impact of losing front teeth on social interaction and confidence
     - Limited social support to enable self- and oral care
     - Stigma and social discrimination experienced by many HIV-positive patients may potentially result in concerns about privacy and access to dental services
   - Medical (see Chapters 4.2, 5.1 and 12.2)
     - Potentially increased bleeding risk due to dual platelet therapy, HIV, MCD, chemotherapy
     - History of myocardial infarction
     - Blood pressure control
     - Comorbidity associated with type 2 diabetes mellitus (e.g. blood glucose control)
     - MCD organ involvement
     - Recent chemotherapy
     - HIV (e.g. opportunistic infection risk, sharps injury, possible drug- and immune-mediated thrombocytopenia)
   - Dental
     - Periodontal disease may be exacerbated in diabetes and HIV infection, and there is a possible association with cardiovascular disease

8) How would you plan the dental extractions?
   - As there is no immediate pain/infection concern, rebook for extraction of the lower central and lateral incisors and select an appointment that is early in the week and in the morning
   - Consider immediate denture construction if the patient has aesthetic concerns; may need to splint the teeth temporarily to reduce the risk of the teeth being inadvertently extracted in the impression material
   - Ensure design of the removal prosthesis is hygienic (due to pre-existing periodontal disease) and reduces trauma to the soft tissues (risk of bleeding)
   - Consider staging the dental extractions appointments (e.g. extracting two teeth at first appointment and two teeth at second appointment)
   - Will need to consider impact on the fitting of an immediate denture

General Dental Considerations

Oral Findings

- Petechiae
- Ecchymoses (Figure 10.5.2)
- Spontaneous gingival bleeding
- Prolonged bleeding after invasive dental procedures

Dental Management

- In general, the rule is not to interrupt antiplatelet therapy (Table 10.5.1)

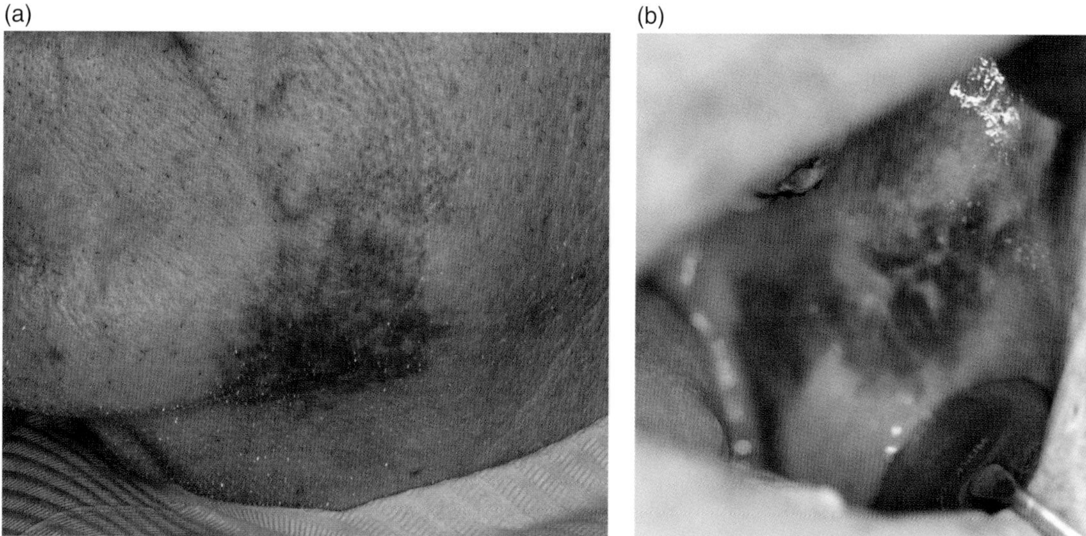

Figure 10.5.2 Ecchymoses associated with dental implant surgery.

Section II: Background Information and Guidelines

Definition

Antiplatelet drugs reversibly or irreversibly inhibit various steps in the platelet activation process, in order to interfere with platelet aggregation (primary haemostasis) (Figure 10.5.3). These are usually prescribed as either single or dual antiplatelet therapy.

Classification and Mechanisms of Action

(Tables 10.5.2 and 10.5.3)

- Cyclo-oxygenase (COX) inhibitors: irreversible inhibitor of COX-1 in platelets and megakaryocytes; subsequently blocks the formation of the potent vasoconstrictor and platelet aggregant thromboxane A2 (TXA2) (e.g. aspirin)
- Phosphodiesterase (PDE) inhibitors: inactivate cAMP (e.g. dipyridamole, cilostazol)
- Thienopyridines: indirect, irreversible ADP $P2Y_{12}$ receptor inhibitors (e.g. clopidogrel, prasugrel, ticlopidine)
- Cyclo-pentyltriazolo-pyrimidines: direct, reversible ADP $P2Y_{12}$ receptor inhibitors (e.g. ticagrelor, cangrelor)
- Glycoprotein (GP) IIb/IIIa receptor inhibitors: block final common pathway for platelet aggregation, preventing fibrinogen and von Willebrand factor from binding to receptors (e.g. abciximab, eptifibatide, tirofiban)
- Protease activated receptor (PAR)-1 inhibitors: inhibit platelet activation through alternative routes, including thrombin-mediated platelet aggregation (e.g. vorapaxar, atopaxar)
- Thienopyridines and cyclo-pentyltriazolo pyrimidines exhibit different mechanisms of action compared to aspirin; as such, these drugs increase aspirin's effects and are usually prescribed in dual therapy

Indications

- Coronary arteries: angina, acute coronary syndromes (ACS) including unstable angina and myocardial infarction
- Heart: atrial fibrillation, heart failure, coronary stent/percutaneous coronary intervention (PCI)
- Veins: venous thromboembolism (VTE)
- Brain: ischaemic stroke/cerebrovascular accident (CVA), transient ischaemic attack (TIA)
- Limbs: peripheral vascular disease (PVD), intermittent claudication

New antiplatelet agents

- For many years, the antiplatelet drugs aspirin and clopidogrel have been widely used to protect against the adverse clinical sequelae of thrombosis
- In recent years, the newer antiplatelet drugs (e.g. prasugrel and ticagrelor) have become increasingly available, providing alternatives for patients who have not responded appropriately to clopidogrel due to variability of the CYP450 enzyme, or those with high risk of ischaemic events
- They are more potent antiplatelet agents with a more rapid onset of action, more predictable absorption and improved efficacy for some outcomes
- As such, they are used in preference to clopidogrel in patients with low bleeding risk or non-ST elevated ACS
- However, clopidogrel remains first line in patients with high bleeding risk

Table 10.5.1 General dental management considerations.

Risk assessment	• Bleeding from surgery and trauma • Rarely of clinical significance and can be managed with local measures • Consider the required dental procedure, other medical conditions that may contribute to bleeding risk, and other prescribed and non-prescribed medications that may contribute to bleeding risk
Criteria for referral	• Dentists should be able to treat the vast majority of patients taking antiplatelet drugs in primary care • If other comorbidities or medications result in additional risks, seek advice from/refer to a more experienced colleague in primary or secondary dental care
Access/position	• Timing of treatment: in morning and early in week • Consider the need to stage invasive treatment to minimise bleeding risk
Communication	• The patient's bleeding history is often more helpful in determining the risk of bleeding • Consult medical practitioner or specialist if patient has other relevant medical complications/is taking other medications which may increase bleeding risk • If antiplatelet drug is prescribed as a time-limited course, consider delaying dental treatment where possible • Patients may independently stop their antiplatelet medication the day before treatment – they should be advised against this due to the risks of rebound coagulation • Furthermore, explain that missing one dose has no clinical benefit
Consent/capacity	• Warn patient of the increased risk of intraoral/postoperative bleeding, and intra/extraoral bruising • Inform the patient of the measures which will be used to reduce bleeding risk
Anaesthesia/ sedation	• Local anaesthesia – Delivered using an aspirating syringe and should include a vasoconstrictor, unless contraindicated – Anaesthetic solution should be delivered slowly to avoid rapid expansion of the soft tissues • Sedation – Intravenous sedation cannulation poses a risk of haematoma formation, though this is rare • General anaesthesia – Hazards of anaesthesia, especially nasal intubation and intramuscular injections
Dental treatment	• Before – Do not interrupt antiplatelet medication – Consider limiting initial treatment area (e.g. perform a single extraction or debride three teeth only initially, and assess bleeding before continuing) – For procedures with higher risk of postoperative bleeding, consider carrying out staged treatment • During – Lubricant/barrier cream used to protect the lips/soft tissue from trauma – Careful manipulation of the cheek and soft tissues – consider the use of gauze when using cheek retractors – Caution with suction to avoid trauma (reduce the volume) and take particular care to avoid trauma in the floor of mouth – Atraumatic extraction technique preferred – Minimal bone removal, teeth sectioned where possible – If a mucoperiosteal flap is required, a buccal approach is best since lingual tissue trauma may open up planes into which haemorrhage may track and endanger the airway – Local haemostatic measures to control bleeding – Bony wound compressed with absorbent gauze – Tranexamic acid 5% mouthwash may be used as an adjunct; this can be soaked in gauze and applied directly over the socket – Haemostatic packing agents: minimise usage to reduce incidence of dry socket; ensure agent of choice is acceptable to patient as some contain animal-based proteins – Suturing: use non-traumatic needle and small number of sutures • After – Extended monitoring – Careful oral cleansing postoperatively – Provide verbal and written postoperative instructions and emergency contact details

(*Continued*)

Table 10.5.1 (Continued)

Drug prescription	• Antiseptics as required (e.g. chlorhexidine rinses) • Antibiotics (e.g. amoxicillin, penicillin V, amoxicillin/clavulanic acid or metronidazole at therapeutic doses) as required • Pain relief (e.g. paracetamol) • Avoid aspirin, ibuprofen and diclofenac as these may increase bleeding risk
Education/ prevention	• Use of fluoride and fissure sealants, oral hygiene education, dietary advice and regular dental visits to minimise dental treatment that may cause bleeding complications

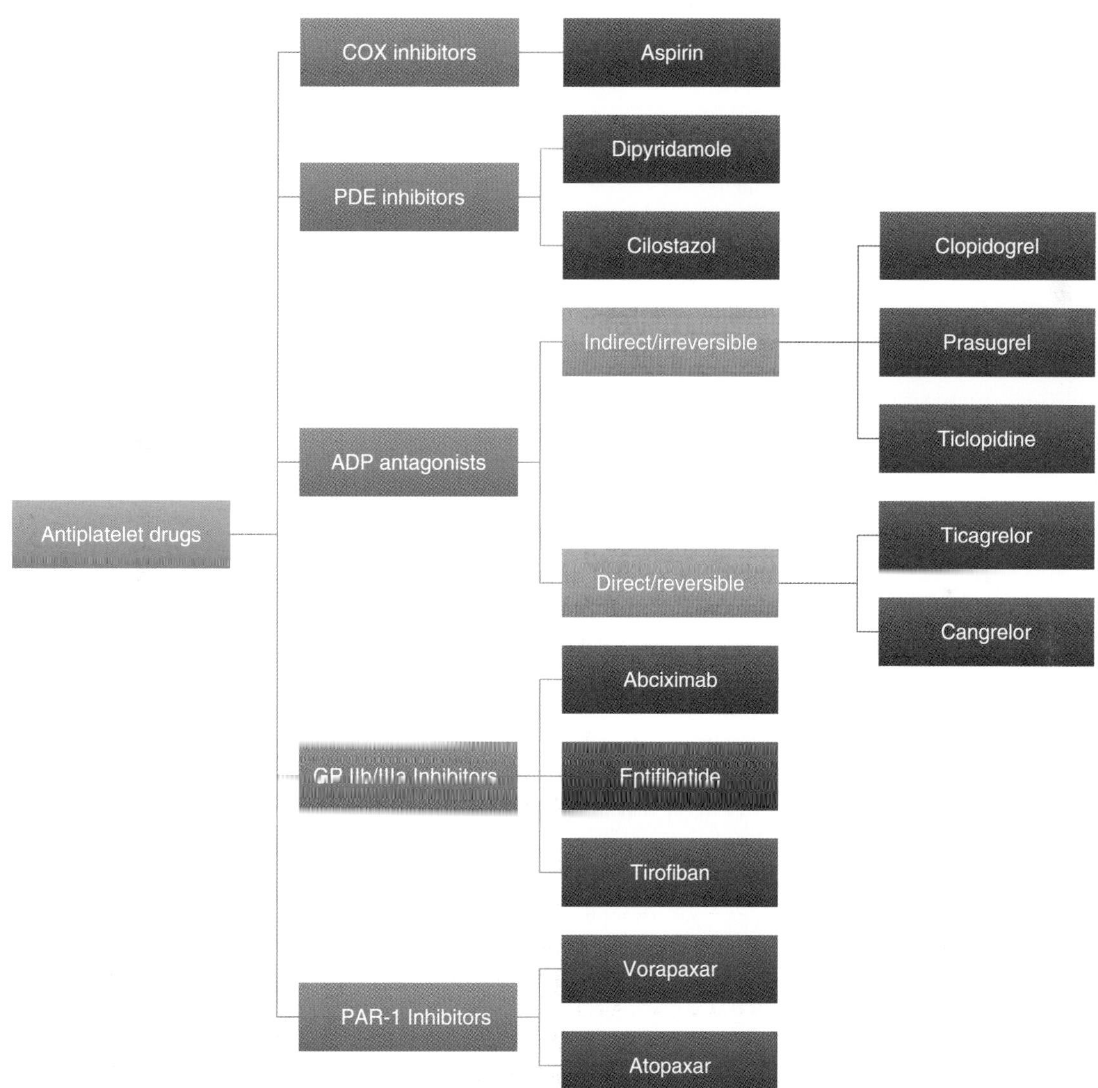

COX: cyclooxigenase; PDE: phosphodiesterase; ADP: adenosine diphosphate; GP: glycoprotein; PAR: protease-activated receptor

Figure 10.5.3 Most common types of antiplatelet drugs.

Table 10.5.2 Antiplatelet medications: drug characteristics.

	COX inhibitors	PDE inhibitors	Thienopyridines (ADP receptor inhibitors)		Cyclo-pentyl-triazolo-pyrimidines (ADP receptor inhibitors)
Drug	**Aspirin**	**Dipyridamole**	**Clopidogrel**	**Prasugrel**	**Ticagrelor**
Mechanism of action	COX-1 irreversible inhibition	Inactivates cAMP	ADP $P2Y_{12}$ receptor irreversible inhibition	ADP $P2Y_{12}$ receptor irreversible inhibition	ADP $P2Y_{12}$ (partly $P2Y_1$) receptor reversible inhibition
Indications	Prevention MI, TIA and CVA Stable angina	Heart valve replacement Prevention CVA combined with aspirin	Prevention and treatment ACS Prevention TIA, CVA and MI Treatment PVD Combined with aspirin following MI or PCI	Secondary prevention PCI and ACS	Prevention TIA and CVA Prevention or treatment ACS Secondary prevention PCI Treatment PVD
Peak plasma concentration	30–40 min	2 hours	1 hour	30 min	1.5 hours
Half-life of active metabolite	20 min	10–12 hours	8 hours	7 hours	7–9 hours
Platelet recovery after drug cessation	7–10 days (30% at 48 hours) Irreversible platelet effect	Reversible but alone has very little antiplatelet effect	7–10 days (40% at 3 days, functional recovery at 5 days) Irreversible platelet effect	7–10 days (functional recovery at 7 days) Irreversible platelet effect	5 days (50% at 24 hours, functional recovery at 2–3 days)
Adverse effects	GI bleeding (1–2/1000 per year) Haemorrhagic stroke (1/1000 per 3 years) GI toxicity Urticaria Hypersensitivity Bronchospasm Tinnitus Alopecia (rare)	GI bleeding GI ulceration Headache Flushing Urticaria Nausea Vomiting Dizziness	Bleeding Abdominal pain Diarrhoea Rash	Risk of intracranial bleeding Nausea Diarrhoea Rash	Bleeding Dyspnoea Bradycardia
Dose / frequency for long-term use	75–325 mg daily	200 mg dipyridamole +50 mg aspirin twice daily	75 mg daily	10 mg daily	90 mg twice daily

(Continued)

Table 10.5.2 (Continued)

	COX inhibitors	PDE inhibitors	Thienopyridines (ADP receptor inhibitors)		Cyclo-pentyl-triazolo-pyrimidines (ADP receptor inhibitors)
Drug	**Aspirin**	**Dipyridamole**	**Clopidogrel**	**Prasugrel**	**Ticagrelor**
Additional information	Antithrombotic effect lasts lifespan of platelet	Repeated dosing or slow-release preparations are required to inhibit platelet function for 24 hours Additional vasodilatory effect	Due to higher costs, reserved for those allergic to aspirin, recurrent atherothrombotic event whilst taking aspirin, or >20% per year absolute risk of serious vascular event	Irreversible effect on 60–70% of platelets (cf. clopidogrel 30%) Must balance stronger antiplatelet effect with increased haemorrhagic side-effects (>75 y, history of stroke/TIA, <60 kg weight)	Contraindicated in cardiac conduction defects Avoid concomitant use of CYP3A4 inhibitors or inducers (e.g. ketoconazole, clarithromycin)
Other antiplatelet drugs (not commonly seen in a dental setting)	Thienopyridines such as ticlopidine Cyclo-pentyl-triazolo-pyrimidines such as cangrelor Glycoprotein IIb/IIIa receptor inhibitors such as abciximab, tirofiban and eptifibatide PAR-1 inhibitors such as vorapaxar and atopaxar				

ACS, acute coronary syndrome; ADP, adenosine diphosphate; cAMP, cyclic adenosine monophosphate; COX, cyclooxygenase; CVA, cerebrovascular accident; GI, gastrointestinal; MI, myocardial infarction; PCI, percutaneous coronary intervention; PDE, phosphodiesterase; PVD, peripheral vessel disease; TIA, transient ischaemic attack.

Table 10.5.3 Indications for antiplatelet therapy.

Medical condition	Commonly used treatments	Treatment duration
• CVA and TIA, in absence of AF	Single or dual antiplatelets	Lifelong
• Stroke prevention, in patients with AF	Antiplatelet therapy is second line (patients intolerant to oral anticoagulants)	Lifelong
• Coronary heart disease – Stable angina – Acute coronary syndromes (unstable angina, MI)	Single antiplatelet, dual antiplatelet, oral anticoagulant, oral anticoagulant with single antiplatelet or heparin	Dual therapy for up to 12 months Single aspirin, warfarin or clopidogrel lifelong
• PHV replacement	Single antiplatelet (tissue valves), oral anticoagulant (mechanical valves)	Long-term
• PCI/coronary stent	Single or dual antiplatelets	Dual therapy for up to 12 months Monotherapy lifelong
• PVD	Single or dual antiplatelets	Lifelong
• Apical, ventricular or mural thrombus	Oral anticoagulant with dual antiplatelets if recent MI	6 months (reviewed after echocardiography)
• Pregnancy, with associated DVT risk factors	Aspirin (or heparin in some high-risk patients)	Until delivery

AF, atrial fibrillation; CVA, cerebrovascular accident; DVT, deep vein thrombosis; MI, myocardial infarction; PCI, percutaneous coronary intervention; PHV, prosthetic heart valve; PVD, peripheral vessel disease; TIA, transient ischaemic attack.

A World/Transcultural View

- Although the popularity of the newer antiplatelet drugs ticagrelor and prasugrel is increasing around the world, worldwide sales of clopidogrel remain higher than those of these new agents
- The treatment costs of aspirin are considerably less than clopidogrel, which in turn are considerably less than for ticagrelor and prasugrel
- Patient affordability across the world may impact on the use of newer antiplatelet drugs in countries where resources are limited and/or patients pay for their own medications

Recommended Reading

Cervino, G., Fiorillo, L., Monte, I.P. et al. (2019). Advances in antiplatelet therapy for dentofacial surgery patients: focus on past and present strategies. *Materials* 12: 1524.

Dézsi, B.B., Koritsánszky, L., Braunitzer, G. et al. (2015). Prasugrel versus clopidogrel: a comparative examination of local bleeding after dental extraction in patients receiving dual antiplatelet therapy. *J. Oral Maxillofac. Surg.* 73: 1894–1900.

Iqbal, A.M., Lopez, R.A., and Hai, O. (2020). Antiplatelet medications. www.ncbi.nlm.nih.gov/books/NBK537062

Napeñas, J.J., Oost, F.C.D., Degroot, A. et al. (2012). Review of postoperative bleeding risk in dental patients on antiplatelet therapy. *Oral Surg. Oral Med. Oral Pathol. Oral Radiol. Endod.* 115: 491–499.

Sáez-Alcaide, L.-M., Sola-Martín, C., Molinero-Mourelle, P. et al. (2017). Dental management in patients with antiplatelet therapy: a systematic review. *J Clin Exp Dent.* 9: e1044–e1050.

Schreuder, W.H. and Peacock, Z.S. (2015). Antiplatelet therapy and exodontia. *J. Am. Dent. Assoc.* 146: 851–856.

Scottish Dental Clinical Effectiveness Programme (2015). *Management of Dental Patients Taking Anticoagulants or Antiplatelet Drugs*. Dundee: SDCEP www.sdcep.org.uk/published-guidance/anticoagulants-and-antiplatelets.

Wahl, M.J. (2014). Dental surgery and antiplatelet agents: bleed or die. *Am. J. Med.* 127: 260–267.

11

Blood Dyscrasias

11.1 Thalassaemia

Section I: Clinical Scenario and Dental Considerations

Clinical Scenario

A 12-year-old girl presents to the dental clinic accompanied by her mother. The patient does not like the appearance of her teeth and feels that the shape of her face is changing.

Medical History

- Beta-thalassaemia major
- Splenomegaly

Medications

- Regular blood transfusion commenced 4 years ago when she moved countries due to her refugee status; prior to this only received transfusions intermittently
- Vitamin B supplementation
- Deferiprone – iron chelating agent

Dental History

- Irregular dental attender; attends only when in pain
- Stopped going due to problems with access and previous traumatic experience
- Often feels tired and forgets to brush her teeth

Social History

- Refugee – originally from Afghanistan; able to communicate in English
- Lives with her mother who does not speak English and relies on her daughter to translate
- Remaining family is in Afghanistan
- Attends school
- Diet includes high quantities of chocolate, biscuits and fizzy drinks

Oral Examination

- 'Chipmunk face' (prominent malar eminence), saddle nose, frontal bossing and anterior open bite (Figure 11.1.1)
- Lips – angular cheilitis
- Soft tissue – pale mucosa
- Gingivae – pale, plaque at cervical margins of teeth
- Hard tissue – maxillary bone expansion/protrusion
- Dentition – class II malocclusion (crowding), mixed dentition with mobility and caries in deciduous teeth (#53, #55, #63, #74, #75 and #84) (Figure 11.1.2)
- Partially erupted teeth #33 and #34

Radiological Examination

- Orthopantomogram undertaken (Figure 11.1.3)
- All teeth of the permanent dentition are present and developing
- Thin mandibular cortex
- Maxillary sinus pneumatisation

Structured Learning

1) How may the presence of a splenomegaly affect how you manage this patient?
   - Progressive splenomegaly may be associated with significant debilitating symptoms including:
     - Early satiety due to pressure on the stomach
     - Abdominal pain, predominantly in the left upper abdomen that may spread to the left shoulder
     - Inactivity and fatigue
     - Portal hypertension
     - Progression of cytopenias due to splenic sequestration may result in more frequent infections, anaemia and increased bleeding
   - In view of these factors, consider:
     - Avoiding a fully supine position if there is abdominal pain
     - Limiting the appointment length due to fatigue
     - Checking the results of a recent full blood count test due to potential cytopenias

A Practical Approach to Special Care in Dentistry, First Edition. Edited by Pedro Diz Dios and Navdeep Kumar.

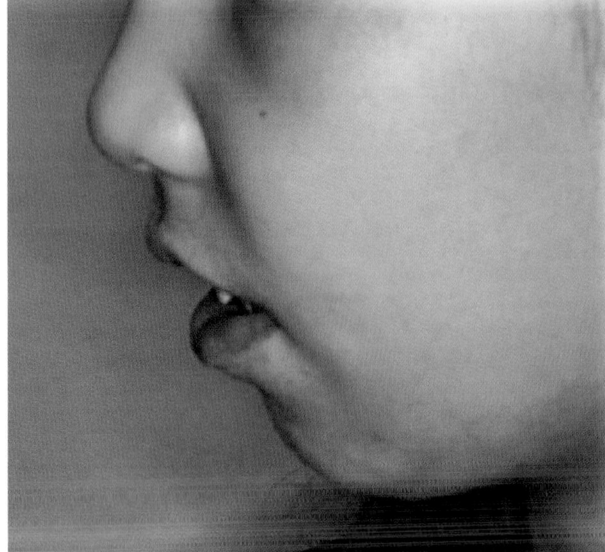

Figure 11.1.1 Lateral view of the face showing malar prominence and anterior open bite.

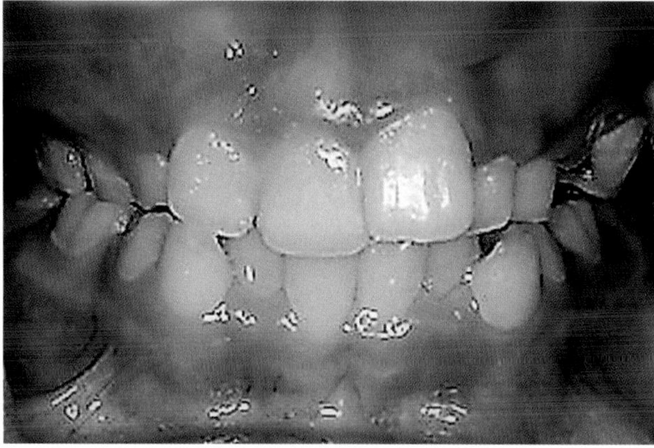

Figure 11.1.2 Mixed dentition with generalised crowding and pale gingivae.

2) What would you need to consider in relation to the regular blood transfusions?
   - Avoid invasive dental care on the same day as the transfusion
     - Transfusions make take up to 4 hours to administer and the patient is often tired
     - The patient may experience side-effects from transfusion, including fever, allergy and more acute reactions such as haemolysis
   - Dental treatment should be planned for the week following a blood transfusion as this will ensure that the patient's blood counts are optimal
   - Determine the presence and extent of transfusion-related iron overload complications and implement precautions as required
3) What factors could be contributing to the patient's perception that her teeth and face are changing in appearance?
   - Thalassaemia-associated changes in the orofacial tissues may be observed in more severe forms of beta-thalassaemia – this patient has the most severe form, namely 'major'
   - These changes are also more likely to present when regular blood transfusions are not given at an early age, as is the case for this patient
   - Many of these are related to expansion of the marrow cavity due to compensatory hyperplasia of bone marrow (extramedullary haematopoiesis)
   - The hyperplasia of bone marrow in the maxilla exceeds that of the mandible, and results in a characteristic appearance known as 'chipmunk face' (Figures 11.1.1 and 11.1.4); this may be associated with spacing of the upper teeth, forward drift of the maxillary incisors and increased overjet

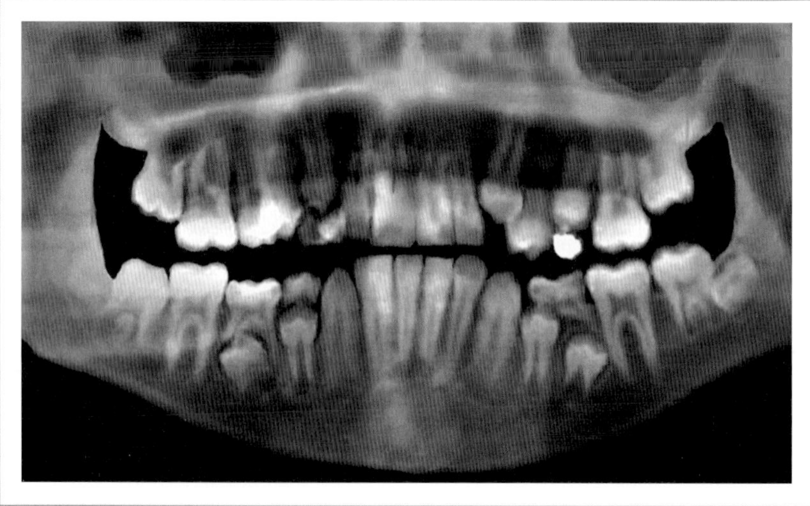

Figure 11.1.3 Orthopantomogram demonstrating mixed dentition, thin mandibular cortex and maxillary sinus pneumatisation.

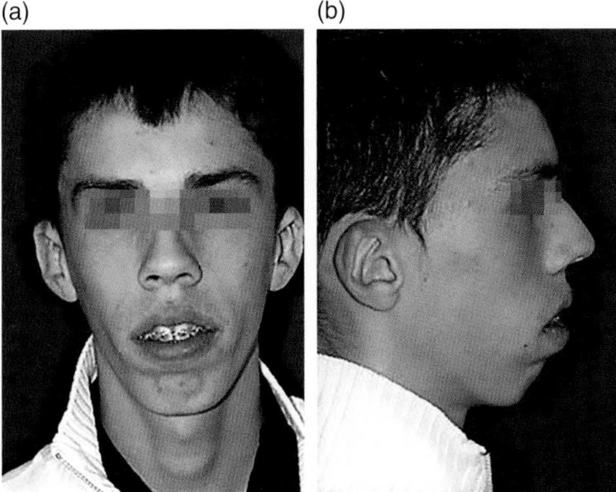

Figure 11.1.4 (a,b) Facial features: frontal bossing, 'chipmunk face', class II malocclusion.

- The patient is also in the mixed dentition stage and undergoing puberty which may also impact on the change in her facial and dental profile

4) What risk factors does this patient have for the development of angular cheilitis?
   - Angular cheilitis is an inflammation at the corners of the mouth, typically caused by infection (bacterial and/or fungal), irritation and/or allergies
   - Risk factors for this patient include:
     - Underlying anaemia due to thalassaemia/splenomegaly
     - Increased risk of infection related to cytopenia caused by splenomegaly
     - Anterior open bite and pronounced Class II skeletal base, resulting in saliva leakage in the corners of the mouth
5) When you discuss the patient's poor dental health with the patient and her mother, they both state that the teeth have deteriorated as they are 'weak' due to the thalassaemia. Are they correct?
   - Tooth deformities (taurodontism) and spacing of teeth may occur in relation to thalassaemia; however, the tooth structure itself is not at more risk of developing dental caries
   - It has been noted that the saliva in patients with thalassaemia contains less phosphorus and IgA, and hence may be less protective
   - Increased dental caries risk is more likely to be due to compliance issues, poor dental attendance, poor oral hygiene and highly cariogenic diet, tendency to eat small amounts of food but frequently (due to splenomegaly)
6) What factors do you need to consider in your risk assessment when planning dental care for this patient?
   - Social
     - Dependent on parents to attend
     - Mother unable to speak English – translator required as it is not appropriate for her daughter to translate for her
     - Past traumatic dental experience
     - Poor self-esteem due to concerns about her facial appearance
     - Potential economic constraints (refugee status)
   - Medical
     - Regular blood transfusions
     - Anaemia
     - Increased risk of bleeding due to hypervascularity of bone (extramedullary haematopoiesis)
     - Risk of blood-borne virus spread
     - Risk of infection (sequestration of cells due to splenomegaly)
   - Dental
     - Past traumatic dental experience
     - Mixed dentition and crowding, may need orthodontic consultation
     - Angular cheilitis – care should be taken not to irritate the fissures
     - Highly cariogenic diet
     - Poor dental attendance
7) The patient asks if there is an operation that she can have to improve her facial appearance by making her top jaw smaller. What would you advise her?
   - Surgical correction of the facial profile may not be stable, particularly as the patient is still growing
   - There is also a significant risk associated with surgical approaches and the maxillary bone in particular is hypervascular (risk of extensive bleeding)
   - The focus should be on preventive approaches and stabilisation of oral health
   - Orthodontic treatment can be initiated as early as possible, once this has been achieved
   - Correction of drifted maxillary anterior teeth and increased overjet should be undertaken to improve aesthetics, reduce susceptibility to trauma, avoid gingival inflammation and improve functional ability

General Dental Considerations

Oral Findings

- Oral manifestations are classified into radiographic changes, skeletal changes and oral changes (Table 11.1.1)

Dental Management

- Dental treatment modifications depend on the type and severity of the patient's thalassaemia (Table 11.1.2)
- Treatment should be modified based on reassessment of the patient on the day of the appointment

Table 11.1.1 Facial features and oral manifestations of thalassaemia.

Type of change	Explanation
Radiographic changes	• Hair-on-end appearance on lateral skull radiographs due to expansion of diploë of skull • Alveolar bone rarefaction produces chicken-wire appearance on radiography due to marrow expansion • Pneumatisation of sinuses is due to the hyperplasia of marrow in frontal, temporal and facial bones
Skeletal changes	• Class II malocclusions (including skeletal and dental features such as increased overjet, maxillary protrusion and anterior open bite) due to bone marrow expansion and mandibular atrophy • Lateral displacement of the orbits due to marrow overgrowth in maxillary bone • 'Chipmunk' face due to malar prominence, saddle nose and frontal bossing • Thin mandibular cortex due to marrow expansion • Brodie syndrome – mandibular arch is telescoped within maxillary arch
Oral changes	• Dental caries due to poor oral hygiene, less phosphorus and IgA in saliva • Mucosal pallor, atrophic glossitis due to decreased haemoglobin • Severe periodontitis if splenectomy performed • Dark gingivae due to high ferritin levels • Generalised tooth spacing due to expansion of marrow • Tooth deformities including short spike-shaped roots, taurodontism and attenuated lamina dura due to growth retardation • Incorporation of bilirubin – a product of haemoglobin breakdown – in the dentinal tubules resulting in yellow discoloration of teeth • Oral ulceration due to chronic anaemia • Necrotising stomatitis which may be linked to agranulocytosis due to iron chelating drugs (deferiprone) • Less commonly: painful swelling of parotids, hyposalivation caused by iron deposition, sore/burning tongue related to folate deficiency

Section II: Background Information and Guidelines

Definition

Thalassaemias are a group of genetically inherited disorders characterised by the reduced synthesis of a globin chain required for the synthesis of haemoglobin (Hb). The most common of these is a reduction in the alpha (alpha-thalassaemia) or beta (beta-thalassaemia) globin chain of the Hb molecule. This leads to production of abnormal Hb production (haemoglobinopathy).

Beta-thalassaemia is prevalent in areas around the Mediterranean, in the Middle East, in Central, South and South-East Asia and in southern China, whereas alpha-thalassaemia is prevalent in South-East Asia, Africa and India. It is estimated that worldwide, 1.5% (80–90 million people) are carriers of beta-thalassaemia and 5% are carriers of alpha-thalassaemia. The high prevalence of alpha- and beta-thalassaemia genotypes in communities with endemic *Plasmodium falciparum* malaria has led to a theory that the thalassaemia gene mutations represent a mechanism of evolutionary protection.

Aetiopathogenesis

- Synthesis of the globin chains required for haemoglobin production is controlled by:
  - Two genes on chromosome 16, namely HBA1 and HBA2, encoding the alpha globins
  - Five genes located on a short region of chromosome 11 encoding the gamma, delta and beta globins
- These clusters are expressed during development to produce different Hb tetramers
  - Foetal haemoglobin: HbF – α2-gamma-2; the role of HbF is to transport oxygen efficiently in a low oxygen environment with levels normally decreasing sharply after birth
  - Adult haemoglobin: HbA – α2-beta-2 and HbA2 – α2-delta-2; over 95% of the haemoglobin in normal red blood cells is adult HbA, with the remaining haemoglobin consisting of 2 minor components, HbA2 and HbF
- In thalassaemia, there is typically an autosomal recessive inheritance of a variant of either the alpha- or beta-globin loci, leading to reduction in HBA levels and significantly increased HbA2 and HbF
- Alpha-thalassaemia: missing alpha chains
  - Typically results from deletions involving the HBA1 and HBA2 genes

Table 11.1.2 Considerations for dental management considerations.

Risk assessment	• Chronic anaemia with associated symptoms • Multiple immune abnormalities, including defective neutrophils and macrophage chemotaxis, have been described • Increased risk of cytopenias if there is significant splenomegaly • Infection associated with splenectomy • Complications of iron overload (e.g. diabetes) • Risk of medication-related osteonecrosis of the jaw in patients under antiresorptive drugs • Change in appearance of the orofacial tissues and teeth • Chronic depression • HBV/HCV/HIV carriage may be complications in repeatedly transfused older patients
Criteria for referral	• Dentists should be able to treat the vast majority of patients, who do not exhibit severe clinical features, in primary care • If necessary, seek advice from/refer to a more experienced colleague in primary or secondary dental care if the patient requires regular blood transfusion, has had a splenectomy and/or exhibits other complications or clinical features
Access/position	• The timing and location of dental treatment need to be considered for blood transfusions • Patients with advanced osteoporosis may have reduced mobility and require assistance/an escort • If there is significant splenomegaly, avoid a fully supine position • Access to the oral cavity may be limited by changes in the mandible and maxilla
Communication	• Consider communication with haematologist for blood transfusion timing
Capacity	• Consider patient's psychological status as some may need support
Anaesthesia/sedation	• Local anaesthesia – Generally safe – Theoretical risk associated with local anaesthetic containing adrenaline if there is associated cardiac disease – Anatomy may be altered for block injections • Sedation – Should be used with caution especially with severe anaemia and risk of respiration depression – Inhalation sedation is safer than intravenous; should be given with oxygen levels not <30% • General anaesthesia – Induction may be complicated by enlargement of maxilla creating intubation difficulties – Chronic severe anaemia and often cardiomyopathy are contraindications
Dental treatment	• Before – Haemoglobin essay/complete blood count should be determined to check the need for blood products and prophylactic antibiotic therapy – Check the need for oxygen supplementation by taking oxygen/pulse oximeter reading – Consider secondary endocrine disorders such as diabetes – check blood glucose – Care should be taken when extracting teeth for patients on antiresorptive medication – Record and monitor any radiographic changes – Orthodontic treatment may be required to correct malocclusion (Figure 11.1.4)

(Continued)

Table 11.1.2 (Continued)

	• During – Lubricant/barrier cream used to protect the lips/soft tissue for trauma – Careful manipulation of the cheek and soft tissues – consider the use of gauze when using cheek retractors – Caution with suction to avoid trauma (reduce the volume) – Atraumatic extraction technique must be used, starting with the simplest extraction to assess the bleeding – Use local haemostatic measures to control bleeding (sutures and haemostatic packs) – Consider local adjuvant use of tranexamic acid 5% if bleeding prolonged • After – Give the patient written postoperative instruction and emergency contact details – Review in 1 week after an invasive dental procedure
Drug prescription	• Drug metabolism/interaction: avoid tetracycline, erythromycin and metronidazole, aspirin/non-steroidal anti-inflammatory drugs; best use paracetamol • Avoid aspirin/non-steroidal anti-inflammatory drugs as they may increase gastric bleeding, thereby worsening anaemia • Consider that the patient may already be on prophylactic antibiotics if they have had a splenectomy – consider dose
Education	• Reinforce meticulous oral hygiene and regular dental visits to prevent caries, periodontal disease and need for future extractions • Inform patients about the oral features and side effects of antiresorptive drugs

 - Four main variants: haemoglobin Bart's hydrops fetalis, HbH disease, alpha-thalassaemia trait and alpha-thalassaemia silent carriers
- Beta-thalassaemia: missing beta chains
  - Over 200 mutations in the beta-globin gene on chromosome 11 have been recognised as linked to the disease
  - Hence beta-thalassaemia can be very variable in presentation and is typically categorised as minor, major or intermedia on the basis of the beta-globin chain imbalance, severity of anaemia and clinical picture at presentation

Clinical Presentation

- Symptoms depend on the type of thalassaemia and can vary from no symptoms to severe manifestations (Table 11.1.3)
- When symptoms are present, these are associated with the presence of chronic haemolytic anaemia, increased infection risk (splenectomy), excess iron accumulation (hemosiderosis) from high gut absorption and repeated blood transfusions, and osteopenia/osteoporosis
- Iron deposits also cause pulmonary hypertension, hepatosplenomegaly, liver cirrhosis/failure, renal failure and/or diabetes
- Depression in relation to lifelong adherence to a complicated medical regimen

Diagnosis

- Diagnosis is made by a combination of clinical findings and specific tests
- Symptoms of haemolytic anaemia, namely paleness and hepatosplenomegaly directly from birth in alpha-thalassaemia or from several months after birth in beta-thalassaemia, indicate a severe form of the disease
- The key sign of minor, intermediate or major thalassaemia is microcytic, hypochromic red blood cells (mean corpuscular volume <70 fL), not responding to iron supplementation
- First-line tests therefore include:
  - Full blood count, including mean corpuscular volume (MCV)
  - Mean corpuscular haemoglobin (MCH)
  - Mean corpuscular haemoglobin concentration (MCHC)
- Second-line tests include:
  - Haemoglobin (Hb) assay
  - Serum iron and ferritin
  - Red cell folate assays
  - Haemoglobin electrophoresis

Table 11.1.3 Clinical presentation of thalassaemia.

Types of thalassaemia	Subtypes	Clinical features
Alpha-thalassaemia	Hb Bart's hydrops fetalis	• Accumulation of excess fluid in the body before birth • Severe anaemia • Hepatosplenomegaly • Heart defects • Abnormalities of the urinary system
	HbH disease	• Mild to moderate anaemia • Hepatosplenomegaly • Jaundice
	Alpha-thalassaemia trait/carriers	• Generally asymptomatic or associated with hypochromic anaemia
Beta-thalassaemia	Beta-thalassaemia major	• Pallor, feeding problems, irritability and hepatosplenomegaly from 3 months of age • If untreated in children: – Severe haemolytic anaemia – Growth retardation – Poor muscular development – Short deviated legs – Pathological fractures – Frontal bossing – Maxillary prominence – Iron overload most importantly in the liver and heart • Chronic anaemia-related complications including cardiomyopathy • Hepatosplenomegaly • Diabetes • Osteoporosis
	Beta-thalassaemia intermedia	• Bone marrow hyperplasia and splenomegaly • Increase of gastrointestinal iron absorption may result in non-transfusional iron overload in the liver but not in the heart
	Beta-thalassaemia minor	• Asymptomatic • Physiological challenge, such as pregnancy, may result in symptoms

Treatment

- Prevention of thalassaemia is focused on raising public awareness of the disease, detection of carriers, genetic counselling and prenatal testing
- Treatment regimens for the management of thalassaemia depend on the type and severity of the disorder
- Asymptomatic carriers do not require specific treatment other than iron supplementation if there is microcytosis
- Patients with beta-thalassaemia intermedia or HbH disease need to be closely monitored for progression of complications induced by chronic haemolytic anaemia; intermittent blood transfusion may be required during periods of rapid growth, infection-associated aplastic or hyperhaemolytic crises and pregnancy
- Beta-thalassaemia major is managed by:
  - Regular blood transfusion (typically every 3 weeks) to maintain a haemoglobin level higher than 9.5 g/dL; the greatest challenge is secondary iron overload with its associated multiorgan morbidity
  - Iron chelation to prevent overload syndrome (chelating agents)
    - Deferoxamine, deferiprone, deferasirox
    - Side-effects include agranulocytosis, hepatitis, renal failure, gastrointestinal bleeding
- Additional management strategies include:
  - Folic acid supplements
  - Ascorbic acid
  - Recombinant erythropoietin/hydroxyurea

  - Splenectomy if hypersplenism is present (with improved drugs and regular transfusion programmes, splenectomies are no longer routinely undertaken)
  - Prophylactic antibiotic therapy after splenectomy
  - Antiresorptive medications if there is significant osteoporosis
  - Management of secondary comorbidities in relation to iron overload
- The only potential cure at the present time is haematopoietic stem cell transplantation; this is undertaken predominantly in selected patients with transfusion-dependent beta-thalassaemia, with outcomes better if it is undertaken at an earlier age

Prognosis

- Hb Bart's hydrops fetalis results in stillborn births/death soon after birth
- Patients with mild thalassaemia can expect a normal life expectancy
- If beta-thalassaemia major is not managed appropriately at an early age with supportive treatment and blood transfusions, life expectancy is less than 5–10 years, with death usually due to cardiac failure
- Survival data derived from large cohort studies have shown that patients undergoing regular transfusion but not chelation can be expected to reach 10–25 years of age, dying of cardiac iron overload
- Patients receiving optimal transfusion and chelation from an early age have a substantially increased survival of more than 40 years
- Bone marrow transplantation may result in complete resolution of the disease

A World/Transcultural View

- Thalassaemia is the world's most common group of hereditary haemolytic diseases
- Although it is mostly prevalent in Asia, India and the Middle East, increasing migration of populations across the world has resulted in increasing prevalence in countries where these diseases are not endemic
- The treatment of thalassaemia major and intermedia has traditionally depended on preventing undesirable outcomes of disease, using transfusion therapy along with iron chelation; however, regular access to these treatments is not uniformly available across the world
- As the world economy improves and the overall infant mortality rate falls, thalassaemia is rapidly emerging as a major economic and health burden in developed and developing countries, since infants with thalassaemia, who would otherwise have died from infection and malnutrition, now survive and require lifelong treatment

Recommended Reading

Elny, S., Ben-Barak, A., Kridin, K., and Aizenbud, D. (2020). Craniofacial deformities in patients with beta-thalassemia: orthodontic versus surgical correction – a systematic review. *J. Pediatr. Hematol. Oncol.* 42: 198–203.

Helmi, N., Bashir, M., Shireen, A., and Mirza Ahmed, I. (2017). Thalassemia review: features, dental considerations and management. *Electron. Physician* 9: 4003–4008.

Kalbassi, S., Younesi, M.R., and Asgary, V. (2018). Comparative evaluation of oral and dento-maxillofacial manifestation of patients with sickle cell diseases and beta thalassemia major. *Hematology* 23: 373–378.

Kumar, N., Hattab, F.N., and Porter, J. (2014). Dental care. *In Guidelines for the Management of Transfusion Dependent Thalassaemia* (TDT). Cappellini, M., Cohen, A., and Porter, J., et al. (eds). 3. Nicosia: Thalassaemia International Federation. www.ncbi.nlm.nih.gov/books/NBK269382/

Movahhedian, N., Akbarizadeh, F., Khojastepour, L. et al. (2020). Assessment of mandibular characteristics in patients affected with beta-thalassaemia major: a retrospective case–control study. *Int. Orthod.* 18: 776–783.

Mulimani, P., Abas, A.B., Karanth, L. et al. (2019). Treatment of dental and orthodontic complications in thalassaemia. *Cochrane Database Syst. Rev.* 8: CD012969.

Ohri, N., Khan, M., Gupta, N. et al. (2015). A study on the radiographic features of jaws and teeth in patients with thalassemia major using orthopantomograph. *J. Indian Acad. Oral Med. Radiol.* 27: 343–348.

Taher, A.T., Weatherall, D.J., and Cappellini, M.D. (2018). Thalassaemia. *Lancet* 391: 155–167.

11.2 Sickle Cell Anaemia

Section I: Clinical Scenario and Dental Considerations

Clinical Scenario

A 25-year-old female presents for an emergency dental appointment following an accidental fall the night before which has resulted in trauma to the lower lip and maxillary anterior teeth. The patient is experiencing acute pain from her traumatised front teeth, making it impossible to eat and drink, with associated bleeding from the adjacent gingivae.

Medical History
- Sickle cell anaemia
  - Blood transfusions intermittently as required; last transfusion 6 months ago
  - Last acute crisis 12 months ago, triggered by cold weather and flu episode
  - Autosplenectomy (spontaneous infarction of the spleen with resulting hyposplenism)
- Mild learning disability – no challenging behaviour
- Mild dental anxiety

Medications
- Folic acid supplement
- Penicillin V

Dental History
- Irregular dental attender; attends only when in pain
- Stopped going due to problems with access and mild dental anxiety
- Brushes her teeth once every other day
- Poor dietary habits (snacks on biscuits and cakes in between meals)
- Previous history of tooth fracture when the patient was young – mother does not recall exact age or date this occurred
- History of periodontal disease

Social History
- Lives at home with her parents and siblings
- Eldest of 6 children
- She is the only one in her family with a learning disability and sickle cell disease – the remaining family members have sickle cell trait
- Attends special education school
- Attends appointments with mother who is also her primary carer

Oral Examination
- Lips
  - Upper lip dry and crusted
  - Lower lip also dry and crusted; mild labial swelling and a traumatic lesion intraorally (Figure 11.2.1)
- Gingiva
  - Generalised plaque, inflammation and oedema
  - Localised bleeding and inflammation associated with both upper lateral and central incisors
- Teeth
  - Grade I mobility and crown fracture of #11; tooth discoloured (Figure 11.2.2)
  - Grade II mobility, buccally displaced, partially extruded #22
  - Crown fracture of #21
  - Localised tooth surface loss on the posterior teeth consistent with attrition and erosion
  - Generalised staining

Radiological Examination
- Limited cooperation/movement impacting on the quality of the images
- Orthopantomogram, upper occlusal and long cone periapical radiographs undertaken of the anterior teeth (Figure 11.2.3)
- Increased periodontal space apically associated with #22
- Radiolucent periapical lesion associated with both the teeth # 11 and #12
- Open apex #11

A Practical Approach to Special Care in Dentistry, First Edition. Edited by Pedro Diz Dios and Navdeep Kumar.

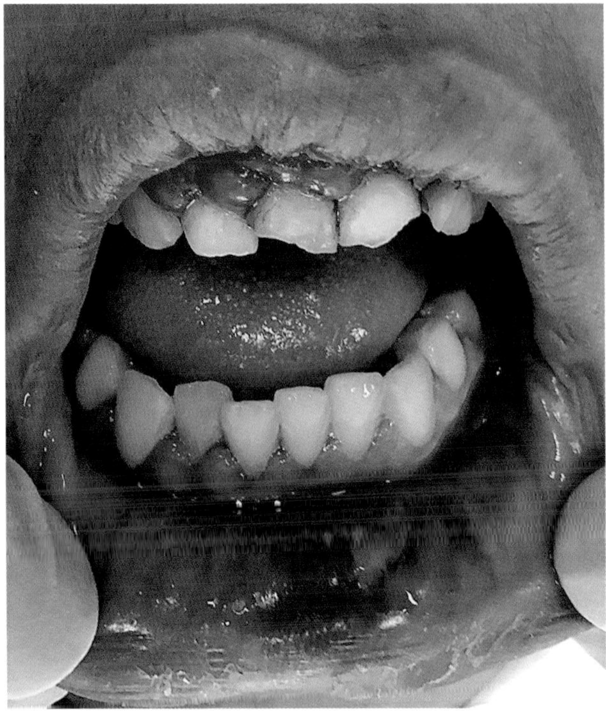

Figure 11.2.1 Lower lip trauma lesion.

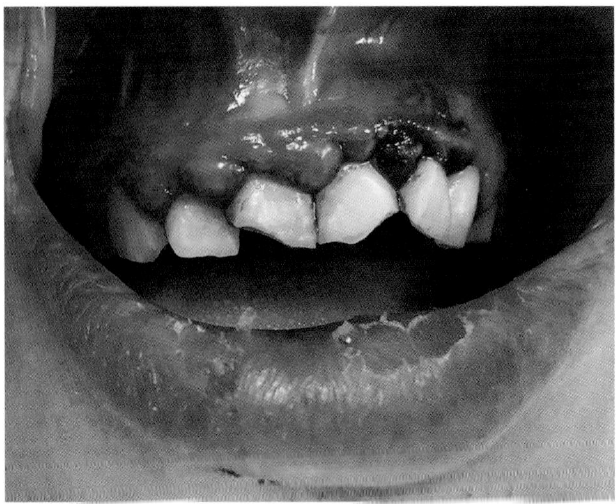

Figure 11.2.2 Fractured crowns #11 and #21, extruded tooth # 21, localised inflammation and bleeding associated with these teeth, lip dryness and crusting.

- Lower lip radiograph is clear from any foreign body/ tooth fragments (Figure 11.2.4)

Structured Learning

1) Why is it particularly urgent to treat this patient's presenting dental complaint?
   - There is a significant risk of dental pain, infection, dehydration and distress triggering a sickle cell crisis
   - This risk may be compounded by the patient's dental anxiety and her learning disability
2) Following a tell–show–do approach, the patient allows you to examine her mouth more thoroughly and consents to emergency management of the dental and lip trauma. What steps would you take?
   - Pain control: ensure that the patient has a supply of analgesics and starts taking this regularly at an appropriate dose; supplement with local anaesthesia in the region of the traumatised teeth to allow stabilisation
   - Infection control: confirm that there are no foreign bodies in the tissue; clean the traumatised lip, gingivae and teeth; consider prescribing antibiotics
   - Dental trauma treatment (Figure 11.2.5)
     - Avulsion treatment: reposition #12 and stabilise the tooth for 2 weeks with a flexible splint
     - Enamel-dentine fracture treatment: tooth fragment can be bonded to the tooth; alternatively, cover any exposed dentine with an adhesive restoration

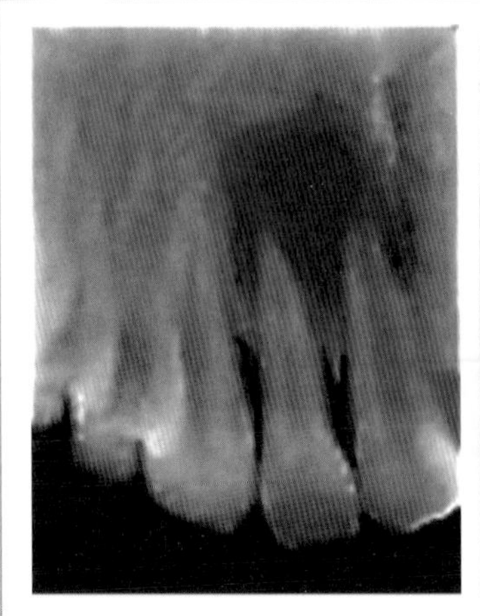
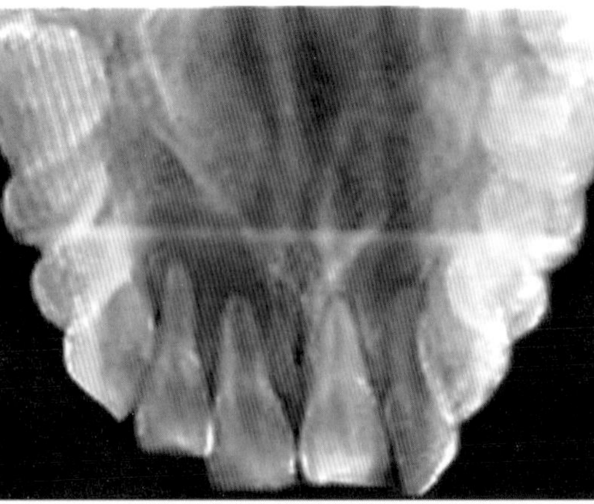
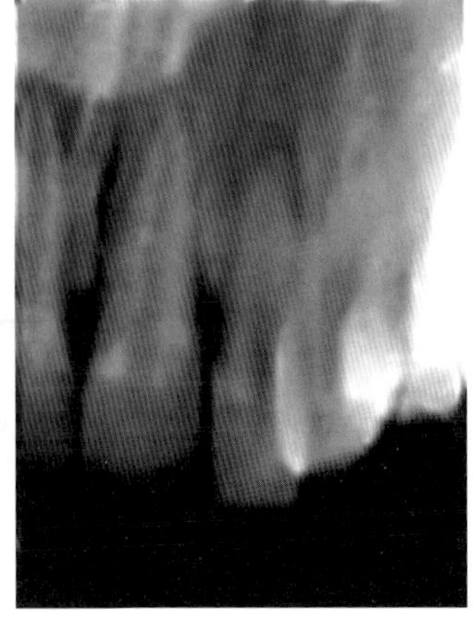

Figure 11.2.3 Upper right and left periapical and upper occlusal radiographs of the teeth involved in trauma.

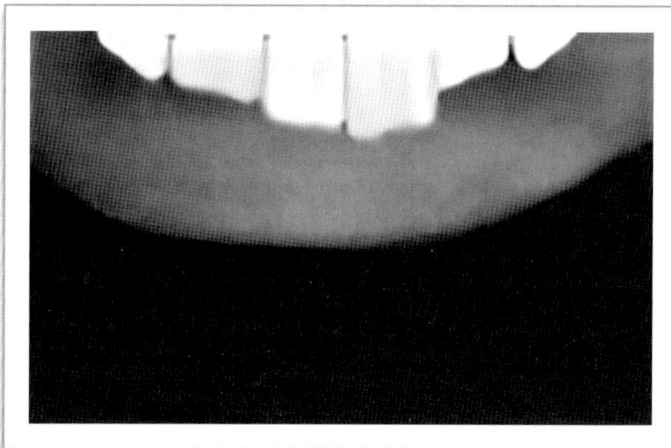

Figure 11.2.4 Lower lip radiograph: no foreign body/tooth fragments.

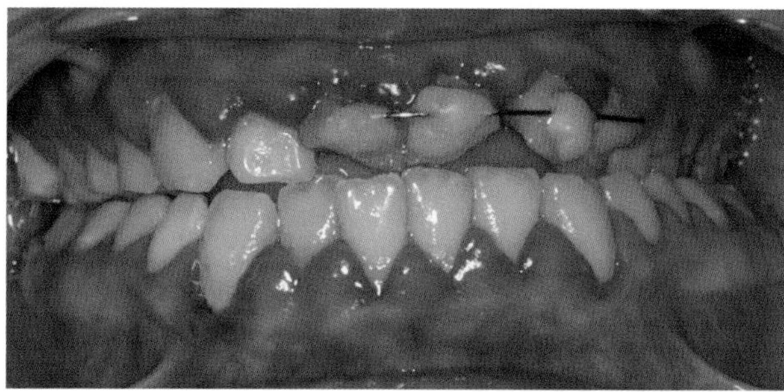

Figure 11.2.5 Splinting of teeth #11–23 with wire and composite splint.

  - For the exposed dentine, placement of calcium hydroxide base and coverage with a glass ionomer is advisable
  - Enamel-dentine-pulp fracture treatment: pulp capping or partial pulpotomy in young patients; root canal treatment in patients with mature apical development, but pulp capping or partial pulpotomy may also be considered

3) What factors do you need to consider in your risk assessment?
   - Social
     - Assessment of capacity in relation to the dental treatment proposed
     - Appropriate communication to ensure that the information is provided in a way that is suitable for the patient
     - Reliant on mother to attend appointments
     - Mild dental phobia
   - Medical
     - Increased risk of a further sickle cell crisis
     - Infection risk due to autosplenectomy
     - Hypoxia risk
   - Dental
     - Poor oral hygiene
     - Previous history of dental trauma
     - Poor dental attendance
     - Cariogenic diet and frequent snacks
4) At the patient's review appointment 10 days later, the pain, swelling and acute infection have resolved. After undertaking vitality testing and confirming that the #11 and #12 are non-vital, you discuss root canal treatment. The patient becomes distressed and states that she cannot cope with this and wants to be sedated. What would you consider?
   - Sickle cell anaemia is a significant risk factor for sedation
   - Intravenous sedation must be used very cautiously because respiratory suppression leads to hypoxia and acidosis, which may precipitate an acute sickle crisis
   - If sedation is being considered, dental care should be delivered in a hospital dental department
   - Consider sedation by an anaesthetist rather than a dental sedationist
5) Further dental treatment under sedation is arranged in a hospital-based dental clinic. What additional steps should be undertaken prior to proceeding with dental treatment?
   - Close liaison with the haematology team is required and any preprocedure interventions must be discussed with them in advance
   - Recent haemoglobin assay/full blood count results are needed
   - Haemoglobin levels should be above 100 g/L
   - Confirmation is required whether an exchange blood transfusion is required before proceeding
   - Ensure that the patient is escorted and that the haematology team are available in case the patient becomes unwell during treatment
   - Perioperative nasal oxygen should be available
   - Pulse oximeter to monitor oxygen saturation
   - Prophylactic antibiotic may be considered
   - Infections that may arise following the trauma need to be treated thoroughly to avoid crises

6) Following stabilisation of the anterior teeth within the hospital-based dental clinic, the patient returns to you for long-term care. What would be your areas of focus?
   - Good oral hygiene and preventive care are very important, because oral infection can lead to a sickle cell crisis and/or osteomyelitis
   - Hence it is important to discuss this with the patient and her family and ensure that the patient receives regular dental care to facilitate preventive measures

such as oral hygiene instructions, diet control and fluoride prescription/applications
- This will also limit the need for invasive dental procedures
- Behaviour management techniques to acclimatise patient to dental treatment without sedation would also be beneficial

General Dental Considerations

Oral Findings

- Many orofacial features have been described but the extent of these findings seen in patients is variable
- Occasionally compensatory hyperplasia and expansion of the bone marrow, including the facial bones, may occur, leading to depression of the nasal bridge, midfacial overgrowth resulting in maxillary protrusion and an increase in the vertical dimension
- There is no direct aetiological link associated with the sickle cell disease process and an increased risk of periodontal disease or dental caries; however, it is known that regular dental attendance in this cohort of patients may be lower, resulting in poorer oral health status
- Delayed eruption of teeth and dental hypoplasia/hypomineralisation and calcified pulp canals have been described (uncommon)
- Painful infarcts in the maxilla/mandible; dental origin of the pain may be incorrectly suspected
- Pulpal infarcts may result in dental pain in the absence of obvious dental disease
- Increased risk of osteomyelitis (due to hypoxia)
- Mental nerve neuropathy (resulting in numbness in the lower lip and chin, hence the term 'numb chin syndrome') can result from vaso-occlusive events
- Bone marrow hyperplasia leading to enlarged haemopoietic maxilla with excessive overjet and open bite
- Delayed skeletal (but not dental) maturation
- Skin/sclera/gingivae may appear yellow due to jaundice
- Oral manifestations of anaemia (e.g. mucosal/gingival pallor, glossitis, oral ulceration)
- Radiographic changes:
  - Dense radiopacities with 'stepladder' trabeculae pattern suggestive of bone infarcts
  - Lamina dura distinct and dense
  - Hypercementosis
  - Skull thickened but osteoporotic with hair-on-end pattern to trabeculae
  - The diploë is thickened, especially in parietal regions, giving tower skull appearance

Dental Management

- Dental treatment considerations should reflect the severity of the underlying disease and secondary complications, as well as the invasiveness of the proposed dental procedure (Table 11.2.1)
- Treatment should be modified based on reassessment of the patient on the day of the appointment

Section II: Background Information and Guidelines

Definition

Sickle cell disease is the name for a group of inherited health conditions that affect the red blood cells. The most serious type is called sickle cell anaemia. People with this disease have atypical haemoglobin molecules called haemoglobin S, which can distort red blood cells into a sickle, or crescent, shape. Carriers are described as having sickle cell trait.

It is particularly common in people of African or Caribbean descent, but is also found in populations originating from India, the Middle East and southern Europe (Mediterranean). The disease has remained prevalent in these regions, as carriers are thought to have some immunity against malaria. It has been postulated that the sickle cells have porous membranes due to their stretched shape, leaking nutrients that the malaria parasite needs to survive. Furthermore, the faulty cells are eliminated, rapidly destroying the parasite at the same time.

Aetiopathogenesis

- This condition has an autosomal recessive inheritance pattern
- A point mutation in the haemoglobin subunit beta (HBB) gene causes the formation of an abnormal version of beta-globin known as haemoglobin S (HbS)
- Other mutations in the HBB gene may lead to additional abnormal versions of beta-globin such as haemoglobin C (HbC) and haemoglobin E (HbE)
- In people with sickle cell disease, at least 1 of the 2 beta-globin subunits in haemoglobin is replaced with haemoglobin S; the other beta-globin subunit is replaced with a different abnormal variant, such as haemoglobin C
- In sickle cell anaemia (also called homozygous sickle cell disease), haemoglobin S replaces both beta-globin subunits in haemoglobin

Table 11.2.1 Dental management considerations.

Risk assessment	• Chronic anaemia with associated symptoms • Risk of sickle cell crisis is increased by factors such as infection, dehydration, hypoxia, acidosis and cold • A crisis may result in significant associated pain and distress • Increased infection risk associated with splenic infarction • Infarction may also result in multiple comorbidities, including stroke, loss of vision, impaired renal, pulmonary and cardiac function and pulmonary hypertension • Consider access to oral cavity due to skeletal changes
Criteria for referral	• Patients with sickle cell anaemia can safely receive routine dental care during non-crisis periods • Dental treatment is best carried out in a hospital setting when the haemoglobin is below 100 g/dL, when the patient is at higher risk of frequent crises or has other comorbid complications related to the disorder
Access/position	• The timing of treatment and location are important to accommodate for anaemia symptoms – i.e. short morning appointments to avoid fatigue, providing oxygen supplementation • Avoid treatment on the same day as a planned transfusion • Reduce triggers such as cold or long, stressful treatments/environments • Ensure that the patient is hydrated and has not rushed to the appointment/missed a meal • Patients may have reduced mobility (due to hypoxia and/or infarction leading to stroke/hip joint deformity) and may require assistance, an escort and/or hospital transport
Communication	• Liaise closely with the haematologist if invasive dental procedures are planned, there is evidence of significant acute oral infection and/or pharmacological adjuncts to manage dental anxiety are being considered
Consent/capacity	• Consider patient's psychological status as the patient may have chronic depression which may impact on their ability to engage in the consent process • Strokes secondary to central nervous system infarcts may also be associated with cognitive changes
Anaesthesia/sedation	• Local anaesthesia – Preferred for pain control – Avoid topical anaesthetics (e.g. benzocaine) and prilocaine, as they may cause methemoglobinemia • Sedation – Relative analgesia safer (at least 30% oxygen needed, provided no respiratory depression or obstruction) – Avoid drugs causing respiratory depression (e.g. benzodiazepines) • General anaesthesia – Ensure anaemia corrected and Hb brought up to at least 100 g/dL – If sickle cell trait – full oxygenation must be maintained and close monitoring postoperatively – Blood should be available for transfusion if Hb falls <30% – If crisis develops, oxygen and bicarbonate infusion is administered by the anaesthetist
Dental treatment	• Before – Ensure that the patient is relatively stable with no signs of a sickle cell crisis – Confirm when the last transfusion was given – Treat dental infections early and aggressively – Prophylactic antimicrobials may be considered for postsplenectomy and autosplenectomy patients – Ensure that the dental surgery is not cold – Check for any secondary comorbidities and plan appropriate adjustments • During – Pulse oximetry monitoring is prudent during invasive dental procedures; oxygen saturation should be above 95% – Terminate the appointment if there are any signs of distress

(Continued)

Table 11.2.1 (Continued)

	• After – Adequate fluid intake should be ensured post appointment to avoid dehydration – Close monitoring and review advisable – If infection occurs post procedure, it must be treated expeditiously – Cellulitis may require hospitalisation for monitoring and intravenous antibiotic administration – If there are any signs/symptoms of a sickle cell crisis, this is a medical emergency and necessitates initiation of emergency protocol and hospital admission
Drug prescription	• Pain relief: avoid aspirin (can cause acidosis and precipitate crisis); use paracetamol and codeine instead; non-steroidal anti-inflammatory drugs should be used cautiously (and for a few days only), if at all, due to risk of exacerbating underlying kidney disease • Be cautious if asked to prescribe additional pain relief as some patients with sickle cell disease become dependent on opioid analgesics
Education	• Reinforce meticulous oral hygiene and regular dental visits to prevent caries, periodontal disease and need for future extractions • Educate patients about the oral features and the need to avoid dental infections as these may trigger a crisis • Discuss the possibility of needing orthodontic treatment

- On deoxygenation, abnormal versions of beta-globin HbS molecules undergo polymerisation (crystallisation), resulting in distortion of red blood cells, which assume a sickle shape
- Initially this shape deformation is reversible with reoxygenation. However, repeated episodes result in progressive damage (loss of water and potassium, and accumulation of calcium), and eventually the sickle shape becomes permanent
- The sickle-shaped red blood cells die prematurely with their lifespan reduced from 120 to 20 days, leading to extravascular haemolytic anaemia
- Sometimes, the inflexible sickle shaped cells obstruct small blood vessels, resulting in serious medical complications due to infarction

Clinical Presentation

- Sickle cell trait (heterozygous HbSA)
  - About 10 times more common than sickle cell anaemia
  - Frequently asymptomatic, but sickle cell crises can be caused by low oxygen tension (general anaesthesia, high altitudes, unpressurised aircraft)
  - Occasionally splenic infarcts and/or renal complications may occur, leading to haematuria
  - Increased risk of a very rare form of renal cancer, renal medullary carcinoma
- Sickle cell anaemia (homozygous HbSS)
  - Usually, a serious disease with numerous complications
  - Frequently becomes apparent in the third month of life as the foetal haemoglobin (HbF) is replaced
  - Chronic anaemia (Hb level typically between 60 and 90 g/dL)
  - Crises may occur from different triggers
    - Painful crisis (i.e. vaso-occlusive crisis): infarcts as a result of sickling are typically triggered by infection, dehydration, hypoxia, acidosis and cold; infarcts form mainly in the bone marrow spaces and in the spleen, but can occur at any site in the body (hand-foot syndrome, central nervous system, eyes, lungs and kidneys)
    - Aplastic crisis: caused by sudden but temporary cessation of erythropoiesis; reticulocytes disappear from blood and the anaemia worsens
    - Haematological crises: caused by parvovirus infection
  - Sequestration syndromes: sequestration of sickle cells in lungs (impeding gas exchange causing chest syndrome), spleen (result in septicaemia), liver (results in bowel dilation)
  - Haemolysis resulting in jaundice due to chronic hyperbilirubinemia, gallstones, reticulocytosis
  - Infections: due to immune defect resulting from splenic infarction and dysfunction (autosplenectomy)
  - Dactylitis: painful osteitis in the hands
  - Skin ulcers: typically on the legs due to interruption of circulation; infection is not uncommon
  - Increased risk of deep vein thrombosis or pulmonary embolism
  - Priapism
  - Delayed puberty/impaired growth
  - Skeletal deformities

Diagnosis

- Screening, prevention and counselling for couples in higher risk groups (Afro-Caribbean) planning to have children
- Prenatal/newborn screening
- Diagnosis is made by a combination of clinical findings and special tests:
  - Haemoglobin assay/complete blood count
  - Mean corpuscular volume (MCV), mean corpuscular haemoglobin (MCH), and mean corpuscular haemoglobin concentration (MCHC)
  - Serum iron and ferritin
  - Red cell folate assays
  - Haemoglobin electrophoresis
  - Sickle solubility tests

Management

- Sickle cell trait
  - Less susceptible to complications but can precipitate crisis if triggering factors are present (e.g. hypoxia)
- Sickle cell disease
  - Main principles in treatment are to prevent trauma, infection, hypoxia, acidosis or dehydration (treat these promptly) and to control pain in association with crises/infarction
  - Regular folic acid in view of the increase in cell turnover due to haemolysis
  - Hydroxyurea to prevent/reduce complications (potential side-effect of leucopenia/thrombocytopenia)
  - In cases where a splenectomy is performed due to splenic infarction and dysfunction, patients are kept on prophylactic phenoxymethyl penicillin
  - Pain control (opioids may be required, leading to dependence)
  - Iron chelation as required
  - Exchange transfusions are given in relation to severe anaemia, acute crises and where the blood profile indicates there are a high number of sickled cells
  - Sometimes blood transfusions are given for cerebrovascular symptoms in early childhood or recurrent pulmonary thromboses; however, they are minimised to reduce the risk of blood-borne infections and iron overload
  - Comprehensive care programmes involving physiotherapy and psychology support
  - Drugs to prevent sickling have been developed but are not widely available: voxelotor, crizanlizumab-tmca
  - Stem cell transplants are the only cure but are associated with inherent risks
  - Gene therapies under development

Prognosis

- Morbidity and early mortality rates high
- Main causes of death: infections and thromboses
- May also die prematurely due to cardiac failure, renal failure, overwhelming infection or stroke

A World/Transcultural View

- Although originating from sub-Saharan Africa, the Arabian Peninsula and the Indian subcontinent, population migration has increased the prevalence of sickle cell anaemia in other regions, such as USA, western and northern Europe
- Hence the World Health Organization now considers the disease to be a global health problem
- It is now the most common inherited blood disorder in the United States, affecting approximately 100 000 Americans, and estimated to occur in 1/500 African Americans and 1/1000–1400 Hispanic Americans
- In the United Kingdom, 1/10 Afro-Caribbean and 1/100 Cypriots and Asians carry sickle cell trait
- It affects millions of people around the globe and is the fourth leading cause of death in children in many developing countries
- In well-[illegible] countries, newborn survival has increased due to early screening and implementing comprehensive care; however, these children face emerging complications and morbidity as they grow older

Recommended Reading

Abed, H., Sharma, S.P., Balkhoyor, A. et al. (2019). Special care dentistry for patients diagnosed with sickle cell disease: an update for dentists. *Gen. Dent.* 67: 40–44.

Acharya, S. (2015). Oral and dental considerations in management of sickle cell anemia. *Int J Clin Pediatr Dent.* 8: 141–144.

Chekroun, M., Chérifi, H., Fournier, B. et al. (2019). Oral manifestations of sickle cell disease. *Br. Dent. J.* 226: 27–31.

Chou, S.T., Alsawas, M., Fasano, R.M. et al. (2020). American Society of Hematology 2020 guidelines for sickle cell disease: transfusion support. *Blood Adv.* 4: 327–355.

Hsu, L.L. and Fan-Hsu, J. (2020). Evidence-based dental management in the new era of sickle cell disease: a scoping review. *J. Am. Dent. Assoc.* 151: 668–677.

Kato, G.J., Piel, F.B., Reid, C.D. et al. (2018). Sickle cell disease. *Nat. Rev. Dis. Primers.* 4: 18010.

Kawar, N., Alrayyes, S., Yang, B., and Aljewari, H. (2018). Oral health management considerations for patients with sickle cell disease. *Dis. Mon.* 64: 296–301.

Mulimani, P., Ballas, S.K., Abas, A.B., and Karanth, L. (2019). Treatment of dental complications in sickle cell disease. *Cochrane Database Syst. Rev.* 12: CD01163.

11.3 Neutropenia

Section I: Clinical Scenario and Dental Considerations

Clinical Scenario

A 29-year-old female diagnosed with type 1b glycogenosis presents to the dental clinic complaining of bleeding gums and mobility of several lower teeth. She reports that her symptoms have worsened in recent weeks.

Medical History

- Type 1b glycogenosis (von Gierke disease), a rare inherited condition caused by mutations in the SLC37A4 gene, characterised by glycogen and fat build-up within the liver and kidneys, that causes:
  - Hypoglycaemic episodes
  - Neutropenia
  - Myeloid cell line dysfunction
  - Recurrent mouth ulcers
  - Hepatomegaly
  - Inflammatory bowel disease
  - Microalbuminuria
- Recurrent epistaxis
- History of hip abscess (8 years earlier)
- History of appendectomy (22 years earlier)

Medications

- Filgrastim (r-metHuG-CSF)
- Mesalazine
- Vitamin D3
- Enalapril

Dental History

- Regular dental attender in your practice; also visits the dental hygienist every 12 weeks
- Meticulous oral hygiene habits; uses a soft toothbrush and does not use interdental brushes as advised by her physician
- Brushes teeth 3 times a day and uses a 0.12% chlorhexidine mouthwash
- History of recurrent, painful and incapacitating mouth ulcers
- Pericoronitis of the mandibular third molar (1 episode)

Social History

- University educated but currently unemployed
- Lives at home with parents
- Attends appointments accompanied by her father, who is a physician by profession

Oral Examination

- Good oral hygiene
- Significant gingivitis
- Generalised bleeding on probing
- Generalised tooth mobility, with grade II mobility of the lower anterior teeth
- Fillings in #15, #25, #35 and #37

Radiological Examination

- Orthopantomogram undertaken (Figure 11.3.1)
- Multiple dental diastemas
- Tooth root resorption of the mandibular incisors
- Impacted tooth #38

Structured Learning

1) Why is this patient on filgrastim (r-metHuG-CSF)?
   - Filgrastim is a recombinant human granulocyte colony stimulating factor (G-CSF) therapy
   - The recombinant protein resembles the natural factor, releasing the neutrophil reservoirs from the bone marrow to the peripheral bloodstream, increasing production and acting as an antiapoptotic factor
   - This can lead to a 10–12-fold increase in the neutrophil count and result in a higher life expectancy for this patient

A Practical Approach to Special Care in Dentistry, First Edition. Edited by Pedro Diz Dios and Navdeep Kumar.

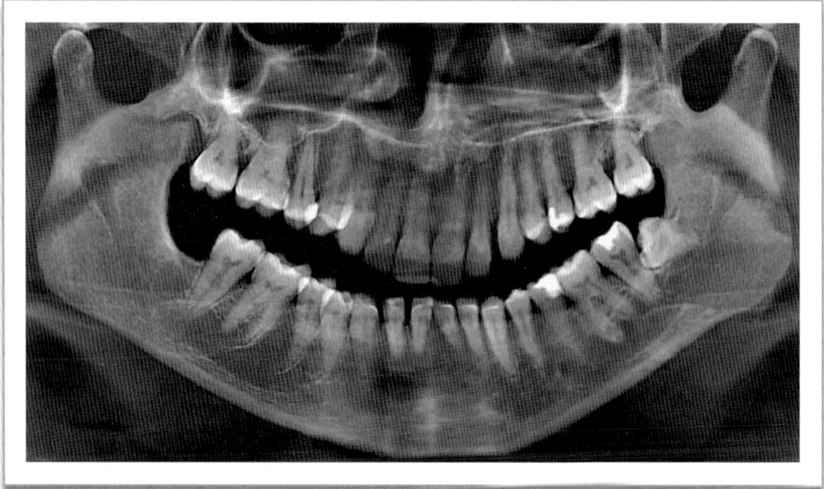

Figure 11.3.1 Panoramic radiography showing tooth resorption of the mandibular incisors and impacted tooth #38.

2) What adverse effects can filgrastim (r-metHuG-CSF) have in the oral cavity?
   - Bleeding gums due to thrombocytopenia
   - Ulcers
   - Swelling (lips and/or tongue)
   - Mucositis
   - Cracked lips
3) The patient is very distressed that her lower teeth are mobile. How would you explain to her why this has happened, despite the fact that she cleans her teeth 3 times a day and visits the dental clinic regularly?
   - Although G-CSF can improve the control of bacterial infections in individuals with neutropenia, many patients still experience these infections such as pneumonia, other respiratory infections, stomatitis and severe persistent gingival inflammation
   - Periodontal manifestations may range from marginal gingivitis to rapidly progressive periodontal disease with advancing bone loss, which may affect both primary and permanent dentition, but primarily the latter
   - Despite her regular toothbrushing, the use of a soft toothbrush, coupled with a lack of interdental cleaning and increased susceptibility to aggressive periodontal disease due to neutropenia, may result in rapid bone loss
4) In the first instance, you recommend a course of periodontal treatment including scaling and root planing. What factors are considered important in assessing the risk of managing this patient?
   - Social
     - The patient has a rare inherited condition and her father is a physician; both are likely to question the knowledge of this condition by the dentist and the awareness of the risks and how to mitigate against these
   - Medical
     - Increased risk of local and focal infection due to neutropenia
     - Risk of hypoglycaemia during and mainly following dental treatment sessions
     - Bleeding tendency based on recurrent epistaxis, potential platelet dysfunction (myeloid cell line dysfunction) and filgrastim administration (decreases platelet count)
   - Dental
     - The patient requires intensive periodontal treatment
     - Mandibular incisors have poor prognosis
     - Assess extraction of tooth #38
5) In order to fully assess the risk of undertaking root planning, preoperative blood tests are advisable. What tests should you request?
   - Full blood count
     - Haemoglobin and haematocrit (risk of anaemia)
     - Red blood cell count (risk of anaemia)
     - Neutrophil count (risk of infection)
     - Platelet count (risk of bleeding)
     - Coagulation study (risk of bleeding due to hepatic dysfunction)
   - Blood biochemistry
     - Blood glucose (risk of hypoglycemia)
     - AST, ALT and GGT (to assess hepatic function)
     - Albumin and creatinine (to assess renal function)
6) The laboratory tests reveal a neutrophil count of 1×10^9/L. After consulting with the patient's physician, they recommend performing the dental treatment in a hospital setting. Why?

- Myeloid dysfunction is common in type 1b glycogenosis; therefore, a sufficient blood cell count (e.g. neutrophils) does not imply that these are functionally adequate and therefore does not ensure that complications will not arise
- Dental treatment can affect oral intake in the subsequent hours/days and, as a result, promote the onset of hypoglycaemic episodes (a complication that can be severe for this patient)

7) If the patient has a new episode of pericoronitis in the third molar (#38), what would you need to consider if prescribing an antibiotic?
   - Empirically, the recommendation is to administer a broad-spectrum antibiotic, although they promote the onset of resistance (especially if taken for an extended period)
   - If the patient takes antibiotics frequently, it is possible that micro-organisms have already undergone a selection process
   - Anytime there is exudate or the treatment response is poor, a sample should be taken for microbiological cultures and antibiogram
   - Assess the need for a concomitant administration of an antimycotic agent if the infection persists
8) In the medium term, the patient will lose the teeth in the anterior mandibular sector. What factors can jeopardise the rehabilitation of the edentulous space with osseointegrated implants?
   - Complications regarding the surgical procedure such as significant bleeding, delayed healing, surgical wound infection and prolonged postoperative pain
   - The history of severe periodontitis (especially if there are still natural teeth remaining)
   - The continuous administration of granulocyte-colony stimulating factors can cause osteopenia/osteoporosis

General Dental Considerations

Oral Findings

- Patients with a quantitative neutrophil deficit
  - Thrush
  - Painful ulcers, with irregular greyish background and no inflammatory halo (Figure 11.3.2)
  - Severe gingivitis (erythematous gingiva and occasionally hyperplastic)
  - Periodontitis with risk of premature tooth loss (Figure 11.3.3)
  - Increased susceptibility to caries and pulp disease (has not been confirmed)
- Patients with a functional neutrophil deficit
  - Mucosal ulcers
  - Recurrent sinusitis
  - Cervical lymphadenopathy
  - Oral candidiasis
  - Gingivitis and aggressive periodontitis (childhood/early adulthood) (Figure 11.3.4)
  - Enamel hypoplasia
  - Delayed tooth eruption

Dental Management

- To prevent complications resulting from dental treatment in patients with moderate to severe neutropenia, it is advisable to conduct a medical consultation to assess the administration of granulocyte-colony stimulating factors and select the most appropriate antibiotic prophylaxis regimen (Table 11.3.1)

(a)

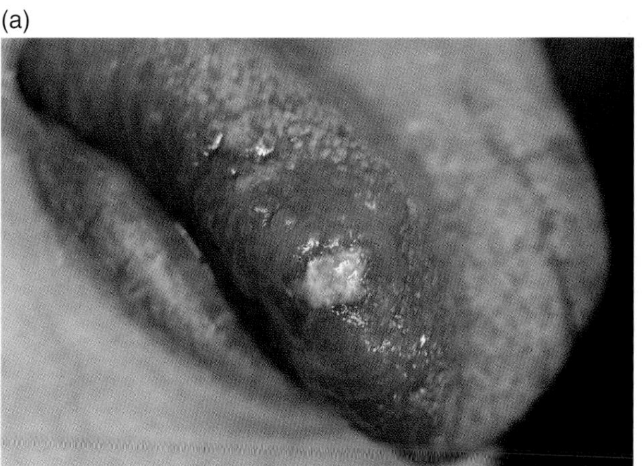

(b)

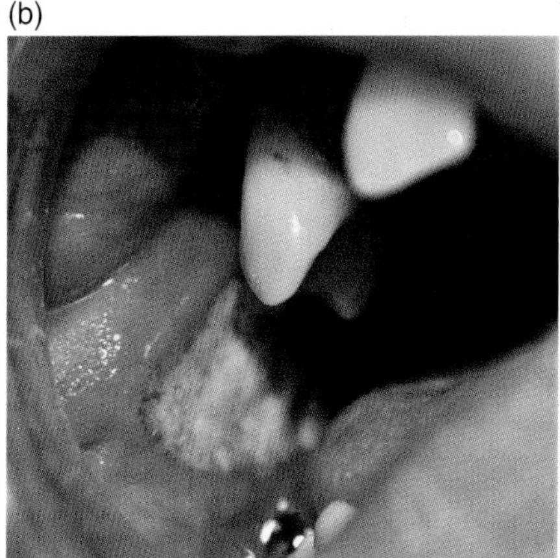

Figure 11.3.2 (a,b) Recurrent oral ulceration in cyclic neutropenia.

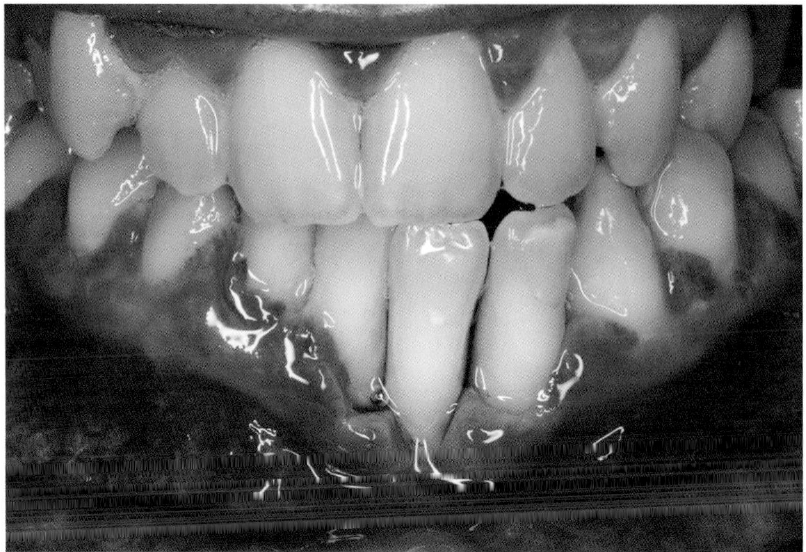

Figure 11.3.3 Severe periodontal disease and early tooth loss related to chronic neutropenia.

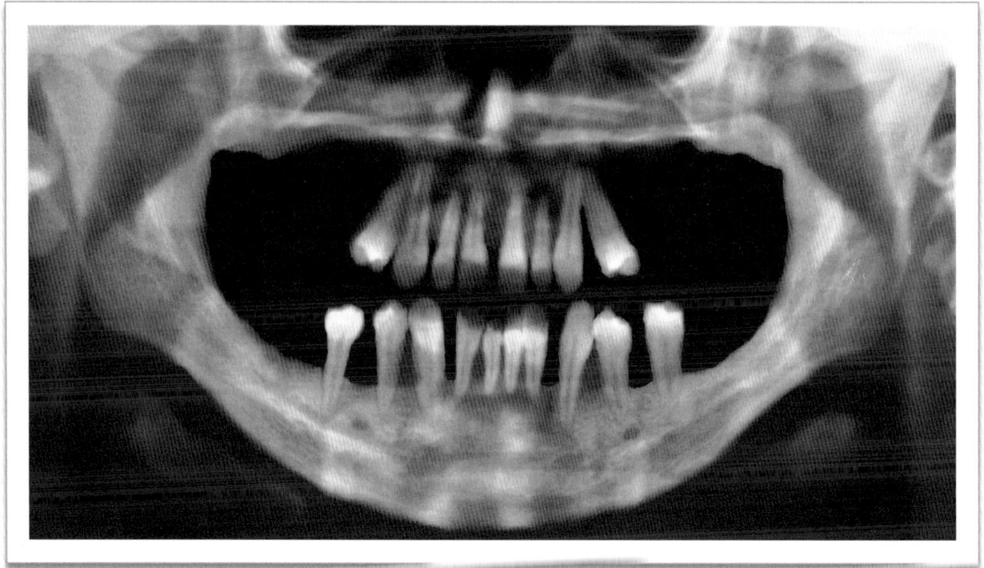

Figure 11.3.4 Aggressive periodontitis in a teenager with DiGeorge syndrome and neutrophil dysfunction.

Section II: Background Information and Guidelines

Definition

Neutropenia is an acute or chronic reduction in the concentration of neutrophils in peripheral blood. In adults, neutropenia is defined as a neutrophil count $<1.5 \times 10^9$/L of blood; a count $<0.5 \times 10^9$/L is considered severe.

The aetiology of neutropenia can be congenital (intrinsic) or acquired (extrinsic), although the most common cause is neutropenia secondary to chemotherapy for cancer (Table 11.3.2). The most severe complication of neutropenia is the dissemination of local infections, commonly bacterial or fungal, which can be life-threatening. The prevalence of neutropenia varies significantly and is based on the underlying disease (e.g. 3–8 cases per million individuals present severe congenital neutropenia, while 20% of cases present febrile neutropenia among patients with cancer).

Aetiopathogenesis

- Reduced neutrophil production (e.g. cytotoxic chemotherapy)
- Displacement of the circulating neutrophil pool to the peripheral tissues (e.g. bacterial infections)
- Increased peripheral destruction of neutrophils (e.g. hypersplenism)

Table 11.3.1 Dental management considerations.

Risk assessment	• Risk of severe local infection and distant spread (bacteraemia/septicaemia) following dental procedures • If antibiotic prophylaxis is to be prescribed for patients with moderate to severe neutropenia, it is advisable to consult with the physician because there can be an overgrowth of resistant micro-organisms
Criteria for referral	• Invasive dental treatments for patients with severe neutropenia ($<0.5\times10^9$ neutrophils/L) should be conducted in a hospital setting
Access/position	• After discontinuing the administration of G-CSF, there is typically a significant reduction in the number of circulating neutrophils (up to 50%) after 1–2 days, with levels normalising 1–7 days later
Communication	• In some patients with chronic neutropenia, maintaining healthy oral hygiene habits and/or motivation for periodically visiting the dental clinic can be difficult, because the prognosis of the teeth is equally problematic, with or without proper care
Consent/capacity	• The consent should reflect the complications resulting from the neutropenia, such as delayed healing and the risk of local and systemic infection • The patient should be explicitly informed of the possibility that dental treatment cannot prevent the progression of the periodontal disease or premature edentulism • The objective and limitations of the protocol for administering G-CSF and antimicrobial prophylaxis need to be specified
Anaesthesia/sedation	• In neutropenic patients there are no special considerations for the use of local anaesthesia, sedation or general anaesthesia
Dental treatment	• Before – In patients with moderate to severe chronic neutropenia, the recommendation is to consult the physician/haematologist – In these cases, the administration of 5 µg/kg/day of G-CSF subcutaneously or intravenously for 3–5 days is usually sufficient to enable invasive dental procedures, such as dental extractions – G-CSF also enable dental procedures that until recently were highly controversial and not recommended; these include scaling and root planing, preprosthetic surgery and the placement of dental implants – To minimise the risk of bacteraemia secondary to invasive dental procedures, prophylactic administration of antibiotics is often considered (e.g. 600 mg clindamycin for a few days before and after the surgery); in addition, the use of antiseptic rinses (0.2% chlorhexidine) prior to any dental manipulation may be advised • During – Where possible, elective dental procedures should be delayed until the absolute neutrophil count rises to $>1\times10^9$ neutrophils/L (normal count 2×10^9 neutrophils/L) – The recommendation is to perform primary closure of the surgical wounds and avoid placing foreign materials (e.g. hemostatic sponges), as the latter can act as a nidus for infection – The type and design of dental prostheses may need to be adapted in relation to the severity and chronicity of neutropenia (avoid mucosal loading, minimise size and extension, ensure easy to clean, minimal risk of trauma) • After – A low incidence of postextraction complications (<10%) has been reported, all of which are relatively minor and manageable (e.g. surgical wound infection, delayed healing and prolonged postoperative pain) – Periodic plaque and calculus removal, the use of antiseptics (0.2% chlorhexidine) and periodontal treatment help maintain periodontal health in most cases – In some patients with neutrophil deficiency, however, periodontitis and tooth mobility inevitably progress despite proper maintenance – Dental implants are not contraindicated, but their prognosis can be jeopardised in patients with premature tooth loss due to severe periodontitis and because the continuous administration of G-CSF can cause osteopenia/osteoporosis

(Continued)

Table 11.3.1 (Continued)

Education/prevention	• The focus of dental care is prevention of oral infection, with the aim of minimising the need for surgical treatment • Conventional prevention measures, such as applying topical fluoride, providing dietary recommendations and promoting oral health, are essential • Eliminating the foci of intraoral infections before haematopoietic transplantation is essential because an odontogenic infection in a patient with severe neutropenia can be life-threatening • It has been suggested that these patients should use soft-bristle toothbrushes to minimise the risk of gingival trauma; this should be balanced with the need to maintain good gingival health • Consider the additional use of antimicrobial mouthwashes (e.g. chlorhexidine)

Table 11.3.2 Classification of neutropenia.

Causes of congenital neutropenia	Causes of acquired neutropenia
• Kostmann syndrome (severe congenital neutropenia) • Benign congenital neutropenia • Cyclic neutropenia • Shwachman–Diamond syndrome • Reticular dysgenesis • Severe chronic neutropenia – Myelokathexis – Associated with immunoglobulinopathy – Associated with phenotypic abnormalities – Associated with metabolic disorders	• Drug induced – Predictable: cytostatics and immunosuppressants – Idiosyncratic: phenothiazides, sulfamides, non-steroidal anti-inflammatory drugs, semi-synthetic penicillins, procainamide, antithyroid agents and others • Postinfection: chickenpox, measles, rubella, hepatitis A and B, mononucleosis, influenza, cytomegalovirus and others • Bone marrow transplantation • Radiation therapy • Nutritional deficiencies – Vitamin B12 – Folates – Copper

Clinical Presentation

- Some patients are asymptomatic
- Fever, asthenia, general discomfort
- Oral ulcers
- Lymphadenopathy
- Pharyngitis, otitis, upper airway infections

Diagnosis

- Full blood count including differential to determine the neutrophil count
- Medical history (risk factors, findings in the physical examination, family history, previous abnormalities in the hemogram)
- Specific diagnoses/tests
  - Neutrophil antibody test for children (e.g. positive in congenital and autoimmune neutropenia)
  - Flow cytometry analysis to assess neutrophil functionality (e.g. positive in large granular lymphocyte syndrome)
  - Antinuclear antibodies (e.g. positive in autoimmune neutropenia)
  - Vitamin B12 and folate levels
  - Genetic sequencing to identify mutations in genes associated with neutropenia (e.g. mutations in neutrophil elastase gene [ELANE] in cyclic neutropenia)
  - Bone marrow examination with differential and cytogenetic cell count (e.g. diagnostic for acute leukaemia and myelodysplasia)

Management

- Broad-spectrum antibiotics
- Granulocyte colony-stimulating factors (G-CSF), glycoproteins that regulate the production and differentiation of myeloid stem cells, as well as the functionality of mature blood cells
  - G-CSFs are contraindicated for Kostmann syndrome with abnormal cytogenetics, for myelodysplastic syndromes and for chronic myeloid leukaemia
  - The use of G-CSFs is recommended for patients with neutrophil levels $<0.5\times10^9$/L with mouth ulcers and gingivitis, recurrent fever, cellulitis, abscesses, sinusitis, pneumonia or perianal infections
  - If the response to G-CSFs is poor, other strategies should be considered, such as haematopoietic transplantation

Prognosis

- The prognosis for neutropenia is determined by the underlying disease (e.g. transient neutropenia usually has a benign and reversible course, while Chédiak–Higashi syndrome is almost invariably fatal)
- Morbidity and mortality increase significantly when neutrophil levels drop below 0.2×10^9/L

A World/Transcultural View

- Benign ethnic neutropenia is the most common form of neutropenia worldwide, given that it affects 25–50% of individuals of African descent and some ethnic groups of the Middle East. In these patients, the fundamental determination is not the neutrophil level in peripheral blood but rather the bone marrow's response capacity. Accordingly, among a number of ethnic groups, neutropenia is considered to exist only when the neutrophil count is $<0.8 \times 10^9$/L
- The protocol for administering granulocyte-stimulating factors varies widely between institutions and countries in terms of indications, dosage, infusion rate and therapy duration

Recommended Reading

Cheretakis, C., Locker, D., Dror, Y., and Glogauer, M. (2007). Oral health-related quality of life of children with neutropenia. *Spec. Care Dentist.* 27: 6–11.

Dale, D.C. (2017). How I manage children with neutropenia. *Br. J. Haematol.* 178: 351–363.

Diz-Dios, P., Ocampo-Hermida, A., and Fernandez-Feijoo, J. (2002). Quantitative and functional neutrophil deficiencies. *Med. Oral.* 7: 206–221.

Fillmore, W.J., Leavitt, B.D., and Arce, K. (2014). Dental extraction in the neutropenic patient. *J. Oral Maxillofac. Surg.* 72: 2386–2393.

Palmblad, J., Nilsson, C.C., Höglund, P., and Papadaki, H.A. (2016). How we diagnose and treat neutropenia in adults. *Expert. Rev. Hematol.* 9: 479–487.

Park, M.S., Tenenbaum, H.C., Dror, Y., and Gloguaer, M. (2014). Oral health comparison between children with neutropenia and healthy controls. *Spec. Care Dentist.* 34: 12–18.

Schmidt, J.C., Walter, C., Rischewski, J.R., and Weiger, R. (2013). Treatment of periodontitis as a manifestation of neutropenia with or without systemic antibiotics: a systematic review. *Pediatr. Dent.* 35: E54–E63.

11.4 Thrombocytopenia

Section I: Clinical Scenario and Dental Considerations

Clinical Scenario

A 18-year-old female patient is referred to your dental clinic from the haematology department regarding her bleeding gums. She is brought to the appointment by her parents and reports that she is feeling depressed about the fact she cannot smile as her teeth and gums are always covered in blood.

Medical History

Bernard–Soulier syndrome

Medications

- Tranexamic acid 500 mg thrice daily during the first 3 days of her menstrual cycle
- Folic acid supplement
- Vitamin C supplement
- Iron supplement

Dental History

- Irregular dental attender due to difficulty with access
- Last dental visit was 4 years ago
- Only brushes her teeth once a day as her gums bleed for ~15 minutes after brushing, leaving a bad taste in her mouth

Social History

- Single, lives with parents
- Student in final year of high school
- Poor dietary habits (snacks frequently on sweets and chocolates)
- Nil alcohol or tobacco consumption reported

Oral Examination

- Pale mucosa (Figure 11.4.1)
- Generalised plaque, calculus, gingival inflammation and spontaneous bleeding
- Generalised tooth surface loss
- Fissured tongue

Radiological Examination

- Orthopantomogram undertaken
- All teeth are present
- Supernumerary tooth in the upper left quadrant behind wisdom tooth (#29)

Structured Learning

1) How may the patient's Bernard–Soulier syndrome be affecting her oral health?
   - It is a rare congenital bleeding disorder (frequency is ~1 per million people)
   - The condition associated with the lack of platelet glycoprotein Ib and characterised by unusually large platelets, reduced platelet adhesion, and thrombocytopaenia
   - Impact on oral health includes:
     - Multiple episodes of spontaneous bleeding gums, exacerbated by toothbrushing, which make it challenging to maintain adequate oral hygiene practices
     - General tiredness resulting from iron deficiency anaemia can lead to general and oral neglect
2) The patient informs you that she did not go back to her previous dentist due to a bad experience. After scaling was undertaken, the patient had to go to the hospital emergency department as her gums would not stop bleeding and she had to be admitted. What would you do to avoid this happening again?
   - Contact the haematology consultant in charge of the patient
   - Explain what dental treatment is planned and liaise with them to confirm whether it is advisable to proceed
   - Detail the patient's previous experience when scaling was undertaken

A Practical Approach to Special Care in Dentistry, First Edition. Edited by Pedro Diz Dios and Navdeep Kumar.

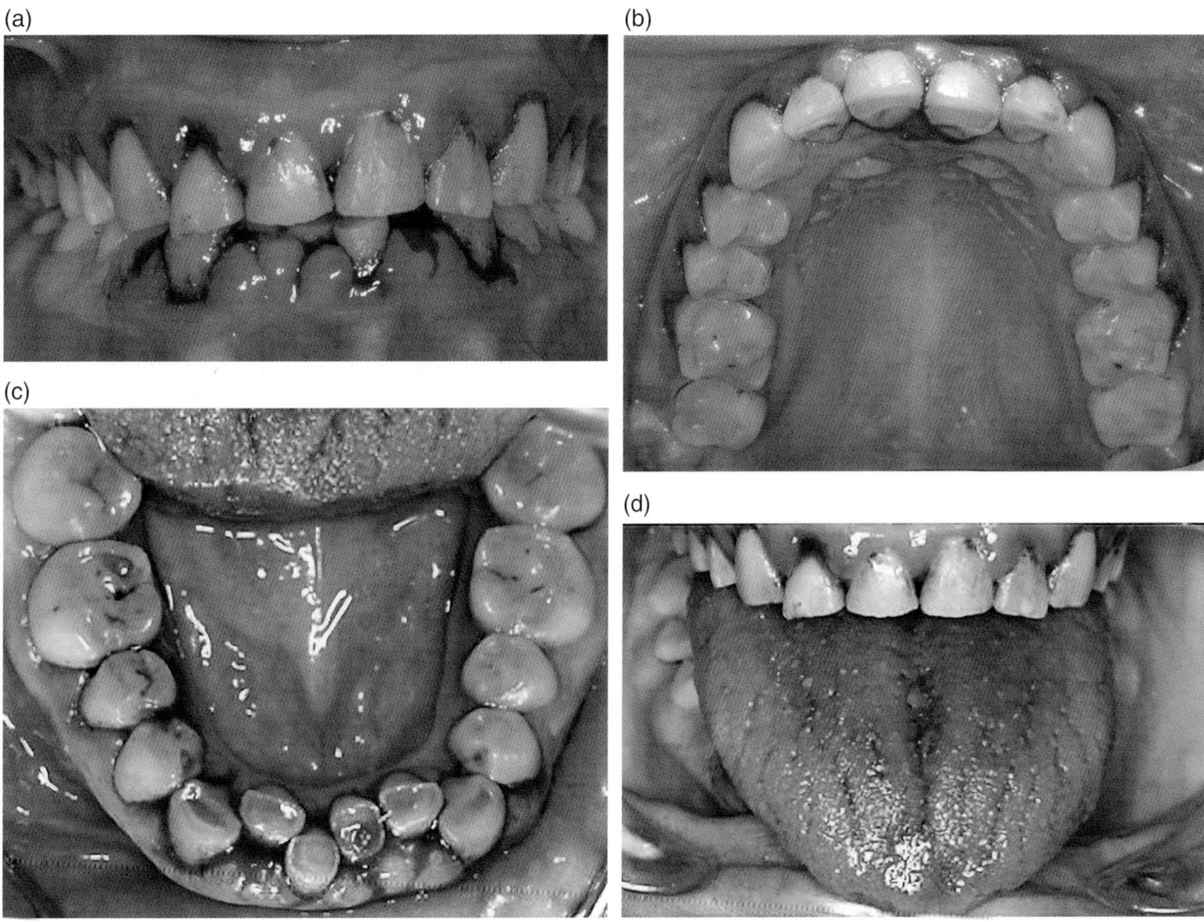

Figure 11.4.1 (a) Dentition: inflamed, hyperplastic, bleeding gingivae; tooth surface loss. (b) Maxillary arch: occlusal tooth surface loss. (c) Mandibular arch: occlusal tooth surface loss, bleeding gingivae. (d) Tongue: fissured and stained with blood.

- Confirm what haematological support should be in place to enable treatment
- Agree the most suitable location for dental care (primary or secondary care)
- Ensure that there is a plan in place to access haematological support should bleeding still persist

3) What other factors do you need to consider in your risk assessment?
   - Social
     - Reliance on parents to attend
     - Low self-esteem due to spontaneous bleeding gingivae
   - Medical
     - Bleeding risk due to bleeding disorder
     - The need for a platelet transfusion and tranexamic acid before and after dental treatment
     - Fatigue from anaemia
   - Dental
     - Excessive gingival bleeding during and after periodontal treatment
     - Inability to maintain her oral health due to excessive bleeding from the gums on toothbrushing
     - Poor dietary habits
4) When discussing the advanced tooth surface loss, you discover that the persistent bleeding from her gums causes her to feel nauseated when she swallows blood. This makes her vomit several times a day. How would you manage this?
   - Inform the haematologist and advise them that the patient may require more haematological support as her persistently bleeding gums are having an impact not only on her well-being but also her oral and dental health
   - Dental support is also necessary – dietary analysis, casts to monitor the tooth surface loss, restorative option depends on changes in occlusal vertical dimension

5) As per the haematologist's advice, the patient is seen for full mouth debridement in your primary care practice, with perioperative tranexamic acid given orally for 5 days preoperatively and 3 days postoperatively. Following scaling, you note that there is bruising in the floor of the patient's mouth. What could be the cause and what is the risk?
   - Due to the patient's increased bleeding risk, trauma from light pressure, including suction, can result in considerable bruising and bleeding
   - The risk is that a sublingual haematoma has formed
   - This is commonly associated with a protruding tongue and respiratory distress
   - If these additional signs are present, this should be treated as an emergency and the emergency services called to secure the airway
6) The patient returns to you 6 months later requesting braces to straighten her lower teeth. What would you consider?
   - Need to confirm that oral hygiene and general oral health have improved
   - Confirm that the patient is committed to regular dental attendance
   - An orthodontic opinion is required as the lower incisor crowding is severe
   - Space creation to align the anterior teeth may require extraction of posterior teeth and extended fixed orthodontic treatment
   - This is associated with risk, namely bleeding due to dental extractions and potential trauma from the orthodontic appliance
   - The orthodontist will need to liaise closely with the physician and adapt their approach to reduce trauma, namely:
     - Use elastomeric modules to secure arch wires rather than metal ligatures
     - Self-ligating brackets are generally more comfortable and associated with less plaque accumulation
     - Clear aligner therapy (CAT)

General Dental Considerations

Oral Findings

- Gingival bleeding
- Blood-filled bullae (Figure 11.4.2)
- Palatal petechiae
- Prolonged bleeding following surgery

Dental Management

- Thrombocytopenia is not an absolute contraindication for dental procedures

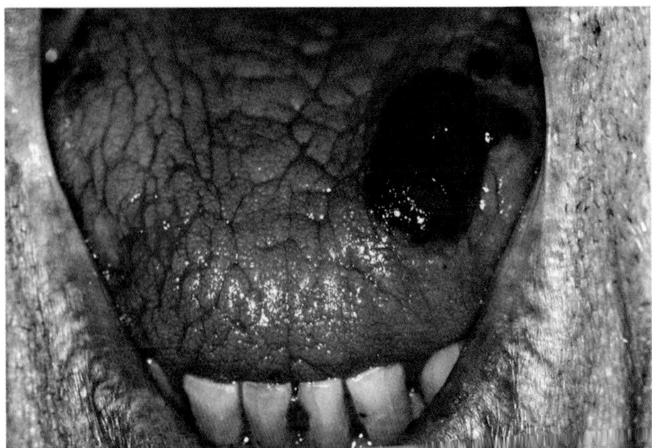

Figure 11.4.2 Spontaneous blood-filled bullae (angina bullosa haemorrhagica) have been described in patients with thrombocytopaenia.

- However, the delivery of dental treatment may need to be modified depending on the associated clinical manifestations, the platelet count and the invasiveness of the proposed dental intervention (Tables 11.4.1 and 11.4.2)
- It is also important to be aware when prescribing drugs, as some may impair platelet function and hence increase bleeding risk (Table 11.4.3)
- There is no evidence to support the long-standing dogma of the need for a platelet count ≥50 000/μL for safe invasive dental procedures
- Platelet transfusion effectiveness for haemostasis support cannot be determined based on currently available data
- Local measures and antifibrinolytics are the mainstay for the prevention and management of bleeding

Section II: Background Information and Guidelines

Definition

A platelet count below 100×10^9/L is termed thrombocytopenia and may be associated with inadequate clot formation, purpura and prolonged bleeding tendency (normal platelet count is 150–450 $\times 10^9$/L).

Aetiopathogenesis

- Altered platelet production caused by:
  - Dehydration
  - Malnutrition (e.g. vitamin B12 and folate deficiency)
  - Bone marrow disease (e.g. aplastic anaemia, myelodysplastic syndromes, radiotherapy, chemotherapy drugs, metastatic disease)

Table 11.4.1 Dental management considerations.

Risk assessment	• Prolonged/excessive bleeding • Splenectomy predisposes to infections (pneumococcal infections of particular risk) • Long-term corticosteroid use complications • Consider the cause of thrombocytopenia and the additional specific risks associated with the conditions • Increased risk of blood-borne virus spread (due to platelet transfusions)
Criteria for referral	• Dentists should be able to provide non-invasive (non-surgical) dental treatment for the vast majority of patients with platelets levels greater than 50×10^9/L in primary care • If necessary, seek advice from/refer to a more experienced colleague in primary or secondary dental care
Access/position	• No special considerations for access to dental clinic, timing of treatment and patient positioning unless related to underlying cause of thrombocytopenia
Communication	• No special considerations unless patients have had a stroke or other cardiovascular disease
Consent/capacity	• No special considerations unless patients have had a stroke or other cardiovascular disease
Anaesthesia/sedation	• Local anaesthesia – Can be given if platelets levels are above 30×10^9/L – Use an aspirating syringe, minimal volume and slow administration – Avoid regional block injections where possible; if unavoidable, ensure platelets above 50×10^9/L • Sedation – Can be given, inhalational preferable – Risk of damaging the vein/haematoma with intravenous sedation • General anaesthesia – Increased risk of submucous bleeding into the airway demands a cautious and experienced approach, with platelet levels ideally above 50×10^9/L
Dental treatment	• Before – Determine the cause and severity of thrombocytopenia and the invasiveness of the type of dental treatment planned to ensure that the appropriate precautions are undertaken – Platelet replacement/supplementation may be given just before surgery to control capillary bleeding, with further available at the end of surgery as required – Local haemostatic measures, use of desmopressin (DDAVP), tranexamic acid or topical administration of platelet concentrate may reduce the need for platelet supplementation – Patients with additional bleeding risks such as liver impairment and/or alcoholism, renal failure, receiving cytotoxic medication, should not be treated in primary care without medical advice; ideally, refer to a hospital-based dental clinic • During – Lubricant/barrier cream used to protect the lips/soft tissue for trauma – Careful manipulation of the cheek and soft tissues – consider the use of gauze when using cheek retractors – Caution with suction to avoid trauma (reduce the volume) – Consider the adjuvant use of tranexamic acid 5% mouthwash or desmopressin if bleeding prolonged – Oral surgery (Table 11.4.2): ○ Minor surgeries can be carried out in primary care (simple extractions from 1 to 3 teeth) ○ For more than 3 extractions multiple visits required ○ Major surgery with platelet levels above 75×10^9/L – Implantology: specialised medical advice mandatory – Conservative dentistry, endodontics, prosthodontics: caution advised – Non-surgical periodontology: minor gingival surgery/dental scaling – caution advised; start in a limited area to assess bleeding – Surgical periodontology: caution advised, may require hospital setting depending on platelet count – Absorbable haemostatic agents may be used to assist clotting (e.g. oxidised regenerated cellulose, synthetic collagen or microcrystalline collagen) • After – Give patient written postoperative instruction and emergency contact details – Review in 1 week after dental procedure

(Continued)

Table 11.4.1 (Continued)

Drug prescription	• Antiseptics (e.g. 0.12–0.2% chlorhexidine) • Paracetamol and codeine are recommended analgesics • Avoid aspirin and non-steroidal anti-inflammatory drugs (reversible effect on platelets, act for up to 48 h) • COX-2 inhibitors can be used because they have no effect on platelets • It is also important to be aware of additional drugs which may impair platelet function and increase bleeding risk (Table 11.4.3)
Education/ prevention	• Prevention and oral hygiene advice to avoid the need for future dental procedures that may require surgery • Inform the patient regarding the side-effects of long-term corticosteroid use • Emphasise the increased risk of infection for those patients who have had a splenectomy

Table 11.4.2 Oral surgery management based on severity of thrombocytopenia.

Severity of thrombocytopenia (platelet count $\times 10^9$/L)	Clinical manifestation	Dentoalveolar surgery	Maxillofacial surgery
Mild (100–150)	• Mild purpura • Slightly prolonged postoperative bleeding	• No platelet transfusion • Local haemostatic measures • Observe	• Mild purpura sometimes • Slightly prolonged postoperative bleeding
Moderate (50–100)	• Purpura • Postoperative bleeding	• Platelets may be needed • Local haemostatic measures • Consider postoperative tranexamic acid mouthwash (3 days)	• Platelets needed • Local haemostatic measures • Postoperative tranexamic acid mouthwash (3 days)
Severe (30–50)	• Purpura • Postoperative bleeding	• Platelets usually needed • Local haemostatic measures • Postoperative tranexamic acid mouthwash (3 days)	• Platelets needed • Local haemostatic measures • Avoid surgery where possible • Postoperative tranexamic acid mouthwash (3 days)
Life threatening (< 30)	• Purpura • Spontaneous bleeding	• Platelets needed • Local haemostatic measures • Avoid surgery where possible • Postoperative tranexamic acid mouthwash (3 days)	• Platelets needed • Local haemostatic measures • Avoid surgery where possible • Postoperative tranexamic acid mouthwash (3 days)

  - Transiently after bone marrow transplant
  - Liver disease
  - Viruses (e.g. human parvovirus B19, rubella, EBV, CMV, HIV)
  - Hereditary syndromes (e.g. congenital amegakaryocytic thrombocytopenia, thrombocytopenia absent radius syndrome, Fanconi anaemia, Bernard–Soulier syndrome, May–Hegglin anomaly, grey platelet syndrome, Alport syndrome, Wiskott–Aldrich syndrome)
- Increased platelet destruction due to:
  - Immune conditions (e.g. thrombotic thrombocytopenic purpura, immune thrombocytopenia, diffuse intravascular coagulation)
  - Haematological disorders (e.g. myeloproliferative)
  - Infections (e.g. malaria, leishmaniasis, EBV)
  - Storage disorders (e.g. Gaucher disease, Niemann–Pick disease)
  - Inflammatory disorders (e.g. systemic lupus erythematosus, Felty syndrome)
- Abnormal platelet distribution:
  - Splenomegaly
  - Transfusion of stored blood

Classification

- Typically, thrombocytopenia is classified according to the platelet count
  - Mild: 100–150 $\times 10^9$/L
  - Moderate: 50–100 $\times 10^9$/L
  - Severe: 30–50 $\times 10^9$/L
  - Life-threatening: <30 $\times 10^9$/L

Table 11.4.3 Drugs that may impair platelet function.

Class	Examples
Alcohol	
Analgesics and other platelet inhibitors	Aspirin Other non-steroidal anti-inflammatory drugs Clopidogrel
Antibiotics	Amoxicillin Ampicillin and derivatives Azithromycin Benzylpenicillin (penicillin G) Carbenicillin Cephalosporins Gentamicin Meticillin Rifampicin Sulfonamides Trimethoprim
Antidiabetics	Tolbutamide
Cardiovascular drugs	Digitoxin Heparin Methyldopa Oxprenolol Quinine
Cytotoxic drugs	Many drugs
Diuretics	Acetazolamide Chlorpromazine Furosemide
General anaesthetic agents	Halothane
Psychoactive drugs	Antihistamines (some) Chlorpromazine Diazepam Haloperidol Tricyclic antidepressants Valproate

Clinical Presentation

- Usually asymptomatic in patients with platelet counts above 50×10^9/L
- Severe thrombocytopenia can cause:
  - Petechiae
  - Ecchymoses
  - Postoperative haemorrhage
  - Spontaneous bleeding in/from inflamed tissue

Diagnosis

- Clinical findings
- Reduced platelet count, as identified from a full blood count test
- Prolonged bleeding time (rarely used)

Management

- Treatment is dependent on the underlying cause
- Platelet transfusions may be given to cover invasive/surgical procedures or to manage uncontrolled bleeding
  - Platelet-rich plasma (PRP): 90% of platelets of 1 unit of blood in half the volume
  - Platelet-rich concentrate (PRC): 50% of platelets of 1 unit of blood in 25 mL; best source of platelets
  - One unit/pack of platelets will only raise the platelet count by ~$10–35 \times 10^9$/L (for an average size adult)
  - Infused platelets are rapidly sequestered/broken down (hence surgery needs to be undertaken as soon as possible after administration)
  - Less effective in immune conditions such as immune thrombocytopenia
  - Risk of infusions: pruritus, isoimmunisation, infection with blood-borne agents and graft versus host disease (rare)
- Tranexamic acid may be given for topical use as a mouthwash, orally or intravenously
- Corticosteroid or immunosuppressive agents may be of value in conditions mediated by an inappropriate immune response (e.g. immune thrombocytopenia)
- Second-line therapies for immune conditions such as immune thrombocytopenia involve the use of thrombopoietin receptor agonists (e.g. eltrombopag, romiplostim, avatrombopag); another option is anti-CD20 antibody, rituximab, which reduces IgG antibody production
- Third-line therapies are used for the small percentage of patients who fail to respond or tolerate first- or second-line treatments; these include dapsone, azathioprine, cyclophosphamide and cyclosporine
- Sometimes splenectomy is required

Prognosis

- About 20% of cases are resistant to treatment
- Prognosis is related to the severity of thrombocytopenia and the underlying disease (e.g. thrombotic thrombocytopenic purpura has a 75% mortality rate)

A World/Transcultural View

- Platelet transfusions and therapies for immune-mediated thrombocytopenia may be expensive and not consistently available across the world
- This can result in inequalities in terms of access to preventive care
- This is particularly true for second- and third-line therapies, such as thrombopoietin receptor agonists used for immune-mediated thrombocytopenia

Recommended Reading

Estcourt, L. J., Malouf, R., Doree, C., Trivella, M., Hopewell, S., and Birchall, J. (2018). Prophylactic platelet transfusions prior to surgery for people with a low platelet count. *Cochrane Database Syst. Rev.* 9: CD012779

Fillmore, W.J., Leavitt, B.D., and Arce, K. (2013). Dental extraction in the thrombocytopenic patient is safe and complications are easily managed. *J. Oral Maxillofac. Surg.* 71: 1647–1652.

Karasneh, J., Christoforou, J., Walker, J.S. et al. (2019). World workshop on oral medicine VII: platelet count and platelet transfusion for invasive dental procedures in thrombocytopenic patients: a systematic review. *Oral Dis.* 25 (Suppl 1). 174–181.

Khammissa, R.A.G., Fourie, J., Masilana, A. et al. (2018). Oral manifestations of thrombocytopaenia. *Saudi Dent. J.* 30: 19–25.

McCord, C. and Johnson, L. (2017). Oral manifestations of hematologic disease. *Atlas Oral Maxillofac. Durg. Clin. North Am.* 25: 149–162.

Provan, D., Arnold, D.M., Bussel, J.B. et al. (2019). Updated international consensus report on the investigation and management of primary immune thrombocytopenia. *Blood Adv.* 3: 3780–3817.

Sandhu, S., Sankar, V., and Villa, A. (2020). Bleeding risk in thrombocytopenic patients after dental extractions: a retrospective single-center study. *Oral Surg. Oral Med. Oral Pathol. Oral Radiol.* 129: 478–483.

11.5 Leukaemias

Section I: Clinical Scenario and Dental Considerations

Clinical Scenario

A 47-year-old male is referred for urgent dental assessment by his haemato-oncology specialist. The patient complains of recurrent pain from a tooth in the upper left quadrant which is typically present 1 week after chemotherapy and then subsides.

Medical History
- Chronic myeloid leukaemia (CML)
  - Diagnosed 2 months ago
  - Already commenced 3 cycles of chemotherapy
  - Due to have cycle 4 in 7 days' time
- Diabetes mellitus type 2

Medications
- Imatinib (3 cycles)
- Vitamin D
- Calcium supplementation
- Metformin
- Long-acting insulin

Dental History
- Irregular dental attender; only attends when in pain due to limited financial resources and lack of access
- Brushes his teeth once a day
- Diet – due to discomfort from his mouth during chemotherapy, can only eat soft food; also has 4 nutritional supplements drinks as advised by his clinical nurse specialist

Social History
- Originally from Bangladesh – has been living and working overseas for 10 years
- Lives with his cousin
- Married; wife and children live in Bangladesh
- Works as a construction worker
- Tobacco consumption: 10 cigarettes daily for 10 years; smokeless tobacco – chews paan 4 times daily for 20 years
- Alcohol consumption: nil

Oral Examination
- Dry lips, mild xerostomia
- Generalised dental plaque, calculus (particularly lingual to lower anterior teeth), staining (Figure 11.5.1)
- Interdental food packing posterior quadrants
- Paan remnants in the lower left buccal vestibule; adjacent white patch on the buccal mucosa; stiffening/banding of the tissue
- Caries in #13, #26 and #27

Radiological Examination
- Orthopantomogram undertaken – demonstrates generalised mild bone loss
- Bilateral bite wing radiographs – extensive caries with likely pulpal involvement #26 (distal) and #27 (mesial) (Figure 11.5.2)

Structured Learning

1) What is the significance of the patient taking imatinib?
   - Imatinib is a targeted cancer therapy drug (biological therapy)
   - It acts as a tyrosine kinase inhibitor, thereby blocking the growth of cancer cells
   - It is taken orally once or twice a day
   - In addition to the general side-effects of cancer therapy, it has been implicated in the development of medication-related osteonecrosis of the jaw (MROJ)

A Practical Approach to Special Care in Dentistry, First Edition. Edited by Pedro Diz Dios and Navdeep Kumar.

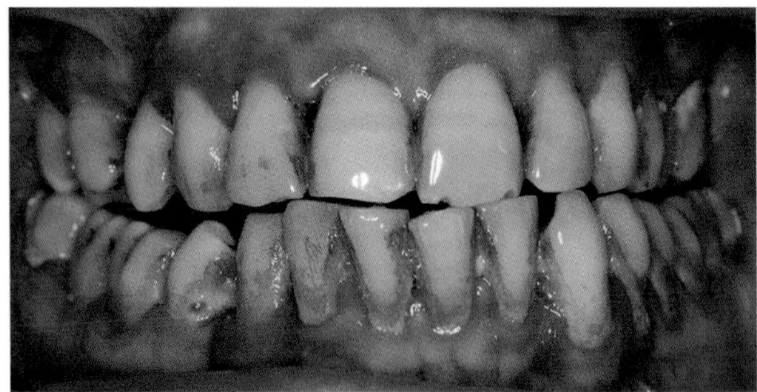

Figure 11.5.1 Generalised dental plaque, calculus and staining.

(a)

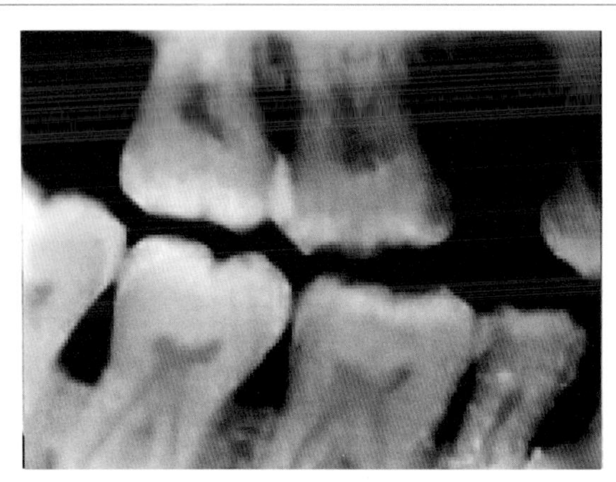

(b)

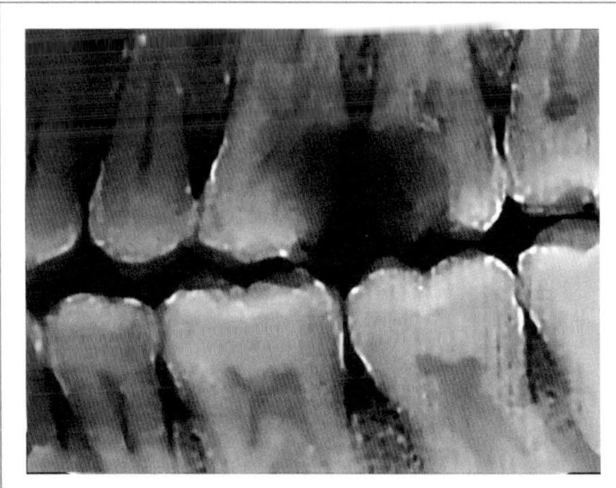

Figure 11.5.2 (a,b) Right and left bitewing radiographs demonstrating extensive caries #26 and #27 and subgingival calculus.

2) What could be the cause of the lesion in the left buccal mucosa?
   - The patient chews paan which is typically composed of areca nut, slaked lime (from limestone or coral) and tobacco wrapped within a betel leaf
   - This is known to be associated with yellow-brown staining of the teeth and mucosal surfaces, the development of white patches (leucoplakia) and oral submucous fibrosis (associated with the areca nut)
3) You advise the patient to stop chewing the paan due to the negative impact on his oral health and the risk of oral cancer. He advises you that it helps him to cope with his chemotherapy and manage his diabetes. What could be the perceived benefits he is referring to?
   - Paan is perceived as a cure for halitosis
   - It is also used by some patients to manage symptoms such as nausea and vomiting associated with chemotherapy
   - Some patients with diabetes also believe that paan helps control the disease
   - However, the perceived health benefits are not proven
   - The risks of continued paan use, particularly when it contains areca nut and tobacco, outweigh any possible benefits
4) Sensibility testing is undertaken on #26 and #27. Both teeth are confirmed to be non-vital. The patient requests root canal treatment as he does not want to lose more teeth. What would you discuss?
   - If the teeth are restorable, endodontic treatment followed by restoration and a full-coverage restoration at a later stage is an option
   - However, consideration should be given to the fact that the patient is receiving active chemotherapy to control his CML
   - Completion of multiroot endodontic treatment and restoration is likely to cause further delays to chemotherapy
   - Furthermore, although the success rate of root canal treatment is 90–95%, a risk of reinfection remains which can cause further delays
   - As the patient is immunocompromised due to both CML and cancer therapy, the success rate is likely to be lower
   - This can pose a further risk during chemotherapy and delay treatment further due to the potential for bacteraemia
5) Following discussion with the haemato-oncologist, dental extraction of #26 and #27 is advised. What factors would you need to take into account?
   - It is ideal to wait at least 10 days post dental extractions before recommencing chemotherapy (to allow for primary healing); hence the next cycle of chemotherapy may need to be delayed (risks and benefits of this should be discussed with the haemato-oncologist)
   - Increased risk of bleeding, infection and delayed wound healing

- This would then need to be followed by further close reviews due to the risk of MRONJ

6) Preoperative blood tests confirm the Hb level is 100 g/dL, platelets 65×10^9/L and neutrophil count 0.5×10^9/L. What are the implications for dental extractions given these blood counts (see Chapter 12.2)?
   - The Hb count is reduced, indicating that the patient is anaemic; this is associated with hypoxia, lethargy and fatigue; supplemental nasal oxygen at 2–3 L/min should be considered during dental extractions
   - Although the platelet levels are low, they are sufficient to proceed with dental extractions under local anaesthesia without platelet supplementation; local haemostatic measures should be used, including sutures and haemostatic agents (sponges and tranexamic acid mouthwash)
   - The neutrophil count is significantly reduced; this is associated with a significant risk of infection; perioperative antibiotic prophylaxis and granulocyte-colony stimulating factor (G-CSF) subcutaneous injections typically given for 5 days prior to surgery, may be advised by the haemato-oncologist; G-CSF stimulates the bone marrow to produce more white blood cells, although it is used with caution as it may stimulate some leukaemic processes; it is currently considered as a safe and effective way to stimulate myelopoiesis and allows for continued imatinib therapy in CML patients at risk for disease progression
7) What other factors do you need to consider in your risk assessment?
   - Social
     - Patient is likely to be fatigued due to CML and chemotherapy
       An escort is desirable
     - When scheduling dental appointments, need to consider the timing and impact of the cancer therapy hospital visits
   - Medical
     - Anaemia, thrombocytopenia and neutropenia are common side-effects of CML treatment
     - Caution when interpreting the haemoglobin A_{1c} levels as anaemia in relation to chemotherapy and/or cancer therapy (anaemia may exaggerate the glycaemic status of the patient)
   - Dental
     - Acute and chronic side-effects of chemotherapy
     - Risk of MROJ
     - Calorific supplement drinks and soft diet increase caries risk
     - Suboptimal oral hygiene habits
     - Compliance issues in daily life
     - Lack of perceived need
     - Irregular dental attender
     - Xerostomia due to chemotherapy and diabetes
     - Increased risk of periodontal disease due to diabetes (bidirectional relationship)
     - Food packing
     - Paan-associated risk of oral submucous fibrosis

General Dental Considerations

Oral Findings

- Oropharyngeal lesions can be the presenting complaint in >10% of cases of acute leukaemia
- Oral bleeding and petechiae/ecchymoses are typical manifestations
- Gingival swelling secondary to infiltration of gingival tissue with leukaemia cells (Figure 11.5.3); this is most commonly seen with acute myeloid leukaemia subtypes (~67% acute monocytic leukaemia, ~18% acute myelomonocytic leukaemia, ~4% acute myelocytic leukaemia). Instances of gingival or palatal enlargement have also been reported in chronic lymphocytic leukaemia
- Herpetic oral and perioral infections are common and troublesome (viruses can also cause encephalitis or pneumonia)
- Candidiasis is particularly common in oral cavity and paranasal sinuses; usually caused by *Candida albicans*
- Aspergillosis and mucormycosis can involve the maxillary antrum and be invasive
- Bacterial infections more common, including *Pseudomonas* spp., *Serratia* spp., *Klebsiella* spp., *Enterobacter* spp., *Proteus* spp. and *Escherichia* spp.; Gram-negative species occasionally cause oral lesions

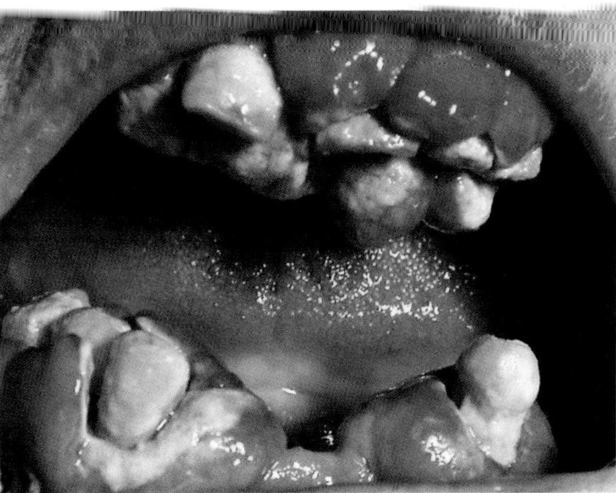

Figure 11.5.3 Infiltration of gingival tissue with leukaemia cells in a patient with acute myeloid leukaemia.

which become a major source of septicaemia or metastatic infections

- In severely immunocompromised patients, over 50% of systemic infections result from oropharyngeal micro-organisms
- Other oral/perioral findings
  - Mucosal pallor
  - Mucosal or gingival ulceration
  - Pericoronitis
  - Cervical lymphadenopathy
  - Tonsillar swelling
  - Paraesthesia (particularly of lower lip)
  - Extrusion of teeth
  - Painful swelling of major salivary glands (Mikulicz syndrome)
- Radiographic changes
  - May be reversible with chemotherapy
  - Destruction of crypts of developing teeth
  - Thinning or disappearance of lamina dura (especially premolar and molar regions)
  - Loss of alveolar crestal bone, and bone destruction near apices of mandibular posterior teeth
- Side-effects of cancer therapy may also be observed (see Chapter 12.2); commonly include mucositis, sometimes with ulceration

Dental Management

- Dental treatment modification depends on the severity of the underlying disease, the intensity and stage of cancer therapy, and the urgency/invasiveness of the proposed dental intervention (Tables 11.5.1 and 11.5.2)
- Treatment should be modified based on reassessment of the patient on the day of the appointment

Section II: Background Information and Guidelines

Definition

Leukaemia is a malignant proliferation of haematopoietic tissue that progressively displaces normal blood-forming elements of the bone marrow.

Aetiopathogenesis

Currently unknown, but predisposing factors implicated include the following:

- Genetics
  - Twins
  - Chromosomal abnormalities (e.g. Down syndrome)

Table 11.5.1 Principles of oral healthcare in leukaemia.

Prior to cancer therapy	During cancer therapy	Following cancer therapy (Long term)
• Oral/dental assessment • Treatment planning • Removal of non-salvageable teeth • Treatment of caries • Advice on potential side-effects, oral hygiene, diet, denture use and hygiene • Periodontal treatment • Removal of trauma • Discontinuation of ongoing long-term dental treatments – orthodontic treatment • Antibiotic prophylaxis • Haematological support • Initiation of fluoride and chlorhexidine prophylaxis	• Continuation of preventive oral healthcare advice in addition to the use of foam swabs, gauze, oral cleansers • Antifungal and antiviral prophylaxis • Monitoring and management of mucositis and xerostomia • Avoidance of elective dental treatment	• Continuation of preventive oral healthcare advice, fluoride supplementation, denture hygiene advice and smoking cessation • Monitor risk of caries, periodontal disease, candidiasis (in denture wearers) • Monitoring of craniofacial and dental development • Management of chronic oral complications • Considerations regarding restorations, orthodontic treatment initiation and dental implant placement • Management and monitoring of medication-related osteonecrosis of the jaw • Discharge to primary care dentist team for long-term review

Table 11.5.2 Dental management considerations.

Risk assessment	• Increased susceptibility to infection • Bleeding tendency • Anaemia • Increased risk of infection and blood-borne viruses spread due to blood transfusions • Susceptibility to HBV, HCV or HIV infection (HIV patients at higher risk of developing acute myeloid leukaemia; higher risk of HBV reactivation; HCV possible cause for certain non-Hodgkin lymphoma) • Corticosteroid treatment-related complications (see Chapter 12.1) • Other factors: disseminated intravascular coagulopathy • Complications of bone marrow transplantation (see Chapter 11.6)
Criteria for referral	• Patients with relatively stable blood counts may be seen in a primary care setting • Patients who require haematological support (e.g. platelets) prior to invasive dental treatment, should preferably be seen in a hospital setting
Access/position	• Ideally patients should be referred for a dental assessment and completion of any urgent dental treatment prior to the commencement of cancer therapy • Schedule essential invasive dental treatment when the effects of any concurrent chemotherapy on the full blood count have diminished (liaise with the haemato-oncologist); commonly, patients receive cycles of 1 week chemotherapy and 3 weeks rest • Defer any non-essential dental treatment until a remission phase • If the patient is admitted in a hospital ward, they may be in isolation (e.g. in a laminar flow room); access to the patient may be limited; if ward visits are permitted in the case of dental emergencies, strict asepsis is indicated • Wheelchair access may be required (patient may be weak, fatigued and hypoxic) • Ensure that the patient is seen in a timely manner – minimise waiting times and exposure to other patients in the waiting room • In order to avoid prolonged disruption of cancer therapy, it may be preferable to plan for a longer dental appointment so that dental assessment, investigations and treatment can be provided on the same day • The patient may need to be kept in a semi-upright position if they are profoundly hypoxic and/or the airway is compromised (e.g. due to mucositis)
Communication	• Consult closely with the haemato-oncologist/physician as dental treatment and timing may be affected by various aspects of leukaemia management and patient's life expectancy • Patients with any cancer may have severe psychological disturbances in view of the nature of the illness • Provide written information to the patient regarding the impact of cancer therapy on the mouth
Capacity/consent	• Discuss the currently available guidance regarding chemotherapy and invasive dental treatment (risks/benefits) with the patient; provide this in a written form and allow the patient to consider the options • Consider psychological well-being as it may affect patient's ability to comprehend, weigh risk and benefits and consent to treatment
Anaesthesia/sedation	• Local anaesthesia – Local anaesthesia with vasoconstriction may be used to control bleeding – Regional block injections may be contraindicated if there is a severe haemorrhagic tendency/significantly low platelet levels – A preoperative antiseptic rinse such as chlorhexidine has been suggested • Sedation – Nitrous oxide is best avoided if a patient is being treated with methotrexate since toxic effects may be exacerbated (largely theoretical) – Consider the severity of anaemia as sedation can cause further hypoxia – Intravenous sedation should be used with caution if platelet counts are low, as cannulation may be complicated by haematoma formation • General anaesthesia – Severe anaemia is a contraindication – Intubation is associated with additional risks if there is associated thrombocytopenia

(Continued)

Table 11.5.2 (Continued)

Dental treatment	• Before – Treatment should be provided in consultation with the multidisciplinary team involved in caring for the patient – Patients receiving palliative therapy must be kept free of active dental disease, although it may not be possible to provide definitive care – The results of a recent full blood count (ideally undertaken on the same day as the dental visit) should be checked – Haematological support should be arranged by the medical team (desmopressin, platelet infusions or blood may be needed preoperatively) – Antibiotic cover may be required for any surgery, particularly for those patients who are neutropenic/have indwelling atrial catheters • During – Surgery ○ Local haemostatic measures should be used ○ Judicious use of packing agents in extraction sockets as they may act as a nidus for infection – Periodontology ○ Full blood and platelet counts checked before scaling and periodontal surgery ○ Teeth with dubious prognosis (periodontal pockets >7 mm) should be extracted prior to chemotherapy ○ An interval of at least 10 days to 2 weeks between extracting the teeth and starting chemotherapy is ideal – Orthodontics ○ Orthodontic bands and appliances contributing to poor oral hygiene or mucosal irritation should be removed before chemotherapy – Paediatric dentistry ○ Mobile primary teeth should be removed (ideally before chemotherapy) – Endodontics/prosthodontics ○ Root canal treatment of restorable anterior teeth may be considered ○ Avoid elective placement of fixed prosthodontics during cancer therapy – Implantology ○ Should be deferred until after cancer therapy/the patient is in remission • After – Liaise with the haemato-oncology team to advise them of the dental treatment outcome – Give patient written postoperative instructions and emergency contact details – Review in 1 week after dental procedure
Drug prescription	• Antiseptics (e.g. 0.12–0.2% chlorhexidine rinses) may be considered • Avoid aspirin and non-steroidal anti-inflammatory drugs which increase the risk of bleeding, may exacerbate a corticosteroid induced peptic ulcer and potentiate the nephrotoxicity of cyclosporine and tacrolimus • Paracetamol is preferred for pain relief but may mask neutropenic fever • Antibiotics may be given until surgical wound healing is complete (penicillin is antibiotic of choice)
Education/prevention	• Educate about the side-effects of chemotherapy and, where relevant, the additional risk of medication-related osteonecrosis of the jaw • Advise the patient to stop smoking and drinking alcohol and to maintain good oral hygiene; this will reduce the oral side-effects of chemotherapy, reduce postoperative complications after invasive dental treatment and reduce the risk of a second cancer • Emphasis on prevention and oral hygiene advice to avoid the need for future dental procedures that may require surgery • Regular warm aqueous chlorhexidine mouthwashes may be considered • Use of a soft nylon toothbrush may be indicated if platelet levels are significantly reduced • Fluoride mouthwash, higher concentration fluoride toothpaste and/or supplements should be considered

- Most patients with chronic myeloid leukaemia have hybrid chromosomes formed between chromosome 22 and 9 (Philadelphia chromosome)
- Immunodeficiency states/acquired haematological disorders (e.g. aplastic anaemia, myeloproliferative disorders and myelodysplastic syndromes)
- Exposure to toxic chemicals (e.g. benzene, petrochemicals, tobacco tar)
- Cytotoxic drugs (e.g. anticancer alkylating agents)
- Ionising radiation
- Viruses (e.g. human T-cell lymphotrophic retrovirus type 1)

Clinical Presentation

- Most common findings arise from the crowding-out of normal blood cells from the marrow by leukaemic cells, leading to:
  - Anaemia resulting in malaise and weakness
  - Thrombocytopenia leading to bleeding
  - Leucocyte defects/neutropenia predisposing to opportunistic infections
  - Lymphadenopathy, especially in lymphatic leukaemias
- When the disease progresses, leukaemic tissue may infiltrate gingivae, testes, liver, spleen, lymph nodes, ears and central nervous system
- Other symptoms include unexplained fever, night sweats, weight loss, nausea and vomiting, headaches, confusion, balance problems, blurred vision, painful lymph node swellings, shortness of breath, abdominal discomfort/swelling, testicular discomfort/swelling, pain in bones/joints, weakness/loss of muscle control, seizures

Classification

- Leukaemias are classified according to the predominant cell type and degree of maturity of the cells involved (Figure 11.5.4; Table 11.5.3); this assists in prescribing the most effective management
- The predominant cell type may be lymphoid (LL) or myeloid (ML)
- The degree of maturity the cells display is acute or chronic
  - Acute (ALL, AML)
    - Primitive blast cells in blood and bone marrow (50% of all malignancies in children)
    - Symptoms develop fairly quickly
    - Complications include secondary malignancy, infertility, endocrine dysfunction, neuropsychological effects, cardiorespiratory sequelae and graft vs host disease
  - Chronic (CLL, CML)

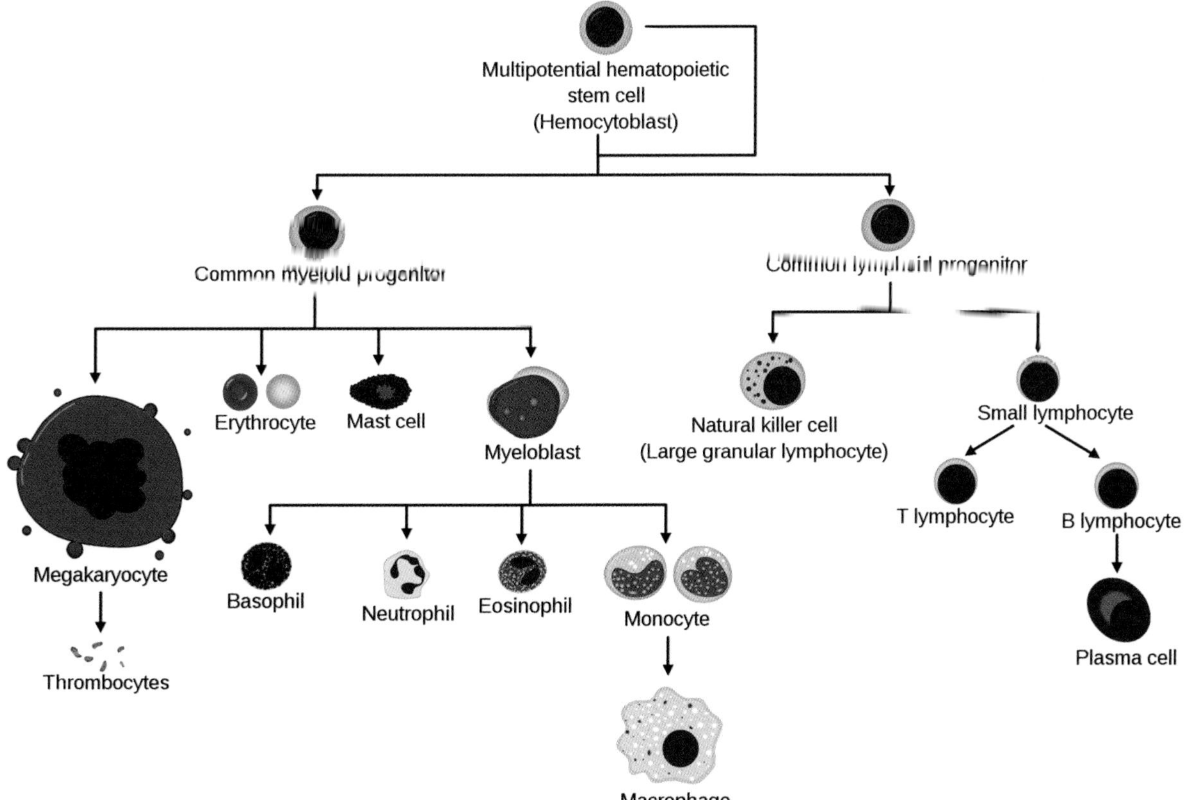

Figure 11.5.4 Formation of blood cells (haematopoiesis). *Source*: A. Rad and M. Häggström. CC-BY-SA 3.0 licence.

Table 11.5.3 Classification of leukaemia.

Types of leukaemia	Variant	Characteristics	Clinical features	Treatment
Acute lymphoblastic (ALL)	• Homogeneous small blast type • Heterogeneous blast cell type • Homogeneous large blast type	• Predominantly affects children (65%) – peak incidence 0–4 years • Central nervous system involvement • No pre-leukaemia phases • Complete remission (combined children/ adults 70–80%) • 2–12 years old >60% cure rate with chemotherapy • Adult 20% cure rate	• Acute serious illness • Infections • Purpura • Gum bleeding on brushing • Bilateral salivary and lacrimal gland swelling (Mikulicz syndrome) • Widespread lymphadenopathy • Cranial nerve palsies • Sensory disturbances	• Chemotherapy, corticosteroids, growth factors, intensive combined treatments • Treatment in isolation • immunocompromised • Prophylactic chemotherapy – radiation/ chemotherapy • Maintenance therapy (consolidation) • Resistant treated with haemopoietic stem cell transplantation (HSCT), with chemotherapy and total body irradiation
Acute myeloid (AML)	• Myeloblastic without differentiation • Myeloblastic with differentiation • Hypergranular • Promyelocytic • Acute myelomonocytic • Monocytic • Erythroleukemia • Megakaryoblastic	• Most common acute leukaemia in male adults – peak incidence young adults/middle age • Central nervous system involvement • 80% complete remission • 10% resistant to disease • 10% mortality	• Oral clinical features more commonly observed (e.g. gingival infiltration, bone infiltration, tooth mobility, neuropathy) • Anaemia-related symptoms and lesions	• Chemotherapy – main treatment • Radiotherapy • Growth factors – increase white blood cells/stem cells • HSCT

(Continued)

Table 11.5.3 (Continued)

Types of leukaemia	Variant	Characteristics	Clinical features	Treatment
Chronic lymphoid (CLL)	• Lymphocytic • Sezary syndrome • Hairy cell • Prolymphocytic • T-cell	• Most common type of leukaemia (~25%) • Almost twice as common as CML • Mostly affects elderly (mean age ≈ 65 years) • 2:1 ratio of males to females • 10% family history • Deranged apoptosis – cells survive abnormally long time and accumulate	• Asymptomatic – 1/3 diagnosed following routine full blood count • Recurrent/severe infections (e.g. shingles) • Lymphadenopathy – painless • Fever • Splenomegaly • Low platelets	• Asymptomatic are monitored (30% patients) • Prompt antibiotics/ antivirals/ antifungals • Chemotherapy (nucleoside analogues, chlorambucil) • Corticosteroids • Radiotherapy • Intravenous immunoglobulin – which reduces recurrent infections • HSCT – for younger patients
Chronic myeloid (CML)	• Granulocytic • Atypical granulocytic • Juvenile • Myelomonocytic • Neutrophilic • Eosinophilic	• ~14% of all leukaemia • Most common in adults (40–60 years) • After 4–5 years, transforms to acute phase similar to AML • CML also classified by phase (chronic, accelerated and blast), defined by number of blasts in blood and bone marrow • Defined by the presence of Philadelphia chromosome (abnormal chromosome 22)	• Pallor • Symptomatic anaemia – shortness of breath • Progressive splenomegaly (>75%) and associated abdominal discomfort • Weight loss • Fever and sweats in the absence of infection • Lymphadenopathy – uncommon, suggests transformation to acute leukaemia • Retinal damage	• Biological therapy (imatinib, nilotinib) • Chemotherapy (hydroxyurea) • Interferon-alpha • HSCT – cure 70% chronic phase

  - Excess of mature leucocytes in blood and bone marrow
  - Mostly disease of adult life
  - May progress to acute leukaemia
  - Symptoms develop gradually (20% do not have symptoms at time of diagnosis)

Diagnosis

- Full blood count with differential – leucocyte count high and platelet/erythrocyte counts low
- Bone marrow biopsy via an aspirate
- Cytogenetics
- Supplemental tests: chest x-ray, computed tomography, nuclear magnetic resonance imaging, lumbar puncture

Treatment

- Chemotherapy
  - Cytotoxic chemotherapy drugs inhibit cell division and/or protein synthesis
  - These may be administered via peripherally inserted central catheter, intrathecal, peritoneal, pleural, topical
  - Administered in 3 phases:
    - Induction – purpose is to kill as many leukaemia cells as possible to achieve remission
    - Consolidation – seek out and kill residual leukaemia cells not destroyed by induction
    - Maintenance – keep numbers of leukaemia cells low (i.e. keep disease in remission); doses of chemotherapy lower than first 2 phases; length up to 2 years
  - General complications include alopecia, bone marrow suppression, hyperuricaemia, mucositis, nausea/vomiting
  - Long-term effects include reproductive function suppression, secondary cancers, pulmonary fibrosis, cardiomyopathy, nerve damage, loss of hearing and renal impairment
  - Advances in chemotherapy include better control of immune effects and side-effects, newer drugs (e.g. taxanes), new techniques (nanoparticles) and adjunctive therapies (hormonal therapy and biological therapy – commonly alpha-interferon, also monoclonal antibodies or interleukins)
- Radiation therapy
  - Treatment of disease with ionising radiation
  - Indications include:
    - Curative or adjuvant cancer treatment
    - Palliative treatment (where cure is not possible, and the aim is for local disease control or symptomatic relief)
    - Total body irradiation is a radiotherapy technique used to prepare the body to receive a bone marrow transplant
- Haematopoietic stem cell transplantation
  - High-dose chemotherapy with total body irradiation to kill the leukaemia cells causes immune system depletion
  - Significant risk of serious life-threatening infections that are treated in sterile, air-filtered marrow transplant rooms
  - Allogeneic stem cells transplanted into vein from healthy, complete blood cell-matched donor (sibling best)
  - Can be pretreated autologous, but far less successful
- Management of symptoms and adverse effects of treatment
  - Control of nausea, infections, haemorrhagic tendencies, anaemia, pain, renal malfunction

Prognosis

- In general, acute leukaemias respond well to treatment and some may be cured
- Chronic leukaemias cannot be cured but can be controlled for long periods
- ALL: best prognosis, especially <10 years old; complete remission is achieved in 95% of children and 75% of adults; relapse risk is greatest in the first 18 months; maintenance therapy is required for 2–3 years
- AML: up to 80% can expect complete remission, and 45% of those can survive 3 or more years
- Chronic leukaemias are usually associated with death in within 3–5 years, although in CLL, the disease is so indolent that an older person with CLL may die from other causes
- After 5 years, 80% of patients without detectable disease are likely to maintain a lifelong remission
- Patients in remission >15 years considered unequivocally cured

A World/Transcultural View

- In 2008 the World Health Organization (WHO) classification of tumours of the haematopoietic and lymphoid tissues was updated
- Since then, there have been numerous advances in the identification and diagnosis of leukaemias
- Substantial racial differences exist in both the incidence and treatment outcome of childhood acute lymphoblastic leukaemia
- Although the survival rate has increased overall, this is not universal across the world as disparities in access to targeted therapies and improved chemotherapy regimens continue to exist
- Asians experienced some of the largest survival improvements during recent years; however, there were no substantial improvements in leukaemia-specific survival among African Americans and the elderly

Recommended Reading

Abed, H., Alhabshi, M., Alkhayal, Z. et al. (2019). Oral and dental management of people with myelodysplastic syndromes and acute myeloid leukemia: a systematic search and evidence-based clinical guidance. *Spec. Care Dentist.* 39: 406–420.

Aggarwal, A. and Pai, K. (2018). Orofacial manifestations of leukaemic children on treatment: a descriptive study. *Int. J. Clin. Pediatr. Dent.* 11: 193–198.

Angst, P.D.M., Maier, J., Dos Santos, N.R. et al. (2020). Oral health status of patients with leukemia: a systematic review with meta-analysis. *Arch. Oral Biol.* 120: 104948.

Bhatnagar, N., Qureshi, A., and Hall, G. (2017). Leukaemias: a review. *Paediatr. Child Health* 27: 489–494.

Cammarata-Scalisi, F., Girardi, K., Strocchio, L. et al. (2020). Oral manifestations and complications in childhood acute myeloid leukemia. *Cancers* (Basel) 12: 1634.

Parra, J.J., Alvarado, M.C., Monsalve, P. et al. (2020). Oral health in children with acute lymphoblastic leukaemia: before and after chemotherapy treatment. *Eur. Arch. Paediatr. Dent.* 21: 129–136.

Royal College of Surgeons of England/BSDH (2018). *The Oral Management of Oncology Patients Requiring Chemotherapy, Radiotherapy and/or Bone Marrow Transplantation – 2018 Updated Guidelines*. London: Royal College of Surgeons of England.

11.6 Lymphoma

Section I: Clinical Scenario and Dental Considerations

Clinical Scenario

A 26-year-old woman is referred by her oncologist for urgent dental assessment. The patient complains of increasing discomfort and mobility of the lower right second molar tooth of 1 week's duration. There is no previous history of symptoms from this tooth.

Medical History

- Hodgkin lymphoma (mediastinal bulky disease) diagnosed 4 years ago with multiple antineoplastic treatment regimens used in the past:
  - ABVD: doxorubicin (also known as adriamycin)/bleomycin/vinblastine/dacarbazine
  - ESHAP: etoposide/methylprednisolone/cytarabine/cisplatin
  - IVAC: ifosfamide/etoposide/citarabine
  - Total body irradiation (40 Gy) delivered to the mediastinal region
- Allogeneic haematopoietic stem cell transplantation (allo-HSCT) undertaken 2 years ago, with several severe complications post transplantation:
  - *Aspergillus fumigatus* sinusitis
  - Cytomegalovirus reactivation
  - Reservoir infection
  - Severe pericardial effusion
  - Septicemia due to *Staphylococcus aureus* and *Streptococcus pneumoniae*
  - Severe neuropathy in lower limbs
  - Thrombocytopenia

Medications

- Brentuximab
- Prednisone
- Fluconazole
- Aciclovir
- Alprazolam
- Magnesium and vitamin B supplements

Dental History

- Irregular dental attender; only attends when in pain
- Brushes teeth 3 times daily using a soft manual toothbrush
- Diet – due to discomfort from her mouth, predominantly eats soft food

Social History

- Lives with her parents and sister; good family support
- Previously worked in the hospitality industry (currently on leave due to ill health)
- Transport: drives her own car
- Alcohol consumption: nil
- Tobacco consumption: nil

Oral Examination

- Good oral hygiene
- Erythematous, friable and tender oral mucosa
- Ulcerated lesion with necrotic background surrounding the cervical region of #47 (Figure 11.6.1)
- Grade III mobility and pain on percussion of molar #47
- Missing tooth #46
- Fillings in #16, #36, #37 and #47

Radiological Examination

- Orthopantomogram undertaken (Figure 11.6.2)
- Severe vertical bone loss in mesial of #47
- #47: radiolucent periapical lesion with ill-defined borders extending to the inferior alveolar nerve canal

Structured Learning

1) What are the differential diagnoses for a in the mouth which has a similar clinical/radiographic appearance as associated with #47?

A Practical Approach to Special Care in Dentistry, First Edition. Edited by Pedro Diz Dios and Navdeep Kumar.

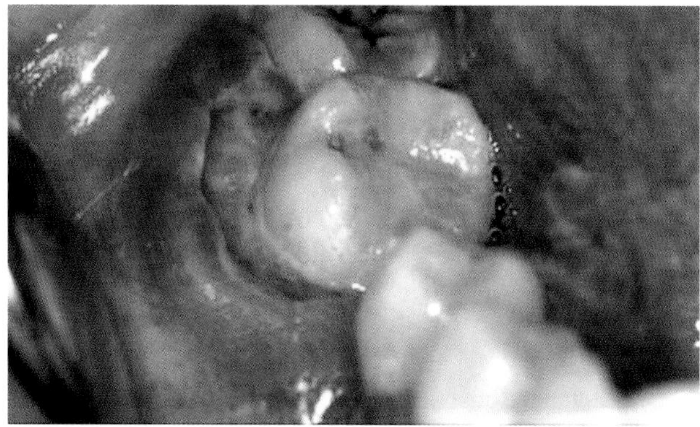

Figure 11.6.1 Extrusion of the lower right second molar and gingival ulcer with necrotic bakground.

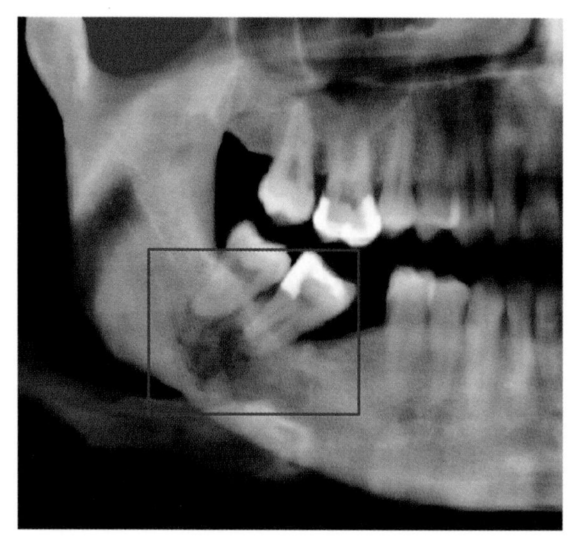

Figure 11.6.2 Orthopantomogram showing #47 radiolucent periapical lesion with ill-defined borders.

- Diffuse periapical infection (atypical presentation)
- Benign lesions: ameloblastomas followed by nasopalatine duct cysts and Stafne bone cavities
- Malignant lesions: metastatic lesions followed by carcinomas

2) Why is medication-related osteonecrosis of the jaw (MRONJ) not included in the differential diagnosis?
   - The patient received radiation therapy which does not meet the MRONJ case definition (see Chapter 16.2)
   - Currently, she is taking brentuximab, an antibody–drug conjugate which at the moment has not been related to the appearance of MRONJ
3) Following electric pulp testing, #47 responds positively and is not hypersensitive to stimulation. What other features indicate that the periapical lesion may be non-dental in origin and could be malignant?
   - Spontaneous tooth mobility and extrusion
   - The patient has a history of lymphoma
   - She is immunosuppressed (radiochemotherapy)
   - Necrotic gingival ulceration
   - Radiolucent periapical lesion with ill-defined borders
4) Given #47 is hypermobile, the patient asks for it to be extracted as she cannot eat on it. What factors do you need to consider in your risk assessment?
   - Social
     - The patient may be fatigued by the cytotoxic treatment and/or the sequelae of radiotherapy and/or sequelae of pericardial effusion
     - Assess whether it is feasible to perform it in the dental chair due to neuropathy of the extremities
     - An escort is recommended
   - Medical
     - A full blood count is needed to rule out anaemia, neutropenia and/or thrombopenia
     - Consider antibiotic prophylaxis as healing is likely to be delayed
     - Assess the need for corticosteroid supplementation (see Chapter 12.1)
     - Complications of allo-HSCT including thrombocytopenia (see Chapters 11.4 and 11.7)
   - Dental
     - Currettage and histological study of the periapical lesion/extracted tooth is mandatory
     - A further biopsy of the oral mucosa is recommended to rule out cytotoxic mucositis, graft-versus-host disease and other causes of erythematous, friable and tender oral mucosa
5) The patient reports feeling slightly anxious and asks if she can have sedation. What would you advise?
   - The patient is regularly taking alprazolam so she may have developed tolerance to benzodiazepines
   - Respiratory function may be impaired due to radiotherapy focused on the mediastinum
   - The blood test results would need to be confirmed as the patient may be anaemic and at increased risk of hypoxia
6) The histopathological report confirms that the currettaged tissue and mucosal biopsy have the features of squamous cell carcinoma. What risk factors does this patient have for this to have developed?
   - The patient has received multiple chemotherapy regimens, including intensive chemotherapy to enable her allo-HSCT

- She remains immunocompromised and is taking systemic steroid long-term

General Dental Considerations

Oral Findings

- Extranodal manifestation of non-Hodgkin lymphoma (Figure 11.6.3)
  - B-cell lymphomas are the most common in the head and neck
  - Oral involvement is more common among HIV-infected patients
  - Painless enlarged cervical nodes
  - Tumour on the gingiva and the palate
  - Ulceration on the gingiva and the palate
  - Parotid, tonsils and cavum (ear) involvement
  - Maxillary bone involvement (16%)
- Extranodal manifestation of Hodgkin lymphoma
  - Very uncommon (~1% of all lymphomas in Waldeyer's ring)
  - Oral manifestations clinically similar to non-Hodgkin lymphoma

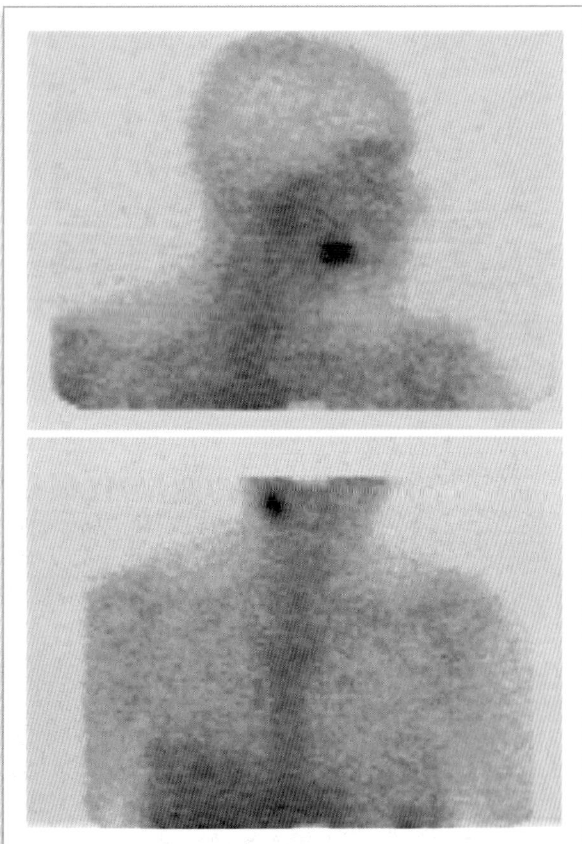

Figure 11.6.3 Radionuclide bone imaging showing mandibular invasion.

- Oral lesions related to immunosuppression (see Chapter 12)
  - Viral, fungal and bacterial infections
- Oral complications related to radiochemotherapy (see Chapter 12)
  - Mucositis, oral ulceration, petechiae, oral paraesthesia, xerostomia
- Oral complications related to bone marrow transplantation (see Chapter 11.7)
  - Mucositis, oral infections, oral ulceration, petechiae, graft-versus-host disease, malignancies (e.g. carcinoma, Kaposi sarcoma, lymphoma)

Dental Management

- Compliance for the delivery of dental care can vary depending on the stage of lymphoma and concurrent cancer therapy
- Treatment should be modified based on reassessment of the patient on the day of the appointment (Table 11.6.1)

Section II: Background Information and Guidelines

Definition

Lymphomas are a heterogeneous group of malignancies that arise from the clonal proliferation of B-cell, T-cell and natural killer (NK) cell subsets of lymphocytes at different stages of maturation. T-cells are programmed for antigen recognition in the thymus whereas B-cells mature in the marrow and encounter foreign antigen for the first time within the lymph node germinal centre (GC). Hence B-cells may be divided into GC or post-GC, with the latter developing eventually into plasma cells, which secrete the soluble form of B-cell receptor, namely immunoglobulin (Ig) or antibody.

Lymphomas represent approximately 5% of malignancies and are broadly classified into Hodgkin lymphoma (HL) and non-Hodgkin lymphoma (NHL). HL is further classified into classic and non-classic types and NHL into B-cell, T-cell and NK cell types (Table 11.6.2). For clinical purposes, lymphoma is termed as aggressive (high grade) and indolent (low grade).

Aetiopathogenesis

- Different environmental, infectious and genetic factors have been identified, which predispose to the development of lymphoma (Table 11.6.3)

Table 11.6.1 Dental management considerations.

Risk assessment	• Similar to leukaemia (see Table 11.5.1) • NHL lesions may present in the oral cavity • Consider infectious organisms which may be implicated in the development of lymphoma and their impact on dental management (e.g. HIV infection) • Patients receiving monoclonal antibody therapy (e.g. rituximab) are considered at risk of developing medication-related osteonecrosis of the jaw (see Chapter 16.2) • Radiation-induced complications (although radiotherapy volume is usually lower for head and neck lymphoma than for other head and neck tumours) • Heart, lung and thyroid disorders (due to mediastinal irradiation), as well as other cancers, can occur secondary to treatment of lymphoma
Criteria for referral	• Similar to leukaemia (see Table 11.5.1)
Access/position	• Similar to leukaemia (see Table 11.5.1) • The patient may need to be kept in a semi-upright position if the airway is compromised due to lymphoma chest involvement or pulmonary irradiation
Communication	• Similar to leukaemia (see Table 11.5.1)
Capacity/consent	
Anaesthesia/sedation	
Dental treatment	
Drug prescription	
Education/prevention	• Similar to leukaemia (see Table 11.5.1) • Any lymph node enlargement, sudden tooth mobility or oral bleeding needs urgent medical consultation

Diagnosis

- Blood tests, including lactate dehydrogenase, full blood counts with differential, urea and electrolytes
- Tissue biopsy with immunohistochemical staining
- Radiographs (Figure 11.6.4)
- PET/CT scans with radiolabelled fluorodeoxyglucose (FDG) to measure the biological activity of lymphoma (Figure 11.6.5)
- Magnetic resonance imaging (MRI) is indicated in certain anatomical areas (e.g. central nervous system, orbits, nose/paranasal sinuses and skull base)
- Bone marrow biopsy
- Cerebrospinal fluid testing

Clinical Presentation

- The clinical features are dependent on the subtype of lymphomas (Table 11.6.2)
- The clinical staging of both HL and NHL is derived from the modified Ann Arbor staging system (Table 11.6.4)

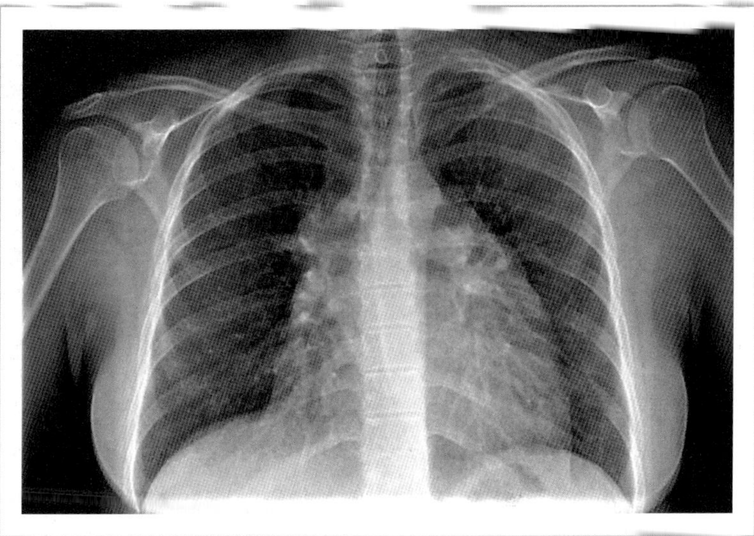

Figure 11.6.4 Mediastinal bulk defined from chest radiograph in Hodgkin lymphoma.

(a)

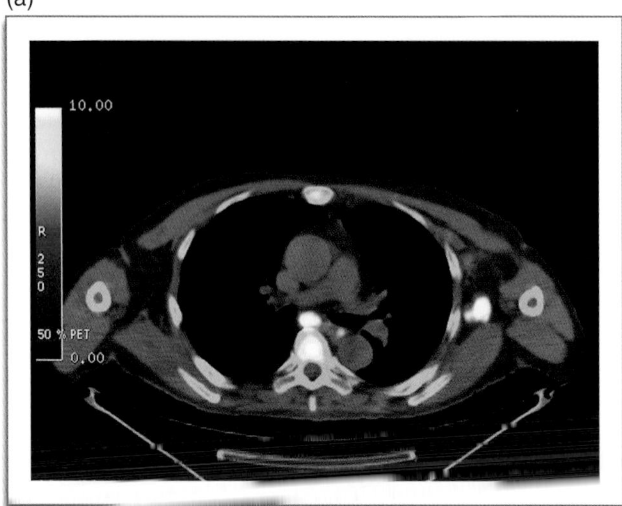

(b)

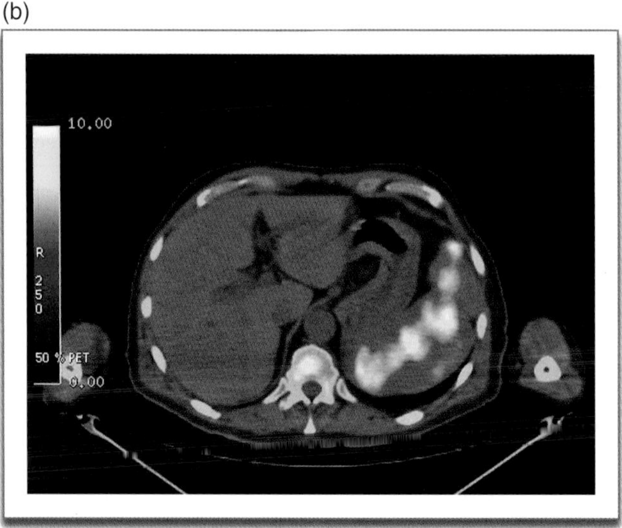

Figure 11.6.5 (a,b) Positron emission tomography/computed tomography (PET/CT) showing lymph nodes, bones and spleen hypermetabolic involvement.

Management

Treatment regimens are specific to the subtype of lymphoma and may include chemotherapy, radiotherapy and haemopoietic stem cell transplantation (Table 11.6.2)

Prognosis

- The prognosis is dependent on the subtype of lymphoma
- Overall survival is estimated to be approximately 70%
- Patients may develop long-term complications
  - Paraneoplastic syndromes (e.g. POEMS syndrome characterised by polyneuropathy, organomegaly, endocrinopathy, monoclonal plasma cell disorder and skin changes)
  - Transformation of indolent forms of NHL such as follicular lymphoma, marginal zone lymphoma into more aggressive NHL (e.g. diffuse large B-cell lymphoma)
  - Chemotherapy complications: pancytopenias, sterility, cardiomyopathy (doxorubicin), pneumonitis (bleomycin), neuropathy (vincristine, brentuximab vedotin) and second primary malignancies (acute myeloblastic and lymphoblastic leukaemias), carcinomas
  - Radiotherapy complications: accelerated atherosclerosis, pericardial fibrosis, second primary cancers (lung, thyroid, breast, soft tissue sarcomas) and hypothyroidism

A World/Transcultural View

- The distribution of lymphomas across the world varies in relation to the associated risk factors

Table 11.6.2 Features of different types of lymphomas.

Main groups of lymphomas	Examples	Typical histopathological characteristics	Clinical features	Treatment
Non-Hodgkin lymphoma (NHL) *(90% of lymphomas)*	• Diffuse large B-cell lymphoma (DLBCL) *(most common NHL; ~20–30% of cases; B-cell)*	• Low-grade lymphomas can develop into high-grade through a transformation of disease into DLBCL • Areas of diffuse involvement by large lymphoid cells that stain positive for B-cell markers CD20 and CD19	• Clinically aggressive • Although it often arises in the lymph nodes, can also present in extranodal sites • The most common complaint is symptomatic, enlarging lymph nodal mass located centrally or peripherally • Can progress with extranodal involvement • ~30% of patients will report B-cell symptoms (unexplained weight loss, fever, night sweats) as well as less specific symptoms of malaise and fatigue	• Aggressive combination chemotherapy can result in long-term disease-free status • R-CHOP • Chemoradiation used for localised disease • Patients with poor performance status are given milder regimes (e.g. R-mini CHOP, R-CVP or single-agent rituximab) • Clinical trials with immunomodulatory agents (lenalidomide) or Bruton's tyrosine kinase inhibitors (ibrutinib) • Anti-CD19 chimeric antigen receptor T-cell therapy • Auto-HSCT • Allo-HSCT • Most disease relapse occurs within 2 years
	• Follicular lymphoma (FL) *(second most common lymphoma; ~20% of cases; B-cell)*	• Originates from the follicular cells in the germinal centre of the lymph node • Overexpression of the antiapoptotic protein BCL-2; due to a translocation 14:18	• Most common presentation is subacute or chronic asymptomatic peripheral lymphadenopathy • Nodal masses are not locally invasive or destructive • Indolent slow-growing, incurable disease • May be asymptomatic, even being untreated, or fluctuate in terms of activity; close monitoring required • Can progress and cause significant symptoms • B-symptoms are seen in less than 20% of patients and can suggest transformation into DLBCL	• If localised, radiotherapy may be given • If more widespread, a single agent such as rituximab may be chosen as first-line therapy • Alternatively, R-Benda has emerged as the most popular treatment • Maintenance chemotherapy often given for 1–2 years • Relapse occurs, with possible transformation to aggressive lymphoma • Overall survival ranges from 8 to 15 years

(*Continued*)

Table 11.6.2 (Continued)

Main groups of lymphomas	Examples	Typical histopathological characteristics	Clinical features	Treatment
	• Marginal zone lymphoma *(~7% of all lymphomas; B-cell)*	• Originates from the mucosa-associated lymphoid tissue (MALT) • Aggregates of small lymphocytes staining positive for CD20 and negative for CD5 and CD10	• Triggered by infection, autoimmune disease or other inflammatory condition • Slow-growing • Presenting symptoms related to the sites of involvement (e.g. stomach, lungs, eyes, bowel, skin) • B-symptoms are rare and should raise suspicion for transformed lymphoma	• Treatment similar to that of follicular lymphomas • For early-stage gastric MALT lymphoma, eradication of *H. pylori* results in tumour regression or remission in 50–80% of patients; where it cannot be eradicated, radiotherapy can be effective • For splenic lesions, surgical splenectomy is indicated, single-agent rituximab therapy is a treatment alternative
	• Mantle cell lymphoma *(~6% of all lymphomas; B-cell)*	• Arises from the postgerminal centre B-cells • Small lymphoid cells staining positive for cyclin D1, a protein involved in cell cycle regulation; results from a translocation 11:14	• Male predominance • Poor prognosis; median survival 5 years • 70–90% of patients present with stage IV/ widespread disease • Bone marrow and gastrointestinal tract involvement are common • Other common sites include spleen and Waldeyer's ring	• R- CHOP or R- Benda, followed by maintenance rituximab • Cytarabine often included as it is particularly effective • Alternating hyper-CVAD with methotrexate/ cytarabine may also be used • Lenalidomide and bortezomib have single-agent activity in cases of relapse • Tyrosine kinase inhibitor, ibrutinib, is now approved in many countries
	• Burkitt lymphoma (BL) *(B-cell; 3 variants: endemic, spontaneous and immunodeficiency associated)*	• Medium to large B-cells with a very high proliferation rate and the classic 'starry sky' appearance • Due to a translocation 8:14, 2:8 or 8:22, of the proto-oncogene C-Myc	• Very aggressive • Endemic BL is prevalent in African children involving the jaw and orbit; it spreads haematogenously to extranodal sites • Sporadic BL presents as a bulky abdominal disease • Immunodeficiency (HIV infection)-related BL usually presents with lymph node involvement	• High proliferation rate requires aggressive chemotherapy regimens • These are associated with complete remission rates of 80–90% and disease-free survival rates of 50–75% • Treatment options include R-hyper-CVAD-methotrexate/cytarabine and R-CODOX-M/IVAC • Recently, DA-R-EPOCH has shown good results

(Continued)

Table 11.6.2 (Continued)

Main groups of lymphomas	Examples	Typical histopathological characteristics	Clinical features	Treatment
	• Peripheral T-cell lymphomas (PTCLs) *(~5–10% of NHL; T- and NK cell; 3 variants: predominantly leukaemic, nodal or extranodal involvement)*	• Diverse and complex histopathology depending on the subtype • Several forms are derived from T-follicular helper cells and are often nodal • Most extranodal T-cell lymphomas are cytotoxic and often arise in mucosa-associated sites	• Leukaemic PTCLs include T-cell prolymphocytic leukaemia, T-cell large granular lymphocytic leukaemia, natural killer/T-cell leukaemia and adult T-cell leukaemia/ lymphoma • Nodal PTCLs include angioimmunoblastic T-cell lymphoma and systemic anaplastic large cell lymphoma • Extranodal PTCLs include mycosis fungoides and cutaneous anaplastic large cell lymphoma	• No consensus on the treatment; depends on subtype • Indolent slow-growing cutaneous T-cell lymphomas can usually be monitored or treated with skin-directed treatments (prednisone, ultraviolet therapy, radiotherapy) or retinoids • For the aggressive PTCLs, chemotherapy with multiple agents is commonly used, such as CHOP • For nasal NK/T-cell lymphoma, radiation therapy in a combined modality therapy results in better outcomes • For CD30-positive lymphomas, the antibody–drug conjugate brentuximab vedotin is effective
Hodgkin lymphoma (HL) *(10% of lymphomas)*	• Classic *(4 variants: nodular sclerosing, mixed cellularity, lymphocyte rich and lymphocyte depleted)* • Non-classic *(only nodular lymphocyte-predominant)*	• Detection of Hodgkin Reed-Sternberg bilobed cells (B-cell origin) on the background of nodular sclerosis, lymphocyte-predominant or depleted stroma • Staining positive for CD30 and CD15 but negative for CD20	• Usually presents as painless swelling of lymph nodes • Later, haematogenous spread occurs • Most patients present with asymptomatic supradiaphragmatic disease: 60–70% cervical and/or supraclavicular lymphadenopathy, 30% axillary disease, 50–60% mediastinal involvement • Only 10–15% of patients have extranodal disease • ~25% of patients with previously undiagnosed HL develop B-symptoms • Other symptoms include severe pruritus and alcohol-induced lymph node pain	• Combined modality therapy, including chemotherapy with antibody–drug conjugates and radiotherapy • Treatment regimens include ABVD, BEACOPP and Stanford V regimen • Overall survival is >80% • Brentuximab vedotin (CD30-targeted antibody–drug conjugate) in combination with AVD chemotherapy for first line treatment of stage III or IV classic HL has been approved • Local radiotherapy may be used for bulky node/ persistent disease • Auto-HSCT/allo-HSCT used in the case of relapse/ resistant disease

R-CHOP: rituximab, cyclophosphamide, doxorubicin, vincristine, prednisone; R-mini CHOP: low-dose CHOP; R-CVP: rituximab, cyclophosphamide, vincristine sulfate, prednisone; HSCT: haematopoietic stem cell transplantation; R-Benda: rituximab-bendamustine; hyper-CVAD: hyperfractionated administration of cyclophosphamide, vincristine, doxorubicin, dexamethasone; R-hyper-CVAD: rituximab-hyper-CVAD; R-CODOX-M/IVAC: rituximab, cyclophosphamide, vincristine, doxorubicin, methotrexate/ ifosfamide, etoposide, cytarabine; DA-R-EPOCH: dose-adjusted etoposide, prednisone, vincristine, cyclophosphamide, doxorubicin, rituximab; ABVD: doxorubicin, bleomycin, vinblastine, dacarbazine; BEACOPP: bleomycin, etoposide, doxorubicin, cyclophosphamide, vincristine, procarbazine, prednisone; Stanford V regimen: doxorubicin, vinblastine, mechlorethamine, vincristine, bleomycin, etoposide, prednisone; AVD: doxorubicin, vinblastine, dacarbazine.

Table 11.6.3 Risk factors associated with the development of lymphomas.

Risk factor	Examples
Genetic	• Characterisation of genetic susceptibility in lymphoma is rapidly evolving • Multiple genetic mutations have been proposed as increasing risk, including mutation in the EZH2 gene (B-cell lymphoma)
Occupational exposure	• Herbicides, pesticides
Infectious organisms	• *Helicobacter pylori* (gastric MALT lymphoma) • *Borrelia burgdorferi* (skin lymphoma) • *Chlamydia psittaci* (ocular lymphoma) • *Campylobacter jejuni* (small intestine lymphoma) • Human T-cell lymphotrophic virus (adult T-cell leukaemia/lymphoma) • Hepatitis C (lymphoplasmacytic lymphoma, diffuse large B-cell lymphoma, marginal zone lymphoma) • Human herpesvirus 8 (primary effusion lymphoma and Castleman disease) • *Plasmodium falciparum* (endemic Burkitt lymphoma) • Persistent viral stimulation of lymph nodes by Epstein–Barr virus (endemic Burkitt lymphoma) and cytomegalovirus (NHL)
Autoimmune diseases	• Inflammatory bowel disease (enteropathy-associated lymphoma) • Rheumatoid arthritis • Hashimoto thyroiditis • Sjögren syndrome (diffuse large B-cell lymphoma)
Immunodeficiency	• Genetic immunodeficiency disorders • HIV infection • Transplant recipients
Drugs	• Tumour necrosis factor-alpha inhibitors (T-cell lymphoma) • Chronic immunosuppression in post-transplant patients (both solid organ transplant and bone marrow transplant recipients)
Geographic location	• Extranodal NK/T-cell lymphoma incidence is high in southern Asia and some parts of Latin America

Table 11.6.4 Modified Ann Arbor staging system for lymphomas.

Stage	Description
Stage I	• Involvement of a single lymph node region or lymphoid structure (e.g. spleen, thymus, Waldeyer's ring) or involvement of a single extralymphatic site (IE)
Stage II	• Involvement of 2 or more lymph node regions on the same side of the diaphragm (II) or • Localised contiguous involvement of only 1 extranodal organ or side and its regional lymph nodes with or without other lymph node regions on the same side of the diaphragm (IIE) Note: The number of anatomical regions involved may be indicated by a subscript (e.g. II3)
Stage III	• Involvement of lymph node regions on both sides of the diaphragm (III), which may also be accompanied by involvement of the spleen (IIIS) or • By localised contiguous involvement of only 1 extranodal organ side (IIIE) or both (IIISE)
Stage IV	• Disseminated (multifocal) involvement of 1 or more extranodal organs or tissues • With or without associated lymph node involvement or isolated extralymphatic organ involvement with distant (non-regional) nodal involvement
Additional designation applicable to any stage	• A: no symptoms • B: fever (temperature >38 °C), drenching night sweats, unexplained loss of more than 10% of body weight during the previous 6 months • X: Bulky disease • E: Involvement of an extranodal site that is contiguous or proximal to the known nodal site

- Estimates indicate that there were over 509 000 NHL and ~79 000 HL cases, with ~248 000 NHL and over 26 000 HL deaths, globally in 2018
- Although new cases of NHL occurred equally in high-income, middle-income and lower-income regions, deaths occurred more frequently in middle- to lower-income countries
- For HL, the vast majority of new cases and deaths occurred in middle- to lower-income regions
- This is despite substantial therapeutic advancements, with the incorporation of rituximab as a standard treatment approach, and reflects inequitable access to care

Recommended Reading

Abed, H., Nizarali, N., and Burke, M. (2019). Oral and dental management for people with lymphoma. *Dental Update* 46: 133–150.

Armitage, J.O., Gascoyne, R.D., Lunning, M.A., and Cavalli, F. (2017). Non-Hodgkin lymphoma. *Lancet* 390: 298–310.

Bagan, J.V., Carbonell, F., Gómez, M.J. et al. (2015). Extranodal B-cell non-Hodgkin's lymphomas of the head and neck: a study of 68 cases. *Am. J. Otolaryngol.* 36: 57–62.

Kaseb, H. and Babiker, H.M. Hodgkin lymphoma. (2021). www.statpearls.com/

Mortazavi, H., Baharvan, M., and Rezaeifar, K. (2020). Periapical lymphoma: review of reported cases in the literature. *J. Stomatol. Oral Maxillofac. Surg.* 121: 404–407.

Mugnaini, E.N. and Ghosh, N. (2016). Lymphoma. *Prim. Care* 43: 661–675.

Völker, H.U., Becker, E., Müller-Hermelink, H.K., and Scheich, M. (2020). Extranodal manifestation of classical Hodgkin lymphoma in the head and neck region (article in German). *HNO* 68: 32–39.

11.7 Bone Marrow Transplantation

Section I: Clinical Scenario and Dental Considerations

A 63 year old male presents to the dental clinic complaining of intermittent mouth ulcers which presented after he had his bone marrow transplantation.

Medical History

- Multiple myeloma diagnosed 3 years ago
- Bone marrow transplant 6 months ago (unrelated, allogeneic)
- Wears a back brace for support and uses a walking cane (Figure 11.7.1)
- Oesophageal spasm
- Chronic obstructive pulmonary disease

Medications

- One year of oral bisphosphonates – ibandronate
- Followed by 2 years of intravenous bisphosphonates 3 monthly – zoledronic acid (ongoing)
- Cyclosporine
- Methotrexate
- Calcium supplementation
- Aciclovir
- Glyceryl trinitrate
- Budesonide and formoterol
- Carbocisteine
- Fentanyl
- Multivitamins
- Omega-3

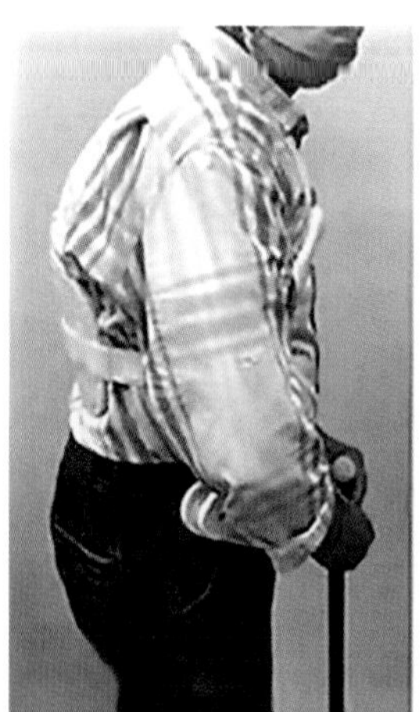
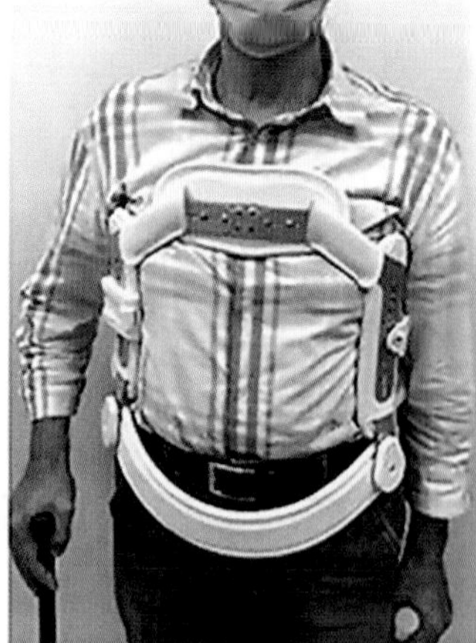

Figure 11.7.1 Back brace for support.

Dental History

- Regular dental attender
- Last dental visit was before the bone marrow transplantation
- Brushes twice daily; uses floss occasionally
- Not using fluoride toothpaste
- Requires frequent sips of water for dry mouth

Social History

- Retired accountant, originally from Jordan
- Lives with wife
- Two adult children who live overseas
- Care-giver support daily
- Private transport
- Twenty-year history of smoking 20 cigarettes a day – stopped prior to transplantation
- Nil alcohol

Oral Examination

- Dry lips
- Healing ulcer in the vestibule close to #26 (Figure 11.7.2)
- Pale palate; small asymptomatic ulcer adjacent to #11 and #12
- Minimal saliva pooling in the floor of mouth (Figure 11.7.3)
- Smooth and atrophic tongue
- Calculus and plaque present in all quadrants
- Pale gingivae, generalised recession, clinical attachment loss consistent with generalised chronic periodontitis
- Class III furcation involvement #46
- Caries in #44, #45 and #46

A Practical Approach to Special Care in Dentistry, First Edition. Edited by Pedro Diz Dios and Navdeep Kumar.

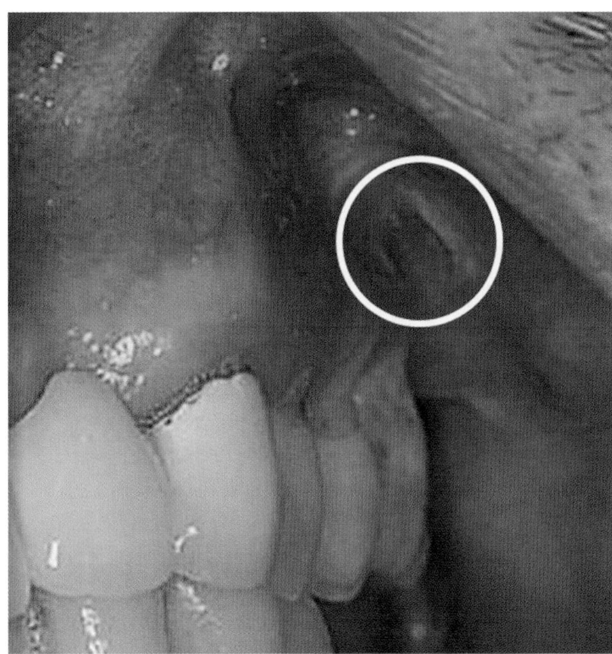

Figure 11.7.2 Mucosa – healing ulcer in the vestibule close to #26.

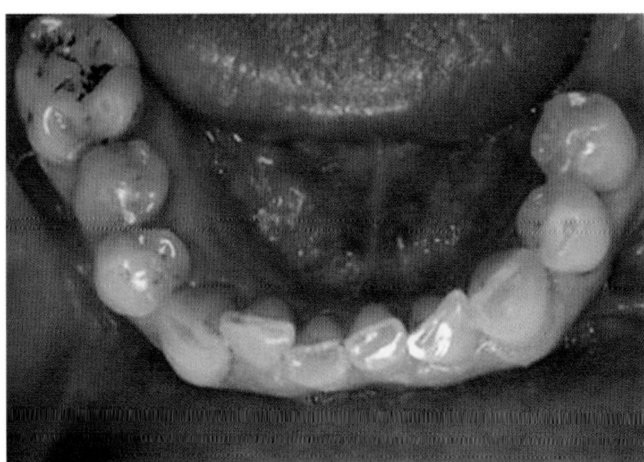

Figure 11.7.3 Floor of mouth – minimal saliva pooling; caries #44, #45 and #46; generalised tooth surface loss.

- Generalised tooth surface loss, predominantly on occlusal surface and buccal surfaces

Radiological Examination

- Orthopantomogram
  - Generalised moderate bone loss
  - Large radiolucent area of poorly defined 'punched-out' lesions in the maxilla and mandible
  - 'Soap-bubble' pattern localised in the left side of the mandibular body
  - Well-defined margins of the extraction socket of #36

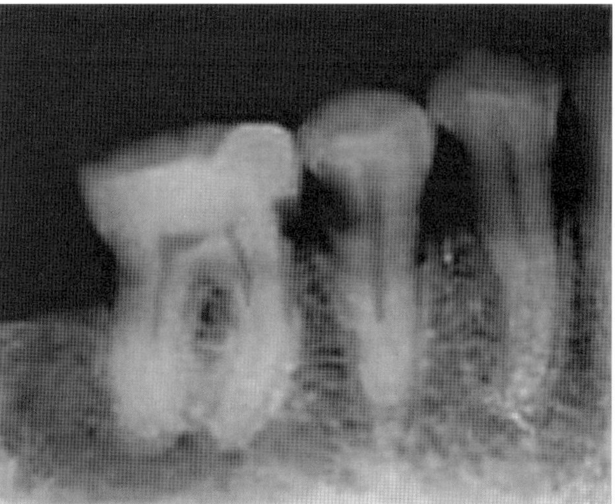

Figure 11.7.4 Periapical radiograph demonstrating caries in #44, #45 and #46.

- Periapical
  - Caries in #44, #45 and #46 (Figure 11.7.4)
  - Intraradicular bone loss in the furcation of #46
  - Horizontal bone loss
  - Large radiolucent area of poorly defined 'punched-out' lesion near the apex of lower right first molar
- Cone beam computed tomography (Figure 11.7.5)
  - Changes in bone density posteriorly but not directly connected to the dentition

Structured Learning

1) What is multiple myeloma (MM)?
   - MM is a plasma cell malignancy
   - Monoclonal plasma cells proliferate in bone marrow, resulting in an overabundance of monoclonal paraprotein (M protein), destruction of bone and displacement of other haematopoietic cell lines
   - It accounts for 15% of blood cancers, mainly affects those over 65 years of age and is more common in men than women
   - Variable presentation from early asymptomatic types to severely symptomatic; signs and symptoms of MM include the following:
     - Bone pain, pathological fractures, spinal cord compression (from pathological fracture)
     - Weakness, malaise
     - Bleeding, anaemia, infection (often pneumococcal)
     - Hypercalcaemia, renal failure
     - Neuropathies

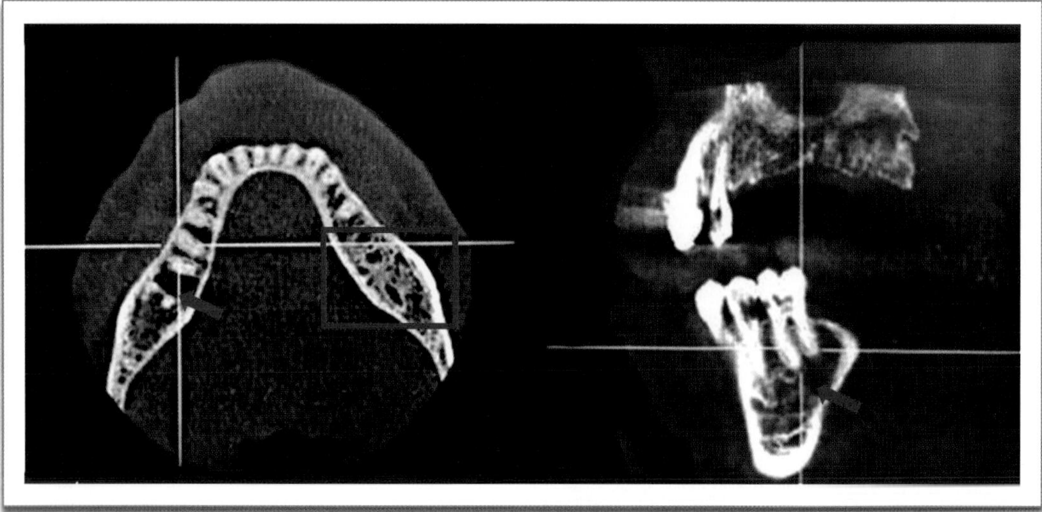

Figure 11.7.5 Cone beam computed tomography images showing a changed bone density in the molar region and a 'punched-out' lesion with a sclerotic margin located near the lower right first molar.

- Although there is no cure, advances in therapy, such as bone marrow transplantation, may help to limit disease progression

2) Given the patient's medical history, what is the most likely reason that the patient is wearing a back brace?
   - Osteolytic disease affecting the spine is common in MM
   - This results in vertebral body compression fractures and is potentially exacerbated by high-dose steroids used in the treatment of MM, further weakening the bone
   - Thoracic kyphosis may also occur, significantly reducing lung function and increasing pulmonary complications
   - In view of this, a back brace is worn to provide support, reduce movement-associated pain and improve posture
3) What are oesophageal spasms and what causes them and how is this relevant to you?
   - These are powerful, irregular and unco-ordinated contractions of the oesophagus that are of unknown cause
   - They are important to keep in mind as symptoms include chest pain that can mimic angina pectoris, difficulty swallowing, the feeling of something stuck in the throat and regurgitation
   - The condition is usually managed by treating any underlying contributing condition such as depression or gastrointestinal reflux disease
   - Muscle relaxants/vasodilators such as glyceryl trinitrate may be used to relieve the symptoms
   - Botulinum toxin injections and surgery (myotomy/peroral endoscopic myotomy [POEM]) may also be considered.
4) What could be the cause of the oral ulceration?
   - Secondary to medication, i.e. methotrexate and cyclosporine (drugs commonly used as graft-versus-host disease [GVHD] prophylaxis)
   - Related to anaemia secondary to MM/immunosuppression
   - GVHD, an immune condition that occurs after transplantation when immune cells present in donor tissue (the graft) attack the host's own tissues – the risk in this patient is higher as he had an unrelated allogeneic bone marrow transplant
5) When you show the patient the dental radiographs and cone beam CT, he asks what is causing the radiographic appearance of the jawbone. What explanation would you provide?
   - The classic MM bone lesion visualised in radiographs is a sharply defined and small lytic lesion with the so-called 'punched-out' appearance
   - Single or multiple well-defined punched-out radiolucencies often present as the first signal of MM with the jawbones affected in 20–30% of cases; it is more common in the mandible than in the maxilla and especially affects the molar region, ramus, angle and condylar process, probably because of the lower amount of haemopoietic marrow in the mandible
   - The cone beam CT scans confirm that the area adjacent to the lower right first molar is not dental in origin

- Differential diagnoses should be considered (e.g. brown tumours, metastatic lesions, chronic osteomyelitis, arteriovenous malformations and Langerhans cell disease)

6) The patient informs you that his previous dentist had confirmed his mouth was healthy prior to bone marrow transplantation. What factors could be contributing to this patient's high level of dental caries?
   - Oral hygiene not optimal (plaque and calculus deposits present, no interdental cleaning); this may have declined due to fatigue/oromucosal discomfort after transplantation (mucositis, oral GVHD)
   - Not using fluoride toothpaste
   - Xerostomia as a side-effect of cancer therapy
   - Loss of protective layer of enamel due to extensive tooth surface loss (may be linked to chemotherapy-related nausea and vomiting)
   - Inhaled beta-2-agonists may lead to reduced salivary flow which has been associated with a reduction in pH, increased food retention and increase in cariogenic bacterial load
   - Dry powder inhalers also contain fermentable carbohydrates, the most common of which is lactose monohydrate which can lead to dental caries
   - Tobacco smoking may be a risk factor for dental caries, as has been demonstrated in some studies (causal link not proven)
7) When you recommend the use of fluoride toothpaste, the patient tells you that he stopped using it as he has read it could make his bones even weaker and cause more pain. How would you respond?
   - It is important to acknowledge that chronic high-level exposure to fluoride can lead to skeletal fluorosis due to accumulation of fluoride in the bones over many years
   - Symptoms of skeletal fluorosis include stiffness and pain in the joints
   - Waters with high levels of fluoride content are mostly found at the foot of high mountains and in areas where the sea has made geological deposits, including a fluoride belt which stretches from Syria through Jordan, Egypt, Libya, Algeria, Sudan and Kenya
   - However, the benefits of topical fluoride supplementation in his case outweigh these risks
8) What other factors do you need to consider in your risk assessment?
   - Social
     - Reduced mobility due to back brace; may not be able to recline fully in the dental chair
     - Reliance on walking cane
     - Fatigue may impact on attendance and ability to cope with dental appointments
     - Psychosocial impact of cancer and chronic pain (related to vertebral collapse)
   - Medical
     - Reduced lung function due to chronic obstructive pulmonary disease and limited thoracic expansion secondary to back brace/kyphosis
     - Need for glyceryl trinitrate to manage oesophageal spasms
     - Corticosteroids – risk of adrenal suppression
     - Immunocompromised – risk of infection
     - Thrombocytopenia – risk of bleeding
     - Oesophageal spasm
     - Drug interactions
   - Dental
     - Medication-related osteonecrosis of the jaw risk due to bisphosphonates
     - Long-term use of steroid inhalers can be associated with oral candidiasis
     - Higher risk of dental caries due to oral dryness, suboptimal oral hygiene, lack of fluoride toothpaste
     - Risk of drug-induced oral ulcerations, mucositis, gingival enlargement
     - Periodontal disease exacerbation
     - Lack of posterior tooth support

General Dental Considerations

Oral Findings

- Significantly increased plaque and gingival inflammation scores have been recorded during the period of intense immunosuppression following allogeneic haematopoietic stem cell transplantation (may be related to oromucosal discomfort, fatigue)
- Mucositis
  - One of the most common and distressing complications, beginning around 5 days post haematopoietic stem cell transplantation infusion and persisting for 2–3 weeks
  - May be a predictor of gastrointestinal toxicity and the onset of hepatic veno-occlusive disease
- Infections
  - Can present within the first month of the transplant (e.g. dental abscess, sinusitis, parotitis)
  - Oral infections, particularly if bacterial, can be lethal and must be treated vigorously
  - Later (2–4 months after transplant), opportunist infections such as herpetic and fungal infections often develop

- Anaemia may manifest as mucosal pallor, burning sensation, oral ulceration
- Thrombocytopenia-associated spontaneous gingival/mucosal bleeding
- Crusting of lips
- The developing dentition may be affected in children who undergo bone marrow transplantation
- Drug-induced complications (e.g. oral ulceration induced by methotrexate and everolimus; cyclosporine-induced gingival swelling)
- GVHD: presents with lichenoid reactions, oral ulceration, xerostomia (Figure 11.7.6)
- Malignancies related to immunosuppressants: lip / oral carcinoma, Kaposi's sarcoma, lymphoma

Dental Management (Table 11.7.1)

- Treatment should be modified based on reassessment of the patient on the day of the appointment
- The immunosuppressive drugs administrated in the post-transplant phase may have a significant impact on the oral cavity

Section II: Background Information and Guidelines

Definition

Bone marrow transplantation (BMT) involves harvesting bone marrow cells from a donor and transplanting them into the recipient by injecting the cells intravenously. It is a life-saving procedure for patients with end-stage diseases and is often the only viable treatment available.

However, it is recognised that there are 2 types of stem cell in the human bone marrow: haematopoietic stem cells (HSCs) and mesenchymal stem cells (MSCs). HSCs primarily maintain haematopoietic functions, while MSCs have the ability to differentiate into various mesodermal and neuroectodermal cells. MSCs are multipotent stromal cells with high proliferative ability that can differentiate into a variety of cell types, including vascular endothelial cells, islet cells and hepatocytes. In view of this, their use in cell and gene therapy, as well as tissue engineering, is a key area of development.

Indications for Haematopoietic Stem Cell Transplantation (HSCT)

- Neoplastic and autoimmune conditions (e.g. leukaemias, lymphomas, myeloproliferative disorders, myelodysplastic syndromes, bone marrow failure syndromes)
- Congenital immunodeficiencies that affect the bone marrow (e.g. CD3 T cell lymphopenia)
- Inborn errors of metabolism/enzyme deficiencies, haemoglobinopathies, primary amyloidosis, POEMS syndrome (polyneuropathy, organomegaly, endocrinopathy, monoclonal protein, skin changes)

Classification

- BMT may include myeloid, erythroid, megakaryocyte, lymphoid and macrophage cells
- It is broadly classified as:
  - Autograft (autologous transplants), from the same person
  - Allograft (allogeneic transplants), from another individual (related/unrelated)
- The cells (either autologous or allogeneic) may be obtained from 3 different sources: bone marrow (BMT), peripheral blood (leukapheresis) or banked cryopreserved umbilical cord or foetal liver blood
- In allografts, the donor cells are best harvested from an identical twin or close relative who is also HLA-matched as

(a)

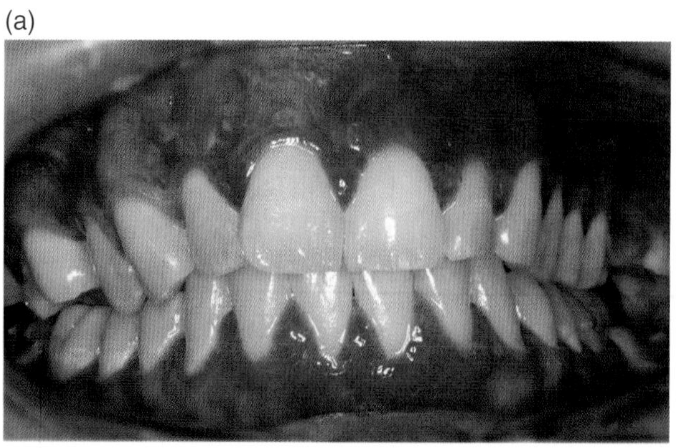

(b)

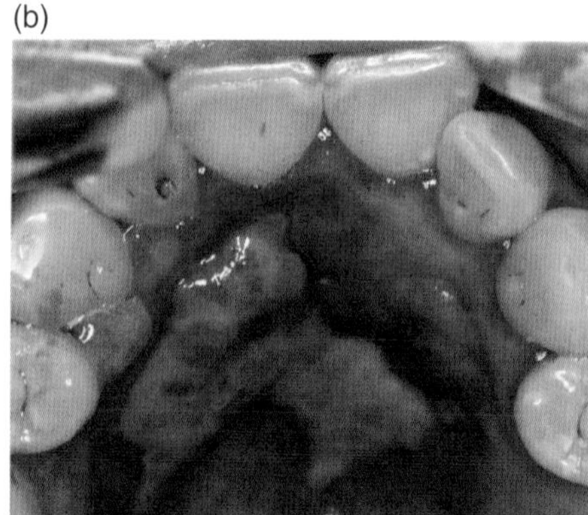

Figure 11.7.6 (a,b) Graft-versus-host disease.

Table 11.7.1 Dental management considerations.

Risk assessment	• Anaemia • Bleeding tendency • Infection risk • Relapse of pre-existing disease • Medical comorbidities • Polypharmacy • Adrenal suppression/risk of crises due to corticosteroids • Long-term side-effects of corticosteroids and immunosuppression • Increased risk of blood-borne infection due to transfusions
Criteria for referral	• Patients who have stable blood counts may be seen in primary care for routine dental assessment and support • Urgent invasive dental treatment within 6 months of a bone marrow transplantation is preferably provided in a hospital-based dental clinic linked to the transplant medical team • Refer to a maxillofacial surgery/oral medicine department if there are oromucosal signs of graft-versus-host disease
Access/position	• Pre-transplant – Oral/dental assessment and urgent dental treatment should be undertaken prior to immunosuppression – Establish optimal oral hygiene, eliminate dental infection and stabilise dental caries – The need for extraction of partially erupted permanent teeth should be evaluated, due to the risk of pericoronitis – If dental extractions under general anaesthesia are required, it may be possible to co-ordinate these with other concurrent procedures, such as bone marrow harvest or placement of the central line – This is particularly advantageous for patients who may not be able to co-operate for treatment under local anaesthesia, and when time available prior to commencement of immunosuppression is limited • Post-transplant – During immediate post-transplant and chronic rejection phases, elective dental care is best deferred for at least 3–6 months; emergency dental care should be provided in a hospital setting – From 6 months to 2 years after transplantation and depending on the success of the bone marrow transplantation and any comorbidities, any elective invasive dental treatment may be undertaken in primary care but close consultation with the physician is required
Communication	• This involves working as a part of the multidisciplinary team and co-ordinating care with the oncologists
Capacity/consent	• Consider patient's psychological status as this may impact on decision making and some may need support
Anaesthesia/sedation	• Local anaesthesia – Consider bleeding and infection risk – A rinse with 0.12–0.2% chlorhexidine mouthwash prior to administration is advisable – Avoid regional block injections where possible • Sedation – Sedative drugs should be avoided, but if unavoidable must only be given in hospital with appropriate expertise and facilities • General anaesthesia – Higher risk of morbidity and mortality

(Continued)

Table 11.7.1 (Continued)

Dental treatment	• Before – Invasive treatment needs consultation with physician with access to recent full blood count tests before invasive dental treatment – Consider the need for steroid cover, antibiotic prophylaxis (particularly during the 6 months after transplantation), precautions to limit excessive bleeding, polypharmacy – Paediatric dentistry: mobile primary teeth and gingival operculum should be removed – Orthodontics: orthodontic bands and appliances that may contribute to poor oral hygiene or mucosal trauma should be removed • During – Limit the extent of treatment provided at each appointment – Careful manipulation of the cheek and soft tissues (lubricant/barrier cream used to protect the lips; consider the use of gauze when using cheek retractors) – Caution with suction to avoid trauma (reduce the volume) – When using matrix band for the placement of restorations, take care not to traumatise the gingivae – Periodontology: cyclosporine may induce gingival enlargement Non surgical periodontal therapy/dental scaling/root planing: start with a limited area to assess bleeding – Consider the adjuvant use of tranexamic acid 5% mouthwash or desmopressin if bleeding prolonged – Prostheses: complex dental prostheses are not indicated in patients with a poor prognosis – Implants: although there is no evidence that immunosuppression is a contraindication to implants, such patients may not be a good risk group and medical advice should be taken first • After – Give patient written postoperative instruction and emergency contact details – Review in 1 week after invasive dental procedures – Routine cancer surveillance is mandatory to assure rapid diagnosis and treatment of any malignancy (secondary to immunosuppression)
Drug prescription	• Consider drug dose alteration in altered metabolism (especially the first 2 years after transplantation) • Cyclosporine, nifedipine and basiliximab may cause impaired healing and infections, and may interact with prescribed drugs (e.g. cyclosporine increases the toxicity of erythromycin and azole antifungals) • There may also be a greater risk from nephrotoxicity with co-trimoxazole, aminoglycosides and quinolones • Avoid aspirin and non-steroidal anti-inflammatory drugs which can potentiate the nephrotoxicity of cyclosporine and tacrolimus, cause a bleeding tendency and exacerbate peptic ulcer particularly if the patient is on corticosteroids
Education/prevention	• The focus of dental care is prevention of oral infection, with the aim of minimising the need for surgical treatment • Conventional prevention measures, such as applying topical fluoride, providing dietary recommendations and promoting oral health, are essential

much as possible to minimise graft rejection; most transplants are made between HLA-identical siblings, though other family members, or matched volunteers, may be involved

Treatment Pathway

- Treatment goals
  - Highest rates of patient and graft survival, to minimise toxicity, infections and malignancy
- Before transplantation
  - Immunological evaluation is undertaken, including ABO blood group determination, human leucocyte antigen (HLA) typing, serum screening for antibody to HLA phenotypes, cross-matching
  - Transplantation across incompatible blood groups may result in a humorally mediated hyperacute rejection
- After transplantation
  - All patients need treatment with immunosuppressive drugs for life to prevent T-cell alloimmune rejection
- Conditioning
  - Unlike organ transplantation, these patients are immunosuppressed before BMT to reduce the chances of graft rejection

  - Intensive immunosuppression is used, often with cyclophosphamide (plus busulfan and total body irradiation in leukaemia) to destroy the malignant cells
  - All conditioning regimens are toxic but those receiving reduced intensity conditioning (busulfan) have lower morbidity and mortality (used in older patients/those with medical comorbidities)
- Transplantation
  - In order to reduce the risk of GVHD, donor stem cells may be treated with antibodies prior to transplant to remove T-lymphocytes
  - The donor marrow is then mixed with heparin and infused intravenously
  - It colonises the recipient marrow and over the next 2–4 weeks, starts to produce blood cells
  - Throughout this time and for the following 3 months or so, the patient is usually provided with an indwelling vascular catheter (Hickman line) to facilitate drug therapy and intravenous fluids
  - Recipients must also be treated with methotrexate, corticosteroids, cyclosporine, intravenous immunoglobulins, tacrolimus, sirolimus or alemtuzumab (anti-CD52 lymphocytes) for 6 months or more to prevent or ameliorate GVHD
  - Since patients are severely immunocompromised until the donor marrow is fully functioning, they must also be isolated and protected from infections, and may require transfusions
  - Antimicrobials may also be needed until the donor marrow is functioning fully
- Maintenance immunosuppression
  - This typically involves the use of corticosteroid-sparing agents (calcineurin inhibitors, e.g. cyclosporine or tacrolimus) and/or corticosteroids, sometimes with antiproliferative agents (e.g. azathioprine, mycophenolate mofetil or rapamycin), inhibitors of mechanistic target of rapamycin (mTOR, e.g. temsirolimus, everolimus, sirolimus or deforolimus), anti-T cytotoxic (anti-Tc, e.g. abatacept, belatacept) or anti-interleukin-2 (e.g. basiliximab, daclizumab) agents, or other biological therapies
  - Many new agents are being trialled, such as eculizumab and bortezomib for treatment of antibody-mediated rejection
  - Prophylaxis for GVHD for allogeneic BMT typically involves the use of cyclosporine or tacrolimus in combination with methotrexate and/or prednisone/prednisolone

Prognosis

- Influenced by factors such as age, general health status, underlying disease or donor cell origin and the immune reactivity of the recipient patient, which may trigger the rejection or reject phenomena
- The life expectancy, survival rate and quality of life after BMT have improved considerably with more accurate genetic matching with donors, prophylaxis for the prevention of infections and improved post-transplant care
- BMTs for patients with non-malignant diseases have a much better success rate, with 70–90% survival with a matched sibling donor and 36–65% with unrelated donors
- The survival rates after transplant for patients with malignant disease are lower, estimated as 55–68% with related donors and 26–50% if the donor is unrelated
- Patients who survive BMT are susceptible to infection, multiorgan failure and acute allograft rejection; in the long term, malignant neoplasms may present
- GVHD remains a serious complication of allograft transplantation where donor cells respond to hystoincompatible antigens to the host; it is more common after BMT than after solid organ transplants
  - Acute GVHD: a syndrome of dermatitis, hepatitis and enteritis (and fever) developing within 100 days
  - Chronic GVHD: also affects skin, liver and gut but describes a more diverse syndrome developing after day 100
  - Can also get 'overlap' syndrome with acute + chronic presentation

A World/Transcultural View

- Disparities by race exist related to BMT
  - Donor availability: people of ethnic origin have a lower likelihood of finding an unrelated donor; race and ethnicity definitions are country-specific and reconciling race data can represent significant challenges to unrelated donor registries worldwide
  - Access: especially where state funding for BMT is not provided, access to autologous and allogeneic BMT is not uniformly available
  - Outcomes: racial disparities in outcomes of BMT are more prevalent among allogeneic HSCT than autologous HSCT recipients, although the reasons for this are not clear
- Transplants may be refused on the basis of religious beliefs such as Jehovah's Witnesses and Orthodox Jews

Recommended Reading

Bollero, P., Passarelli, P.C., D'Addona, A. et al. (2018). Oral management of adult patients undergoing haematopoietic stem cell transplantation. *Eur. Rev. Med. Pharmacol. Sci.* 22: 876–887.

Brennan, M.T., Hasséus, B., Hovan, A.J. et al. (2018). Impact of oral side effects from conditioning therapy before haematopoietic stem cell transplantation: protocol for a multicenter study. *JMIR Res. Protoc.* 7: e103.

Elad, S., Raber-Durlacher, J.E., Brennan, M.T. et al. (2015). Basic oral care for hematology-oncology patients and haematopoietic stem cell transplantation recipients: a position paper from the joint task force of the Multinational Association of Supportive Care in Cancer/International Society of Oral Oncology (MASCC/ISOO) and the European Society for Blood and Marrow Transplantation (EBMT). *Support Care Cancer* 23: 223–236.

Haverman, T.M., Raber-Durlacher, J.E., Raghoebar, I.I. et al. (2020). Oral chronic graft-versus-host disease: what the general dental practitioner needs to know. *J. Am. Dent. Assoc.* 151: 846–856.

Hansen, H.J., Estilo, C., Owosho, A. et al. (2021). Dental status and risk of odontogenic complication in patients undergoing haematopoietic stem cell transplant. *Support. Care Cancer* 29: 2231–2238.

Khaddour, K., Hana, C.K., and Mewawalla, P. (2021). Haematopoietic Stem Cell Transplantation (Bone Marrow Transplant). www.statpearls.com/

Royal College of Surgeons of England/BSDH. *The Oral Management of Oncology Patients Requiring Chemotherapy, Radiotherapy and/or Bone Marrow Transplantation – 2018 Updated Guidelines.* (2018) London: Royal College of Surgeons of England

Samim, F., Ten Böhmer, K.L., Koppelmans, R.G.A. et al. (2019). Oral care for haematopoietic stem cell transplantation patients: a narrative review. *Oral Health Prev. Dent.* 17: 413–423.

12

Immunosuppression

12.1 Systemic Corticosteroids

Section I: Clinical Scenario and Dental Considerations

Clinical Scenario

A 65-year-old male presents to your dental clinic for an emergency appointment. He complains of a left-sided, painful facial swelling. His symptoms commenced 3 days ago and have increased significantly over the last 12 hours.

Medical History
- Systemic lupus erythematosus (SLE) diagnosed at the age of 39 years
- Lupus arthritis
- Arterial hypertension
- Peripheral arterial disease
- Hyperuricaemia
- Personality disorder
- Severe obesity (BMI = 38 kg/m^2)
- History of thyroidectomy (9 years earlier)
- History of saphenectomy to remove varicose veins (14 years earlier)

Medications
- Prednisone (30 mg/day)
- Pimecrolimus (topical)
- Mometasone (topical)
- Methotrexate
- Hydroxychloroquine
- Vitamin D
- Folinic acid
- Candesartan/hydrochlorothiazide
- Allopurinol
- Omeprazole

Dental History
- Irregular dental attender – only visits the dentist when in pain as he feels poorly motivated/chronically tired
- Does not brush his teeth regularly as often feels tired/lethargic
- Diet: consumes large amounts of carbonated drinks, chocolate, biscuits

Social History
- Pensioner (lives alone and with limited financial resources)
- Reduced mobility; using a cane as required
- Largely sedentary lifestyle
- Poor compliance with medical/dental treatment; often stops taking prescribed medication if he feels reasonably well
- Ex-smoker (30 cigarettes/day until 8 years ago)

Oral Examination
- Bilateral facial erythema (Figure 12.1.1)
- Poor oral hygiene
- Buccal abscess/swelling in left canine fossa region
- Fractured crown of #15 and #44
- Caries in #25, #43, #46 and #48
- Missing teeth: #16, #17, #23, #34–37, #45 and #47
- Tooth surface loss, more advanced in association with the anterior teeth

Radiological Examination
- Orthopantomogram undertaken (Figure 12.1.2)
- Generalised bone loss due to periodontal disease
- Retained root #23 (related to the abscessed area)
- Advanced tooth surface loss

Structured Learning

1) What is the most likely cause of the bilateral facial erythema (Figure 12.1.1)?
   - The presence of a bilateral butterfly rash is present in 45–65% patients with SLE (an autoimmune disease that can affect the skin, joints, kidneys, brain and other organs, with oral involvement)

A Practical Approach to Special Care in Dentistry, First Edition. Edited by Pedro Diz Dios and Navdeep Kumar.

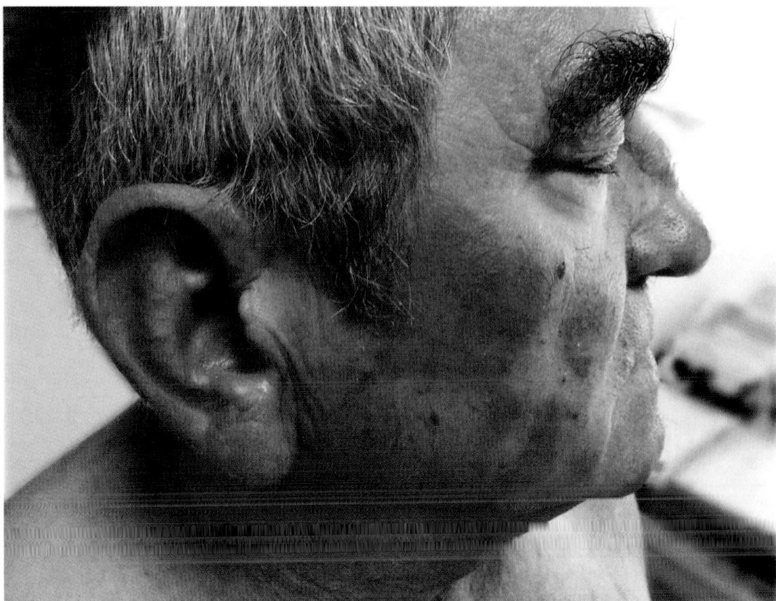

Figure 12.1.1 Malar rash (butterfly rash).

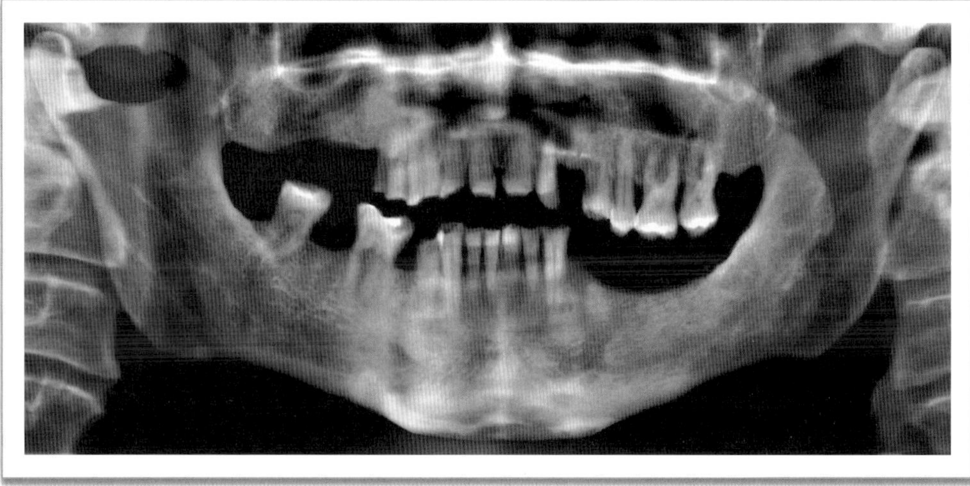

Figure 12.1.2 Orthopantomogram demonstrating generalised bone loss, retained root #23, severe tooth surface loss.

- Typically, the butterfly rash appears in a malar distribution across the nose and cheeks
- Other oral manifestations of SLE include oral ulceration, raised keratotic plaques, non-specific erythema, purpura, petechiae and cheilitis

2) In addition to SLE, what other conditions should be included in the differential diagnosis of facial erythema?
   - Rosacea: a chronic inflammatory acneiform disease, pathogenesis uncertain, not associated with systemic illness
   - Erysipelas: painful and well-circumscribed skin infection with systemic symptoms, including fever, chills and malaise
   - Cellulitis: skin infection, less well demarcated than erysipelas with little or no oedema that does not usually have systemic symptoms
   - Polymorphous light eruption: common form of primary photosensitivity, mainly affecting young women in spring/summer months
   - Drug-induced photosensitivity: photosensitising medications cause unexpected dermatitis on sun-exposed skin (e.g. fluoroquinolones)
   - Other: diseases such as sarcoidosis, pellagra (related to lack of vitamin B3), dermatomyositis appear less frequently

3) What factors could be contributing to the advanced tooth surface loss?
   - Attrition
     - Loss of posterior occlusal support causing increased loading on the remaining dentition
     - Bruxism more common in chronic pain conditions such as SLE-associated arthritis
   - Erosion
     - Diet: high consumption of acidic fizzy drinks
     - Gastro-oesophageal reflux disease likely (related to obesity – patient is taking omeprazole)
     - Xerostomia secondary to prednisone (less effective protection from saliva)
   - Abrasion
     - Unlikely cause in this patient as he brushes his teeth infrequently
4) You determine that the infected retained root #23 is the cause of this patient's acute facial swelling. What factors increase his risk of oral infection?
   - Poor oral hygiene
   - SLE
     - Genetic factors predisposing to SLE include genes related to lymphocyte signalling, the innate immune response (type I interferon and nuclear factor kappa B signalling), apoptotic cell death and defective clearance of immune complexes
     - SLE is known to be associated with primary immunological abnormalities, such as lymphopenia and low production of interleukin-2 (IL-2)
   - Immunosuppression related to medication
     - Prednisone (systemic steroid)
     - Immunosuppressants (methotrexate; pimecrolimus which if used in high doses and frequently may be absorbed)
5) What factors are considered important in assessing the risk of managing this patient?
   - Social
     - Escort advisable due to reduced mobility and personality disorder
     - Informed consent may be affected by the underlying personality disorder; behaviour can further be affected by the side-effect of systemic steroids
   - Medical
     - Poor compliance with medical care, including medication
     - Access and position in the dental chair will be affected by the patient's lupus arthritis, peripheral arterial disease and obesity (see Chapter 16.4)
     - There is a risk of a hypertensive crisis due to arterial hypertension (see Chapter 8.1)
     - Risk of an adrenal crisis due to corticosteroid medication
     - Drug adverse effects and interactions
   - Dental
     - Acute presentation of dental infection
     - Poor oral hygiene
     - Poor motivation/infrequent dental attender
     - Highly cariogenic diet
     - Advanced tooth surface loss
     - Limited financial resources
6) The abscess relating #23 needs to be drained urgently. The patient has taken 30–40 mg/day of prednisone over the last 8 years. Can you proceed?
   - The procedure is considered low risk, because it is relatively simple (will last less than 1 hour), will be performed with local anaesthesia, and there are no other factors that would predict significant bleeding (except arterial hypertension)
   - Hence corticosteroid supplementation is not routinely given as drainage of a dental abscess is not considered as surgically stressful as a dental extraction
7) During the dental procedure, the patient complains that his head hurts, he feels nauseated and he is confused. What should you do?
   - Stop the procedure
   - Measure the patient's blood pressure to distinguish between an adrenal crisis (generally accompanied by abrupt hypotension) and a hypertensive crisis (the patient has hypertension)
   - Take appropriate action
8) The patient stabilises and you are able to proceed with draining the buccal abscess. Due to the extent of infection and the fact the patient is immunosuppressed, you prescribe an antibiotic postoperatively. What drug interactions should you take into account?
   - Beta-lactams (e.g. ampicillin and amoxicillin) reduce the excretion of methotrexate, enhancing its toxicity (see Chapter 12.2)
   - The rate of skin rashes caused by ampicillin and amoxicillin increases when combined with allopurinol
   - Moxifloxacin (a quinolone) is contraindicated for patients who take hydroxychloroquine
   - The risk of tendonitis and Achilles tendon rupture secondary to the administration of quinolones (e.g. levofloxacin and ciprofloxacin) can increase if combined with corticosteroids
9) What analgesic would you recommend?
   - For patients who take corticosteroids, non-steroidal anti-inflammatory drugs increase the probability of gastrointestinal haemorrhages

- The risk of haematological and gastrointestinal toxicity of methotrexate is increased with non-steroidal anti-inflammatory drugs (see Chapter 12.2)
- Non-steroidal anti-inflammatory drugs attenuate the effect of some antihypertensives such as angiotensin-converting enzyme inhibitors (see Chapter 8.1)
- Accordingly, paracetamol should be prescribed because corticosteroids already have an anti-inflammatory effect

10) When planning dental extraction of #23, what local complications related to the patient's medications should you discuss when obtaining informed consent?
    - Corticosteroids can cause delayed healing and promote superinfection of the surgical wound (Figure 12.1.3)
    - Methotrexate promotes local infections (leucopenia and neutropenia) and bleeding (thrombopenia and hepatotoxicity) and has been involved in the development of medication-related osteonecrosis of the jaw (see Chapter 12.2)

General Dental Considerations

Oral Findings

- Predisposition to infections
  - Herpes virus
  - Varicella zoster virus
  - Candidiasis
  - Bacterial infections
- Hairy leucoplakia
- Kaposi sarcoma
- Lymphoma

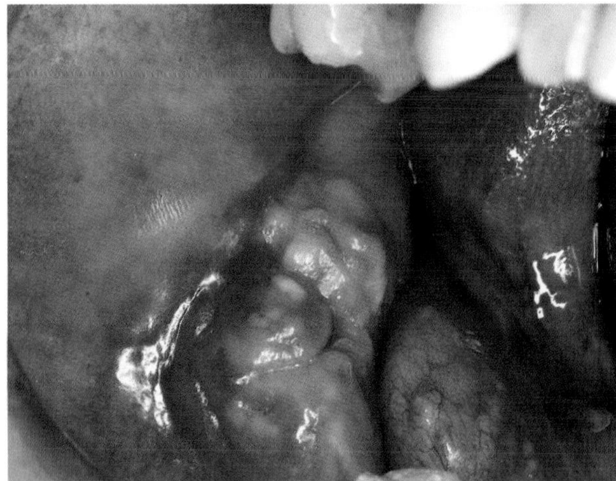

Figure 12.1.3 Delayed wound healing and bacterial infection following tooth extraction in a patient under systemic corticosteroids.

- Delayed healing of wounds and infections
- Loss of bone mineral density in the jawbones
- Edentulism

Dental Management

- Dental management modifications include (Table 12.1.1):
  - The systemic disease for which the consumption of corticosteroids is indicated, as well as the presence of comorbidities
  - The adverse effects and drug interactions of corticosteroids
  - The risk of adrenal crisis
- Steroid supplementation should be considered for invasive dental procedures in patients taking ≥ 10 mg of prednisone (or equivalent) in the last 3 months (Table 12.1.2)

Section II: Background Information and Guidelines

Definition

Endogenous corticosteroids (glucocorticoids) are a series of natural hormones whose production is governed by the hypothalamic–pituitary–adrenal axis. Partial changes in the chemical structure of natural corticosteroids have led to synthetic corticosteroid analogues, which are mainly involved in carbohydrate, fat and protein metabolism and have anti-inflammatory, immunosuppressive, antiproliferative and vasoconstrictor effects. Immunosuppressive actions include downregulation of cytokine gene expression in lymphocytes, antagonisation of macrophage differentiation and inhibition of neutrophil adhesion.

Glucocorticoids are classified based mainly on the duration of their action and their relative potency (Table 12.1.3).

Mechanism of Action

- Corticosteroids cross the cell membrane and bind to the glucocorticoid receptor in the cytoplasm
- Once activated, there are 2 mechanisms of action which result in an anti-inflammatory effect:
  - Genomic
    - The activated glucocorticoid receptor bound to its ligand induces the transcription of anti-inflammatory genes (transactivation) or inhibits the transcription of inflammatory genes (transrepression), causing the production of proinflammatory cytokines, cell adhesion molecules and other key enzymes involved in the host's inflammatory response

Table 12.1.1 Dental management considerations.

Risk assessment	• The continuous administration of exogenous steroids suppresses the hypothalamic–pituitary–adrenal axis, compromising cortisol production in response to a stress situation such as invasive dental procedures • This can cause the patient to have acute adrenal insufficiency (adrenal crisis) • Patients are considered to be at risk of an adrenal crisis if they have the following 3 factors in relation to their regular corticosteroid therapy: – Continuous administration (daily) – Prolonged administration (>3 months) – High doses (≥10 mg/day of prednisone or its equivalent) • Patients taking above 50 mg prednisolone are close to the innate maximum cortisol level seen in patients when stressed and may not require further supplementation • Supplementation is considered unnecessary with intermittent oral administration regimens (e.g. alternating days) • High doses of inhaled steroids such as fluticasone and budesonide (e.g. 1500 μg) may potentially cause adrenal suppression; however, steroid supplementation is typically not considered for patients who inhale corticosteroids or apply them topically • Most authors consider supplementation unnecessary for preventive, restorative or rehabilitative dental procedures • The current tendency is to consider steroid supplementation before surgical procedures • The invasiveness of the procedure should be assessed • The trend now appears to be to reserve supplementation only for sessions conducted with the patient under general anaesthesia, for patients with an impaired general health condition and for patients who are taking drugs that interfere with cortisol (e.g. ketoconazole, sodium valproate, bromocriptine)
Criteria for referral	• Dentists should be able to treat the vast majority of patients in primary care • However, those patients who have had a previous episode of adrenal crisis and/or have complex medical comorbidities should be referred to secondary care • A patient's ability to cope with a dental procedure cannot be predicted by the dosage and duration of the corticosteroid therapy or the demonstration of adrenal suppression (through stimulation tests) – it is multifactorial; psychological factors/dental anxiety may have an impact • Patients with underlying Addison disease who require life-long steroid supplementation should be considered at higher risk (dental procedures have been identified as a risk factor in ~8% of cases) – referral to a hospital setting for invasive procedures is advisable
Access/position	• Schedule sessions for early in the morning, when endogenous cortisol levels are higher • Assess the risk of fractures secondary to osteoporosis during the transfer and positioning manoeuvres in the chair
Communication	• Confirm that the patient has no visual deficit caused by the corticosteroids (e.g. glaucoma and cataracts) • Rule out the presence of adverse psychiatric effects from the systemic corticosteroids (e.g. depression, mood swings, psychosis)
Consent/capacity	• The consent form should include the complications resulting from the long-term administration of systemic corticosteroids, such as delayed healing and the risk of infection • The possibility of an adrenal crisis should be specified, emphasising the risk factors, symptoms and potential consequences • The corticosteroid supplementation protocol and its objective should be explicitly explained
Anaesthesia/sedation	• Local anaesthesia – Local anaesthesia may be employed, applying the routine precautions • Sedation – Conscious sedation may be employed, applying the routine precautions; it is important to consider the underlying disease • General anaesthesia – Administer corticosteroid supplementation – In cases of minimal surgery, 25–50 mg of hydrocortisone should be administered during the induction – In cases of moderate surgery, 25–50 mg of hydrocortisone should be administered during the induction and 100 mg 24 hours after the surgery

(Continued)

Table 12.1.1 (Continued)

Dental treatment	• Before – Assess the need for corticosteroid supplementation and the impact of the underlying medical condition for which it is being taken – For those patients with significant underlying disease (e.g. Addison disease), contact the patient's physician to confirm the appropriate perioperative steroid supplementation regime and the supply of oral and injectable hydrocortisone that should be available before commencing surgery – In some cases, the patient/their family may have at their disposal emergency steroid injections for emergency situations (e.g. 4 mg injection of dexamethasone) – Dental implants are not contraindicated – It has been suggested that systemic corticosteroids can promote tooth movement during orthodontic treatment • During – Monitor blood pressure – Clinical presentation of an adrenal crisis: ○ Headaches ○ Vomiting ○ Sudden hypotension ○ Progressive loss of consciousness ○ Lethargy and coma – Managing medical emergency: ○ Contact for emergency medical assistance ○ Place the patient horizontally with the legs elevated ○ Monitor the vital signs (blood pressure) ○ Administer hydrocortisone (200 mg intramuscularly; check local guidelines) ○ Administer oxygen (15 L/min) • After – Regular review after surgery due to delayed healing and increased risk of infection – The results of orthodontic treatment may be less stable
Drug prescription	• Azole antifungals (ketoconazole, itraconazole, voriconazole) and some macrolides (erythromycin, clarithromycin) increase plasma glucocorticoid levels and the onset of adverse effects • Non-steroidal anti-inflammatory drugs have a synergistic anti-inflammatory action with glucocorticoids but increase the risk of gastrointestinal injury • A risk of tendon rupture has been reported with the concomitant administration of glucocorticoids and quinolones (e.g. ciprofloxacin), especially in elderly patients
Education/prevention	• The patient should be made aware that the steroid therapy should not be abruptly discontinued in relation to dental treatment, due to the risk of causing an adrenal crisis • The use of a warning bracelet/card is recommended – reinforce to the patient that this should be available at dental appointments so that the information can be checked and the dose of steroids taken over the last 3 months confirmed • In general, it is advisable that patients undergoing corticosteroid treatment follow a low-calorie, low-fat, low-sodium, protein-rich, potassium-rich and calcium-rich diet – this may also reduce the dental caries risk • Dental care professionals should reinforce the health advice that tobacco use should be avoided, and regular physical exercise should be performed • Oral health education should include the increased risk of infection and delayed healing after invasive dental procedures

Table 12.1.2 Corticosteroid supplementation regimen for patients undergoing invasive dental treatment and who are taking/have taken ≥10 mg of prednisone (or its equivalent) within the last 3 months.

Level of risk associated with the dental procedure	Corticosteroid supplementation regime
Low risk	
• Minor oral surgery undertaken with local anaesthesia and completed < 60 mins • Includes simple tooth extractions, periodontal surgery limited to up to 2 teeth, mucosal biopsies and placement of up to 2 dental implants (provided complex bone regeneration, sinus lifting, pre-prosthetic surgery and/or other additional invasive techniques are not required) • Excludes simple procedures such as drainage of a dental abscess	• Double the morning oral dose or administer 25–50 mg of hydrocortisone (or its equivalent) intravenously prior to the surgery • Following surgery, continue with the standard steroid dosage
Moderate risk	
• Significant oral surgery, such as multiple tooth extraction, extraction of impacted teeth, single-quadrant periodontal surgery and osteotomies • Procedures lasting longer than 60 mins • Procedures performed under general anaesthesia • Conditions and procedures in which significant bleeding is expected	• Double the morning oral dose and administer 25–50 mg of hydrocortisone (or its equivalent) intravenously on the day of surgery • Repeat 24 hours after the surgery • Then, continue with the standard dosage

Source: Adapted from Gibson, N. and Ferguson, J.W. (2004).

Table 12.1.3 Classification of glucocorticoids.

Glucocorticoids	Equivalent doses (mg)	Daily dose limit for which there is a risk of adrenal suppression (mg)	
		Men	Women
• **Short-acting**			
Cortisone	50	25–30	20–30
Hydrocortisone	40	20–30	15–20
• **Intermediate-acting**			
Methylprednisolone	8	7.5–10	7.5
Prednisolone	10	7.5–10	7.5
Prednisone	10	7.5–10	7.5
Triamcinolone	8	7.5–10	7.5
• **Long-acting**			
Betamethasone	1.2	1–1.5	2.5–5
Dexamethasone	1.6	1–1.5	1–1.5

- Non-genomic
  - Immediate action as a result of physical–chemical interactions
  - The mechanisms are due to the activation of intracellular signalling cascades mediated by kinases with anti-inflammatory effects, such as interference with the metabolism of arachidonic acid, induction of apoptosis and reduction in leucocyte maturation

- The prescription of corticosteroids for longer than 7 days requires a gradual reduction regimen for discontinuing the treatment and monitoring the potential adverse effects

Indications

- The first patients treated successfully with glucocorticoids were diagnosed with rheumatoid arthritis
- Currently, the indications for treatment with corticosteroids are numerous and are based mainly on their anti-inflammatory and immunosuppressive properties (Table 12.1.4)

Contraindications

- Epilepsy, psychosis, congestive heart failure, severe arterial hypertension, thromboembolism, systemic infections (e.g. tuberculosis), glaucoma, myasthenia gravis, decompensated diabetes, kidney failure and peptic ulceration

Adverse Effects

- Systemic corticosteroids can cause numerous adverse effects, which entail significant morbidity and mortality (Table 12.1.5)

Table 12.1.4 Most common therapeutic indications for systemic corticosteroids.

Medical specialty	Disease
Allergies	Asthma
	Allergic rhinitis
	Urticaria/angio-oedema
	Atopic dermatitis
	Anaphylaxis
Pulmonology	Pneumonitis due to hypersensitivity
	Sarcoidosis
	Eosinophilic pneumonia
	Interstitial lung disease
	Chronic obstructive pulmonary disease
Dermatology	Pemphigus vulgaris
	Contact dermatitis
Endocrinology	Suprarenal failure
	Congenital adrenal hyperplasia
Gastroenterology	Ulcerative colitis
	Crohn's disease
	Autoimmune hepatitis
Haematology	Lymphoma/leukaemia
	Haemolytic anaemia
	Idiopathic thrombocytopenic purpura
Rheumatology/ immunology	Rheumatoid arthritis
	Systemic lupus erythematosus
	Polymyalgia rheumatica
	Polymyositis/dermatomyositis
	Polyarteritis
	Vasculitis
	Scleroderma
Ophthalmology	Uveitis
	Keratoconjunctivitis
Others	Multiple sclerosis
	Organ transplantation
	Nephrotic syndrome
	Cerebral oedema

Table 12.1.5 Most common adverse effects of systemic corticosteroids.

System	Adverse effect
Musculoskeletal	Osteoporosis
	Myopathy
	Avascular necrosis
Endocrine/metabolic	Hyperlipidaemia
	Hyperglycaemia
Cardiovascular	Hypertension
	Heart failure
	Ischaemic heart disease
Neuropsychiatric	Behavioural disorders
	Cognitive disorders (including psychosis)
Gastrointestinal	Gastritis
	Peptic ulcer
	Gastrointestinal haemorrhage
Dermatological	Acne and hirsutism
	Striae
	Skin atrophy
	Purpura and ecchymosis
Ocular	Glaucoma
	Cataracts
Immune	Predisposition to infections
	Pneumonia by *Pneumocystis carinii*
	Latent tuberculosis
	Invasive mycosis

A World/Transcultural View

- Glucocorticoids are one of the most widely prescribed drugs in the world, especially in the elderly
- However, the dose and duration of these drugs remain variable
- Due to the numerous side-effects associated with long-term use, treatment alternatives are being explored but are not widely available

Recommended Reading

Chilkoti, G.T., Singh, A., Mohta, M., and Saxena, A.K. (2019). Perioperative "stress dose" of corticosteroid: pharmacological and clinical perspective. *J. Anaesthesiol. Clin. Pharmacol.* 35: 147–152.

Gibson, N. and Ferguson, J.W. (2004). Steroid cover for dental patients on long-term steroid medication: proposed clinical guidelines based upon critical review of the literature. *Br. Dent. J.* 11: 681–685.

Henderson, S. (2014). What steroid supplementation is required for a patient with primary adrenal insufficiency undergoing a dental procedure? *Dent. Update* 41: 342–344.

Ngeow W Ch, Lim D, Ahmad N. (2017). *66 Years of Corticosteroids in Dentistry: and We Are Atill at a Cross Road?* IntechOpen. www.intechopen.com/books/corticosteroids/66-years -of-corticosteroids-in-dentistry-and-we-are-still-at-a-cross-road-

Oray, M., Abu Samra, K., Ebrahimiadib, N. et al. (2016). Long-term side effects of glucocorticoids. *Expert Opin. Drug Saf.* 15: 457–465.

Spies, C.M., Strehl, C., van der Goes, M.C. et al. (2011). Glucocorticoids. *Best Pract. Res. Clin. Rheumatol.* 25: 891–900.

Yong, S.L., Coulthard, P., and Wrzosek, A. (2012). Supplemental perioperative steroids for surgical patients with adrenal insufficiency. *Cochrane Database Syst. Rev.* 12: CD005367.

12.2 Antineoplastic Agents (Chemotherapy)

Section I: Clinical Scenario and Dental Considerations

Clinical Scenario

A 50-year-old woman is referred by her haematologist for an urgent dental assessment. The patient reports that the lower left first molar has been acutely painful on 2 occasions, 3 months and 1 month ago. These episodes coincided with intensive chemotherapy, which had to be discontinued.

Intravenous antibiotics were given at the time and the tooth is currently asymptomatic. The haematology team are keen to avoid further interruption of chemotherapy.

The dental appointment has been postponed twice due to febrile neutropenia complicating the patient's chemotherapy.

Medical History

- B-cell acute lymphoblastic leukaemia diagnosed 5 months ago
- Steroid-induced type 2 diabetes mellitus
- Gastro-oesophageal reflux disease
- Heart murmur
- Vitamin D deficiency

Medications

- Currently undergoing alternating cycles of chemotherapy (methotrexate, cytarabine, methylprednisolone) and immunotherapy (blinatumomab)
  - Commenced 4 months ago, with 4 months planned
  - Peripherally inserted central catheter line in situ
- Platelet transfusions weekly
- Intravenous immunoglobulin replacement every 3–4 weeks
- Trimethoprim/sulfamethoxazole
- Posaconazole
- Famciclovir
- Pantoprazole
- Ranitidine
- Metoclopramide
- Ondansetron
- Metformin
- Amlodipine
- Cholecalciferol
- Potassium chloride

Dental History

- Regular dental attender: attends every 6 months; has had same general dentist for decades
- Brushes teeth twice daily using sensitive toothpaste and soft manual toothbrush
- Previously flossed daily and used electric toothbrush until she was instructed to stop upon commencing chemotherapy
- Diet: low sugar contact, predominantly drinks water

Social History

- Occupation: teacher (currently on extended sick leave)
- Lives alone, has support of friends
- Alcohol: 1 glass of wine per week prior to chemotherapy; nil now
- Tobacco consumption: nil

Oral Examination

- Wearing a headscarf due to complete hair loss
- Facial and oral tissues appear pale
- Oral ulceration predominantly affecting the lower labial mucosa
- Lower left first molar (#36): large disto-occlusal composite restoration in situ, negative to cold sensibility testing, mild tenderness to percussion, buccal tenderness on palpation
- Good oral hygiene and gingival health on visual inspection
- No caries detected

A Practical Approach to Special Care in Dentistry, First Edition. Edited by Pedro Diz Dios and Navdeep Kumar.

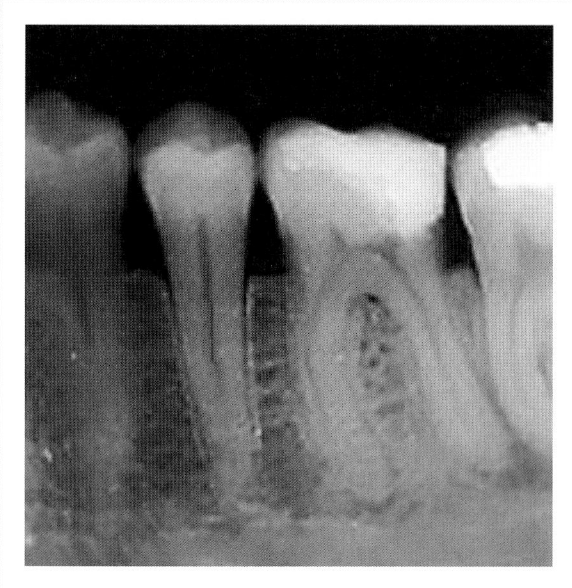

Figure 12.2.1 Long cone periapical radiograph #36 demonstrating associated periapical radiolucencies.

Radiological Examination

- Long cone periapical radiograph #36 (Figure 12.2.1) and orthopantomogram undertaken
- #36: mesial and distal periapical radiolucencies present; small distal deficiency present under the restoration; large restoration with close proximity to the pulpal chamber

Structured Learning

1) What further information would you require from the oncology team?
   - Timing of each alternate chemotherapy and immunotherapy cycle, and length of breaks between each cycle
   - Most recent full blood count and profile
   - Frequency of platelet transfusions and immunoglobulin replacement
   - Platelet count levels normally achieved post transfusion, and the possibility of achieving higher platelet counts post transfusion ($>50 \times 10^9$/L)
   - Dose of corticosteroid administered with chemotherapy, and risk of adrenal suppression
   - Need for antibiotic prophylaxis with invasive dental procedures
   - Likelihood of requiring haematopoietic stem cell transplant
   - Overall long-term prognosis
2) What are the treatment options for managing the lower left first molar (#36)?
   - Continued pain and infection control with antibiotics if the tooth becomes symptomatic again
     - Advantages: obviates the need for a chemotherapy break; may be preferred if there is a narrow window of time to maximise the therapeutic effects of chemotherapy; avoids potentially invasive dental procedures in a patient with persistently low blood counts; avoids loss of the tooth, allowing definitive treatment (e.g. endodontics) to be provided after the course of chemotherapy is completed
     - Disadvantages: the tooth may pose an infection risk with the risk of repeated infection, local spread and bacteraemia, leading to further cessation in chemotherapy
   - Elective dental extraction
     - Advantages: removes the risk of repeated dental infection and related cessation of chemotherapy; of particular benefit if stem cell transplant is planned
     - Disadvantages: dental treatment will require a chemotherapy break; additional haematological support (platelets ± intravenous immunoglobulin) will need to be discussed and implemented; healing may be delayed; prophylactic antibiotics often indicated; permanent loss of tooth
   - Root canal treatment
     - Advantages: reduces (but does not eliminate) the risk of repeated dental infection; allows the patient to keep the tooth
     - Disadvantages: risk of suboptimal outcomes (patient fatigue and hence ability to tolerate longer treatment appointments, low blood counts may affect the success rate); stem cell transplants, particularly allogeneic, require a more critical approach (i.e. dental extraction preferred)
3) What factors are considered important in assessing the risk of managing this patient?
   - Social
     - Escort advisable due to likely fatigue
     - Need to be empathetic to the psychosocial impact of cancer (e.g. depression)
   - Medical
     - Increased risk of infection due to leukaemia and chemotherapy
     - Hypoglycaemia risk related to type 2 diabetes mellitus (see Chapter 5.1)
     - Cause of heart murmur (if significant, may impact on dental management/the need for antibiotic prophylaxis)
     - Vitamin D deficiency increases the risk of osteopenia
     - Risk of an adrenal crisis due to corticosteroid medication
     - Drug adverse effects and interactions

- Dental
  - Dental erosion risk due to gastro-oesophageal reflux disease
  - Discomfort/secondary infection risk related to the oral ulceration – likely to be related to chemotherapy
  - Pale mucosa likely to be related to underlying anaemia – may be associated with burning mouth/discomfort

4) The patient wishes to have the #36 extracted as she does not want to risk further infection. The haematologist is in agreement and withholds chemotherapy to allow you to proceed. Blood test results on the day of planned dental extraction are as follows: haemoglobin 98g/L, platelets 19×10^9/L, neutrophils 1.05×10^9/L, lymphocytes 0.79×10^9/L.
What are the risks?
   - Anaemia
     - Hypoxia can cause fatigue and lethargy, patient may appear poorly motivated; dental care should be adapted according to her tolerance of the planned procedure on the day of treatment
     - Additional increased risk of angular cheilitis, oral ulceration, altered taste, glossitis
   - Thrombocytopenia
     - Bleeding risk
   - Neutropenia and lymphocytopenia
     - Infection risk

5) What are the minimum blood counts (FBC) to allow you to proceed with extraction of #36?
   - Anaemia
     - There is no universal threshold of haemoglobin concentration at which transfusion of red blood cells is appropriate for all patients
     - However, the general consensus is that red blood cell transfusion is not indicated when haemoglobin concentrations are >100g/L
     - Transfusion of red blood cells is indicated at a haemoglobin concentration of < 70g/L
     - The correct strategy for transfusion of patients with haemoglobin concentrations between 70–100g/L is less clear; clinical judgement plays a vital role in the decision to transfuse red cells or not
     - Perioperative nasal oxygen should be considered
   - Thrombocytopenia
     - There is variation in literature regarding the recommended minimum platelet counts to allow for invasive dental procedures (Table 12.2.1)
     - In general, platelet counts $>50 \times 10^9$/L (>50 000 cells/mm^3) are considered acceptable, although this depends on the complexity and site of surgery
     - Where treatment is urgent, platelet transfusions can be given on the same day as treatment
   - Neutropenia
     - Similarly, there is variation in the recommended minimum neutrophil counts to allow for invasive dental procedures (Table 12.2.1)
     - In general, neutrophil counts $>1.0 \times 10^9$/L (1000 cells/mm^3) are considered acceptable, although this is again affected by the complexity and site of surgery
     - Recombinant human granulocyte-colony stimulating factor (G-CSF; filgrastim and pegylated filgrastim) and granulocyte-macrophage colony stimulating factor (GM-CSF; sargramostim) may be used to reduce the duration and degree of neutropenia but require ~5 days of treatment to raise the counts
     - The haematologist will advise on the appropriate regime and whether it is suitable (in a small subset of patients G-CSF may act as a driver for leukaemic cell production)
     - Postoperative antibiotics should be considered

6) Ideally, when should you have been involved in the pathway of care for this patient?
   - The dental team should have been involved in the patient's care pathway prior to commencement of cancer therapy so that issues such as the periapically involved #36 could have been identified and this tooth removed (Table 12.2.2)

General Dental Considerations

Oral Findings

- The mucosa that covers the oral cavity and the entire gastrointestinal tract is especially susceptible to the toxic effects of chemotherapy due to its high rate of cell renewal
- Oral complications of chemotherapy are common and should be considered before, during and after treatment
- They are commonly described as acute and chronic changes and can significantly impact on the quality of life for these patients (Tables 12.2.3 and 12.2.4)
- One of the most significant side-effects is mucositis, as this can be so debilitating as to result in cessation of chemotherapy; in view of this, grading systems have been developed to monitor its severity (Figure 12.2.2; Table 12.2.5)

Table 12.2.1 Guidelines for minimal haematological values for performance of invasive dental procedures.

Guideline, date	Platelet count	Neutrophil count
American Academy of Pediatric Dentistry, 2018	• >75 000 cells/mm^3: without additional support • 40 000–70 000 cells/mm^3: platelet transfusion may be considered in the preoperative and 24 h later	• >1000 cells/mm^3: no need for antibiotic prophylaxis. Some authors suggest prophylaxis if values 1000–2000 cells/mm^3 • <1000 cells/mm^3: postpone dental treatment. If emergency, discuss antibiotic prophylaxis with the medical team. Hospitalisation may be required
US National Cancer Institute, 2016	• >60 000 cells/mm^3: no additional support • 30 000–60 000 cells/mm^3: optional transfusion for non-invasive procedure. Consider administering preoperatively and 24 h later for surgical treatment • <30 000 cells/mm^3: platelets should be transfused 1 h before procedure. Transfuse regularly to maintain counts >30 000–40 000 cells/mm^3 until the start of healing. Consider local haemostatic agents and aminocaproic acid	• > 2000 cells/mm^3: no antibiotic prophylaxis • 1000–2000 cells/mm^3: American Heart Association antibiotic prophylaxis recommendations (low risk). If infection present, more aggressive antibiotic therapy may be indicated • <1000 cells/mm^3: amikacin 150 mg/m^2 and ticarcillin 7 mg/kg 1 h before surgery. Repeat both 6 h postoperative
Royal College of Surgeons of England and British Society of Disability and Oral Health, 2018 (additional comments to US National Cancer Institute guidelines)	• >60 000 cells/mm^3: major surgery may require platelet supplementation • 30 000–60 000 cells/mm^3: liaise with oncologist. Platelet requirements also depend on extent of treatment required and need for block injections. Utilise local haemostatic techniques • <30 000 cells/mm^3: tranexamic acid rather than aminocaproic acid	• 1000–2000 cells/mm^3: liaise with oncologist • <1000 cells/mm^3: liaise with oncologist. An amoxicillin/clindamycin antibiotic regimen is more often recommended

Table 12.2.2 Dental treatment planning prior to chemotherapy.

- Care pathway
  - Early pretreatment oral assessment, including radiographs
  - Liaison with oncology team to determine the current condition of the patient, type of treatment planned and overall prognosis
- Formulate dental treatment plan
  - An aggressive approach is required to stabilise oral health prior to cancer treatment
  - Time constraints as well as medical condition itself may require modification of the plan
- Remove infectious and traumatic dental/oral foci
  - Surgery: teeth with dubious prognosis should be removed no less than 10 days (preferably 3 weeks) prior to commencement of cancer therapy. Remove mobile primary teeth. Evaluate need to remove partially erupted teeth and gingival operculum
  - Periodontics: professional debridement of plaque/calculus deposits to stabilise periodontal disease. Extract teeth with doubtful prognosis (periodontal pockets >6 mm)
  - Endodontics: treat decayed teeth with risk of pulpal involvement or suspicious periapical lesions early. If not possible, consider extractions. Treatment of asymptomatic chronic periapical lesions may be delayed
  - Restorative: if time permits, definitively restore carious teeth
  - Orthodontics: discontinue orthodontic treatment and remove fixed orthodontic appliances
- Antibiotic prophylaxis/haematological support: may be warranted prior to invasive dental procedures. Liaise with the oncologist
- Oral hygiene: establish an adequate standard of oral hygiene to meet the increasing challenges during cancer therapy
- Dentures: if a removable prosthesis is worn, ensure it is clean and well adapted to tissue (consider soft liners)

Table 12.2.3 Acute oral side-effects of chemotherapy and oral care management.

Mucositis

- **Oral side-effects**
  - Acute mucosal inflammation, white/yellow fibrinous slough, often with ulceration
  - Painful to speak/eat/swallow/eat
  - Portal for microbial entry (septicaemia risk with neutropenia)
- **Background**
  - Onset typically 7 days after drug initiation
  - Degree of mucositis dependent on patient's age, nutritional status, oral hygiene, salivary function, chemotherapeutic agent
  - Typically resolves 2 to 3 weeks post completion of cancer therapy
  - Develops in 20–40% of patients undergoing chemotherapy (80% in radiochemotherapy)
  - Higher for 5-fluorouracil (5-FU) and cisplatin
- **Prophylaxis**
  - Oral cryotherapy (e.g. cooling with ice chips for 30 minutes before administration of 5-FU, methotrexate or melphalan)
  - Folinic acid, levofolinic acid or disodium folinate before administration of 5-FU or methotrexate
- **Symptomatic relief/treatment**
  - Viscous lidocaine 2%
  - Opioid analgesics – 2% morphine mouth rinse, fentanyl dermal patches
  - Special diet or tube feeding
  - Intravenous recombinant human keratinocyte growth factor 1 (palifermin 60 μg/kg/day intravenously)
  - Areas of research: low-level laser (He-Ne); biological response modifiers; anti-inflammatory drugs; colony-stimulating factors (GM-CSF), cytoprotective agents; angiogenesis inhibitors

Blood changes

- **Oral side-effects**
  - Crusting lips, oral ulceration, glossitis, mucosal pallor, burning sensation, oral infections
- **Background**
  - Anaemia, neutropenia, thrombocytopenia due to myelosuppressive effect of chemotherapy and some cancer processes (e.g. haematological malignancies)
  - Hepatotoxic and nephrotoxic effects of chemotherapy may further increase bleeding and anaemic risk
  - Onset from treatment commencement until 4 weeks post-therapy
- **Management**
  - Careful handling of soft tissues
  - Liaise with the oncology team if invasive treatment is planned

Immunosuppression

- **Oral side-effects**
  - Acute gingivitis
  - Exacerbates pre-existing periodontal disease
  - Pericoronitis in children
  - Periapically involved teeth can become a medical emergency
  - Fungal infections usually caused by *Candida* spp.
  - Viral infections usually herpes simplex or zoster viruses
- **Background**
  - Increases susceptibility to bacterial/fungal/viral infection
  - Periodontal disease exacerbated by oral flora changes, mucositis, hyposalivation and immunosuppression
  - Oral lesions can be portals for Gram-negative rapid systemic spread
  - Acute herpetic gingivostomatitis and *Candida* spp. infections with systemic involvement in children
- **Management**
  - Ensure scrupulous oral hygiene
  - Alcohol-free chlorhexidine mouthwash (diluted 1:1 to warm water for comfort)
  - Antibiotics for acute oral bacterial infections (in liaison with oncology team) to reduce risk of rapid systemic spread
  - Professional scaling and debridement, depending on blood counts; if periodontal disease uncontrolled, identification of atypical/resistant pathogens and antibiotics prescription (in liaison with oncology team)
  - Topical/systemic antifungals for oropharyngeal candidiasis: nystatin (100 000 units/mL suspension), miconazole (2% gel), fluconazole (50–100 mg daily for 7–14 days)
  - Herpes simplex or zoster virus infections: prophylactic or therapeutic administration of aciclovir (5% cream or 200–400 mg 5 times daily for 5–10 days)

(*Continued*)

Table 12.2.3 (Continued)

- **Nursing action**
  - Use tongue scrapers if coating developing on dorsum of tongue
  - Remove and clean dentures after each meal (at least twice daily)
  - Prescribed antifungals may be applied to denture fitting
  - Remove dentures nightly; soak in chlorhexidine or sodium hypochlorite solution (Milton's diluted 1:80) if no metal components
  - Microwave disinfection of complete dentures found to be effective

Changes in salivary flow/composition

- **Oral side-effects**
  - Saliva becomes thick, viscous, acidic
  - Hyposalivation (less common in children)
  - Acute ascending sialadenitis (most common in children)
- **Background**
  - Onset within 12–24 hours of cancer therapy
  - Saliva flow usually returns to normal within 2 months
- **Management**
  - Sip water frequently
  - Sugar-free chewing gum
  - Artificial saliva substitutes (ideally containing fluoride, and not acidic) and pilocarpine can provide certain symptomatic relief from xerostomia
  - Oral gel/lubricant to coat and protect lips/soft tissues
  - Bethanechol significantly increases the salivary flow in these patients (25 mg tablets, 3 times a day)
  - The efficacy of amifostine has not been definitely confirmed, and its use is only palliative
  - Areas of research: acupuncture, electrostimulation
  - Antimicrobials as required for acute sialadenitis

Dysgeusia/hypogeusia

- **Background**
  - Onset on treatment commencement
  - Associated with hyposalivation and direct damage to taste buds
  - Develops in 50% of patients receiving chemotherapy
  - Sense of taste often returns (not always), with unpleasant interim period of altered taste (e.g. metallic or bitter)
- **Management**
  - Dietary advice
  - Zinc sulfate 220 mg tablets twice daily
  - Avoid compensating for taste loss by consuming sweet food/drink
    Artificial sweeteners (e.g. xylitol)

Dysphagia

- **Background**
  - Due to mucositis and hyposalivation
  - Can be very severe due to severe ulceration
  - It usually disappears in a few months
- **Management**
  - Close monitoring, in liaison with oncology team and dietitian (especially if patient losing weight)
  - If dental treatment required, protect the airway, seat patient upright and minimise aerosols due to aspiration risk
  - Rinse mouth with analgesic mouthwash prior to eating (e.g. benzydamine HCl)
  - Eat moist food, have water with food
  - Eat high-energy food

(Continued)

Table 12.2.3 (Continued)

Tooth sensitivity/pain

- **Background**
  - May begin weeks or months after chemotherapy (notably vincristine and vinblastine)
  - Increased risk of tooth surface loss due to bruxism, vomiting and hyposalivation
  - Gingival recession may contribute
  - Increased risk of dental decay
  - May be related to leukaemic infiltration of dental pulp tissue and jaw
  - Toothache-like or mandibular jaw pain related to neurotoxicity of vincristine administration (usually subsiding 1 week after chemotherapy)
  - Leucopenia can cause chronic dental infections to become acute and painful
- **Management**
  - Recommend bicarbonate rinses (1 tsp bicarbonate soda dissolved in 200 mL water), mainly following episodes of vomiting to reduce dental erosion risk
  - Sensitive toothpaste
  - Consider topical fluoride application
  - Assess the need for conventional dental procedures (e.g. fillings or endodontics)

Table 12.2.4 Chronic oral side-effects of chemotherapy (management as for acute changes).

Blood changes
- Prolonged by maintenance chemotherapy or persistent haemato-oncology disease

Prolonged immunosuppression
- Increased susceptibility to viral infections and candidiasis
- Herpes labialis may be a chronic problem

Periodontal/gingival disease
- Can continue to be exacerbated by hyposalivation, oral flora changes and maintenance chemotherapy

Adrenal suppression
- Can occur due to corticosteroid therapy

Craniofacial maldevelopment
- Delayed development or abnormalities in craniofacial skeleton, jaws and dentition in children
- Early specialist involvement essential to ensure good outcomes

Medication-related osteonecrosis of the jaw (see Chapter 16.2)
- May occur as a result of non-conventional drugs used in the treatment of some cancers (e.g. bisphosphonates, RANKL inhibitors, VEGF inhibitors and tyrosine kinase inhibitors)
- Prevalence when these drugs are given in cancer patients is reported as 0.8–12%.
- Risk is approximately 1% (range 0.2–6.7%) following dental extraction if antiresorptive agents are administered for cancer treatment
- Recent case reports of association with rituximab and methotrexate

Increased risk of malignancy
- Routine surveillance for development of further malignancies

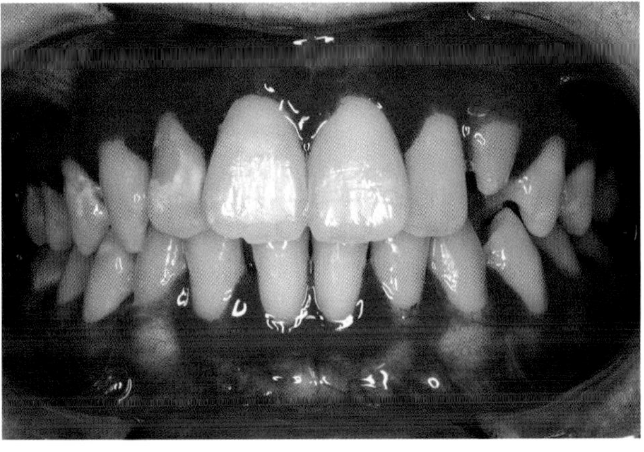

Figure 12.2.2 Acute mucositis secondary to the administration of 5-fluorouracil.

Dental Management

- Dental risk assessment for patients receiving chemotherapy varies according to the drug regimen and related side-effects
- It is important to consider the psychosocial effect of chemotherapy side-effects such as alopecia, as this can have a significant impact on the patient's ability to cope with further intervention, including dental treatment (Figure 12.2.3)
- In all instances, it is essential to liaise closely with the haematology/oncology teams to ensure appropriate support and treatment modifications are in place (Table 12.2.6)

Table 12.2.5 Oral mucositis scales.

Scale	Grade 0	Grade I	Grade II	Grade III	Grade IV	Grade V
WHO	None	Erythema and soreness; no ulcers	Oral erythema; ulcers; solid diet tolerated	Oral ulcers; liquid diet only	Not able to tolerate a solid or liquid diet	N/A
OMAS[a]	None	Ulceration <1 cm^2; erythema (mild/moderate)	Ulceration 1–3 cm^2; severe erythema	Ulceration >3 cm^2	N/A	N/A
NCI-CTCAE v5.0	None	Asymptomatic or mild symptoms; intervention not indicated	Moderate pain or ulcer; modified diet indicated	Severe pain; interfering with oral intake	Life-threatening consequences; urgent intervention indicated	Death

WHO, World Health Organization; OMAS, Oral Mucositis Assessment Scale; NCI, National Cancer Institute; CTCAE, Common Terminology Criteria for Adverse Events; N/A: not applicable.

[a] The value of OMAS is obtained by summing the ulceration/pseudomembrane and erythema subscores at each site (range 0–5), and then averaging these scores across all 8 anatomical sites.

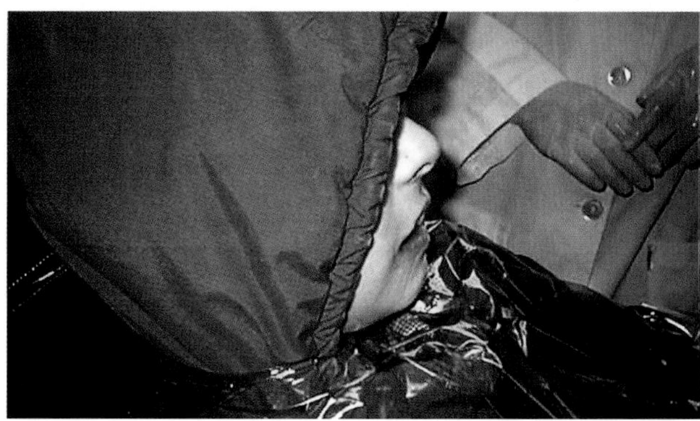

Figure 12.2.3 A child wearing a hood due to alopecia.

Section II: Background Information and Guidelines

Definition

Chemotherapy, or 'chemical treatment'. As the treatment of cancer began in the 1940s with the use of nitrogen mustard. The term is used most often to describe drugs that kill cancer cells directly. These are sometimes referred to as 'anti-cancer' drugs or 'antineoplastics'.

More than 100 chemotherapy drugs are now available to treat cancer, with even more still under development and investigation. Chemotherapy drugs may also be used in lower doses for the management of autoimmune disorders such as rheumatoid arthritis, multiple sclerosis and systemic lupus erythematosus.

Conventional chemotherapy drugs are increasingly being replaced by other drugs, which work in different ways to treat cancer. These include biological response modifiers, hormone therapy and monoclonal antibodies.

Chemotherapy Regimens

- Chemotherapy treatment may involve a single drug or more than one drug as part of a combination chemotherapy regimen (often with high-dose steroids)
- Combination chemotherapy works on the principle that 2 or more agents have greater response than when used alone as they may act in different phases of the cell cycle and have synergistic effects to overcome drug resistance
- The approach to chemotherapy depends on treatment intent (Table 12.2.7)
- Chemotherapy may be used as monotherapy or in combination with other treatments, including surgery, radiotherapy, hormonal therapy and targeted therapy/immunotherapy
- Immunotherapy uses the immune system to detect and attack cancer cells, often with targeted therapy
- Hormonal therapy alters the production or activity of particular hormones to treat hormone-dependent cancers (e.g. breast and prostate cancer)

Types of Chemotherapy Drugs

- Chemotherapy uses cytotoxic drugs that act mainly by interaction with the cancer cell DNA or RNA, affecting some phase of the cell's life cycle
- Some cytotoxic drugs exert their action in a specific phase of the cell's life cycle (cell cycle-specific drugs), whilst others (cell cycle-non-specific drugs) exert cytotoxic

Table 12.2.6 General dental management considerations.

Risk assessment	• Common side-effects of chemotherapy include anaemia, thrombocytopenia and neutropenia • Some patients may be taking anticoagulant medication to reduce thromboembolic risk associated with both the disease process and some antineoplastics (see Chapters 10.2–10.4) • Significant psychosocial impact of cancer and its treatment
Criteria for referral	• Patients receiving intensive chemotherapy with associated reduction in blood counts should be seen in a secondary care setting • Patients with dental infections during chemotherapy should be referred to secondary care
Access/position	• The patient may feel fatigued or unwell due to chemotherapy so may need to cancel appointments • Consider inpatient or outpatient status and need for hospital transport • Escort requirements • Reduce time in waiting room with other patients, especially if the patient is neutropenic • Liaise closely with the medical/oncology team regarding timing of proposed treatment and co-ordination of visits with other medical appointments • Elective treatment should be avoided wherever possible during cancer therapy. Ideally perform dental treatment prior to or after recovery from chemotherapy • Some dental treatment may require an interruption to chemotherapy – typically 10 days recovery is required after dental extractions • Position: consider a semi-reclined position if the patient is breathless or nauseated/vomits frequently
Communication	• Close liaison with the oncology team is required • Close liaison with the patient and escort to confirm attendance on the day
Consent/capacity	• Discuss the risks and benefits of treatment options with patient, in light of current and foreseeable medical status • Consider the impact of fatigue and emotional distress on decision making • Provide information in an appropriate format (e.g. there may be ototoxicity or blurred vision secondary to chemotherapy)
Anaesthesia/sedation	• Local anaesthesia – Check platelet count before administering – Regional block injections should be avoided for patients with platelet counts $<50 \times 10^9$/L – Should include vasoconstrictor • Sedation – Caution due to the risk of anaemia/respiratory depression – Cannulation may result in extended bruising/bleeding • General anaesthesia – Avoid in case of severe anaemia – A thorough prior medical consideration is mandatory
Dental treatment	• Before – Check the recent blood test results – Confirm the need and arrangements for supportive measures such as timing of platelet transfusions and immunoglobulin replacement – Confirm the need for antibiotic prophylaxis or corticosteroid supplementation (see Chapter 12.1) – Be sensitive that the patient may be wearing a wig/scarf/hat due to alopecia, which they may feel uncomfortable removing unless absolutely necessary

(*Continued*)

Table 12.2.6 (Continued)

	• During – Consider the need for perioperative nasal oxygen if the patient is anaemic or has secondary cardiotoxicity (2–3 L/min) – Avoid shining the dental light into the patient's eyes as blurred vision/photosensitivity may be present as a side-effect of chemotherapy (use dark eye protection safety glasses) – Sterile surgical environment and procedure (including gown/gloves) recommended for all invasive procedures – Lubricant/barrier cream to protect lips/soft tissue from trauma – Careful manipulation of cheek and soft tissues (oral mucositis, increased risk of bruising/bleeding) – Consider acute oral side-effects of chemotherapy (Table 12.2.2) • After – Consider adjuvant use of tranexamic acid 5% mouthwash if bleeding prolonged – Wound healing may be impaired and there is a higher risk of postoperative infection (consider antiseptics ± antibiotics)
Drug prescription	• Antiseptics: 0.12–0.2% alcohol-free chlorhexidine mouthwashes • Antibiotics: consult with oncologist regarding most appropriate prescription • Pain relief: paracetamol • Caution with drug selection and dosages if there is secondary nephrotoxicity or hepatotoxicity • Contraindications: avoid aspirin/non-steroidal anti-inflammatory drugs due to increased risk of bleeding and increased risk of gastric ulcers in combination with corticosteroids • Drug interactions: check before prescribing (e.g. aspirin enhances methotrexate toxicity)
Education/prevention	• If mouth is too painful to clean with a soft toothbrush, consider use of oral sponges or gauze moistened with alcohol-free chlorhexidine mouthwash • If severely thrombocytopenic, advise cessation of flossing • Dietary advice to reduce risk of dental decay provided in liaison with dietitian • Increased risk of gout which may reduce dexterity for oral hygiene • Prescribe 2800 or 5000 ppm high fluoride toothpaste and consider fluoride supplements (mouthwash daily, varnish twice yearly). Do not use during acute episodes of mucositis • Ongoing smoking and alcohol cessation support • Consider chronic oral side-effects of chemotherapy (Table 12.2.4)

action during both the cycling and G_0 resting phase of the cell cycle

- Chemotherapeutic drugs are divided into several broad categories depending on their principal mode of action (Table 12.2.8)

Routes of Administration

- Topical: creams, gels (typically for skin cancers)
- Oral: tablets, capsules
- Subcutaneous: injection
- Intramuscular: injection
- Intravenous: cannula, implantable port (e.g. Port-A-Cath), central or peripheral line (e.g. Hickman, peripherally inserted central catheter) (Figure 12.2.4)
- Intracavitary: intraperitoneal (abdomen), intrapleural (chest), intravesical (urethra)
- Intrathecal: lumbar puncture into cerebrospinal fluid
- Direct application: during surgery (e.g. wafer disc placed near tumour; injection into cancer-supplying artery or vein)

General Side-Effects of Chemotherapy Drugs

The potential associated toxicities of chemotherapy drugs are varied and broadly associated with their mechanism of action (Table 12.2.9)

A World/Transcultural View

- Worldwide, the global cancer burden is rising due to population growth and ageing, and the changes in social and economic development
- One in 2 people are expected to have a form of cancer in their lifetime

Table 12.2.7 Chemotherapeutic treatment intents.

• Primary chemotherapy	Sole treatment for cancer, primarily for haematological cancers
• Neo-adjuvant chemotherapy	Prior to surgery or radiotherapy, to reduce the size of large tumours
• Chemoradiation	At same time as radiotherapy, to preferentially sensitise tumour cells to its cytotoxic effects ('radiosensitising')
• Adjuvant chemotherapy	After surgery or radiotherapy, to reduce the chance of relapse by treating any remaining cells
• Palliative chemotherapy	Shrinking/controlling a cancer to relieve symptoms in advanced end-stage tumours
• Cytoreductive conditioning	In preparation for bone marrow transplant or haemopoietic stem cell transplant

Table 12.2.8 Drugs used in treatment of malignant disease.

Drug class	Main drug types and examples
• **Conventional chemotherapeutic (cytotoxic) drugs**	
Alkylating agents	Oxazaphosphorines: cyclophosphamide, ifosfamide Nitrogen mustards: chlorambucil, melphalan Alkylsulfonate: busulfan Hydrazine: temozolomide Platinum-based agents: carboplatin, cisplatin, oxaliplatin
Antimetabolites	Adenosine deaminase inhibitors: cladribine Antifolates: methotrexate, pemetrexed Purine analogues: 6-mercaptopurine, 6-thioguanine Purine antagonists: fludarabine Pyrimidine antagonists: 5-fluorouracil, capecitabine, cytarabine, gemcitabine Ribonucleotide reductase inhibitors: hydroxyurea (hydroxycarbamide)
Antitumour antibiotics	Anthracyclines: daunorubicin, doxorubicin, idarubicin Chromomycins: dactinomycin (actinomycin D), mithramycin Others: bleomycin, mitomycin
Mitotic inhibitors	Taxanes: docetaxel, paclitaxel Vinca alkaloids: vinblastine, vincristine
Topoisomerase inhibitors	Topoisomerase I inhibitors: irinotecan, topotecan Topoisomerase II inhibitors: etoposide, teniposide
• **Other drugs used in cancer therapy**	
Monoclonal antibodies	Bevacizumab, nivolumab, rituximab, cetoxumab, trastuzumab
Growth factor inhibitors	Hedgehog pathway blockers Histone deacetylase inhibitors mTOR inhibitors: everolimus, sirolimus PI3K inhibitors Proteasome inhibitors: bortezomib, carfilzomib
Angiogenesis inhibitors	Thalidomide derivatives: lenalidomide, pomalidomide, thalidomide Tyrosine kinase inhibitors: sunitinib VEGF inhibitors: aflibercept, bevacizumab
PARP inhibitors	Olaparib, rucaparib, niraparib
Enzymes	L-asparaginase

(*Continued*)

Table 12.2.8 (Continued)

Drug class	Main drug types and examples
Hormones	Androgens: fluoxymesterone Oestrogens: ethinyloestradiol, diethylstilboestrol, fosfestrol Progestogens: norethisterone
Hormone antagonist	Aromatase inhibitors: anastrozole, exemestane, letrozole Selective oestrogen receptor modulators: tamoxifen, toremifene Gonadotrophin-releasing hormone analogues: buserelin, goserelin, leuprorelin, triptorelin
Recombinant interleukin-2	Aldesleukin
Somatostatin analogues	Lanreotide, octreotide
Others	Adoptive cell transfer/T-cell therapy, gene therapy, nanoparticles, vaccines, virus therapy

PARP, poly-ADP-ribose polymerase; VEGF, vascular endothelial growth factor.

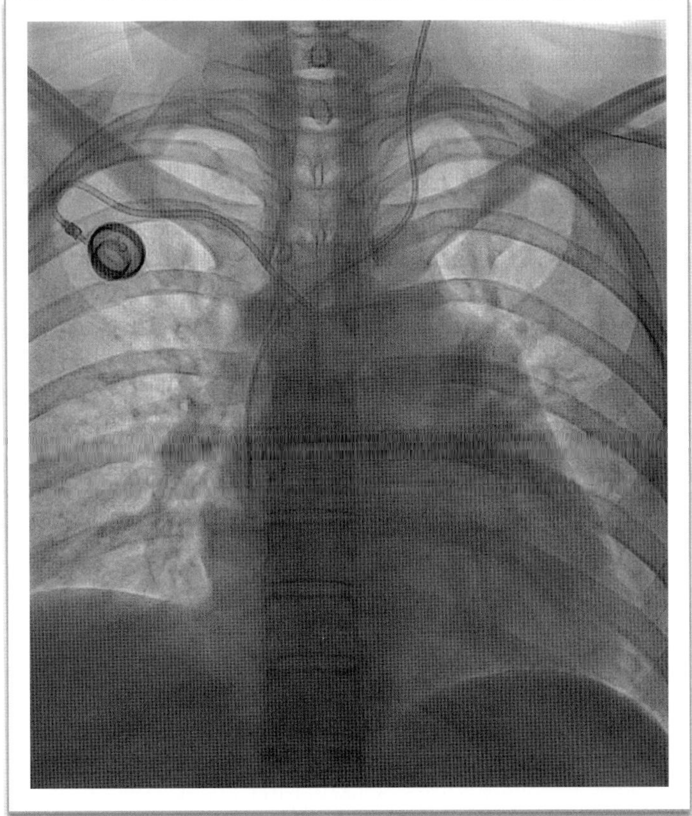

Figure 12.2.4 Chest radiograph showing a left single-lumen central venous catheter and a right subcutaneous port catheter for delivery of chemotherapeutic agents.

Table 12.2.9 Adverse effects and toxicities of various chemotherapeutic agents.

Early complications	
Cutaneous	Alopecia Erythema Exfoliative dermatitis Hyperpigmentation Maculopapular eruptions Photosensitivity Stevens–Johnson syndrome
Gastrointestinal	Constipation Diarrhoea Emesis Mucositis Nausea Oesophagitis
Hepatotoxicity	Biliary stricture Cholestasis Fibrosis/cirrhosis Hepatitis Steatosis Veno-occlusive disease
Musculoskeletal	Muscle wasting Osteoporosis
Myelosuppression (bone marrow)	Anaemia Leucopenia Thrombocytopenia
Nephrotoxicity	Electrolyte abnormalities Glomerular disease Hypertension Hyperuricaemia, hypercalcaemia, proteinuria Thrombotic microangiopathy Tubulointerstitial damage
Neurotoxicity	Central and peripheral neuropathies Centrally induced emesis Convulsions Pain
Ototoxicity	Hearing loss Tinnitus Vertigo
Late complications	
Cardiotoxicity	Cardiomyopathy Congestive heart failure Supraventricular tachycardia
Reproductive	Spermatogenesis/oogenesis inhibition (infertility) Menstrual cycle disturbance Teratogenicity
Pulmonary toxicity	Interstitial pneumonia Pulmonary fibrosis
Bone marrow	Myelodysplasia Secondary malignancy (leukaemia)

- The number of people who will need chemotherapy is predicted to rise steadily over coming decades, two-thirds of which will be from low- and middle-income countries
- In 2040, the most common indications for chemotherapy worldwide are predicted to be lung cancer, breast cancer and colorectal cancer

Recommended Reading

American Academy of Pediatric Dentistry (2018). Dental management of pediatric patients receiving immunosuppressive therapy and/or radiation therapy. *Pediatr. Dent.* 40: 392–400.

Brennan, M.T., Woo, S.-B., and Lockhart, P.B. (2008). Dental treatment planning and management in the patient who has cancer. *Dent. Clin. North Am.* 52: 19–37.

Busenhart, D.M., Erb, J., Rigakos, G. et al. (2018). Adverse effects of chemotherapy on the teeth and surrounding tissues of children with cancer: a systematic review with meta-analysis. *Oral Oncol.* 83: 64–72.

Carvalho, C.G., Medeiros-Filho, J.B., and Ferreira, M.C. (2018). Guide for health professionals addressing oral care for individuals in oncological treatment based on scientific evidence. *Support. Care Cancer* 26: 2651–2661.

King, R., Zebic, L., and Patel, V. (2020). Deciphering novel chemotherapy and its impact on dentistry. *Br. Dent. J.* 228: 415–421.

Kumar, N., Burke, M., Brooke, A., et al. (2018). *The Oral Management of Oncology Patients Requiring Radiotherapy, Chemotherapy and / or Bone Marrow Transplantation*. London: Royal College of Surgeons of England/British Society for Disability and Oral Health. www.rcseng.ac.uk/dental-faculties/fds/publications-guidelines/clinical-guidelines

PDQ® Supportive and Palliative Care Editorial Board. (2016). *PDQ Oral Complications of Chemotherapy and Head/Neck Radiation*. Bethesda, MD: National Cancer Institute. www.cancer.gov/about-cancer/treatment/side-effects/mouth-throat/oral-complications-hp-pdq

Shimada, Y., Nakagawa, Y., Ide, K. et al. (2017). Importance of eliminating potential dental focal infection before the first cycle of chemotherapy in patients with hematologic malignancy. *Support. Care Cancer* 25: 1379–1381.

12.3 Immunosuppressants (Solid Organ Transplantation)

Section I: Clinical Scenario and Dental Considerations

Clinical Scenario

A 47-year-old male has been referred by his nephrologist for management of 'loose teeth'. The patient reports he pulled out a lower incisor and upper right molar himself using his fingers. The patient believes it may be best to have all his teeth removed.

Medical History

- History of renal failure secondary to bilateral polycystic kidney disease
- Right kidney transplant 9 years ago
- Hypertension
- Osteopenia
- Absolute polycythaemia diagnosed three years ago
- Obstructive sleep apnoea (moderate severity)

Medications

- Mycophenolate mofetil
- Tacrolimus
- Prednisolone (5 mg daily)
- Trimethoprim/sulfamethoxazole
- Irbesartan
- Calcium and vitamin D
- Pantoprazole
- Intermittent venesections (phlebotomy)

Dental History

- Last dental visit 9 years ago for pretransplant work-up
- Did not return as had no dental pain
- Good compliance: all previous dental treatment under local anaesthetic in the dental chair
- Reports brushing twice per day; does not use interdental brushes

Social History

- Caucasian origin
- Married, lives with wife and two daughters
- Ceased tobacco smoking when he had the renal transplant, previously smoked seven cigarettes per day for 23 years
- Alcohol: Two to three bottles of beer per month

Oral Examination

- Halitosis
- Poor oral health
- Carious retained roots #17, #35, #45 and #46
- Caries in #26 distal and #36 mesial
- Generalised severe gingivitis with generalised extensive supra- and subgingival calculus (Figure 12.3.1)
- Multiple teeth with 4–7 mm periodontal pockets
- Multiple mobile teeth, notably grade III mobility of #26 and #48

Radiological Examination

- Orthopantomogram undertaken showing advanced bone loss, subgingival calculus and retained roots #17, #35, #45 and #46
- Right bitewing radiograph: horizontal bone loss; calculus; retained roots #17, #45 and #46 (Figure 12.3.2)
- Left bitewing radiograph: horizontal bone loss; calculus; retained root #35

Structured Learning

1) Why is this patient taking mycophenolate mofetil, tacrolimus and prednisolone?
   - All three drugs are immunosuppressive agents that act to prevent transplant T-cell alloimmune rejection
   - Mycophenolate mofetil

A Practical Approach to Special Care in Dentistry, First Edition. Edited by Pedro Diz Dios and Navdeep Kumar.

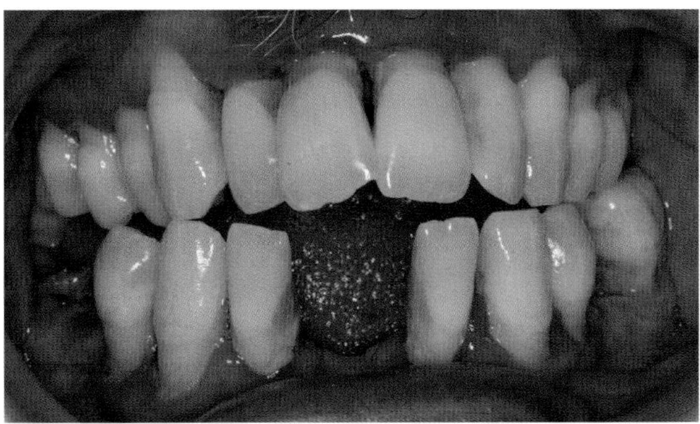

Figure 12.3.1 Anterior view of the dentition showing generalised hard and soft deposits and gingival recession.

(a)

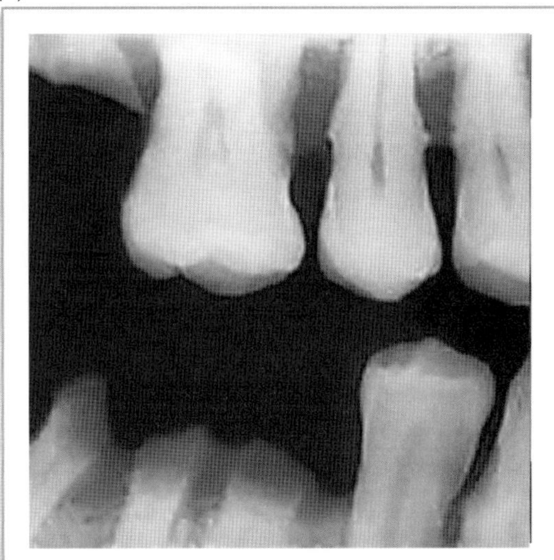

(b)

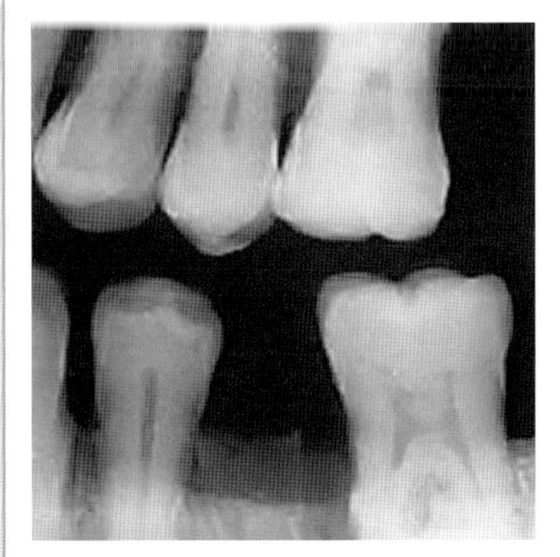

Figure 12.3.2 (a,b) Bite-wing radiographs showing horizontal bone loss, subgingival calculus and retained roots #17, #45, #46 and 35.

  - Antiproliferative agent that inhibits purine biosynthesis (selective for lymphocytes)
  - Common adverse effects include gastrointestinal disturbances and myelosuppression
- Tacrolimus
  - Calcineurin inhibitor that inhibits IL-2 production
  - Highly potent immunosuppressant that has nephrotoxic, hepatotoxic, neurotoxic, diabetic and hypertensive side-effects
- Prednisolone
  - Corticosteroid used for its immunosuppressive effects, as well as to treat other inflammatory and endocrine disorders

2) What oral changes may be associated with mycophenolate mofetil and tacrolimus?
   - Mycophenolate mofetil: stomatitis, petechiae/gingival bleeding, dental erosion
   - Tacrolimus: oral ulceration, circumoral paraesthesia
   - Both: opportunistic infections (candidiasis, herpes simplex virus, varicella zoster virus, cytomegalovirus, oral hairy leucoplakia caused by Epstein–Barr virus), impaired wound healing, increased malignancy risk
3) The patient feels that his periodontal disease and related tooth mobility have worsened after his renal transplantation. Could he be correct?
   - Recipients of the new organ (except when the donor and the recipient are identical twins) undergo immunosuppressive therapy throughout life to prevent the rejection process
   - As this patient is immunosuppressed, his periodontal disease activity may have accelerated
   - Other factors will also have had an impact, namely his irregular dental visits and poor oral health
4) Conversely, could this patient's periodontal disease affect the survival of the renal transplant?
   - There is evidence of an association between periodontal status and worsening of graft function and systemic health among kidney transplant recipients
   - In view of this, it is especially important to manage the patient's periodontal disease and remove this risk
5) What factors are considered important in assessing the risk of managing this patient?
   - Social
     - History of smoking
     - Lack of motivation for oral health maintenance
     - Possible fatigue
   - Medical
     - Bleeding (renal impairment, myelosuppression, absolute polycythaemia)

- Thrombotic tendency (thromboembolism and myocardial infarction risk)
- Hypertension in relation to polycythaemia
- Blood glucose level monitoring (e.g. corticosteroids, calcineurin inhibitors)
- Risk of an adrenal crisis due to corticosteroid medication
- Drug interactions and metabolism
- Increased risk of secondary malignancy (e.g. squamous cell carcinoma, Kaposi sarcoma, lymphoma)

- Dental
  - Dental erosion risk (due to emesis)
  - Impaired wound healing
  - History of irregular attendance
  - Mouth breathing (obstructive sleep apnoea)
  - Oral side-effects of immunosuppressants (e.g. oral ulceration and stomatitis)

6) Given the poor status of the patient's remaining teeth, he consents for dental extraction of multiple teeth, namely the retained roots #17, #35, #45, #46, teeth with very poor periodontal prognoses #26, #48 and non-functional periodontally involved teeth #16, #36, #38. Would you consider antibiotic prophylaxis when undertaking these dental extractions?
   - Due to increased risk of infection in the immunosuppressed transplant patient, many transplant centres recommend antibiotic prophylaxis for dental procedures that may produce a transient bacteraemia
   - However, no data exist to indicate whether this is effective practice, and protocols vary between different countries
   - Selection of the best antibiotic is difficult since the oral flora is altered by both immunosuppression and repeated/background antibiotic prophylaxis
   - Furthermore, drug interactions between immunosuppressants and multiple antibiotics exist
   - Given the lack of scientific evidence regarding any benefit from antibiotic prophylaxis, usage should be determined on an individual patient basis in consultation with the transplant team

General Dental Considerations

Oral Findings

- Fungal infection (candidiasis most common)
- Viral infection (herpes simplex virus, varicella zoster virus, cytomegalovirus)
- Oral hairy leucoplakia (Epstein–Barr virus)
- Petechiae, gingival bleeding
- Reduced salivary flow
- Oral ulceration and stomatitis (Figure 12.3.3)
- Mucosal pallor, angular cheilitis, glossitis, fissured/burning tongue, ulcers (anaemia)
- Impaired healing
- Dental erosion
- Progressive gingivitis and periodontitis (indication of immunosuppression)
- Gingival hyperplasia (cyclosporine) (Figure 12.3.4)
- Dysgeusia (mTOR inhibitors)
- Circumoral paraesthesia (tacrolimus, cyclosporine)

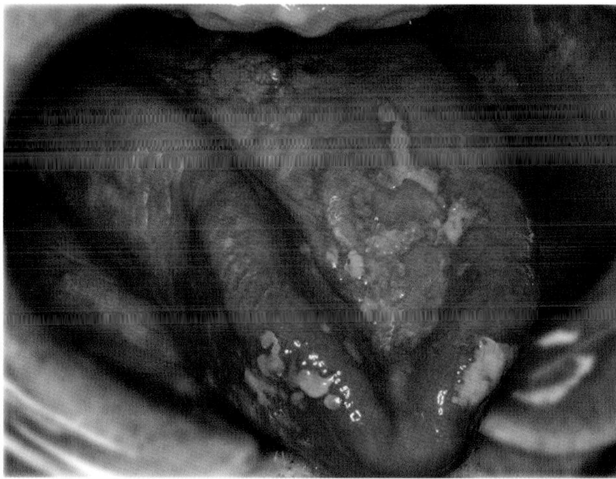

Figure 12.3.3 Sirolimus-induced oral ulceration.

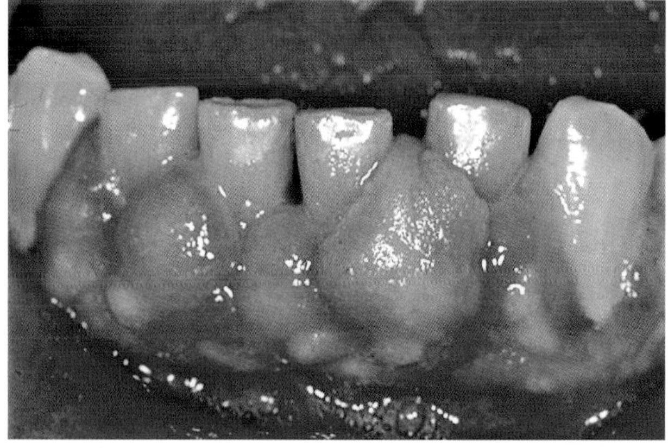

Figure 12.3.4 Cyclosporine-induced gingival hyperplasia.

- Medication-related osteonecrosis of the jaws (mTOR inhibitors, bone-altering medications prescribed secondary to corticosteroid osteoporosis, possibly methotrexate)
- Graft-versus-host disease-related side-effects

- Malignancy
  - Virally driven: carcinoma of skin/lip (human papillomavirus), Kaposi sarcoma (human herpes virus-8), lymphoma (Epstein–Barr virus)
  - Cutaneous: squamous cell carcinoma, melanoma, basal cell carcinoma
  - Post-transplant lymphoproliferative disorder (ranging from benign B-cell hyperplasia to immunoblastic malignant lymphoma); incidence ~2%; most cases develop within the first year post-transplant; association with Epstein–Barr virus; rapidly progressive and often fatal

Dental Management

- Patients who receive organ transplantation are immunosuppressed to prevent organ rejection; in view of this they are at increased risk of local and systemic infections
- Since these infections can be life-threatening, maintenance of good oral care and aggressive treatment of odontogenic infections are crucially important, with dental management considerations summarised in Table 12.3.1
- In addition, there are specific risks which need to be considered in relation to the specific type of organ transplant and immunosuppressive agents used post-transplant (Tables 12.3.2 and 12.3.3)

Section II: Background Information and Guidelines

Definition

A solid organ transplant is a highly effective treatment for advanced organ failure via transplantation of a healthy organ. Transplanted solid organs may come from a living or deceased donor, with clinical and ethical guidelines for organ transplantation developed in many countries. Organs from deceased donors are retrieved after either brain death or circulatory death (cadaveric).

The first documented successful kidney transplantation was performed between living identical twins in Boston, USA, by Joseph Murray and John Merrill in 1954. However, it was not until the 1980s that transplantation survival rates showed significant improvement. This was linked to the development of antimicrobial agents, prophylaxis strategies, enhancement in monitoring methods and advancement of immunosuppressive induction and maintenance agents.

Transplant activity data reported in 2017 to the World Transplant Registry (in partnership with the World Health Organization) showed that ~135 860 solid organ transplants were performed worldwide: 89 823 kidney transplants (40% from living donors), 30 352 liver transplants (19% from living donors), 7626 heart transplants, 5497 lung transplants, 2342 pancreas transplants and 220 small bowel transplants. Solid organ transplantation can save lives affected by terminal organ failure and also improve quality of life.

Classification

- The most common organs, tissues and cells transplanted include kidneys, hearts, lungs, pancreas, liver and small bowel; bone marrow, cornea, bone and skin; and cells of muscle, bone and pancreas
- Types of transplants include autografts, allografts and isografts (Table 12.3.4)
- Most solid organ transplants are allografts, whereas autografts are more commonly used in haemopoietic stem cell transplantation or bone marrow transplantation
- Due to the shortage of organs for transplantation, the focus has been on stem cell research to enable healthy organs to be grown outside the human body
- One such method, called blastocyst complementation, has already produced promising results. These have been injected with stem cells from a normal donor, not necessarily of the same species. The stem cells then differentiate to form the entire missing organ in the resulting animal. The new organ retains the characteristics of the original stem cell donor, and can thus potentially be used in transplantation therapy

Indications

- Limited life expectancy
- Untreatable end-stage disease
- Substantial limitation of daily activities
- Ambulatory patient with rehabilitation potential
- Acceptable nutritional status
- Satisfactory psychosocial profile and emotional support system
- Absence of other severe concomitant underlying diseases

Immunosuppression

- Given most organ transplants are allografts, and as such have an element of mismatch, the recipient needs to be

Table 12.3.1 General dental management considerations.

Risk assessment	• Infection, bleeding, anaemia risk • Adrenal suppression • Secondary diabetes • Oral complications (e.g. mucositis, dental erosion, medication-related osteonecrosis of the jaw) • Increased risk of malignancy • Risks related to type of organ transplantation (Table 12.3.2)
Criteria for referral	• Patients about to undergo organ transplantation may be managed by primary care dentists prior to the operation • If necessary, seek advice from/refer to secondary dental care • In the immediate post-transplant period or chronic rejection period, refer to secondary dental care (consider hospital setting)
Access/position	• Immediate post-transplant period (first three months) – Elective dental treatment should be delayed at least three months and ideally until 6 months after transplant – If emergency dental treatment required: ○ Close medical consultation ○ Conservative selection of treatment ○ Consider treating in hospital setting • Stable post-transplant period – Six months may be required before transplant recipient deemed stable enough to receive dental treatment – Confirm that blood counts, coagulation and blood chemistry profiles are satisfactory • Book surgical appointments in the morning and early in week (bleeding risk)
Communication	• Close liaison with the patient's transplant team regarding dental treatment plan • Fatigue may affect the patient's ability to engage and communicate
Consent/capacity	• May be impacted by fatigue and lethargy
Anaesthesia/sedation	• Local anaesthesia – Bleeding and infection risk – Use an aspirating syringe and include a vasoconstrictor, unless contraindicated • Sedation – Not recommended due to anaemia, potential drug interactions with immunosuppressants and potentially impaired clearance – If needed, advise the patient's transplant team • General anaesthesia – Not recommended (as above)
Dental treatment	• Before The specific risks in relation to the type of organ failure should be assessed (Table 12.3.2) – Close liaison with physician/transplant team regarding the dental treatment plan and need for antibiotic prophylaxis – Consider the need for preoperative blood tests • During – Lubricant/barrier cream used to protect the lips/soft tissue from trauma – Careful manipulation of the cheek and soft tissues (e.g. caution with suction) – Consider bleeding risk • After – Consider the use of tranexamic acid 5% mouthwash if bleeding prolonged – Postoperative chlorhexidine mouthwashes for 1–2 weeks after invasive procedures

(Continued)

Table 12.3.1 (Continued)

Drug prescription	• Antiseptics: 0.12–0.2% chlorhexidine mouthwashes • Antibiotics: consult with transplant team regarding most appropriate prescription • Pain relief: paracetamol
Education/prevention	• Need for life-long oral health maintenance in view of the medically compromised status • Maintain effective oral hygiene procedures • Initiate active recall programme, with appointments 3–6 monthly • Consider the need for fluoride supplementation and use of chlorhexidine mouth rinses • Constant surveillance for malignancy (e.g. squamous cell carcinoma, Kaposi sarcoma, lymphoma)

Table 12.3.2 Risk assessment and modifications in relation to specific organ failure/transplantation.

Heart transplant	• Adequate pain and anxiety control to reduce cardiac stress • Bleeding risk (anticoagulant or antiplatelet medications) • Caution with intravascular injection of adrenaline (consider adrenaline-free solutions) • Consider antibiotic prophylaxis especially if infective endocarditis risk • Side-effects of antihypertensive medications (see Table 8.1.1) • Pacemakers and electromagnetic interference • 'Silent' myocardial infarction may occur without angina (lack of cardiac innervation)
Lung transplant	• Mouth breathing before transplant may lead to dry mouth and related exacerbation of periodontal disease • Caution with respiratory depressant drugs (e.g. opioid analgesics) • Consider semi-reclined position • Consider airway protective measures (e.g. rubber dam, high-volume suction, minimisation of aerosols) • Consider preoperative chlorhexidine rinse to reduce oral bacterial load • Pulse oximetry may be of benefit
Kidney transplant	• Consider any residual renal impairment and its impact • Nephrotoxic drugs should be avoided (e.g. non-steroidal anti-inflammatory drugs) • Bleeding risk (thrombocytopenia, platelet dysfunction, defective vWF, reduced thromboxane) • Altered bone metabolism (medication-related osteonecrosis of the jaw risk if prescribed antiresorptive drugs)
Liver transplant	• Nutritional deficiencies (risk of angular cheilitis, glossitis, fissured tongue, ulceration) • Bleeding risk (reduced coagulation factors, thrombocytopenia) – Petechiae, ecchymosis, gingival bleeding – Preoperative complete blood count, coagulation studies – Local haemostatic measures • Avoid liver metabolism agents and hepatotoxic drugs
Pancreas transplant	• Often performed with kidney transplant • Hypoglycaemia (especially pretransplant or in rejection phase) – Preoperative blood glucose levels – Patients can experience sudden alterations in blood glucose levels leading to insulin shock – Immunosuppressed patients may have intermittent or temporary elevations in glucose, particularly in those with acute rejection

Table 12.3.3 Immunosuppressive agents used in organ transplantation and dental management implications.

Drug class and examples		Mechanism of action	Dental management implications and drug interactions
Corticosteroids	Prednisolone Methylprednisolone Hydrocortisone	Block transcription of cytokine genes, IL-1, IL-2, IL-3, IL-5, IL-6, TNF-alpha and interferons	• Impaired wound healing • Opportunistic infections • Steroid supplementation • Increased risk of medication-related osteonecrosis of the jaw • Avoid aspirin and non-steroidal anti-inflammatory drugs (gastrointestinal bleeding)
Calcineurin inhibitors	Cyclosporine	Inhibits IL-2 production and stimulates TGF-beta production	• Impaired wound healing • Gingival hyperplasia • Circumoral paraesthesia • Bleeding • Avoid clarithromycin, ketoconazole
	Tacrolimus	Inhibits IL-2 production	• Oral ulceration • Circumoral paraesthesia • Avoid clarithromycin, aciclovir, azole antifungals, non-steroidal anti-inflammatory drugs
Antiproliferative (antimetabolite) agents	Azathioprine	Inhibits purine synthesis and CD28 signalling	• Stomatitis • Opportunistic infections • Bleeding • Emesis (dental erosion risk) • Avoid muscle relaxants
	Mycophenolate mofetil	Inhibits purine synthesis and glycosylation	• Stomatitis • Opportunistic infections • Bleeding • Emesis (dental erosion risk) • Avoid aciclovir
	Methotrexate	Inhibits purine and pyrimidine synthesis	• Oral ulceration • Bleeding • Medication-related osteonecrosis of the jaw risk • Avoid non-steroidal anti-inflammatory drugs (may be fatal) and beta-lactam antibiotics
Polyclonal antibodies	Antithymocyte globulins (ATG) Antilymphocyte globulins (ALG)	Complement-mediated lysis, opsonisation and clearance blockade of cell surface receptors	• Bleeding • Opportunistic infections

(*Continued*)

Table 12.3.3 (Continued)

Drug class and examples		Mechanism of action	Dental management implications and drug interactions
Monoclonal antibodies	Muromonab -CD3 (OKT-3)	Complement-mediated lysis, opsonisation and clearance blockade of CD3 receptor	• Emesis (dental erosion risk) • Wound infection
	Alemtuzumab	CD52-specific depletion of T- and B-lymphocytes, natural killer cells and monocytes	
	Basiliximab Daclizumab	Block IL-2 receptor on activated T-lymphocytes	
mTOR inhibitors	Everolimus Sirolimus	Block IL-2-induced cell cycle progression (from G1 to S phase)	• Oral ulceration • Dysgeusia • Impaired wound healing • Medication-related osteonecrosis of the jaw risk • Bleeding • Emesis (dental erosion risk) • Avoid macrolide antibiotics, azole antifungals

Table 12.3.4 Types of transplants.

Type of graft	Procedure	Source
Autograft	Autologous	Self
Allograft	Allogeneic	Genetically different individual of the same species
Isograft	Syngeneic	Genetically identical individual (i.e. monozygotic twin)
Xenograft	Xenogeneic	Different species

immunosuppressed for life to prevent transplant T-cell alloimmune rejection

- Most immunosuppressive drugs target T-lymphocytes, which are the primary mediators of the rejection process
- Immunosuppressant drugs have a narrow therapeutic index. Treatment aims must balance the need to prevent rejection of the organ to allow patient and graft survival, whilst minimising the side-effects of toxicity, infections and malignancy
- There are typically three types of immunosuppressive regimens used: induction, maintenance and rejection treatment (Table 12.3.5)
- There is no consensus as to the single best protocol, with each programme using slightly different regimens
- An individualised approach is required, along with therapeutic drug monitoring
- General risks of immunosuppressant drugs include bone marrow suppression, infections, nephrotoxicity, hepatotoxicity, cardiovascular disease and malignancy
- Moreover, there are specific side-effects associated with the various classes of drugs (Table 12.3.6)
- Patients are regularly monitored for adequacy of their blood counts, liver function, kidney function, blood glucose and lipids, immunosuppressant drug levels and other transplant complications

Prognosis

- Complications following organ transplantation include:
  - Recurrent organ and multiorgan disease
  - Solid organ transplant rejection
    - Hyperacute: within minutes to hours, due to recipient's pre-existing antibodies against donor tissue HLA
    - Acute rejection: usually after one week to three months, caused by cellular and humoral immunity
    - Chronic rejection: develops over months to years, with multiple episodes of acute rejection
  - Non-immunological graft dysfunction
    - Surgical complications, comorbidities, infectious, drug-related side-effects, vascular complications

Table 12.3.5 Immunosuppressive regimens.

Immunosuppressive regimen	Description	Drugs commonly used
Induction	Treatment begun before, at the time of or immediately after transplantation Intended to deplete or modulate T-cell responses at the time of antigen presentation Doses not continued long-term (usually <three months)	• Corticosteroids • Cell-depleting (lytic induction) drugs[a] (e.g. alemtuzumab, antithymocyte globulin, antilymphocyte globulin, muromonab) or cell-surface receptor blockers/non-cell-depleting drugs[b] (e.g. basiliximab, daclizumab)
Maintenance	Long-term treatment to prevent acute rejection and deterioration of graft function Either combination therapy or monotherapy Combination therapy aims to minimise side-effects whilst maintaining adequate overall immunosuppression Doses usually reduced 2–4 months after transplantation (lower acute rejection risk)	• Monotherapy – Calcineurin inhibitors (e.g. cyclosporine, tacrolimus) • Combination therapy – Calcineurin inhibitors or mTOR inhibitors (e.g. sirolimus, everolimus) – Antiproliferative agents (e.g. mycophenolate, azathioprine) – Corticosteroids[c]
Rejection	Treatment of acute rejection due to immune response of host to destroy graft Mediated by cellular and/or humoral responses	• Cellular rejection – High-dose corticosteroids – Lymphocyte-depleting antibody (e.g. antithymocyte globulin) or muromonab • Antibody-mediated rejection – Corticosteroids – Plasma exchange – Intravenous immunoglobulin – Anti-CD20 antibody (rituximab) – Lymphocyte-depleting antibody – Rejection episodes – Mycophenolate

[a] Lytic induction agents have increased potency and lower rates of acute rejection, but increased incidence of infectious and malignant complications (used if high immunological risk).
[b] First-line therapy.
[c] Steroid-free protocols exist to avoid side-effects of corticosteroids.

  - Immunosuppression-related complications
    - Infection (viral, fungal, bacterial)
    - Malignancy (>50% cutaneous, also lymphoma and virally induced)
    - Bone marrow suppression and cytopenia
  - Side-effects of immunosuppressant drugs (Table 12.3.5)
  - Post-transplant lymphoproliferative disorders
  - Graft-versus-host disease (unusual)
  - Immune reconstitution syndrome
- Nevertheless, survival rates following solid organ transplantation have significantly improved in the last 10 years (Table 12.3.7)
- The best reported outcomes have been seen after adult kidney transplantation. Receiving a cadaveric graft doubles a patient's chances of survival, and a living donor graft quadruples them, in comparison with those who remain on the waiting list
- The success of repeat kidney, liver or heart transplantation is reduced, particularly for repeat liver transplantation, which only adds 1.5 life-years per recipient
- Graft-versus-host disease (GvHD)
  - Immunological rejection remains a major barrier to organ transplant success
  - Incompatibility is measured by evaluation of immunological parameters:
    - Tissue-type matching of human leucocyte antigen (HLA) – number of antigens mismatched at each HLA locus
    - Degree of humoral sensitisation to HLA antigens – presence of anti-HLA antibodies against those of the organ donor (negative cross-match required for transplant)

Table 12.3.6 Relative potency and side-effects of immunosuppressant drugs.

	Cyclosporine	Tacrolimus	Sirolimus	Azathioprine	Mycophenolate	Corticosteroids
Immunosuppressive potency	+++	+++±	++±	+	++	+
Nephrotoxicity	++	++	–	–	–	–
Hepatotoxicity	±	±	+	+	–	–
Neurotoxicity	+	++	–	–	–	–
Marrow suppression	–	–	+	+	+	–
Diabetes	+	++	–	–	–	++
Diarrhoea	–	–	+	–	++	–
Skin rash	–	–	+	–	–	–
Hirsutism/hypertrichosis	++	–	–	–	–	++

- No effect; + mild (or low incidence) toxicity/potency; ++ moderate toxicity/potency; +++ high toxicity/potency; ++++ extreme toxicity/potency. *Source*: Adapted from Taylor, A.L., Watson, C.J.E., and Bradley, J.A. (2005). Immunosuppressive agents in solid organ transplantation: mechanisms of action and therapeutic efficacy. *Crit. Rev. Oncol. Hematol.* 56: 23–46.

Table 12.3.7 Transplanted organs, source and graft/patient survival.

		Graft survival[b]		Patient survival[a]	
Organ	**Donor source**	**1-year**	**5-year**	**1-year**	**5-year**
Heart	Deceased	90.6%	85.4%	90.0%	78.6%
Lung	Deceased or living (rare)	92.3%	73.5%	85.8%	56.1%
Kidney	Deceased or living	94.4%	83.6%	97.3%	89.7%
Liver	Deceased or living	91.8%	84.6%	89.3%	76.5%
Pancreas	Deceased or living (rare)	93.4%	87.2%	96.4%	88.3%
Intestine	Deceased or living (rare)	Insufficient data	Insufficient data	75.2%	55.5%

[a] Organ Procurement and Transplantation Network (OPTN) and Scientific Registry of Transplant Recipients (SRTR) (2019). OPTN/SRTR 2017 Annual Data Report. *Am. J. Transplant.* 19 (S2): 1–516.
[b] ANZOD Registry 2019 Annual Report, Section 12: Deceased Organ Transplant Outcome Data. Adelaide: Australia and New Zealand Dialysis and Transplant Registry; 2019. www.anzdata.org.au/anzod/reports/annual-reports

  - ABO blood group – whether patient is a potential target of recipient circulating preformed anti-ABO antibody (resulting in hyperacute rejection)
- The acute or fulminant form of the disease (aGvHD) is traditionally described as occurring within the first 100 days post-transplant and is a major challenge to transplants owing to associated morbidity and mortality; it is characterised by severe intestinal inflammation, sloughing of the mucosal membrane, severe diarrhoea, abdominal pain, nausea and vomiting. Skin GvHD is associated with a diffuse red maculopapular rash and oral GvHD resembles lichen planus, with a higher risk of malignant transformation
- The chronic form of the disease (cGvHD) normally occurs after 100 days; moderate to severe cases of cGVHD can adversely influence long-term survival (Figure 12.3.5)
- It is important to note that the conventional 100-day division between acute and chronic GvHD has been challenged by the recognition that signs of acute and chronic GvHD may occur outside these designated periods; this observation has led to the increased use of clinical findings, rather than a set

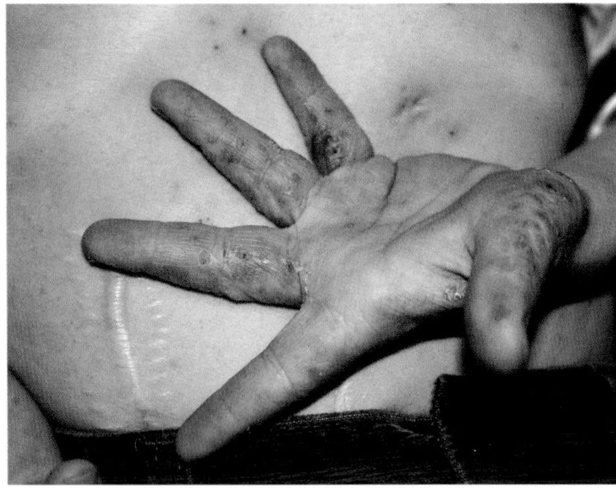

Figure 12.3.5 Cutaneous chronic graft-versus-host disease following kidney transplantation

time period, to differentiate between acute and chronic GvHD, namely:

- Classic acute GvHD – cases present within 100 days of transplantation and display features of acute GvHD. Diagnostic and distinctive features of chronic GvHD are absent
- Persistent, recurrent, late-onset acute GvHD – cases present greater than 100 days post transplantation with features of acute GvHD. Diagnostic and distinctive features of chronic GvHD are absent
- Classic chronic GvHD – cases may present at any time post transplantation. Diagnostic and distinctive features of chronic GvHD are present. There are no features of acute GvHD
- Overlap syndrome – cases may present at any time post transplantation with features of both chronic GvHD and acute GvHD. On occasion, this is colloquially referred to as 'acute on chronic' GvHD

A World/Transcultural View

- Worldwide, the number of patients who may potentially benefit from organ transplantation is far greater than the number of organs donated. On the other hand, there are huge geographical differences in transplant activity, ranging from >70 per million population in developed countries to 0–2.4 per million population in developing countries. As such, careful medical and ethical decision making regarding the allocation and transplantation of donated organs is critical
- Donation schemes and eligibility criteria for organ donation/receipt vary between countries. Schemes include organ donor registration, directed living donations (e.g. to friends and relatives), paired/pooled living donation programmes and altruistic donor chains. In some countries, people must 'opt out' of the organ donation register rather than 'opt in' as part of a legal consent framework to raise organ donation rates
- The 'Declaration of Istanbul on Organ Trafficking and Transplant Tourism' (updated 2018) has been developed to unite member states engaged in combating unethical practices in organ transplantation. It is also important to note that transplantation may be refused by some Jehovah's Witnesses and Orthodox Jews

References

Organ Procurement and Transplantation Network (OPTN) and Scientific Registry of Transplant Recipients (SRTR) (2019). OPTN/SRTR 2017 Annual Data Report. *Am. J. Transplant.* 19 (S2): 1–516.

Recommended Reading

Abed, H., Burke, M., and Shaheen, F. (2018). The integrated care pathway of nephrology and dental teams to manage complex renal and post-kidney transplant patients in dentistry: a holistic approach. *Saudi J. Kidney Dis. Transpl.* 29: 766–774.

Carlos Fabuel, L., Gavaldá Esteve, C., and Sarrión Pérez, M.G. (2011). Dental management in transplant patients. *J. Clin. Exp. Dent.* 3: 43–52.

Guggenheimer, J., Eghtesad, B., and Stock, D.J. (2003). Dental management of the (solid) organ transplant patient. *Oral Surg. Oral Med. Oral Pathol. Oral Radiol. Endod.* 95: 383–389.

Haverman, T.M., Raber-Durlacher, J.E., Raghoebar, I.I. et al. (2020). Oral chronic graft-versus-host disease: what the general dental practitioner needs to know. *J. Am. Dent. Assoc.* 151: 846–856.

National Institute of Dental and Craniofacial Research. (2011). *Dental Management of the Organ Transplant Patient*. Bethesda: US Department of Health and Human Services, National Institutes of Health. www.in.gov/isdh/files/OrganTransplantProf.pdf

Weinberg, M.A., Segelnick, S.L., Kay, L.B., and Nair, V. (2013). Medical and dental standardization for solid organ transplant recipients. *N. Y. State Dent. J.* 79: 35–40.

Ziebolz, D., Hraský, V., Goralczyk, A. et al. (2011). Dental care and oral health in solid organ transplant recipients: a single center cross-sectional study and survey of German transplant centers. *Transpl. Int.* 24: 1179–1188.

13

Head and Neck Cancer

13.1 Surgery

Section I: Clinical Scenario and Dental Considerations

Clinical Scenario

A 78-year-old patient with a history of oral cancer presents to the dental clinic complaining of poorly located dull pain from the teeth in the lower left quadrant. The discomfort commenced several days earlier and is exacerbated when drinking or eating. No painkillers or antibiotics have been taken.

Medical History

- T1N0M0 oral squamous cell carcinoma of the gingivae adjacent to the lower molar teeth diagnosed 6 years earlier
  - Surgical treatment included tumour removal and marginal mandibulectomy
- Recurrence of the oral carcinoma 3 years earlier with a T3N1M0 presentation
  - Partial glossectomy
  - Segmental mandibulectomy; reconstructive surgery not undertaken; plates in situ
  - Ipsilateral lymph nodes removal (neck dissection)
  - Postsurgical sequelae include dysglossia and occasional episodes of choking
  - Postoperative radiotherapy received but discontinued at the fifth session (10 Gy) due to the onset of severe mucositis
  - Chemotherapy not planned due to the presence of comorbidities
- Ischaemic heart disease (coronary stents)
- Atrial fibrillation
- Arterial hypertension
- Type 2 diabetes

Medications

- Acenocoumarol
- Nitroglycerine
- Enalapril
- Atenolol
- Furosemide
- Metformin

Dental History

- Soft diet since carcinoma recurrence
- Only attends the dentist when in pain
- Brushes teeth only at night
- Anxious about choking when brushing his teeth
- Patient requested a dental prosthesis but was told it was not feasible

Social History

- Widowed and lives alone
- Active life (walks 2 hours daily)
- Does not drive but can travel independently
- Ex-smoker (15 cigarettes/day until 12 years ago)
- Alcohol: rarely (<2 units/week)

Oral Examination

- Poor oral hygiene
- Numerous lost teeth
- Buccal caries in teeth #14, #25, #34, #35 and #36
- Retained root #22
- Periodontal disease with associated gingival recession
- Grade II mobility of teeth #34 and #36
- Trauma to the buccal mucosa bilaterally from the unopposed upper third molar teeth
- Surgical scars on the oral mucosa in relation to the mandibulectomy have resulted in sulcus obliteration

Radiological Examination

- Orthopantomogram undertaken (Figure 13.1.1)
- Right-sided segmental mandibulectomy
- Osteosynthesis plate to bridge the bone defect and another to reinforce the marginal mandibulectomy area
- Generalised advanced alveolar bone loss; exposed furcation #36

A Practical Approach to Special Care in Dentistry, First Edition. Edited by Pedro Diz Dios and Navdeep Kumar.

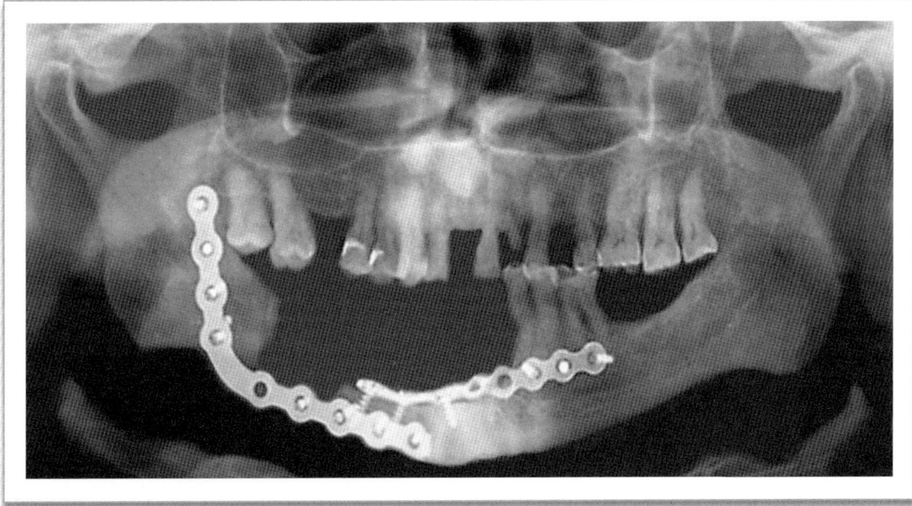

Figure 13.1.1 Orthopantomogram showing segmental mandibulectomy reconstructed with an osteosynthesis plate and severe periodontal disease.

Structured Learning

1) What is the likely cause of this patient's oral pain?
   - The most likely cause is in relation to the advanced periodontal disease and gingival recession associated with the 3 remaining lower teeth, #34, #35 and #36
   - However, in view of the patient's cancer history, it is important to exclude recurrence of the oral squamous cell carcinoma, particularly as he did not complete the full course of postsurgical radiotherapy and did not receive chemotherapy
2) Following discussion of the oral findings, which teeth would you recommend for extraction?
   - Extraction of teeth associated with a poor prognosis/infection risk: #34, #35, #36 and #22 retained root
   - Elective extraction of the #18 and #28 should also be discussed as they are associated with mucosal trauma, are non-functional and are difficult to reach for cleaning
3) What factors are considered important in assessing the risk of managing this patient?
   - Social
     - Lives alone/need to identify a suitable escort
     - Lack of perceived importance of dental care when compared with the systemic problems/oral cancer
     - Impaired communication due to partial glossectomy
     - Fear of tumour recurrence
     - Psychosocial impact of cancer and the disfigurement caused by surgical removal
   - Medical
     - Risk of tumour recurrence
     - Sequelae of cancer treatment, including dysphagia
     - Risk of an ischaemic heart disease episode (see Chapters 8.2 and 8.6)
     - Bleeding tendency due to acenocoumarol see (see Chapter 10.3)
     - There is a risk of a hypertensive crisis due to arterial hypertension (see Chapter 8.1)
     - Hypoglycaemia/hyperglycaemia, increased risk of infection and poor wound healing related to diabetes (see Chapter 5.1)
     - Drug interactions
   - Dental
     - Poor oral hygiene and irregular dental attendance
     - Sequelae of the surgical therapy can hinder dental management (e.g. partial glossectomy in this patient is associated with an altered cough reflex, choking and aspiration risk)
     - Oral rehabilitation is more challenging as there is no bony reconstruction of the mandible
4) What specific precautions should be implemented for this patient when dental extractions are undertaken?
   - Confirm preoperative international normalised ratio (INR) because the patient is taking acenocoumarol
   - Confirm diabetic control (haemoglobin A_{1c}) and blood glucose due to diabetes
   - Monitor vital signs (oxygen saturation, blood pressure and pulse) due to the ischaemic heart disease and arterial hypertension
   - Avoid a fully reclined position and limit irrigation during the procedure due to aspiration risk
5) Following completion of the dental extractions and healing, the patient asks for a lower denture. What factors would you need to consider when assessing him for this?

- Lack of bone reconstruction after segmental mandibulectomy
- Lack of sulcus depth in the region of the resection due to surgical scarring
- Position of the osteosynthesis plates/screws
- Volume and morphology of the remaining mandibular bone
- Degree of lateral mandibular deviation
- Number and condition of the remaining natural teeth

6) It is determined that there is insufficient support and access for construction of a mandibular prosthesis. The patient asks if dental implants can be placed instead. What would you discuss?
   - Osseointegrated dental implants can provide stability to a dental prosthesis
   - Radiation therapy does not worsen the prognosis, because the patient was administered a very small dose, and the implants would be located distant to the radiation field
   - However, there are several other factors to consider, including:
     - Poor oral hygiene
     - Periodontal disease
     - Degree of diabetes control
     - Cancer prognosis (recurrent tumour; not having undergone adjuvant therapy)

General Dental Considerations

Sequelae of Surgical Treatment

- Primary tumour resection
  - Postoperative difficulties in feeding/chewing (Figure 13.1.2)
  - Aesthetic disfiguration with psychological implications

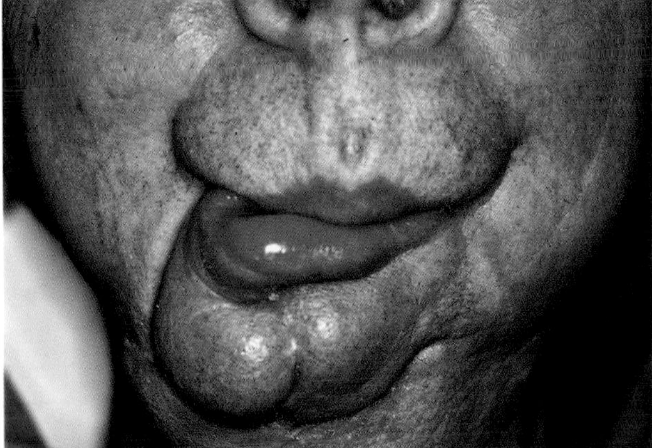

Figure 13.1.2 Surgical sequelae of a lower jaw carcinoma. Reconstruction of soft tissues is essential to recover oral functionality.

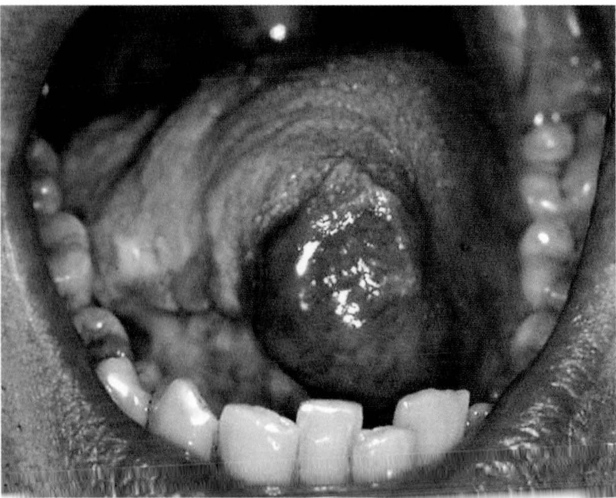

Figure 13.1.3 The mobility of the residual tongue determines the functional sequelae of a partial glossectomy.

  - Dysarthria
  - Organic dyslalia/dysglossia and dysphagia; extent dependent on the location of the tumour (the further back, the greater the functional repercussions), the extent of the resected area and the mobility of the residual tissues/tongue (Figure 13.1.3)
  - Difficulties breathing
- Cervical dissection
  - Dysfunctional shoulder
  - Pain in the neck and/or shoulder
  - Cervical contour abnormalities
  - Difficulty swallowing
  - Lymphoedema

Dental Management

- The dental treatment plan for these patients is determined by the tumour prognosis, the presence of comorbidities and local factors such as the location and extent of the resected area, the reconstruction technique and the condition of the remaining oral structures (Table 13.1.1)

Section II: Background Information and Guidelines

Definition

Head and neck cancer is the sixth most common cancer worldwide. Surgery is the therapeutic procedure of choice for oral squamous cell carcinoma (OSCC). Depending on the size, position and extent of the lesion, surgery may need to be supplemented by radiation therapy and/or adjuvant chemotherapy.

Table 13.1.1 Dental management considerations.

Risk assessment	• Risk of dental treatment before/during cancer surgery will be determined by: – Potential limitations to oral access depending on the site/size of the oral cancer lesion – Presence of medical comorbidities – Concurrent smoking and alcohol use • Following cancer surgery, risks associated with dental treatment are dependent on: – Location and extent of the resected area – Reconstruction technique for bone defects and soft tissues – Concomitant administration of radiation and/or chemotherapy – Tumour prognosis – Presence of comorbidities
Criteria for referral	• Most patients can be seen in primary care following surgical cancer therapy • Patients with severe surgical sequelae (e.g. impaired swallowing), severe comorbidities or advanced stages of oncological disease should be seen in a hospital setting
Access/position	• When there is airway impairment, dysphagia and an aspiration risk, it is important to keep the dental chair in a more vertical position • Although rubber dam may be used to further protect the airway, it may paradoxically also obstruct the entry of air
Communication	• Alteration in facial aesthetics often negatively impacts upon socialisation and quality of life, and may be associated with depression • Altered/limited tongue movement may hinder communication because it compromises the intelligibility of the speech
Consent/capacity	• Before cancer surgery – Explain that the need to avoid any delay in cancer treatment may require a modified dental treatment plan – Confirm that the main objective is to eliminate the infectious intraoral foci to minimise complications resulting from the cancer treatment – Inform the patient of the complications resulting from cancer therapy and the importance of maintaining proper oral hygiene • After cancer surgery – The consent should reflect the medical and oncological factors that could determine the success of the dental procedures and increase the risk (e.g. dysphagia) – Anticipate the cancer treatment-related complications that could occur in the long term and the measures that can be adopted to minimise them – Emphasise the importance of periodic follow-up
Anaesthesia/sedation	• Local – Local infiltration of anaesthesia can be challenging in patients with altered sensory perception or an unusual location for innervation (postoperative sequelae) • Sedation – Consideration should be given to altered anatomy which may impact on the airway, particularly for inhalational sedation – Ensure oversedation is avoided, particularly when there is a risk of dysphagia/aspiration • General anaesthesia – In some cases intubation may be difficult because of altered anatomy following cancer surgery, restricted neck mobility

(Continued)

Table 13.1.1 (Continued)

Dental treatment	• Before – Eliminate potential foci of dental and periodontal infection (extraction of teeth with a poor prognosis, removal of active caries, scaling and root planing) – Taking measurements (radiographs and intraoral silicone impressions/digital scanner) can facilitate postsurgical prosthetic rehabilitation – Promote oral hygiene instructions (adapt in relation to the individual patient/tumour/planned surgery) • During – Obturators: these are used to close palatal defects after a maxillectomy; support may be requested by the surgeon to construct a provisional obturator which may be placed at the time of surgery (minimises postoperative trauma) – Osseointegrated implants: can be inserted at the time of cancer surgery; can provide retention and stability to the dental prosthesis or to support an obturator, overdenture, fixed prosthesis or facial prosthesis; preferentially be inserted into the remaining healthy bone, away from the surgical site if this underwent radiation therapy (can also be placed in the bone graft) • After – In patients who have undergone a partial maxillectomy, prepare a provisional dental prosthesis at 3–4 weeks, which will be used for 4–6 months – Factors that determine the success of the definitive upper jaw dental prosthesis in terms of retention and stability include: ○ Size/weight of the prosthesis ○ Bone and soft tissues morphology/reconstruction ○ Condition of the remaining teeth (possibility of placing dental implants) ○ Adaptability (rubber obturators and tissue conditioners are recommended) ○ Patient's motivation – Factors that determine the success of the definitive lower jaw dental prosthesis include: ○ Extent and morphology of the remaining bone ○ Degree of mandibular deviation ○ Number and condition of the remaining teeth (possibility of placing dental implants) ○ Bone and soft tissue defects reconstruction
Education/prevention	• The elimination of intraoral infectious foci significantly decreases the degree of inflammation in the postoperative period • The dentist should encourage smoking cessation, because this habit affects postsurgical healing, jeopardises tissue perfusion and alters neutrophil functionality, favouring the onset of infectious complications

Cancer staging is critical to ensure that the correct approach to cancer therapy is used (Table 13.1.2). Major modifications and additions to staging head and neck cancer became effective in 2018:

- Oral cavity cancers now incorporate depth of invasion as a criterion for T designation
- A novel staging system has been introduced for high-risk HPV-associated oropharyngeal cancers (HPV+ tumours tend to be associated with better treatment outcomes)
- Pathological staging of high-risk HPV oropharyngeal cancers differs from clinical staging by exclusively using node number

Surgical Approaches

- Resection of the tumour
  - This involves removal of the lesion with a safety margin of surrounding healthy tissue
- Neck dissection
  - Involves elective or therapeutic removal of cervical lymph nodes (cervical dissection)
  - Classic radical neck dissection removes all the ipsilateral lymph nodes, the submandibular salivary gland, sternocleidomastoid muscle, internal jugular vein and spinal accessory nerve; however, it is associated with significant functional and cosmetic deformities
  - Multiple modifications now exist which can variably preserve structures such as the spinal accessory nerve, internal jugular vein and sternocleidomastoid muscle
  - Sentinel lymph node biopsy is proposed as an effective alternative to elective neck dissection (through nanocolloid lymphoscintigraphy) (Figure 13.1.4)

Table 13.1.2 TNM staging system for oral cancer.

Tumour size (T)	TX	The primary tumour cannot be evaluated
	Tis	Describes a stage called carcinoma (cancer) *in situ*; this is a very early cancer where cancer cells are found only in 1 layer of tissue
	T1	The tumour is ≤2 cm at its greatest dimension, and it has invaded nearby tissues to a depth of ≤5 mm
	T2	The tumour is ≤2 cm, and the depth of invasion is 5–10 mm; or the tumour is 2–4 cm, and the depth of invasion is ≤10 mm
	T3	The tumour is >4 cm, or it is any tumour with a depth of invasion >10 mm
	T4	T4a (lip): the tumour began on the lip but has invaded bone or spread to the inferior alveolar nerve in the mouth, the floor of the mouth or the skin of the face T4b (oral cavity): the tumour has invaded nearby structures in the mouth, such as the jaw, sinuses or skin of the face T4c: the tumour has invaded the muscles and bones that form the mouth or the base of the skull, and/or it encases the internal arteries
Lymph nodes – clinical (N)	NX	The regional lymph nodes cannot be evaluated
	N0	There is no evidence of cancer in the regional lymph nodes
	N1	The cancer has spread to a single lymph node on the same side as the primary tumour, and the cancer found in the node is ≤3 cm or smaller; there is no extranodal extension (ENE)
	N2a	Cancer has spread to a single lymph node on the same side as the primary tumour and is >3 cm but not >6 cm; there is no ENE
	N2b	Cancer has spread to more than 1 lymph node on the same side as the primary tumour, and none measures >6 cm; there is no ENE
	N2c	Cancer has spread to more than 1 lymph node on either side of the body, and none measures >6 cm; there is no ENE
	N3a	The cancer is found in a lymph node and is >6 cm; there is no ENE
	N3b	There is ENE in any lymph node
Metastasis (M)	M0	Cancer has not spread to other parts of the body
	M1	Cancer has spread to other parts of the body

- Reconstruction
  - Recovering oral aesthetics and functionality following tumour resection is increasingly considered part of the routine surgical planning
  - Reductions that only affect the free portion of the tongue have minimal functional repercussions, provided the remaining tongue preserves its mobility
  - In the anterior portion of the floor of the mouth, soft tissue reconstruction is essential to prevent chronic functional sequelae
  - Palatine defects can be repaired using a local, regional or microvascularised flap or an obturator prosthesis
  - Mandibular osteosynthesis with titanium plates is indicated for reinforcing marginal mandibulectomies, for bridging bone defects after segmental mandibulectomy and for fixing bone grafts
  - The reconstruction of large defects in the oral cavity requires the use of pedicled or free flaps which may be local, regional or microvascular free flaps (e.g. RFF – radial forearm flap; DCIA – deep circumflex iliac artery flap)
- Advances in surgery
  - Reconstructive surgery has substantially improved with the incorporation of new technologies such as computer-assisted preoperative planning, the preparation of individual surgical guidelines and the preparation of grafts with three-dimensional (3D) printing technology
  - One-stage microvascular replacement of missing tissue and bone and the use of innervated flaps are increasingly common
  - Significant advances have also been made in facial reanimation
  - Consideration of placement of osseointegrated dental implants at the time of cancer surgery allows earlier dental rehabilitation postoperatively
  - Robotic surgery enables access for resection of tumours and reconstruction with free flap in the

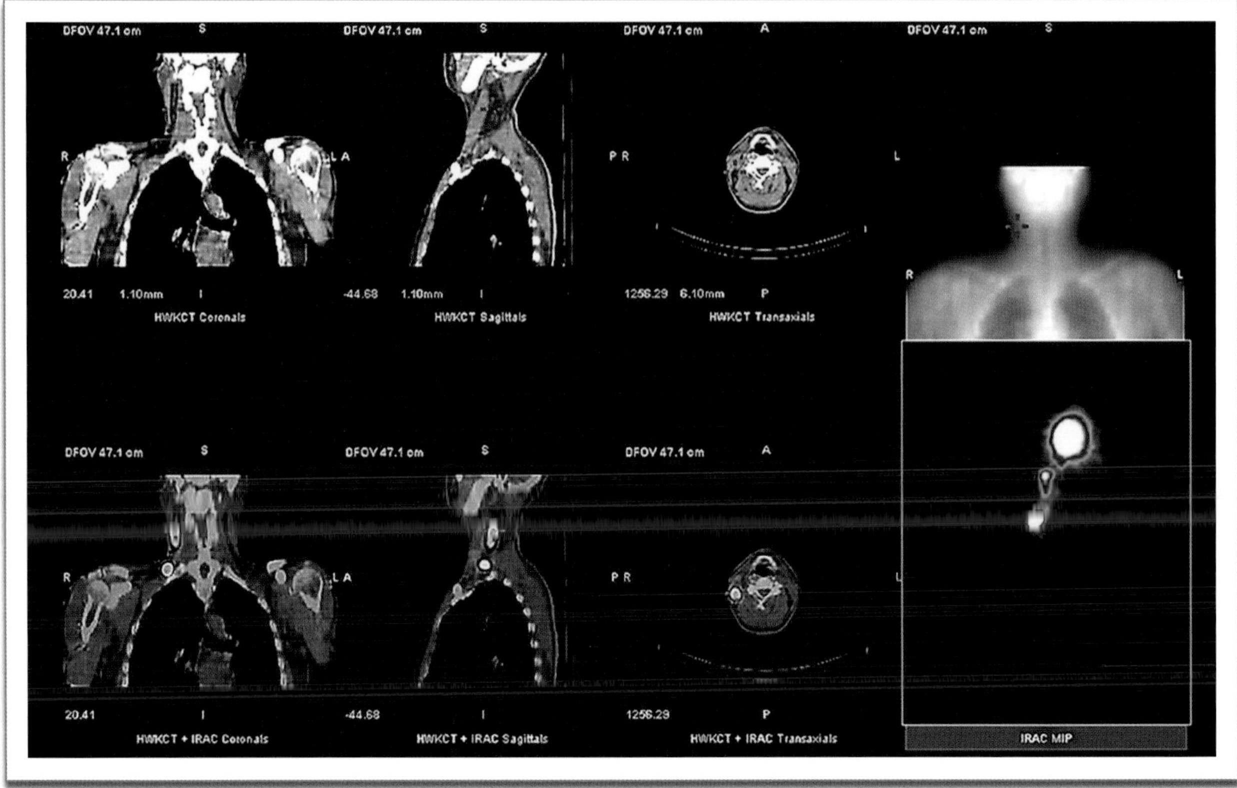

Figure 13.1.4 Lymphoscintigraphy for sentinel lymph node detection in patients with oral cavity squamous cell carcinoma.

deep oropharynx, obviating the need for mandibulotomy
  - Advances in immunosuppressant therapies have made it possible to reconstruct composite facial anatomical units with allotransplant in a single surgery, along with sensory and motor recovery
  - Research is ongoing into stem cell and tissue engineering to regenerate tissues and avoid the need for autologous tissue flaps

Limitations of Surgery

- Patient comorbidities (e.g. cardiac and pulmonary complications may reduce the feasibility of surgical approached for head and neck cancer)
- Large neoplasms (primary location)
- Regional expansion (cervical lymph nodes)
- The tumour invades critical structures
  - Carotid artery
  - Cranial nerves
  - Eye socket
  - Skull base
  - Intracranial cavity

Prognosis

- While surgery has demonstrated superior local control rates, overall survival of surgical versus non-surgical therapy remains similar for many head and neck cancers
- It has been reported that 40% of patients with squamous carcinoma of the oral cavity and pharynx present with regional metastases to the cervical lymph nodes
- Metastasis to the regional lymph nodes reduces the 5-year survival rate by 50% compared with that of patients with early-stage disease

A World/Transcultural View

- In the surgical treatment of oral cancer, the main differences between countries lie in the extent of the safety margins and in the surgical technique, both in resective and reconstructive surgery
- The technology necessary for sentinel lymph node biopsy and reconstructive surgery using digital workflow systems is still not available in many countries

Recommended Reading

Brown, J.S., Barry, C., Ho, M., and Shaw, R. (2016). A new classification for mandibular defects after oncological resection. *Lancet Oncol.* 17: e23–e30.

Schilling, C., Shaw, R., Schache, A. et al. (2017). Sentinel lymph node biopsy for oral squamous cell carcinoma. Where are we now? *Br. J. Oral Maxillofac. Surg.* 55: 757–762.

Shah, J.P. and Gil, Z. (2009). Current concepts in management of oral cancer – surgery. *Oral Oncol.* 45: 394–401.

Shanti, R.M. and O'Malley, B.W. (2018). Surgical management of oral cancer. *Dent. Clin. North Am.* 62: 77–86.

Shaw, R.J., O'Connell, J.E., and Bajwa, M. (2020). Basic surgical principles and techniques. In: *Textbook of Oral Cancer: Prevention, Diagnosis and Management* (eds. S. Warnakulasuriya and J.S. Greenspan), 254–282. Basel: Springer Nature Switzerland AG.

Suarez-Cunqueiro, M.M., Schramm, A., Schoen, R. et al. (2008). Speech and swallowing impairment after treatment for oral and oropharyngeal cancer. *Arch. Otolaryngol. Head Neck Surg.* 134: 1299–1304.

Yao, C.M.K.L., Chang, E.I., and Lai, S.Y. (2019). Contemporary approach to locally advanced oral cavity squamous cell carcinoma. *Curr. Oncol. Rep.* 21: 99.

13.2 Radiation Therapy

Section I: Clinical Scenario and Dental Considerations

Clinical Scenario

A 54-year-old male with a head and neck cancer history presents to the dental clinic complaining that his teeth keep 'crumbling' and he is finding it difficult to eat.

Medical History

- Stage III nasopharyngeal carcinoma (NPC) diagnosed 10 months earlier
  - Radiation therapy (60 Gy) completed
  - Induction and adjuvant chemotherapy with cisplatin and 5-fluorouracil
  - Persistent disease confirmed on imaging and managed with oral capecitabine twice daily
  - Chronic serous otitis media
- Gastro-oesophageal reflux due to incompetence of the gastric cardia
- Familial dyslipidaemia
- Benign prostatic hypertrophy

Medications

- Capecitabine
- Omeprazole
- Rosuvastatin
- Tamsulosin

Dental History

- Previous regular attender
- Had numerous dental extractions of posterior teeth prior to cancer therapy
- Has not attended after cancer treatment
- Recurrent dental problems in the past 6 months
- Brushes teeth 3 times a day and uses a 0.12% chlorhexidine mouthwash
- Due to profound xerostomia, sucks lemon sweets to stimulate saliva flow

Social History

- Married; lives with wife and 2 adult children
- Physician by profession
- Hearing loss due to chronic otitis
- Difficulty talking for long periods due to the xerostomia
- Ex-smoker (20 cigarettes/day until 15 years ago)
- Alcohol: nil (mouth too uncomfortable)

Oral Examination

- Limited mouth opening (20 mm interincisal distance)
- Severe xerostomia
- Good oral hygiene
- Multiple cervical carious lesions
- Fillings in #14, #22, #23 and #33
- Crown fractures of #31, #32, #41 and #42

Radiological Examination

- Orthopantomogram and periapical radiographs undertaken (Figure 13.2.1)
- Multiple failed dental fillings with extensive caries
- Retained roots (root filled) #24 and #25
- Extensive caries in teeth #33 and #34

Structured Learning

1) This patient currently resides in Spain but is of mixed heritage, with the maternal side of his family originally from China. How is this relevant to his diagnosis of NPC?
   - Although NPC is rare in most parts of the world, it is relatively common in South-East Asia
   - Chinese populations, living either in mainland China or elsewhere, have the highest incidence of this tumour worldwide

A Practical Approach to Special Care in Dentistry, First Edition. Edited by Pedro Diz Dios and Navdeep Kumar.

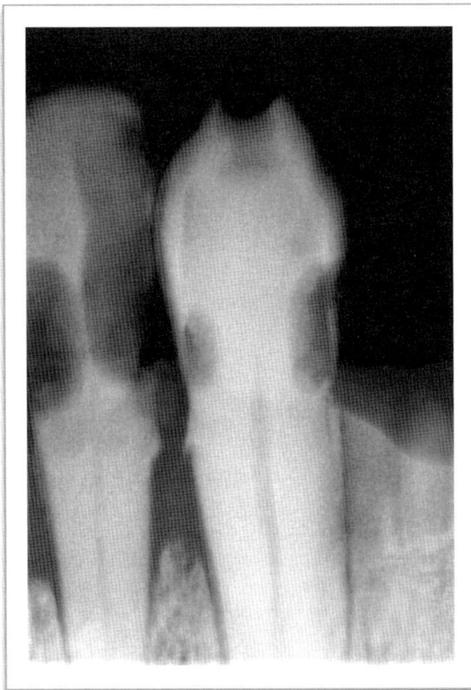

Figure 13.2.1 Periapical radiograph showing extensive cervical caries #33 and #34.

2) What is the most likely cause of this patient's limited mouth opening?
   - Radiotherapy of NPC typically delivers a considerable radiation dose to the temporomandibular joint (TMJ) region and related muscles
   - Trismus results mainly due to fibrosis of muscles of mastication; reduction in the TMJ disc thickness has also been noted
   - This does not present immediately but occurs progressively as mucositis subsides
   - The severity of trismus is dependent on the radiation source, dose and number of fields radiated
   - This patient received 60 Gy of radiotherapy – this is a considerable dose, despite the likelihood that intensity-modulated radiotherapy was used
3) How is the diagnosis of trismus confirmed and what is the treatment of choice?
   - Diagnosis of trismus is clinical; it is typically made when the maximum interincisal distance between the incisal edges of the maxillary and mandibular incisors is <40 mm, regardless of its aetiology
   - For edentulous patients, the distance is measured between the maxillary and mandibular alveolar ridges
   - Some authors have graded trismus according to visual assessment of restricted mouth opening (mild/moderate/severe or grades 1–3)
   - Imaging adjuncts may be useful to establish its aetiology and determine the articular involvement of the TMJ
   - Computed tomography may be useful to identify traumatic aetiologies, including haematomas or facial and mandibular fractures when suspected
   - This condition can be managed by adapting the diet (softer foods cut into smaller pieces), jaw exercises, physical therapy devices (e.g. Therabite®), using drugs (e.g. muscle relaxants, pain relievers, anti-inflammatory medication, botulinum toxin) or, in advanced cases, surgery
4) The patient reports difficulties with eating and occasionally chokes on his food; this has been more pronounced in recent months. Fibreoptic laryngoscopy has demonstrated food residues in the oropharynx, reaching the entry to the airways. What is the most likely diagnosis and what complications can this lead to?
   - Late radiation-induced dysphagia
   - This condition is due to progressive fibrosis caused by the ionising radiation that was absorbed by the cricopharyngeal muscle and oesophagus
   - The condition can cause malnutrition, an increased risk of aspiration, anxiety and depression and deterioration in quality of life
5) The patient has severe xerostomia. What is the impact of this and how would you manage it?
   - Xerostomia has promoted the onset of caries, affected oral function and consequently reduced the patient's quality of life (QoL) (Figure 13.2.2)
   - Acknowledge the physical and psychosocial impact and implement supportive strategies

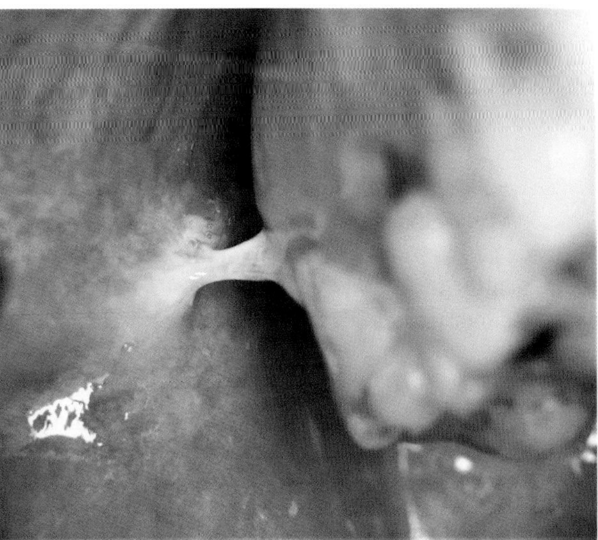

Figure 13.2.2 Hyposalivation and thick and sticky saliva are common acute complications of radiotherapy.

- Advise the patient to stop using lemon sweets to stimulate flow as these will promote further tooth surface loss/caries
- Prescribe fluoride toothpaste to help stabilise the teeth
- A saliva substitute should be administered that provides symptomatic relief, such as hydroxyethyl cellulose, hydroxypropyl cellulose or carboxymethyl cellulose
- Consider systemic salivary stimulants, such as pilocarpine (5–10 mg/8 h)
- Consider referral for psychological support if there is significant depression/negative impact on QoL

6) What factors are considered important in assessing the risk of managing this patient?
   - Social
     - The information provided to the patient should be adapted to take into account his medical training
     - Hearing impairment
     - Psychosocial impact of cancer diagnosis and complications of cancer therapy
   - Medical
     - Sequelae of radiotherapy and chemotherapy
     - Poor prognosis of NPC – stage III NPC has an overall 5-year survival rate as low as 30% (compared to 60–85% for patients with stage I or II NPC)
     - Capecitabine-associated side-effects
     - Appropriate selection of drugs
   - Dental
     - Postradiotherapy sequelae: oropharyngeal dysphagia with occasional choking, profound xerostomia, trismus
     - High risk of dental caries due to xerostomia, use of acidic lemon sweets to stimulate flow, and gastro-oesophageal reflux
     - Multiple carious lesions and deteriorating dentition (Figure 13.2.3)
     - Determine the prognosis for the remaining teeth and design a treatment plan which considers his reduced likelihood of long-term survival

7) The #33 and #34 are non-vital and have extensive subgingival caries. What are the considerations for management of these teeth?
   - Capecitabine is an antimetabolite chemotherapy drug and may be associated with side-effects such as leucopenia, thrombocytopenia and anaemia, in addition to nausea, vomiting and fatigue
   - A full blood count test result is required prior to proposed dental treatment
   - Depending on the results and general profile, haematological support (e.g. platelets) and antibiotic prophylaxis may be considered

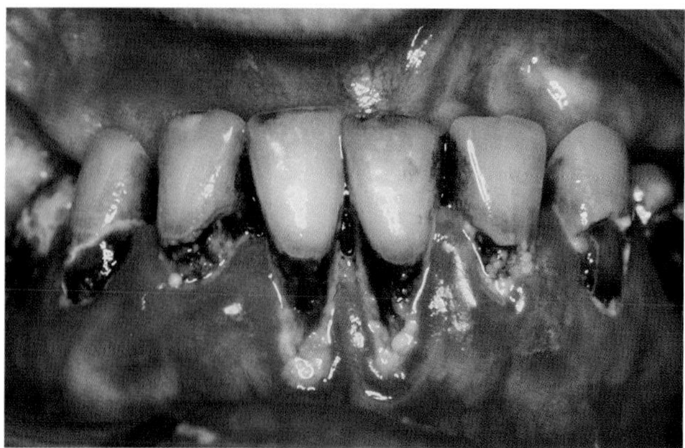

Figure 13.2.3 Rampant caries ('radiation caries') is a delayed complication of radiotherapy.

   - The success rate for endodontic treatment is poor due to limitations in access, inability to create a good coronal seal and potential complications of bleeding and increased infection risk; crown lengthening may be considered to improve restorability but the patient may not be able to tolerate this additional procedure
   - However, dental extractions are associated with the additional risk of osteoradionecrosis (ORN) (Figure 13.2.4); this is a significant risk for this patient as he has received a high dose of radiotherapy, namely 60 Gy; however, the anterior teeth may have received a lower dose and it is important to confirm the field/dose in this region
   - It is also important to consider tooth replacement options if #33 and #34 are extracted and discuss the challenges of both fixed and removable prosthodontic solutions given the limited mouth opening, deteriorating dentition and xerostomia

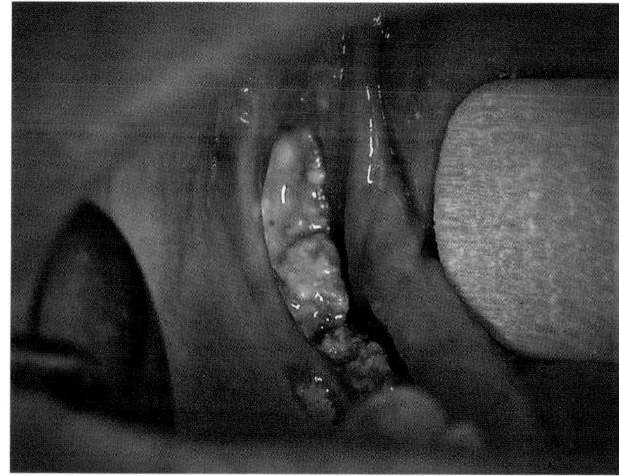

Figure 13.2.4 Clinical findings highly suggestive of osteoradionecrosis in a patient who received radiation therapy for oral cancer.

8) What antibiotics and analgesics should be avoided for this patient?
    - Macrolides alter statin metabolism and increase the risk of rhabdomyolysis
    - Acetylsalicylic acid and other non-steroidal anti-inflammatory drugs favour the onset of oesophageal erosions in patients with gastro-oesophageal reflux
    - Opioid analgesics can cause urinary retention in patients with benign prostatic hypertrophy

General Dental Considerations

Oral Findings

- Complications of radiotherapy may be acute and chronic (Tables 13.2.1 and 13.2.2)
- Starting in the second week of radiation therapy, mucositis and taste disorders occur
- By the third week, the patient experiences dry mouth, followed by delayed complications, which may include trismus, rampant caries and ORN
- ORN of the jaw is defined as an area of exposed necrotic bone in a region previously irradiated that fails to heal over a period of 3–6 months; however, cases with radiological evidence of necrosis with intact mucosa have been described; variable incidence of 2–22% reported, with a reduction in association with advances in radiotherapy techniques
- Risk factors for the development of ORN
    - Local: tumour site (mandible more common), tumour stage, proximity of the tumour to bone, radiation field, dose of radiation, poor oral hygiene and associated trauma, such as dental extraction/surgery before or after radiotherapy
    - Systemic: comorbidities, smoking and drinking alcohol, immunodeficiency status and infection

Dental Management (Table 13.2.3)

- The most appropriate dental approach for these patients is determined by tumour-related factors (e.g. location and size), dose and field of radiotherapy, concurrent cancer therapy (e.g. surgery and/or chemotherapy) and the patient themselves (e.g. toxic habits and comorbidities)
- Additional considerations for patients who have had surgery and/or chemotherapy should be considered (see Tables 13.1.1 and 12.2.6)

Section II: Background Information and Guidelines

Definition

Radiation therapy is the administration of ionising radiation for therapeutic purposes, employing high-energy particles or waves that damage the cancer cells' DNA and destroy their ability to divide and grow. Typically, it is combined with surgery and is administered postoperatively. Head and neck cancers are generally sensitive to radiotherapy, which is being increasingly used with the

Table 13.2.1 Acute oral complications of radiation therapy in head and neck cancer.

	Characteristics	Prevention/treatment
Mucositis	Prevalence of 75% The most common and disabling complication Can affect nutrition, favour the onset of infections and require a reduction in radiation therapy dose or even a discontinuation of therapy	• The pain can be mitigated with 0.2% morphine rinses every 3 h (6 times a day) • Palifermin, a recombinant derivative of the human keratinocyte growth factor, is currently the only drug approved for reducing the incidence and severity of mucositis (60 μg/kg/day intravenously)
Hyposalivation (xerostomia)	Prevalence of ~70–90% Reaches its maximum expression 1–3 months after completing the radiation therapy Above 55 Gy, the glandular dysfunction is usually irreversible	• Amifostine is the only drug approved for protecting glandular acini against radiation therapy (200 mg/m^2 intravenously 15–30 min before each session) • Pilocarpine is effective in treating hyposalivation (5–10 mg tablets every 8 h)
Dysgeusia	Prevalence of 66% Its onset is determined by the radiation dose Mainly affects salty and bitter tastes	• Can be treated with zinc sulfate (220 mg tablets every 8 h); limited evidence, hence specialised dietary advice may be more helpful

Table 13.2.2 Delayed oral complications of radiation therapy in head and neck cancer.

	Characteristics	Prevention/treatment
Trismus	Prevalence of 25% It is important to differentiate whether the trismus is caused by postsurgical scarring, is a radiotherapy sequela or is an initial sign of recurrence Has a negative impact on feeding, oral hygiene, articulation and quality of life	• May be managed with drugs (e.g. pentoxifylline + tocopherol), physical therapy or, in rare cases, surgery; however, none of these techniques is clearly superior to the others
Dental caries	Prevalence of 25% Has been related to the radiation dose received by the major salivary glands Radiation caries affects atypical dental surfaces (cusps, smooth surfaces and tooth necks), can affect various surfaces simultaneously (circular caries) and has a greater risk of recurrence	• See Table 13.2.3
Osteoradionecrosis	Prevalence <10% Defined as the presence of exposed and necrotic bone associated with ulceration or necrosis of the neighbouring soft tissues, which persists for more than 3 months in a previously irradiated area and that is not caused by tumour recurrence The risk is high for doses >60 Gy, especially in the mandible and in the first 2 years after radiation therapy, although the risk decreases with time	• Support measures should be applied, such as the elimination of trauma, ensuring appropriate nutritional intake and eliminating the consumption of tobacco and alcohol • The proposed surgical approach is sequestrectomy and/or resection of the necrotic tissue • Topical antibiotics, antiseptics and pentoxifylline with tocopherol can help resolve the lesions • The administration of hyperbaric oxygen (20–30 sessions with 100% oxygen at 2–2.5 atm of pressure) has been proposed as adjuvant therapy in selected high-risk cases that do not respond to conservative therapy or surgical resection; however, the evidence regarding its efficacy remains poor

rising prevalence of human papillomavirus-positive (HPV+) squamous cell carcinoma.

New developments in radiotherapy and concurrent improvements in imaging have helped to improve the outlook for patients with head and neck cancers. They have allowed radiation oncologists to escalate the dose of radiation delivered to tumour and minimise the dose delivered to surrounding normal tissue, thereby reducing the side-effects.

Indications

- The main indications for radiation therapy are advanced stage tumours, regional lymph node infiltration, perineural or perivascular invasion and incomplete surgical resection of tumour margins
- Radiotherapy may also be combined with chemotherapy for head and neck cancer either as an adjuvant approach for advanced stage tumours as induction therapy or for maintenance/palliative care

Radiation Therapy Modalities

- Hyperfractionated radiation therapy
  - The total dose is distributed across a large number of smaller doses
  - Improves the efficacy, but adverse effects persist or are more severe
- Accelerated fractionation
  - The treatment is completed in a very short period
  - Can reduce the recurrence rate but increase the adverse effects
- Three-dimensional conformal radiation therapy
  - The volume of the field to irradiate is established based on the images obtained with computed tomography
  - The radiation beams are transmitted from several angles that converge on the tumour
  - Damage is reduced to the surrounding healthy tissue penetrated by the radiation
- Intensity-modulated radiation therapy (IMRT)
  - This advanced three-dimensional radiation therapy modality uses x-ray linear accelerators to administer specific radiation doses to malignant tumours or to specific areas within the tumour (distributed in several small volumes)

Table 13.2.3 Dental management considerations.

Risk assessment	• Complications related to comorbidities and risk factors (e.g. alcohol and tobacco) • Complications due to sequelae of previous resective surgery (e.g. impaired swallowing or altered cough reflex) • For patients who undergo radiation therapy, increased risk of delayed wound healing, infection and osteoradionecrosis
Criteria for referral	• Avoid elective dental treatment during the administration of radiation therapy or chemotherapy • After radiation therapy or radiochemotherapy, most patients can be managed in a primary care setting • Treatment in a hospital setting should be assessed for patients with an advanced stage cancer, significant comorbidities and/or significant complications of radiation therapy
Access/position	• Liaise closely with the surgical/oncology team regarding timing of the proposed treatment and co-ordination of visits in relation to the radiation therapy sessions • Ideally, perform dental treatment prior to or after recovery from chemotherapy • Elective treatment should be avoided wherever possible during cancer therapy • The patient may feel fatigued or unwell due to radiotherapy/its sequelae so may need to cancel appointments • Consider escort requirements • Consider inpatient or outpatient status and need for hospital transport • Consider a semi-reclined position if the patient has airway impairment due to the cancer or radiotherapy sequelae and/or is nauseated/vomits frequently
Communication	• Consult the radiation oncologist and surgeon before undertaking any invasive dental treatment • Speech intelligibility can be impaired by the sequelae of radiation therapy (e.g. mucositis, xerostomia and trismus)
Consent/capacity	• Inform the patient that dental treatment in the different phases of the cancer therapy aims to prevent complications (emphasise the importance of maintaining proper oral hygiene), manage the adverse effects of radiotherapy and, ultimately, rehabilitate oral functionality • Discuss the risks and benefits of treatment options with patient (should consider prognosis, i.e. limit invasive treatment for palliative care patients to dental treatment which is necessary to manage pain/acute infection as definitive care may not be possible) • Explain that some factors related to the cancer process and its treatment sequelae might require changes in the ideal dental treatment plan • The consent should reflect the medical and oncological factors that could determine the success of the dental procedures • Consider the impact of fatigue and emotional distress on decision making
Anaesthesia/sedation	• Local anaesthesia – Avoid local anaesthetics with epinephrine (risk of osteoradionecrosis) – The intraligamentary technique is not recommended (risk of osteoradionecrosis) • Sedation – No specific considerations due to radiotherapy • General anaesthesia – Intubation can be difficult for patients with limited mouth opening (trismus)
Dental treatment	• Before radiation therapy – Perform preprosthetic surgery (e.g. alveolar ridge contouring) at least 6 weeks prior to radiotherapy – Perform extractions and periodontal treatment at least 10–14 days prior to radiotherapy – Remove teeth with a poor prognosis (minimise the surgical trauma and achieve primary closure) – Conservative treatment of restorable teeth should be focused on stabilising teeth – Eliminate potential causes of trauma (removing fixed orthodontic appliances and readjusting removable prostheses)

(*Continued*)

Table 13.2.3 (Continued)

	• During radiation therapy – No elective dental treatment should be conducted – If an urgent procedure needs to be performed, consult the oncologist – Prevention measures and treatment of the acute oral complications of radiation therapy – Prevention of radiation caries using 1% sodium fluoride (NaF) gels administered with individualised cuvettes for 5 minutes a day and toothpaste with 5000 ppm of NaF twice daily (mouthwashes with 0.05% NaF may also be prescribed) – The effectiveness of protective splints has not been definitively proven – Oral hygiene instructions adapted to the situation • First 6 months after radiation therapy – Avoid extractions and other oral surgery procedures – Assessment for the placement of dental implants should be delayed – Non-surgical periodontal treatment may be performed 6 weeks after the radiation therapy – Root canal is preferable to extraction (lower risk of osteoradionecrosis), even in non-restorable teeth – Removable dental prostheses may once again be employed 6–12 weeks after the radiation therapy (readjust them if necessary) – Orthodontic treatment is not recommended – Prevention measures and treatment of the chronic oral complications of radiation therapy should be the area of focus – Silver diamine fluoride can be useful for postradiation caries (low level of evidence available)
Education/prevention	• Dietary counselling – Reduce sugar and fermentable carbohydrate intake – Avoid acidic drinks • Adapt oral hygiene instructions as appropriate – Toothbrushes with extra-soft nylon bristles – Electrical and ultrasonic toothbrushes and dental floss can be too uncomfortable to use – Adjuvant use of alcohol-free chlorhexidine rinses (0.12–0.2%) should be considered • Specific advice should be given in relation to the management of the oral complications of radiotherapy (Tables 13.2.1 and 13.2.2) • Withdraw the removable dental prostheses for as long as possible (at least at night), avoid the use of adhesives, and do not use in the case of mucositis • The dentist should encourage smoking cessation and alcohol abstinence (increased risk of osteoradionecrosis and recurrent/secondary cancer risk)

  - The technique maximises the dose applied to the tumour while minimising the dose to adjacent healthy tissues, reducing the adverse effects
- Brachytherapy
  - This 'internal' radiation therapy modality places radioactive material directly within the tumour
- Radiopharmaceuticals
  - Radioisotopes drugs may be administered intravenously or orally or placed in a body cavity; although more commonly used in small amounts for imaging tests, larger doses can be used to deliver radiotherapy (e.g. for the treatment of thyroid cancer)
  - Radiolabelled monoclonal antibodies are a further area of development which specifically target cancer cells and hence limit damage to adjacent tissues

Extraoral Complications

- The rate and severity of adverse effects are dependent on the type, dose and field of radiotherapy
- Complications are more significant when radiation therapy and chemotherapy are combined
- Common side-effects include fatigue, hair loss, nausea, vomiting, skin changes, headache and blurred vision
- When radiotherapy is used to manage metastatic head and neck cancer, fields may extend to include other tis-

sues and organs, resulting in additional side-effects including problems with fertility, urinary and bladder changes

A World/Transcultural View

- More than 90% of the population in low-income countries lack access to radiation therapy services
- In many sub-Saharan countries, there is an almost complete lack of facilities with this treatment modality
- Conversely, the prevalence of cancer is increasing in low-income countries, which often have no access to radiotherapy or palliative care
- Even in countries with adequate treatment capacity (such as Brazil, Australia and Canada), the facilities tend to be grouped in large urban centres, creating geographical barriers for equitable access in remote scarcely populated areas

Recommended Reading

Kumar, N., Burke, M., Brooke, A., et al. (2018). *The Oral Management of Oncology Patients Requiring Radiotherapy, Chemotherapy and / or Bone Marrow Transplantation*. London: Royal College of Surgeons of England/British Society for Disability and Oral Health. www.rcseng.ac.uk/dental-faculties/fds/publications-guidelines/clinical-guidelines.

Levi, L.E. and Lalla, R.V. (2018). Dental treatment planning for the patient with oral cancer. *Dent. Clin. North Am.* 62: 121–130.

Lin, A. (2018). Radiation therapy for oral cavity and oropharyngeal cancers. *Dent. Clin. North Am.* 62: 99–109.

PDQ® Supportive and Palliative Care Editorial Board. (2016). *Oral Complications of Chemotherapy and Head/Neck Radiation*. Bethesda: National Cancer Institute. www.cancer.gov/about-cancer/treatment/side-effects/mouth-throat/oral-complications-hp-pdq

Shah, B.A., Yan, S.X., Concert, C. et al. (2020). Chemoradiotherapy in oral cavity cancer. In: *Textbook of Oral Cancer: Prevention, Diagnosis and Management* (eds. S. Warnakulasuriya and J.S. Greenspan), 292–301. Basel: Springer Nature Switzerland AG.

Sroussi, H.Y., Epstein, J.B., Bensadoun, R. et al. (2017). Common oral complications of head and neck cancer radiation therapy: mucositis, infections, saliva change, fibrosis, sensory dysfunctions, dental caries, periodontal disease, and osteoradionecrosis. *Cancer Med.* 6: 2918–2931.

Villa, A. and Akintoye, S.O. (2018). Dental management of patients who have undergone oral cancer therapy. *Dent. Clin. North Am.* 62: 131–142.

13.3 Oral Cancer Survivor

Section I: Clinical Scenario and Dental Considerations

Clinical Scenario

A 79-year-old man with a history of oral cancer presents to your dental clinic requesting a replacement upper denture. Although he has worn a removable maxillary prosthesis for the last 4 years, it is unstable and he cannot chew properly. In addition, when he drinks fluids, drops of liquid escape through his nose.

Medical History

- Right-sided palatal T2N2aMx adenoid cystic carcinoma (detected 5 years earlier)
- Cancer therapy included surgery, radiation therapy (60 Gy) and chemotherapy with cisplatin
- Primary biliary cholangitis
- Arterial hypertension
- Hiatus hernia
- Inguinal hernia surgery (4 years earlier)

Medications

- Ursodeoxycholic acid
- Fenofibrate
- Losartan/hydrochlorothiazide
- Omeprazole

Dental History

- The patient reports that many of his teeth were in poor condition and hence extracted before the radiation therapy
- In recent years, the patient has had several fillings under local anaesthesia
- His dental prosthesis has been adapted on 2 occasions since it was made but he is still unhappy with it
- Brushes his prosthesis and remaining teeth 3 times a day
- Diet: low cariogenic potential, balanced with good quantities of fruits and vegetables

Social History

- Retired (worked as a sailor)
- Lives with his wife
- No mobility issues, independent, drives his own car
- Ex-smoker (10 cigarettes/day until 20 years ago)
- Alcohol: nil

Oral Examination

- Significant oral–nasal communication (surgical sequelae)
- Edentulous maxilla
- Maxillary bulb obturator with poor stability
- Remaining natural teeth #35–45 with several fillings
- Good oral hygiene

Radiological Examination

- Cone beam computed tomography (CBCT) undertaken
- Reveals 2 retained roots in the remaining maxillary alveolar bone crest on the right side; right-sided palatine defect 40 × 25 mm; good bone volume in the maxillary upper left quadrant

Structured Learning

1) What is an adenoid cystic carcinoma (ACC) and what does the staging of T2N2aMx mean?
   - ACC is an uncommon type of malignant tumour that arises within glandular tissue (type of adenocarcinoma), most commonly the major and minor salivary glands of the head and neck region; other sites include the trachea, lacrimal gland, breast, skin and vulva
   - It has a relatively indolent but relentless course; although disease-specific survival is 89% at 5 years, it falls to 40% at 15 years due to a higher rate of recurrence/progression

A Practical Approach to Special Care in Dentistry, First Edition. Edited by Pedro Diz Dios and Navdeep Kumar.

- Although it seldom metastasises to regional lymph nodes, distant metastasis, particularly to the lung, is the more common; perineural invasion is also a characteristic feature and is indicative of a poor prognosis
- T2N2aMx confirms the staging of the tumour (see Table 13.1.2)
  - T2: tumour measuring 2–4 cm with an invasion depth ≤10 mm or measuring ≤2 cm with an invasion depth of 5–10 mm
  - N2a: metastasis in an ipsilateral lymph node measuring 3–6 cm in diameter, with negative extranodal extension
  - Mx: distant metastasis cannot be assessed

2) What is primary biliary cholangitis?
   - It is a chronic, autoimmune disease in which the bile ducts in the liver are slowly destroyed, causing cholestatis and eventually hepatic cirrhosis
   - Common symptoms are fatigue, pruritus and, in advanced cases, jaundice
   - Complications include portal hypertension secondary to cirrhosis, fat malabsorption and osteoporosis/osteomalacia
3) What factors are considered important in assessing the risk of managing this patient?
   - Social
     - Psychosocial state in response to cancer diagnosis and therapy
     - Managing expectations
   - Medical
     - Although the patient has reached 5 years after cancer therapy and is currently disease free, recurrence of ACC should be considered
     - Bleeding tendency (liver cirrhosis secondary to primary biliary cholangitis)
     - Avoid drugs metabolised in the liver
     - There is a risk of a hypertensive crisis due to arterial hypertension (see Chapter 8.1)
     - Drug interactions
   - Dental
     - Sequelae of oral cancer surgical treatment (e.g. risk of choking)
     - Chronic and late complications of radiation therapy (e.g. radiation caries and osteoradionecrosis)
     - Large oroantral/nasal defect with limited support for a maxillary prosthesis
4) What are the considerations for extracting the retained roots in the upper right quadrant?
   - A risk–benefit analysis should be undertaken as there are occasions when leaving the roots is the most prudent clinical decision
   - Risks:
     - The patient has received high-dose radiation therapy (60 Gy) which is associated with a higher risk of osteoradionecrosis (ORN) (see Chapter 13.2)
     - The retained roots are on the right alveolar ridge which is likely to have been in the field receiving the highest dose of radiotherapy
     - The roots may displace into the oroantral/nasal communication during extraction, particularly if a surgical approach is required (fluid/debris may also be displaced)
     - The retained roots may become problematic at a later date, particularly if a new maxillary prosthesis is constructed and the area is loaded
   - Benefits:
     - The retained roots were a coincidental finding and they are likely to have been in place for at least 5 years when the precancer dental extractions were undertaken (with a recovered immune system, the likelihood of infection is low)
     - Submergence of dental roots has been shown to maintain alveolar bone for prosthodontic purposes
     - Implants have been shown to successfully integrate around dental root fragments with cementum
5) Although the retained maxillary roots are not clinically visible and are covered by mucosa, further examination confirms they are palpable. The decision is made to extract the retained roots prior to further prosthodontic procedures. Other than the dose of radiation therapy, what other factors need to be considered when assessing the risk of postoperative ORN?
   - It has been more than 2 years since he finished the radiation therapy
   - The patient has not smoked since the age of 59 years
   - Alcohol consumption is nil
   - Good oral health
   - Balanced diet/good nutritional status
   - There are no infectious foci in relation to the retained roots or the remaining teeth
   - The roots are located in the maxilla which is generally more vascular (ORN incidence is higher in the mandible)
6) Following successful extraction of the retained roots and confirmed healing at 3 months, it is determined that insertion of dental implants as anchoring elements is the best option for constructing a stable and functional prosthesis. The CBCT confirms that the quantity and quality of the bone in the left maxillary ridge region are sufficient for dental implant placement (Figure 13.3.1). What precautions should be taken when inserting the dental implants?

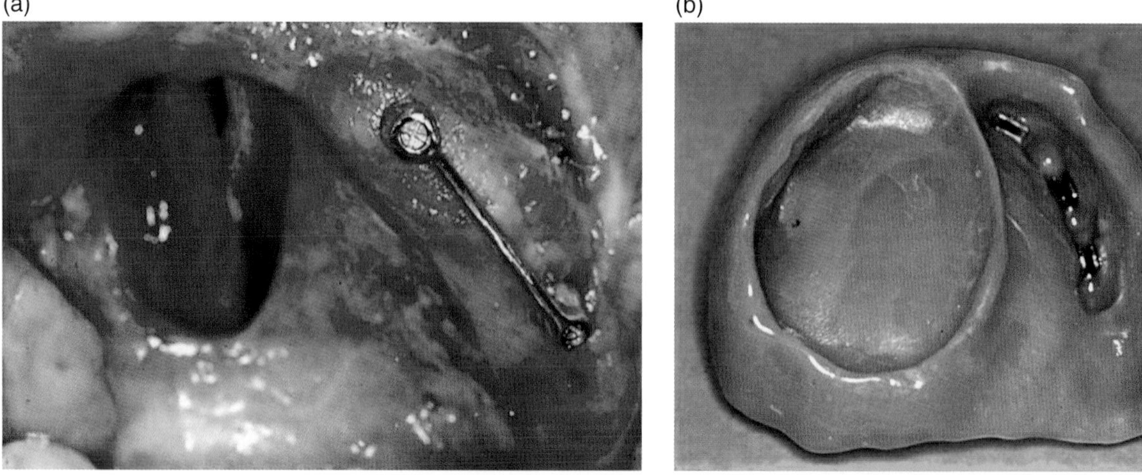

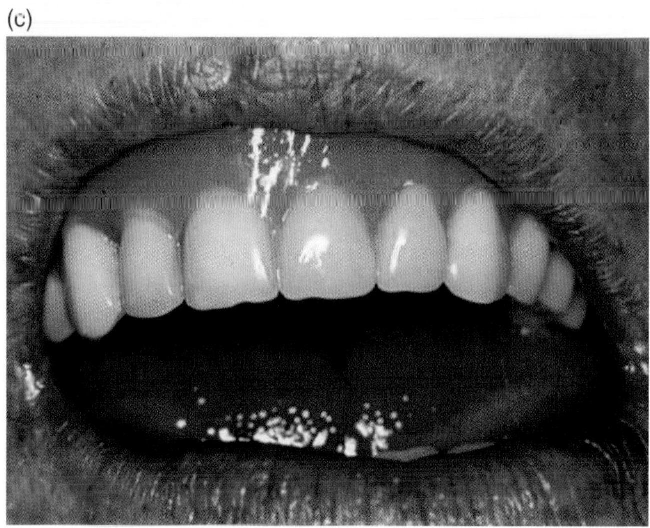

Figure 13.3.1 (a–c) Implant-supported prosthetic rehabilitation after surgical resection of a carcinoma of the palate and radiation therapy administration.

- Consider the increased risk of bleeding due to liver disease/arterial hypertension:
  - Coagulation tests and platelet counts should be performed to assess the need for haematological support
  - Blood pressure reading should be taken before starting the procedure
  - Bleeding is typically controlled with local haemostasis measures
- Ensure that placement is as far from the maximally irradiated area as possible (liaise with the radiation oncologist to determine field/dose delivered)
- Insert the minimum number of implants possible
- Consider administering antibiotic prophylaxis
- Do not fully recline the patient due to the risk of fluid/debris escaping via the oroantral/nasal fistula; use gauze/a barrier to protect this area

General Dental Considerations

Oral Findings

- Anatomical and functional sequelae of surgical treatment
- Longer term complications of radiation therapy in the oral cancer survivor are typically described as:
  - Early complications of radiation therapy that become chronic (xerostomia and dysgeusia)
  - Late complications of radiation therapy that become chronic (trismus, late dysphagia, rampant caries) (Figure 13.3.2)
  - Late complications of radiation therapy of deferred onset (ORN)

Dental Management

- Studies have confirmed high levels of post-traumatic stress for many years following the diagnosis, both in patients and their companions

(a)

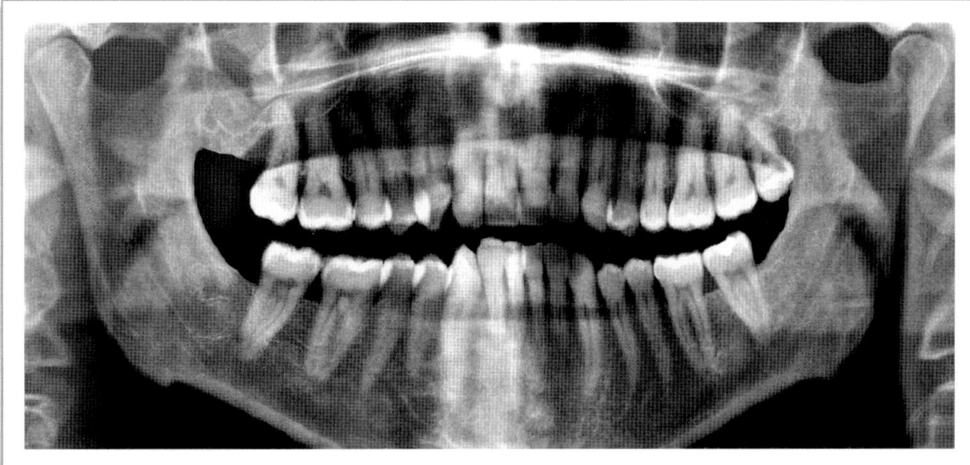

(b)

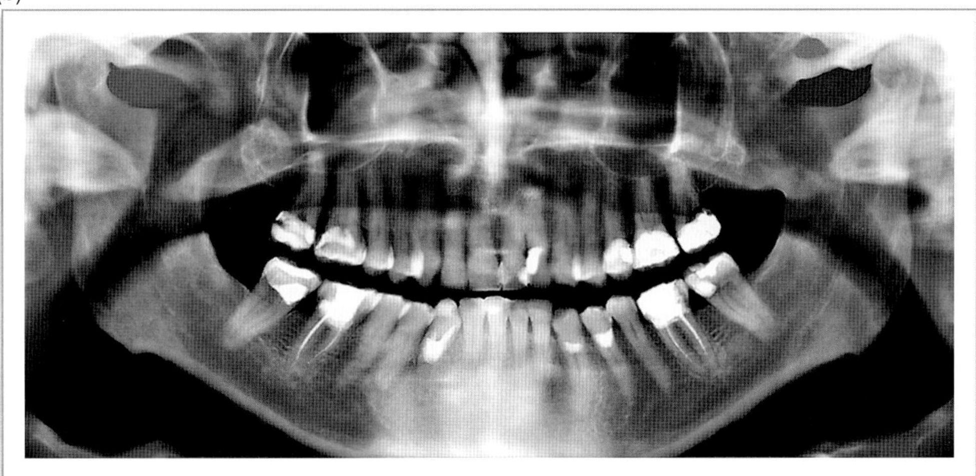

Figure 13.3.2 (a,b) Oral health status in a patient with nasopharyngeal carcinoma. Orthopantomograms before cancer treatment and 7 years after completing radiochemotherapy, demonstrating significant dental intervention/decline in dental health

- Dental management plans need to consider the patient's emotional state, given that some psychological disorders, such as anxiety, depression and self-blame, are particularly prevalent in oral cancer survivors (Table 13.3.1)
- In addition, consideration should be given to the location and extent of the resected area, the concomitant administration of radiation and/or chemotherapy and the disease prognosis
- The primary objective of prevention, treatment and oral rehabilitation strategies is to improve quality of life (Figure 13.3.3)
- To this end, dentists need to be part of a multidisciplinary team that enables a comprehensive approach for the patient; this should consist of the oncologist, primary care physician, psychologist, nutritionist, speech therapist and physiotherapist, among others (Table 13.3.2)

Section II. Background Information and Guidelines

The survival rate for oral squamous cell carcinoma (OSCC) has increased significantly in the past 2 decades and is currently approaching 60% at 5 years. One-year net survival amongst all head and neck cancer subtypes is highest in cancers of the salivary glands and lowest in hypopharyngeal cancer. Increased survival rates are thought to be related to the advances in diagnostic tools (especially imaging techniques) and therapeutic procedures, although the results also accentuate the differences between countries.

Healthcare Demands of Cancer Survivors

- Care-giver social support
- Physical and daily life needs

Table 13.3.1 Dental management considerations.

Risk assessment	• Complications related to comorbidities and risk factors (e.g. alcohol and tobacco)
	• Psychosocial impact of cancer diagnosis/therapy and post-traumatic stress
	• Presence/severity of side-effects of cancer therapy:
	– Limited mouth opening as a sequela of radiation therapy
	– Painful and fragile oral mucosa following radiation therapy or radiochemotherapy
	– Increased risk of aspiration and choking in patients with sequelae of resective cancer surgery
	– Risk of osteoradionecrosis for patients who underwent radiation therapy
	– High risk of caries recurrence and increased risk of failure of the dental treatment following radiation therapy
	– Unstable prosthetic rehabilitation risk related to location, extent and reconstruction technique of the resected area
	• Unrealistic patient expectations (mainly in those with persistent oral dysfunction)
Criteria for referral	• Most oral cancer survivors can be seen in a primary care setting
	• Referral to a hospital-based dental setting should be considered for patients with severe and/or poorly controlled comorbidities or those with significant late/chronic complications of cancer therapy (e.g. osteoradionecrosis)
	• Specialist input should also be requested (e.g. maxillofacial surgeon) if there is a clinical or radiological suspicion of a recurrence/secondary tumour
Communication	• Consult the radiation oncologist before undertaking any invasive dental treatment (to determine radiation dose/fields)
	• Speech intelligibility can be permanently impaired by the sequelae of the surgery or by the chronicity of complications of the radiation therapy (e.g. xerostomia)
Consent/capacity	• The consent should reflect the medical factors that could affect the success of the dental procedures
	• Explain that some factors related to the cancer process and its treatment sequelae might require changes in the ideal dental treatment plan
	• Anticipate the cancer treatment-related complications that can occur in the long term
	• Discuss that the patient's previous oral health state can limit the expectations for the dental treatment
	• Emphasise the importance of periodic follow-up and maintaining appropriate oral hygiene
	• Consider the impact of depression/psychosocial factors on decision making
Anaesthesia/ sedation	• Local anaesthesia
	– In areas that have received significant doses of radiation therapy, the recommendation is to reduce the use of local anaesthetics with epinephrine and avoid the intraligamentary technique (risk of osteoradionecrosis)
	• Sedation
	– No sedation technique is contraindicated
	• General anaesthesia
	– For procedures under general anaesthesia, intubation can be difficult for patients with a persistent limited mouth opening
Dental treatment	• Before
	– Dental extractions
	○ If possible, delay extractions to 24 months after the radiation therapy
	○ Antibiotic prophylaxis is recommended from 24 hours before the procedure up to 4 weeks after (e.g. clindamycin 300 mg/8 h)
	○ There is little evidence as to the efficacy of the prophylactic administration of hyperbaric oxygen
	– Implantology
	○ Delay for at least 6–12 months after radiation therapy
	○ Antibiotic prophylaxis is recommended from 24 hours before the procedure up to 4 weeks after (e.g. clindamycin 300 mg/8 h)
	○ Little evidence as to the efficacy of the prophylactic administration of hyperbaric oxygen
	○ Chemotherapy does not affect the success of dental implants

(*Continued*)

Table 13.3.1 (Continued)

- Periodontal therapy
  - The recommendation is to avoid surgical procedures
  - Antibiotic prophylaxis is recommended from 24 hours before the procedure
- Prosthetic rehabilitation
  - Wait 6–12 months after the cancer treatment to prepare the definitive prosthesis
  - Removable prostheses are generally preferable, with their improved access for hygiene and for monitoring the onset of new tumours

- During
  - Dental extractions
    - In cases of a high risk of osteoradionecrosis, consider root canal treatment and crown amputation as an alternative to extraction
    - Limit the number of extractions per session
    - Perform alveolectomy and primary closure with a mucoperiosteal flap
  - Implantology
    - Avoid the placement of implants in the irradiated bone; placing them in the remaining healthy bone is preferable (can also be placed in bone reconstruction graft)
    - Insert the minimum number of implants possible
  - Periodontal therapy
    - Perform periodontal treatment by sextant and extend the interval between sessions
  - Dental caries treatment
    - Consider the use of remineralisation products such as amorphous calcium phosphate
    - For patients who are administered fluoride on a regular basis, the recommendation is to use composite resin or resin-modified glass ionomers rather than conventional glass ionomers, although there is no scientific evidence to support this proposal
  - Prosthetic rehabilitation
    - Avoid zinc oxide and plaster as impression materials as these can be very uncomfortable
    - Intraoral 3D scanners can be useful for taking recordings, designing and manufacturing the prosthesis
    - Design prostheses with short arches and teeth with flat cusps (non-anatomical) to minimise occlusal trauma
- After
  - Caries prevention
    - The recommendations should be based on a previous assessment of the risk of caries (e.g. Caries Management By Risk Assessment – CAMBRA protocol)
    - Prescribe high-fluoride toothpaste (e.g. 2800 or 5000 ppm NaF for use twice daily)
    - In high-risk cases, mouthwashes with 0.05% NaF may also be prescribed
    - Professional application of 5% NaF coating (22 600 ppm every 3 months)
  - Periodontal and implant maintenance
    - Maintenance care is mandatory for the long term success of periodontal and implant treatment

Education/ prevention

- The oral health of survivors of oral cancer is broadly similar to that of the general population and is affected by age, income level, educational level, smoking and cancer treatment sequelae
- The loss of teeth in these patients has been associated with poorer physical functionality and emotional control, as well as dyspnoea, insomnia, loss of appetite, nausea/vomiting and bowel habit disorders
- The dentist should encourage smoking cessation and alcohol abstinence (increased risk of osteoradionecrosis); the persistent complications of radiation therapy, such as dry mouth, thick mucus and tooth and gum problems, are more severe for those who smoke
- Toothbrushing has a significant positive effect on the quality of life of cancer survivors
- Dental follow-up
  - More frequent check-ups for the first 2 years, when recurrence is more common; urgent referral for any suspicious lesion
  - Then every 3–6 months for the rest of the patient's life
  - Continue using fluoride indefinitely

(a)

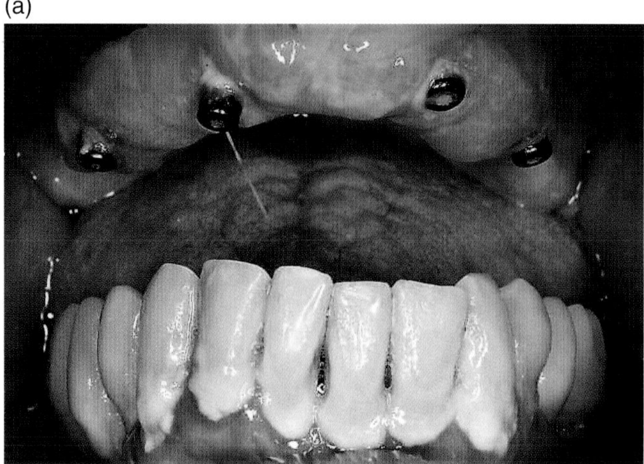

(b)

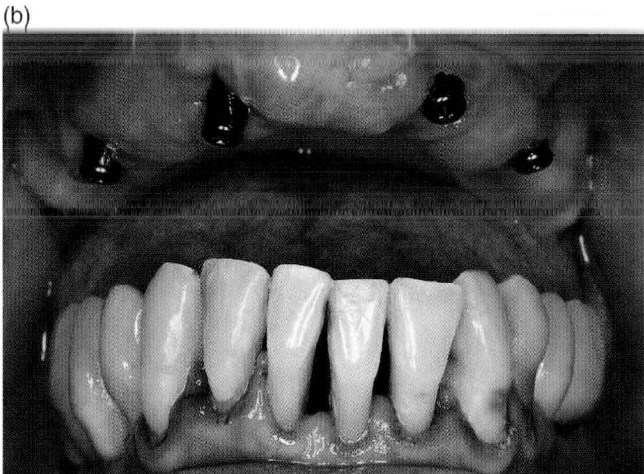

Figure 13.3.3 (a,b) Maintenance care is mandatory for the long-term success of periodontal and implant treatment in cancer patients.

- Access to the health system
- Demand for information
- Psychological support
- Occupational counselling and rehabilitation for returning to work activities

Health-Related Quality of Life (HRQL)

- Quality of life is a multidimensional concept that includes the patient's self-perception of their own existence, in a social-cultural context and the context in which they live, and in relation to their objectives, expectations, standards and concerns
- The HRQL of survivors of oral cancer is generally poorer than that of the general population and is determined by factors such as:
  - Tumour size and, accordingly, treatment complexity. The HRQL of survivors who only underwent surgery is better than that of survivors who underwent multimodal therapy or adjuvant radiation therapy
  - Permanent disfiguration and functional limitations as a result of the surgical resection
  - The delayed complications and persistent sequelae of radiochemotherapy
  - The sensory disorders and presence of chronic pain
  - Psychological/emotional state
  - Socio-economic factors such as income and marital status
- The dental treatment for oral cancer survivors should be conducted within the framework of a multidisciplinary approach, designing an individualised plan and respecting the patient's social, cultural and religious preferences

A World/Transcultural View

- The differences in mortality rate are obvious not only between north and south and between east and west but also between regions (e.g. between Scandinavian countries and old Soviet republics)

Table 13.3.2 Multidisciplinary approach for survivors of head and neck cancer.

Specialties involved	Activities
The oncology team (surgeon, radiation therapist and oncologist)	Determining the prognosis The follow-up The assessment of recurrence The need for adjuvant therapy
The primary care physician	Responsible for managing the comorbidities
The psychologist/psychiatrist	Conducting a psychological/emotional assessment If necessary, planning psychotherapy meetings Specific drugs prescription
The nutritionist and dysphagia units	Analysing feeding difficulties Establishing individualised treatment plans (e.g. suitability of percutaneous endoscopic gastrostomy)
The speech therapist	Assisting in treating dysglossia and swallowing problems Improving the mobility of the remaining anatomical structures
The physiotherapist	Controlling impaired swallowing, irregular breathing and painful shoulders
The dental team	Maintaining the oral health condition Managing the sequelae of cancer therapy Preventing the onset of delayed complications Conducting comprehensive oral rehabilitation that is functional and aesthetically acceptable Screening for a recurrence/new lesion

- Anecdotally, the highest mortality rate was recorded in Papua New Guinea (17.7 cases per 100 000 age-standardised population rate)
- These substantial differences between countries are attributable to the persistence of certain risk factors, lifestyles, socio-economic conditions, diagnostic delay, limited access to specialised therapy facilities and the presence of comorbidities

Recommended Reading

Cocks, H., Ah-See, K., Capel, M., and Taylor, P. (2016). Palliative and supportive care in head and neck cancer: United Kingdom National Multidisciplinary Guidelines. *J. Laryngol. Otol.* 130: S198–S207.

Diz Dios, P. and Diniz Freitas, M. (2020). Supportive and palliative care for patients with oral cancer. In: *Textbook of Oral Cancer: Prevention, Diagnosis and Management* (eds. S. Warnakulasuriya and J.S. Greenspan), 344–358. Basel: Springer Nature Switzerland AG.

Epstein, J.B., Güneri, P., and Barasch, A. (2014). Appropriate and necessary oral care for people with cancer: guidance to obtain the right oral and dental care at the right time. *Support. Care Cancer* 22: 1981–1988.

Kondo, T., Sugauchi, A., Yabuno, Y. et al. (2019). Performance status scale for head and neck scores for oral cancer survivors: predictors and factors for improving quality of life. *Clin. Oral Investig.* 23: 1575–1582.

Lee, M.S., Nelson, A.M., Thompson, L.M., and Donovan, K.A. (2016). Supportive care needs of oral cancer survivors: prevalence and correlates. *Oral Oncol.* 53: 85–90.

Petrovic, I., Rosen, E.B., Matros, E. et al. (2018). Oral rehabilitation of the cancer patient: a formidable challenge. *J. Surg. Oncol.* 117: 1729–1735.

Valdez, J.A. and Brennan, M.T. (2018). Impact of oral cancer on quality of life. *Dent. Clin. North Am.* 62: 143–154.

Yan, R., Chen, X., Gong, X. et al. (2018). The association of tooth loss, toothbrushing, and quality of life among cancer survivors. *Cancer Med.* 7: 6374–6384.

14

Neurological Disorders and Strokes

14.1 Alzheimer Disease

Section I: Clinical Scenario and Dental Considerations

Clinical Scenario

A 68-year-old male is referred by his neurologist for dental assessment as requested by the patient's wife. She has noticed that her husband has bad breath, gets food trapped between his back molars and finds it difficult to clean his teeth. The patient has not complained of any dental pain or gum swelling. He does not understand why he needs a dental visit and he believes his teeth are healthy.

Medical History
- Alzheimer disease (middle stage)
- Stroke
- Hypertension

Medications
- Rivastigmine
- Aspirin
- Amlodipine
- Candesartan
- Citicoline and *Gingko biloba* supplements

Dental History
- Irregular dental attender
- Independently brushes his teeth using a manual toothbrush; does not like electric toothbrushes; his wife usually supervises his brushing routine
- Uses 1450 ppm fluoride toothpaste

Social History
- Lives with his wife, son and daughter-in-law
- Stopped working more than 5 years ago
- Uses a wheelchair but can transfer and walk short distances with assistance
- Tobacco and alcohol consumption: nil

Oral Examination
- Fully dentate
- #11 chipped incisal edge (Figure 14.1.1)
- #17 extensive distal subgingival caries
- Generalised attrition
- Maxillary anterior teeth palatal erosion (Figure 14.1.2)
- Moderate plaque retention
- Localised gingivitis
- Food impaction areas bilaterally (molars) (Figure 14.1.3)
- Xerostomia

Radiological Examination
- Limited co-operation; unable to tolerate/remaining still for an orthopantomogram
- Long cone periapical radiograph taken demonstrating extensive distal subgingival caries #17

Structured Learning

1) Why does this patient's perception of his oral health differ from reality?
   - Alzheimer disease results in a progressive decline in cognition
   - The patient is less able to recognise the signs of deteriorating oral health, such as bad breath
   - Deterioration of memory and executive functioning may result in poor recall of any signs or symptoms associated with dental disease
2) The patient's wife reports that he has always had very good oral health in the past. What factors could have contributed to the decline?
   - Dementia: reduced ability to self-care, tendency for an increase in cariogenic diet, irregular visits to the dentist, xerostomia secondary to medication
   - Stroke: reduced mobility may have an impact on ability to self-care

A Practical Approach to Special Care in Dentistry, First Edition. Edited by Pedro Diz Dios and Navdeep Kumar.

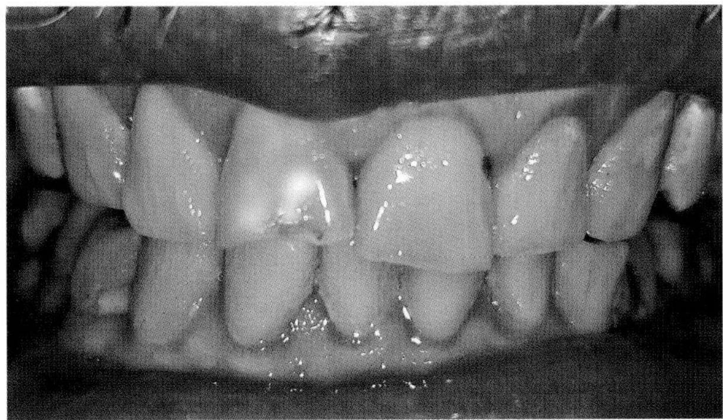

Figure 14.1.1 Anterior dentition: marginal gingivitis; #11 chipped incisal edge.

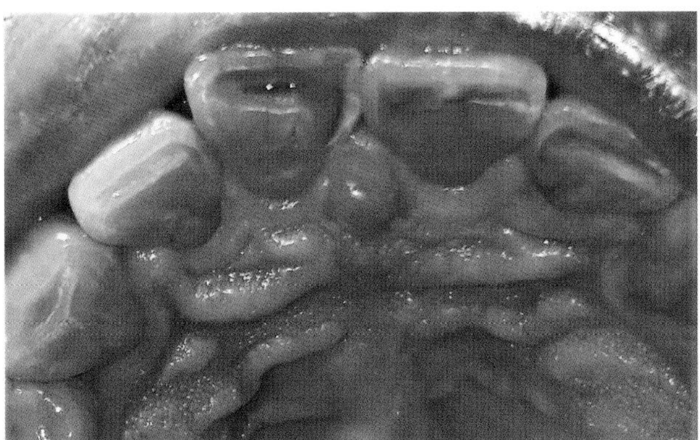

Figure 14.1.2 Palatal aspect of the upper anterior teeth: palatal erosion and xerostomia.

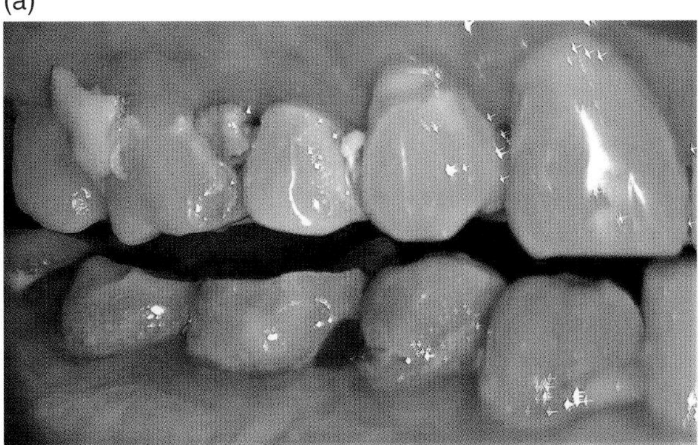

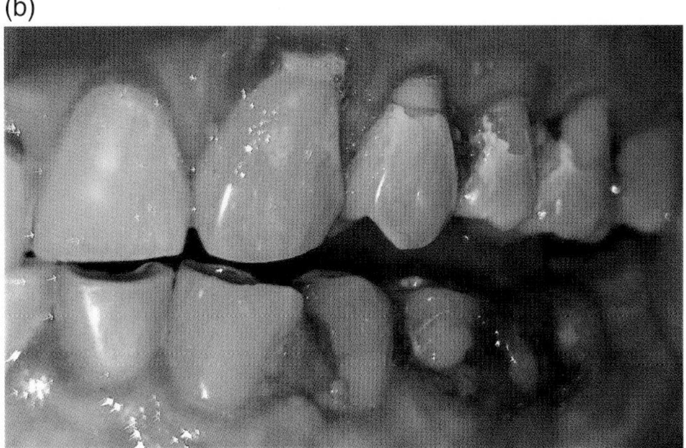

Figure 14.1.3 (a,b) Food packing posteriorly.

3) Dietary analysis reveals that the patient increasingly consumes large quantities of high-sugar foods. Why is this?
   - People with dementia often experience sudden changes in appetite preferences and an increase in unhealthy cravings
   - As the disease progresses, taste buds diminish, insulin in the brain can drop and some people experience intense cravings for high-calorie foods
   - This leads to an intake of food with stronger flavours and increased sweetness
   - As appetite declines, adding sugar to foods may encourage eating
4) The patient has also noticed that her husband's teeth are becoming more worn down and that #11 has recently chipped. What factors may be contributing to the tooth wear?
   - Attrition: awake/diurnal bruxism secondary to Alzheimer disease (present in ~4% of patients); nocturnal bruxism (sleep-related disorder) may also be present
   - Erosion: increasingly acidic diet
   - Abrasion: due to repetitive toothbrushing action
   - Trauma: due to falls which may have caused #11 edge to fracture
5) What are the risks of leaving untreated dental disease in this patient?
   - Progression of dental disease can cause significant pain or discomfort
   - This can worsen confusion associated with dementia and translate to aggression or agitation
   - Poor oral health can also contribute to perceived stress and has a negative impact on quality of life, in particular self-esteem, dignity, social integration and nutrition
   - Patient management in the dental setting will be more complicated as the disease progresses
   - There is also a potential relationship between poor oral health and cognitive decline, particularly in memory and executive functioning
6) Due to the extensive soft deposits/interdental food packing, you advise the patient that he needs further assistance from his wife with his toothbrushing, particularly with interdental cleaning. What practical steps would you recommend?
   - Break mouthcare tasks into small steps

- Stand behind
- Distraction – music, talking, stroking arm, another object to hold
- Bridging – person holds same implement as carer
- Hand-over-hand – carer guides person's hands
- Cueing – polite, one-step commands
- Visual prompts, gestures and mime
- Mirror – person watches mouthcare in mirror
- Rescuing – replacement of his wife with his son when care-resistant behaviours escalate

7) Although the patient does not report any pain associated with #17, the ability to recall symptoms may be associated with his decline in memory and cognition. What other signs may indicate dental pain?
   - Inability to chew food
   - Refusal of food
   - Grimacing when tooth is touched
   - Frequently holding onto face, cheeks or mouth
   - Scratching or rubbing the tooth with his fingernail
   - Refusal to brush the teeth in the area of #17
   - Inability to sleep at night or disruption in sleep because of dental pain
   - Increasingly withdrawn or aggressive behaviour (compared to baseline behaviour)

8) What other factors do you need to consider in your risk assessment?
   - Social
     - Availability of an escort
     - Capacity may be impaired
     - Wheelchair access required, transfer arrangements to the dental chair
     - Stroke leading to reduced mobility and ability to self-care
   - Medical
     - Potential risk of aspiration due to stroke
     - Hypertensive crisis risk and bleeding tendency
     - Bleeding risk due to aspirin
   - Dental
     - Xerostomia
     - Bruxism
     - Poor oral health
     - Inability to accurately report dental pain/symptoms

9) When discussing the need to extract #17 under local anaesthesia, how would you ensure that the patient understands and has the capacity to proceed?
   - Always start from the assumption that the person has the capacity to make the decision in question
   - Demonstrate that you have made every effort to encourage and support the person to make the decision themselves
   - Undertake a capacity assessment to determine if the patient can:
     - Understand the information given to them
     - Retain that information long enough to be able to make the decision
     - Weigh up the information available to make the decision
     - Communicate their decision – this could be by talking, using signs, including hand signals
   - Depending on the outcome of the capacity assessment, obtain informed consent or make a best interest decision

General Dental Considerations

Oral Findings

- Neglected mouth
- Poor oral hygiene/increased plaque/calculus deposits with associated halitosis
- Multiple carious lesions/retained roots
- Periodontal disease with associated halitosis
- Dental trauma due to fall
- Xerostomia
- Sialorrhoea/drooling related to cholinesterase inhibitors intake
- Bruxism
- Tooth wear and fracture
- Loss of taste
- Tardive dyskinesia secondary to antipsychotic medications (e.g. fenotiacine)
- Dysphagia
- Losing dentures often/inability to tolerate them

Dental Management

- Deterioration of oral health is common, with 75% of patients with Alzheimer disease needing frequent dental attention
- Comprehensive oral rehabilitation and full-mouth diagnostic radiographs should be undertaken as early as possible since the patient's ability to co-operate during dental treatment diminishes with advancing disease. Clinical holding may be required (training, risk assessment, and consent/best interest decision required) (Figure 14.1.4)
- Treatment modifications are related to the stage of dementia (Table 14.1.1)

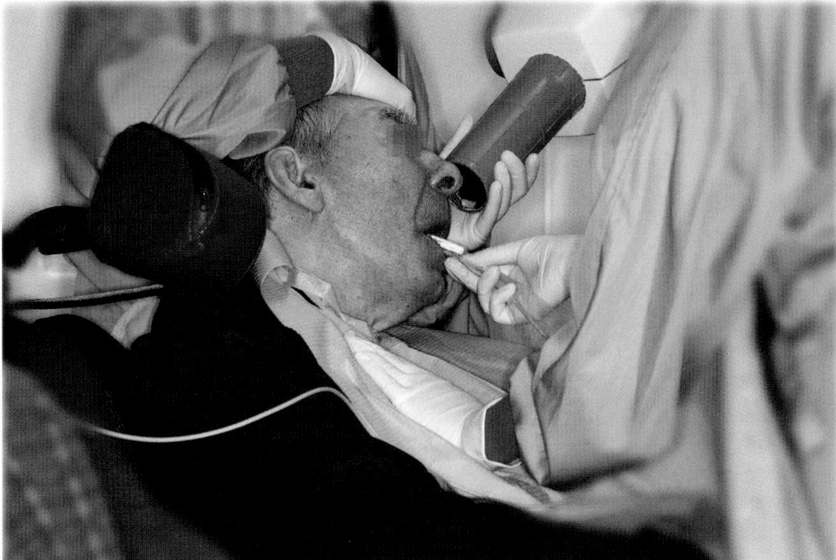

Figure 14.1.4 Co-operation during radiological examination diminishes with advancing disease; clinical holding may be required.

Section II: Background Information and Guidelines

Definition

Alzheimer disease (AD) is the most prevalent neurodegenerative disorder in elderly people, affecting an estimated 26.6 million people worldwide. Without a major therapeutic breakthrough, the prevalence of AD is expected to increase to more than 100 million by 2050.

Alzheimer disease is also the most common cause of dementia. It is caused by progressive accumulation of proteins known as amyloid plaques which damage the neurons, producing changes in parts of the brain involved in thinking, learning, memory or cognition

Aetiopathogenesis

- Changes within the brain structure may include:
  - Accumulation of protein fragments called beta-amyloid (beta-amyloid plaques) outside the neurons and protein tau (tau tangles) inside
  - Beta-amyloid plaques cause cell death by interfering with neuron-to-neuron communication at synapses
  - Tau immunoreactive neurofibrillary tangles block transportation of nutrients and essential molecules inside the neurons
  - Brain changes such as inflammation and atrophy are responsible for the continuous decline in function
- The cause of AD is thought to be multifactorial involving genetic, environmental and biological risk factors (Table 14.1.2)
- The main risk factor is age
  - The majority of people who develop the disease are over 65 years of age
  - People over 85 years of age have a sixfold increase of developing the disease (14.7% prevalence)
  - Only 5% of people are diagnosed when they are younger than 65 years old – this variant is known as early-onset Alzheimer's
- Women have a 1 in 5 chance of developing AD compared to a 1 in 11 chance for men (exact cause not known; potential impact of oestrogen)
- Rare forms of early-onset familial AD are strongly linked to causal gene mutations, namely mutations in amyloid precursor protein (APP) and presenilin (PSEN1/2) genes
- In contrast, late onset sporadic AD is a multifactorial disorder in which age-related changes, genetic risk factors, such as allelic variation in apolipoprotein E (Apo E) and many other genes, vascular disease, tobacco/alcohol and risk factors associated with diet, the immune system, mitochondrial function, metal exposure and infection have been implicated
- In addition to AD, there are several other types of dementia:
  - Vascular dementia
    - Second most common dementia, 17% of cases
    - Neuron damage or death is caused by the decreased oxygen supply to the brain due to the blockage of blood vessels
    - Often happens after a stroke and can progress through time

Table 14.1.1 Dental management considerations.

Risk assessment	• May miss appointments due to memory loss • Reduced compliance and co-operation • Fear and anxiety heightened • In later stages may become physically and verbally aggressive • Capacity may be impaired
Criteria for referral	• Patient should ideally continue dental care with a dentist who is familiar with their dental history and has seen them regularly before diagnosis of Alzheimer disease • Referral to a specialised clinic or hospital centre is determined by factors that significantly limit access for dental procedures (e.g. significantly reduced co-operation in late stages of the disease which may require sedation/general anaesthesia to deliver dental care)
Access/position	• Ensure the patient/escort is contacted to remind them of any appointments • Determine the preferred time of the day for the appointment (e.g. late afternoon may be more suitable if the patient is asleep earlier in the day) • Consider initial domiciliary visit – assessing a patient in a familiar, less threatening environment may be beneficial • The stage of disease and complexity of the dental treatment will determine if the patient can be treated in the dental clinic, a hospital setting or at home • Confirm access/transfer requirements (i.e. transport, parking, wheelchair, escort, toilet) • Ensure that the dental environment is appropriate – Easy-to-read information in large font – Appropriate space in waiting area with bright distinguishable colours for furniture – Noise reduction – Even lighting – Matt, even-coloured flooring (shiny floor surface can appear wet/slippery) – Clear signage with picture on doors – ideally large pictures to demonstrate the purpose of each room • Ideally, avoid keeping the patient waiting on arrival as this may cause agitation • Shorter appointments starting with the least complex procedure if possible • Patients with dysphagia may need a more upright position during procedures • Even without dysphagia, many patients refuse to be in a backward position • Clinical holding may be required
Communication	• Additional information may be required from the physician to determine the stage of the dementia as this can impact on dental treatment planning • Explain the treatment in short words and simple sentences • Avoid covering your mouth with a mask • Give the patient time to process the information and to respond; ask 'yes' or 'no' questions slowly and repeat their answer to ensure they have understood • Consider other communication methods if the patient has aphasia or is non-verbal
Consent/capacity	• Capacity to give informed consent may be impaired • A decision-specific capacity assessment should be undertaken • Family/carer may be involved in a best interest decision • Provide a clear written treatment plan and rediscuss at each appointment
Anaesthesia/sedation	• Local anaesthesia – Co-operation may be limited • Sedation – Oral sedation prior to the dental visit may improve compliance – Co-operation for the mask used for inhalational sedation may be limited; caution also required as this method suppresses the gag reflex and compounds the risk of aspiration where there is dysphagia – Co-operation for cannulation for intravenous sedation may be reduced; risk of aspiration due to respiratory depression • General anaesthesia – Risk of postoperative cognitive decline with further deterioration in quality of life – Considered if all the other available options are not feasible and there is a dental emergency/significant oral pain and infection

(Continued)

Table 14.1.1 (Continued)

Dental treatment	• Before – Identify teeth with poor prognosis, little functional or aesthetic value that may be better extracted than restored – Consider a shortened dental arch which may be easier to maintain and access in the longer term – Early intervention is recommended to prevent extensive dental problems – Consider decline in self-care/oral hygiene and dependence on others in the future when determining the type of restorative material/finalising the treatment plan – Choose self-cleansing or easily maintained restorations – Atraumatic restorative techniques and silver diamine fluoride can be used to arrest enamel-dentine caries – Assess the need for clinical holding, record and obtain informed consent • During – Approach and communicate with the patient from the front, as coming from behind may startle or frighten the patient – Avoid quick and jerky movements – Slowly recline the dental chair to avoid startling the patient – A familiar person in the room during the appointment to accompany the patient may be helpful – Use simple language and repeat information and instructions • After – For patients with advanced dementia, explain to carers changes in behaviour that can indicate any sign of dental pain – Give verbal and written postoperative instructions
Drug prescription	• Non-steroidal anti-inflammatory drugs may increase risk of gastrointestinal bleeding when taken with cholinesterase inhibitors • Scopolamine patches counteract the effect of cholinesterase inhibitors (e.g. sialorrhoea)
Education/prevention	• Frequent recall visits, ideally 3–4 times a year • Comprehensive preventive programme must be implemented especially in the early stages of the disease to reduce the need for invasive dental treatment in later stages • Use of fluoride varnish and fissure sealants, oral hygiene education, dietary advice • Minimum of 1450 ppm fluoride toothpaste to be used twice daily during toothbrushing; for patients with higher caries risk, prescribe 2800 or 5000 ppm toothpaste – be aware of aspiration risk • May need to educate carers regarding supervision and assistance with daily oral care (depends on the stage of dementia and motor skills of the patient) • Aspiration risk: use of suction or aspirating toothbrushes may help for patients in late-stage dementia; using gauze to wipe off excess toothpaste may be undertaken for persons who cannot spit out any more; consider non-foaming toothpaste • Denture must be kept out of the mouth during bedtime, and cleaned before and after use

    - Can also be caused by subcortical vascular dementia where the small vessels deep in the brain are affected
- Frontotemporal dementia
    - 2% of diagnosed cases
    - Abnormal proteins accumulating in neurons can cause personality and behaviour changes. Symptoms like difficulty in speech and difficulty with the meaning of words depend on whether the frontal or temporal lobe of the brain is affected
- Dementia with Lewy bodies
    - 4% of cases
    - Closely related to Parkinson disease with the same movement difficulty symptoms
    - Involves abnormal structures called Lewy bodies accumulating in the brain which disrupt neurotransmission and eventually cause cell death of neurons
- Mixed dementia
    - 10% of dementia cases
    - More than one cause of dementia
    - Increased likelihood with age and more common with people aged 85 and older
- Parkinson dementia
    - 2% of cases
    - When Parkinson disease progresses, accumulation of alpha-synuclein in the cortex of the brain or the

Table 14.1.2 Alzheimer disease – potential risk factors.

Category	Risk factor
Demographic	Age Gender Education Race Social environment
Genetics	Amyloid precursor protein (APP) Presenilin 1 and 2 (PSEN1/2) Apolipoprotein E (APOE) ATP-binding cassette transporter A1 (ABCA1) Adaptor protein evolutionarily conserved signalling intermediate in Toll pathway (ECSIT) Clusterin gene (CLU) Oestrogen receptor gene (ESR) Fermitin family homologue 2 gene (FERMT2) Glyceraldehyde 3 phosphate dehydrogenase (GAPDH) Histocompatibility locus antigen (HLA class III) mtDNA haplotype (H, V, U, K, J, T, others) Transferrin gene (Tf) Triggering receptor expressed on myeloid cells 2 (TREM 2) Vascular protein sorting-10 domain (VpS10) genes Vitamin D receptor gene (VDR) Epigenetic factors
Lifestyle	Alcohol Lack of exercise Lack of cognitive activity Malnutrition Poor diet Smoking
Medical	Cancer Cardiovascular disease Congestive heart failure Immune system dysfunction Microinfarcts Obesity Poor cholesterol homeostasis Poorly controlled type 2 diabetes Stroke Traumatic brain injury
Psychiatric	Depression Early stress
Environmental	Air pollution Calcium deficiency Geographic location Metals (especially aluminium, copper, zinc) Organic solvents Occupation Vitamin deficiency
Infection	Bacteria Fungi Viruses Chronic dental infections (periodontal disease)

further accumulation of beta-amyloid and tau tangles can cause further damage to neurons, resulting in dementia

Diagnosis

- Diagnosis by exclusion; need to exclude underlying treatable conditions such as abnormal thyroid function, normal pressure hydrocephalus or a vitamin deficiency that may result in cognitive difficulties
- Cognitive and neuropsychological tests are used to assess memory, problem solving, language skills, maths skills and other abilities related to mental functioning
- Laboratory tests to exclude other causes
- Brain scans (CT/MRI/PET) – to identify strokes, tumours and other brain-occupying lesions that may be responsible
- Psychiatric evaluation to determine if there is a mental health condition such as depression that may be contributing to the symptoms
- Genetic tests (rarely used)

Clinical Presentation

- AD is a progressive disorder which is often diagnosed late as early signs are typically attributed to ageing (Table 14.1.3)
- Patients may live with the symptoms of memory loss and language problems for years, affecting their ability to remember, understand, reason and communicate
- The common clinical presentation before diagnosis is irritability and repetitive speech
- As the disease progresses, there is also a decline in performing activities of daily living and social interactions
- In late stages, parts of the brain that are responsible for bodily functions such as walking, breathing and swallowing are affected
- Dysphagia with the associated risk of aspiration is common in the latter stages of disease

Table 14.1.3 Alzheimer disease – clinical presentation.

Stage	Clinical features
• **Early (mild) stage** – 'preclinical'	Memory loss – mostly for short-term events
	Challenges in planning or problem solving
	Confused and disoriented
	Difficulty with solving problems and carrying out tasks
	Aphasia
	Language difficulties
	Problems with communication
	Change in mood/personality
• **Middle (moderate) stage** – mild cognitive impairment	Impaired short-term memory
	Confused about night and day
	Easily gets upset or angry
	Communication difficulties
	Repetitive speech
	Delusions or hallucinations
	Object agnosia – difficulty judging distances or confused with shiny surfaces with reflections
	Restlessness
	Disoriented with unfamiliar environment
	Begins to be dependent with activities of daily living
• **Late (severe) stage** – established dementia	Apathy and disorientation
	Major behavioural and psychiatric symptoms including increasing anxiety, agitation, aggression, psychosis and depression
	Failure to recognise family members
	Inability to remember details of personal history
	Decreased articulation
	Decreased facial expressions/reactions
	Unsteady balance and shuffling gait
	Urinary and faecal incontinence
	Dysphagia
	Needs assistance with activities of daily living
	Sleep disturbance

Management

- There is currently no cure for AD, with treatment regimens focusing on symptom management
- Non-pharmacological therapy
  - Support the person and carer
  - Planning ahead after the diagnosis
  - Talking therapies
  - Cognitive behavioural therapy
- Pharmacological treatment
  - Approved drugs are cholinesterase inhibitors such as rivastigmine, galantamine, donepezil and tacrine
  - N-methyl-D-aspartate inhibitors such as memantine and memantine with donepezil
  - Drugs available do not slow down or stop the damage and destruction of the neurons but temporarily improve symptoms
  - Medications to treat behavioural symptoms – antidepressants, anxiolytics and antipsychotics
  - Areas of research: statins, disease-modifying antirheumatic drugs (DMARDs), oestrogen replacement

Prognosis

- AD is a progressive disease, eventually making the person lose his personality, memories and functional capabilities
- As the person loses motor skills, they will eventually become fully dependent on carers and family to perform oral hygiene care
- Aggression towards carers may contribute to poor compliance to enable care, and there is an inability to articulate pain

A World/Transcultural View

- Globally, 50 million people are diagnosed with dementia, 60% of which are from low- and middle-income countries
- From 1990 to 2015 there was an increase in prevalence of AD in high-income countries such as North America, high-income Asia Pacific, east Asia, south Asia, the Caribbean, and southern sub-Saharan Africa, but a decrease noticed elsewhere
- In the past 25 years there has been a doubling of people worldwide who die from AD

Recommended Reading

Armstrong, R.A. (2019). Risk factors for Alzheimer's disease. *Folia Neuropathol.* 57: 87–105.

Faculty of General Dental Practice (UK). (2017). *Dementia-Friendly Dentistry: Good Practice Guidelines*. www.fgdp.org.uk/publication/dementia-friendly-dentistry

Foltyn, P. (2015). Ageing, dementia and oral health. *Aust. Dent. J.* 60: 86–94.

Friedlander, A.H., Norman, D.C., Mahler, M.E. et al. (2006). Alzheimer's disease: psychopathology, medical management and dental implications. *J. Am. Dent. Assoc.* 137: 1240–1251.

Marchini, L., Ettinger, R., Caprio, T., and Jucan, A. (2019). Oral health care for patients with Alzheimer's disease: an update. *Spec. Care Dentist.* 39: 262–273.

Peters, R., Booth, A., Rockwood, K. et al. (2019). Combining modifiable risk factors and risk of dementia: a systematic review and meta-analysis. *BMJ Open* 25; e022846.

So, E., Kim, H.J., Karm, M.H. et al. (2017). A retrospective analysis of outpatient anesthesia management for dental treatment of patients with severe Alzheimer's disease. *J. Dent. Anesth. Pain Med.* 17: 271–280.

14.2 Parkinson Disease

Section I: Clinical Scenario and Dental Considerations

Clinical Scenario

An 81-year-old female presents to the dental clinic, accompanied by her daughter and carer. The patient reports that she finds it increasingly embarrassing to communicate, socialise and go to public places. In part, she feels that this is related to her excessive drooling and the fact that food persistently accumulates in her mouth (Figure 14.2.1).

Medical History

- Parkinson disease (PD) diagnosed 25 years ago
- Rheumatic heart disease following rheumatic fever 21 years ago
- Prosthetic mitral valve replacement placed 20 years ago
- Stage II colon cancer with hemicolectomy 10 years ago
- Subdural haematoma 9 years ago, due to fall from the bed; craniotomy undertaken
- Severe osteoporosis causing the patient to stoop forward – diagnosed around 4 years ago

Medications

- Carbidopa/levodopa
- Ropinirole
- Amantadine
- Risperidone
- Warfarin
- Digoxin
- Trimetazidine
- Atorvastatin
- Denosumab – twice a yearly infusion; last infusion 3 months ago
- Calcium carbonate
- Vitamin D

Dental History

- Irregular dental attender due to her mobility issues; last visit 2 years ago
- Brushes her own teeth with a handheld toothbrush and 1450 ppm fluoride toothpaste twice daily
- Soft diet as finds it difficult to chew hard food

Social History

- Widowed; lives with her daughter
- Care-giver support daily due to frequent falls
- Can walk limited distances with assistance; uses a wheelchair for longer distances
- Tobacco and alcohol consumption: nil

General/Oral Examination

- Haematoma observed on the right side of the forehead (Figure 14.2.2)
- Partially edentate with loss of posterior occlusal support (Figure 14.2.3)
- #34 extensive distal-buccal subgingival caries
- Plaque-induced gingivitis
- Gingival recession
- Multiple cervical abrasion lesions
- Moderate plaque and calculus deposits
- Food impaction area on tooth #17

Radiological Examination

- Long cone periapical radiograph showing tooth #34 with subgingival distal caries into the pulp (Figure 14.2.4)

Structured Learning

1) Following further questioning regarding the haematoma on the right side of the patient's forehead, you determine that she fell over in the bathroom at home that morning. What additional questions would you ask and why?

A Practical Approach to Special Care in Dentistry, First Edition. Edited by Pedro Diz Dios and Navdeep Kumar.

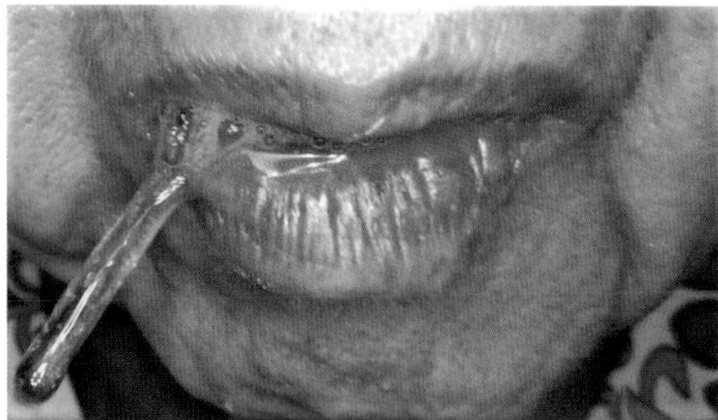

Figure 14.2.1 Excessive drooling (sialorrhoea, hypersalivation).

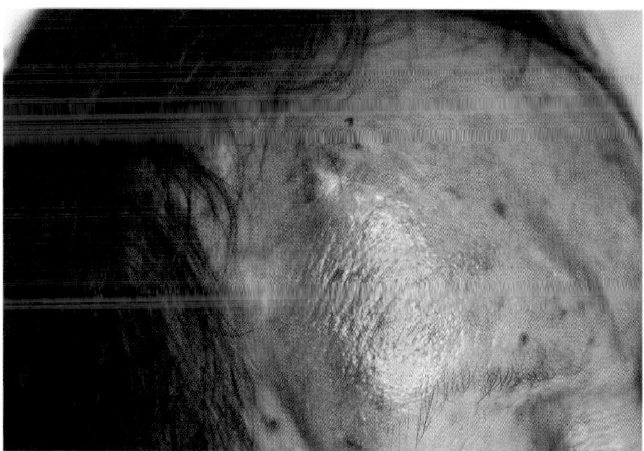

Figure 14.2.2 Haematoma on the right side of the forehead due to a fall.

- In view of the risk of a traumatic brain injury, it is important to enquire if there was any loss of consciousness, any amnesia before or after the injury, persistent headache, drowsiness or any vomiting episodes since the injury; the patient may require urgent referral to the emergency services if any of these are present; this patient is particularly at risk of an intracranial bleed as she is anticoagulated (see Chapter 10.3) and hence should be alerted that if any of these signs do appear later, she should seek urgent medical attention
- Further details regarding how the fall occurred are also important as these may highlight safeguarding issues (inadequate support/supervision in the bathroom, possible non-accidental injury)

2) Following further assessment of the patient, you determine that she appears stable (Glasgow Coma Scale 15) and there are no safeguarding concerns. The patient wishes to proceed with the dental appointment and asks what could be causing the worsening of her drooling. What would you discuss?
   - Up to 85% of patients experience sialorrhoea (drooling) in advanced PD

(a)

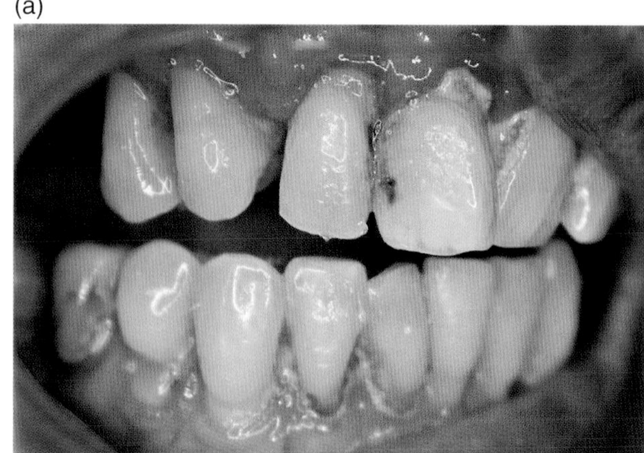

(b)

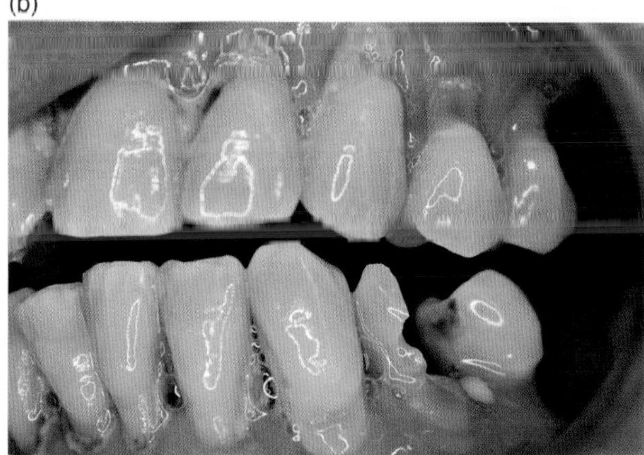

Figure 14.2.3 (a,b) Partially edentate, plaque-induced gingivitis, moderate calculus deposits, multiple cervical abrasion lesions, and #34 carious with extensive fracture of the distal buccal wall.

   - This is in relation to reduced muscle control, which results in swallowing dysfunction, oropharyngeal dysphagia, poor oral musculature control and forward flexed positioning of the head
   - Treatment options include botulinum toxin injected to the parotid and submandibular glands usually through ultrasound guidance or palpating the gland; the duration of its effects can range from 6 weeks to 6 months with the usual side-effect being xerostomia. Speech therapy and physical therapy may also be helpful

3) In addition to drooling, what other factors make it difficult for the PD patient to communicate and socialise in public?
   - A mask-like facial appearance and reduced movements of the small muscles of the face (hypomimia) are perceived by others as staring blankly or responding flatly

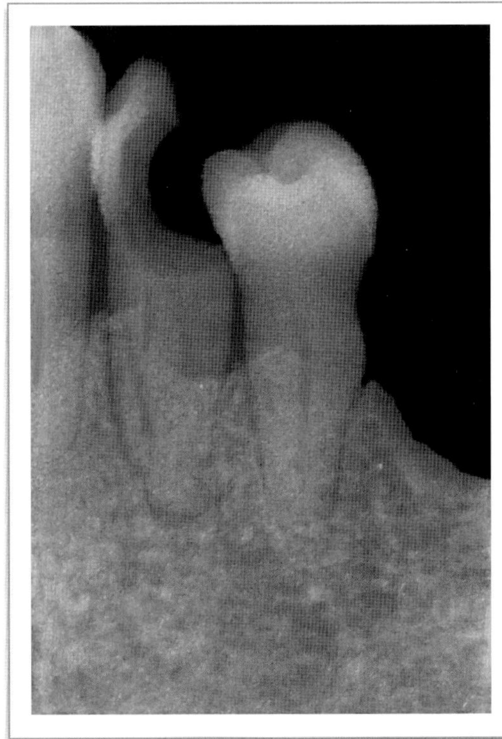

Figure 14.2.4 Long cone periapical radiograph demonstrating extensive caries in the #34.

- The quality of speech deteriorates along with disease progression, with hypophonia and even whispering in the later stages
- Patients may fear not being understood or interrupted in a conversation with several people
- The patient may also experience altered emotions or mood swings that vary day to day and may be associated with depression

4) The patient also asks why food is accumulating in her mouth and if this is causing the deterioration in her oral health. What would you discuss?
   - Bradykinesia can affect chewing, slowing down the clearance of food in the oral cavity
   - Poor bolus formation with reduced tongue movement make propulsion of food down the oral cavity difficult
   - In the latter stages of disease, there is weakened pharyngeal motor control, causing dysphagia and making swallowing certain foods more difficult, if not impossible, causing them to remain in the oral cavity
   - A forward/drooped head position can also make swallowing worse
   - Tremors, loss of fine muscle control and impaired manual dexterity make it increasingly difficult for the patient to brush her teeth efficiently; an electric toothbrush/adapted brush with suction may help
   - Depression also contributes to the low motivation in self-care and difficulty in performing oral hygiene care regularly
5) The patient reports that #34 is not painful, although there was a gingival swelling in the adjacent gum for which the doctor prescribed antibiotics 3 months ago. Why is this of particular concern in this patient?
   - The tooth should be managed urgently as it is grossly carious, with further episodes of infection likely
   - There may be associated bacteraemia with the associated risk of infective endocarditis as the patient has a prosthetic heart valve (see Chapter 8.5)
6) What other factors do you need to consider in your risk assessment when planning extraction of #34?
   - Social
     - Escort availability
     - Consider positioning the chair to accommodate the patient's forward bent position
     - Access and transfer from the wheelchair (a wheelchair recliner may be required)
     - Particular caution if transferring the patient due to history of frequent falls
   - Medical
     - PD-associated complications such as tremor, communication and swallowing problems
     - Prosthetic heart valve/infective endocarditis risk (see Chapter 8.5)
     - Bleeding risk related to INR range (see Chapter 10.3)
     - Osteoporosis: hyperkyphotic posture, increased fragility of bone (see Chapter 7.1)
     - Drug interactions/side-effects: benzodiazepines used in conscious sedation may reduce effect of levodopa/carbidopa; antihypertensive medication may increase the risk of orthostatic hypotension
   - Dental
     - Antibiotic prophylaxis prior to invasive dental surgery (see Chapter 8.5)
     - Medication-related osteonecrosis of the jaw risk due to denosumab (see Chapter 16.2)
     - Haemostatic measures to control bleeding after surgery and at home
     - May require assistance for oral care
7) Following stabilisation of her oral health, the patient returns to you 6 months later for a routine review. She informs you that she has had a deep brain stimulator (DBS) placed. What are the dental implications of a DBS that you should be aware of in case the patient requires dental treatment in the future?

- When exposed to strong electrical fields, a DBS system can transmit unintended electrical energy that can cause brain injury even if the system is turned off
- Close liaison with the neurologist is required; the advice is often that the DBS device should be turned off prior to all invasive surgery
- Electric dental drills, ultrasonic probes, wires and grounding plates should not be placed near the neurostimulator, extension connecting wire or implant site on the scalp
- Diathermy should not be used as it can cause neurostimulation, brain tissue damage, stroke and even death
- Avoid electrocautery as it may also cause interference in patients with a DBS device
- Due to an increased risk of intracranial infection, prophylactic antibiotics may be advisable in relation to invasive dental treatment

General Dental Considerations

Oral Findings

- Sialorrhoea may be due to inefficient swallowing, poor oromuscular control and forward bend position of the head; some neuroleptic agents may also cause sialorrhoea; the pooling of saliva contributes to the risk of aspiration and developing pulmonary infection
- Medication-related side-effects
  - Xerostomia (e.g. levodopa/carbidopa, amantadine, benztropine, cabergoline, rasagiline, ropinirole)
  - Dysgeusia (e.g. levodopa, carbidopa, selegiline)
  - Tongue dyskinesia and grimacing (e.g. levodopa)
  - Reddish saliva (e.g. levodopa)
- Burning mouth syndrome
- Dysphagia
- Decreased oral clearance of food
- Reduced tongue movements (may increase swallowing problems and food pouching)
- Tremor and rigid orofacial muscles may produce orofacial pain
- Temporomandibular joint pain or discomfort
- Bruxism exacerbated by parkinsonian tremors
- Difficulty in retaining dentures
- Impaired oral hygiene due to poor manual dexterity or loss of fine movements may increase risk of plaque retention, dental caries/root caries and periodontal disease
- Falls and injuries, which may involve the orofacial region

Dental Management

- Dental treatment should be modified depending on the stage and severity of PD, the patient's cognitive ability and other comorbidities (Table 14.2.1)
- Denture construction and fitting may pose a challenge because of motor changes affecting the oral musculature, especially with the presence of muscle rigidity and facial dyskinesia

Section II: Background Information and Guidelines

Definition

Parkinson disease is a chronic, progressive neurodegenerative disease characterised by decreased dopamine release due to damage/loss of neurons in the substantia nigra of the brain. It is the second most common neurodegenerative disorder, following Alzheimer disease.

Aetiopathogenesis

- The cause of PD is still unknown but it may arise from interaction of predisposing genetic factors, accidental injuries to the head and environmental factors (e.g. herbicides, pesticides)
- The most common genetic variant linked to PD is a change in the LRRK2 gene; in the UK, around 1 in 100 people with PD carry it and it is more common in North African and Jewish populations; people who carry this variant may develop the condition later in life and have around a 70% chance of being diagnosed by the age of 80
- People diagnosed with PD at a younger age are more likely to have a genetic predisposition related to genetic changes in alpha-synuclein, parkin, PINK1, DJ-1, ATP13A2, PLA2G6, FBXO7 and VPS35
- Lewy body proteins (seen in Lewy body dementia) have also been found to accumulate in the substantia nigra of patients with PD
- The loss of neurons depletes the neurotransmitter in the striatum of the basal ganglia, affecting the ability to produce smooth and co-ordinated body movements, typically resulting in:
  - Parasympathetic cholinergic failure (dry mouth, constipation, urinary retention)
  - Sympathetic cholinergic failure (decreased sweating)
  - Sympathetic noradrenergic failure (orthostatic hypotension)

Table 14.2.1 Dental management considerations.

Risk assessment	• Fear and anxiety heightened • Tremors/gait instability increase the risk of falls/traumatic injury • In later stages there is a risk of aspiration due to dysphagia • Tremor and rigidity may reduce oral access; may also cause orofacial pain and temporomandibular joint discomfort during prolonged periods of opening the mouth • Orthostatic hypotension
Criteria for referral	• Most patients can be managed by primary care dentists • If multiple comorbidities are present, specialist care may be required • Severe uncontrolled motor symptoms may require referral for sedation or general anaesthesia
Access/position	• Late morning or afternoon appointments may be better to give the patient time to mobilise due to slow movements earlier in the day • A vacuum-formed pillow to position the head of the patient comfortably can be used; a pillow to support the hands and legs to decrease tremors • Wheelchair recliners can be used if available to avoid distress/additional risk when transferring from the wheelchair to the dental chair • Orthostatic hypotension can be avoided by slow repositioning of the dental chair • Additional protective aprons, napkins and/or suction equipment may be required if there is excessive drooling
Communication	• Hypophonia may impact on communication; background noises in the clinic should be reduced; provide the patient with non-verbal 'stop' cues if a break is required • Ensure that the PD-associated mask-like expression is not misinterpreted as the patient not responding; facial reactions to pain may also be present and it is important to establish alternative ways of communicating this • Speak directly to the patient; explain slowly and give the patient enough time to respond
Consent/capacity	• Tremors can make it difficult to sign a consent form; a witness may need to record the patient's consent • Dementia in more advanced stages of the condition may impact on the patient's capacity to give consent; in this case a best interest decision is required
Anaesthesia/sedation	• Local anaesthesia – May be problematic to deliver if there are uncontrolled movements; caution is advised – Contraindicated for those taking monoamine oxidase inhibitors (MAOIs) • Sedation – Tremors and anxiety may be controlled with the use of conscious sedation – Sedation is contraindicated when there is significant risk of dysphagia/aspiration – Hypoxia is not uncommon and respiratory rate should be monitored closely – It is especially important to check the airway for trapped salivary secretions and use the suction regularly to prevent coughing or aspirating – Concomitant use of MAOIs can increase risk of respiratory depression • General anaesthesia – Particular caution when monitoring the patient while in recovery to reduce aspiration risk – General anaesthesia can cause confusion and hallucinations which can last for days
Dental treatment	• Before – Urinary frequency and incontinence are quite common; especially for long procedures, ensure the patient has gone to the toilet prior to treatment – Morning medication to be taken prior to treatment to decrease rigidity and tremors – Determine if the patient has deep brain stimulation; liaise with the neurologist regarding any planned invasive dental treatment, need to switch the device off and antibiotic prophylaxis requirement

(*Continued*)

Table 14.2.1 (Continued)

	• During – Limit to short appointments and break down treatment plan to avoid fatigue – Restoring teeth must be attempted especially in the early stages of the disease when co-operation, tolerance and cognition are better – Atraumatic restorative techniques can be useful to arrest enamel-dentine caries at a very early stage – Self-cleansing restorations and fluoride-releasing materials are ideal especially for root caries that can easily be maintained by the patient – Teeth that are not restorable or have a poor prognosis must be extracted to prevent complicated infection and trauma to soft tissues when the patient is less able to tolerate treatment – Long-duration treatments such as root canal treatment, aesthetic restorations or crown preparations may not be tolerated in the later stages of disease; in these cases, dental extractions may be indicated instead – Use of high-vacuum suction is essential – Rubber dam should be used where possible to decrease aspiration risk – Ultrasonic scaling, electrocautery and diathermy may cause interference in patients with implanted microelectrodes for deep brain stimulation – Implant-supported prostheses can improve retention and help a patient retain a denture better, eventually improving chewing abilities; however, maintenance is likely to be compromised as the disease progresses; the design should reflect this to ensure it is simple and can be adapted/removed easily if required • After – Explain to the patient that saliva pooling with blood from surgical sites can make bleeding look exaggerated – Denture wearing can be a problem due to poor oral musculature control, rigidity of the oral musculature and change in the quality of saliva
Drug prescription	• Benzodiazepines used in conscious sedation may reduce effect of levodopa/carbidopa • Avoid macrolides as they can increase the levels of bromocriptine and cabergoline
Education/prevention	• Modifying the type of toothbrush such as an electric toothbrush with wide handles or with hand grips to make independent brushing easier for patients whose hands are affected with tremors and bradykinesia; 3-sided toothbrushes may also be of benefit • Oral hygiene practices that require fine motor hand movements such as flossing or interdental brushing may be difficult; assistance from a carer may be required; water irrigators can be an alternative if there is no risk of aspiration or choking • Patients in the advanced stages who have swallowing problems or dysphagia should be advised to use non-foaming fluoride toothpaste with the minimum 1450 ppm fluoride concentration • Fluoride varnish applied 2–4 times yearly depending on the dental caries risk of the patient • It has been suggested that early and periodic dental scaling decreases the risk of PD

PD, Parkinson disease.

Diagnosis

- The UK Parkinson's Disease Society Brain Bank clinical diagnostic criteria are used to make clinical diagnosis accurate and objective (Table 14.2.2)
- Brain structural imaging via either computed tomography (CT) or magnetic resonance imaging (MRI); MRI is preferred over a CT scan to view the substantia nigra region
- Dopamine transporter (DAT) imaging with single-photon emission computed tomography (DAT-SPECT) is useful in dopamine functional imaging
- Pathological diagnosis is confirmed after death by dopaminergic neuron loss in the region of the substantia nigra and presence of intraneuronal Lewy bodies

Clinical Presentation

- PD is progressive, presenting with worsening motor and non-motor signs and symptoms
- Motor symptoms
  - Generalised weakness
  - Postural instability
  - Parkinsonian tremors characterised as 'pill-rolling' of thumb and fingers
  - Resting tremors, which are less evident during purposeful movements, may involve legs, face, tongue and jaws
  - Dyskinesia
  - Bradykinesia

Table 14.2.2 Diagnostic criteria for Parkinson' disease (UK Parkinson's Disease Society Brain Bank clinical diagnostic criteria).

Step 1	**Diagnosis of parkinsonian syndrome** • Bradykinesia • At least 1 of the following: – Muscular rigidity – 4–6 Hz rest tremor – Postural instability not caused by primary visual, vestibular, cerebellar or proprioceptive dysfunction
Step 2	**Exclusion criteria for Parkinson disease** • History of repeated strokes with stepwise progression of parkinsonian features • History of repeated head injury • History of definite encephalitis • Oculogyric crises • Neuroleptic treatment at onset of symptoms • More than 1 affected relative • Sustained remission • Strictly unilateral features after 3 years • Supranuclear gaze palsy • Cerebellar signs • Early severe autonomic involvement • Early severe dementia with disturbances of memory, language and praxis • Babinski sign (positive sign when the big toe bends up and back to the top of the foot and the other toes fan out) • Presence of cerebral tumour or communication hydrocephalus on imaging study • Negative response to large doses of levodopa in absence of malabsorption • MPTP (1-methyl-4-phenyl-1,2,3,6-tetrahydropyridine) neurotoxin exposure
Step 3	**Supportive prospective positive criteria for Parkinson disease** • Three or more required for diagnosis of definite PD in combination with step 1: – Unilateral onset – Rest tremor present – Progressive disorder – Persistent asymmetry affecting side of onset most – Excellent response (70–100%) to levodopa – Severe levodopa-induced chorea – Levodopa response for 5 years or more – Clinical course of 10 years or more

PD: Parkinson disease.

  - Akinesia or muscular rigidity evident in decreased facial expressions, blinking and swallowing (i.e. 'mask-like' appearance) (Figure 14.2.5)
  - Rigidity of muscles (i.e. cogwheel-like movements)
  - Gait disturbance (i.e. stooped head, bent and leaning posture, difficulty in initiating walking characterised as short/shuffling movement with a tendency to walk faster to prevent themselves from falling)
- Non-motor symptoms
  - Dysautonomia (e.g. orthostatic hypotension, cardiac dysrhythmia, excessive sweating, urinary incontinence, sexual dysfunction, bowel dysfunction)
  - Neuropsychiatric (e.g. apathy, anxiety, depression, hallucinations, cognitive deterioration/dementia)
  - Sleep disorders (e.g. nocturnal akinesia, insomnia, rapid eye movement, behaviour disorder, restless leg syndrome, daytime sleepiness)
  - Hypophonia (soft speech or whispering) or monotonous speech
- The social impact of PD is significant, affecting a person's ability to perform activities of daily living, to work and communicate; this can lead to social isolation and increasing depression

Management

- There is currently no cure for PD, with treatment regimens focusing on symptom management

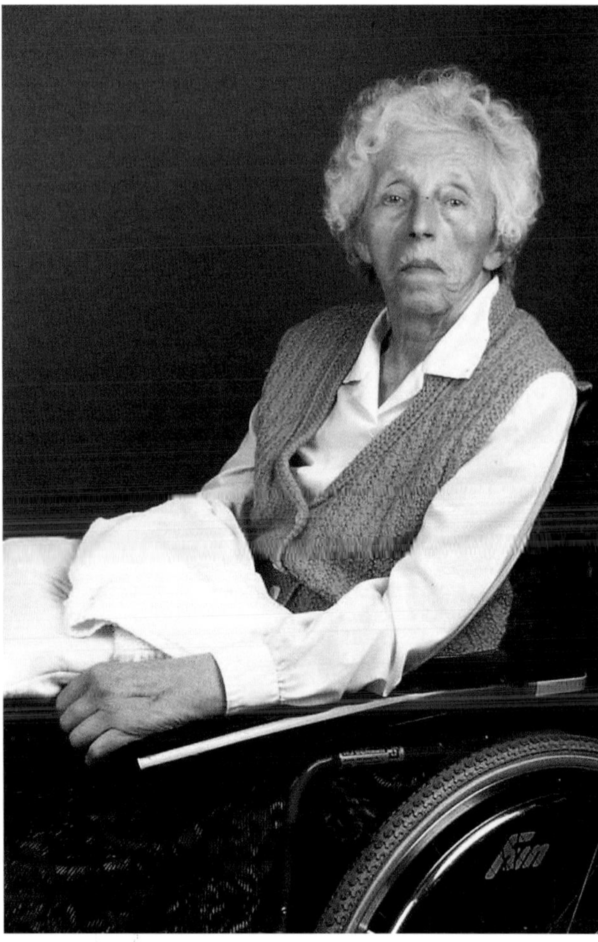

Figure 14.2.5 Advanced Parkinson disease showing mask-like appearance, tremor of the right arm (immobilised with a cloth) and use of a wheelchair.

- Non-pharmacological therapy of motor and non-motor symptoms
  - Physiotherapy for balance and motor function problems
  - Occupational therapy for difficulties in activities of daily living
  - Speech and language therapy addressing difficulties in communication, swallowing, training oromuscular function; strategies to minimise risk of aspiration – expiratory muscle strength training
  - Deep brain stimulation of the subthalamic nucleus or globus pallidus interna
    - Where available, offered to patients with symptoms that are not well controlled with medical therapy and those with advanced PD
    - Found to be effective in reducing motor fluctuations and dyskinesia
    - Electrodes are placed in brain tissue, with electrical impulses initiated by an impulse generator usually placed in the chest, with an insulated wire under the skin leading to the electrode tips
    - Caution: need for antibiotic prophylaxis; risk of induction of electrical surge or current in the insulated wires; overheated tissue injury with diathermy, electrocautery and laser use; lithotripsy and MRI damage of electrical components
- Pharmacological treatment
  - Dopamine precursor (e.g. levodopa): effective treatment for motor symptoms especially in the early stage
    - 'ON/OFF' signs appear 3–5 years after starting levodopa treatment, but can begin much earlier
    - 'OFF' episodes are a generally predictable recurrence of motor or non-motor symptoms that precedes a scheduled dose and usually improves with antiparkinsonian medication; it can also be caused by gastroparesis and/or by *Helicobacter pylori* infection, which delays delivery of levodopa
    - 'OFF' episodes can be offset using lower levodopa doses where possible, incremental dose increases and combinations of levodopa with other pharmacological agents
    - In addition, pen injector, intranasal and inhaled dosing systems may provide relief via non-intestinal routes
  - Synergistic medications (e.g. levodopa/carbidopa); considered the gold standard; adding carbidopa to levodopa helps prevent levodopa from breaking down before it crosses into the brain; also helps reduce side-effects such as nausea and vomiting, intrajejunal levodopa/carbidopa gel infusion into a percutaneous enteral tube has been indicated for reduction of off-time or to reduce dyskinesia
  - Dopamine agonist (e.g. cabergoline, pramipexole, ropinirole)
  - Decarboxylase enzyme inhibitor (e.g. carbidopa)
  - Drugs to increase dopamine release (e.g. amantadine)
  - Anticholinergic drugs (e.g. benztropine, trihexyphenidyl)
  - Disease-modifying therapy with monoamine oxidase inhibitors (MAOIs, e.g. rasagiline, selegiline)
  - Subcutaneous apomorphine injection for treatment of acute 'OFF' episodes

Prognosis

- 10–30% in the advanced disease process meet the criteria for dementia
- The positive effects of pharmacotherapy diminish as the disease progresses

- With the general increase in life expectancy of the population, there is an expected longer disease duration for patients with PD which means there will be more patients living with advanced stages of disease

A World/Transcultural View

- Amongst all the neurological disorders, PD is the fastest growing in terms of prevalence – highest in high-income regions and lowest in the sub-Saharan African regions, Latin America and Australasia
- Globally, there was a 74% increase in the last 25 years
- Its estimated worldwide prevalence is 6.1 million
- There is a male predominance, with a male to female ratio of 3:2
- Death rates related to PD were lowest in higher income countries and highest in middle-income countries

Recommended Reading

Friedlander, A., Mahler, M., Norman, K.M., and Ettinger, R.L. (2009). Parkinson disease: systemic and orofacial manifestations, medical and dental management. *J. Am. Dent. Assoc.* 140: 658–669.

Gosnell, R., Lazear, J., Hemphill, J.C., and Dotson, D. (2019). Development of guidelines for improving oral health in individuals with Parkinson's disease. *Gerodontology* 36: 229–235.

Grimes, D., Fitzpatrick, M., Gordon, J. et al. (2019). Canadian guideline for Parkinson disease. *CMAJ.* 191: E989–E1004.

Jeter, C.B., Rozas, N.S., Sadowsky, J.M., and Jones, D.J. (2018). Parkinson's disease oral health module: interprofessional coordination of care. *MedEdPORTAL.* 14: 10699.

Kobylecki, C. (2020). Update on the diagnosis and management of Parkinson's disease. *Clin. Med.* 20: 393–398.

Kojima, Y., Kojima, M., Nohara, K., and Sakaguch, Y. (2018). Dental treatment effect on deep brain stimulation system in Parkinson's disease. *Bull. Tokyo Dent. Coll.* 59: 133–137.

Srivanitchapoom, P., Pandey, S., and Hallett, M. (2014). Drooling in Parkinson's disease: a review. *Parkinsonism Relat. Disord.* 20: 1109–1118.

van Stiphout, M.A.E., Marinus, J., van Hilten, J.J. et al. (2018). Oral health of Parkinson's disease patients: a case–control study. *Parkinsons Dis.* 2018: 9315285.

14.3 Multiple Sclerosis

Section I: Clinical Scenario and Dental Considerations

Clinical Scenario

The husband of a 29-year-old female presents at the dental clinic, concerned about the oral health of his wife. He requests a home visit as his wife is unable to attend in person due to a relapsing episode of multiple sclerosis and they do not have access to appropriate transport to bring her to the dental clinic. You arrange a domiciliary visit. The patient reports that her teeth are brittle and break easily, with additional intermittent pain in the upper right quadrant, especially when food gets caught.

Medical History

- Multiple sclerosis (MS) diagnosed 7 years ago with associated:
  - Irregular bowel movement, mostly constipated and bloated
  - Frequent mood changes
  - Right side lower limb loss of sensation in higher temperature environments
  - Left side lower limb weakness and paraesthesia

Medications

- Baclofen
- Gabapentin
- Prednisone daily with recent increase in dose due to MS relapse; reducing dose over 4 weeks from 60 to 10 mg currently; normal maintenance dose 2.5 mg daily

Dental History

- Irregular dental attender due to her mobility issues and unavailable escort/transport
- Usually brushes her own teeth with a handheld brush and 1000 ppm fluoride toothpaste twice daily but when tired, sometimes forgets
- Wears an upper removable partial denture which is 5 years old, worn at night as finds it difficult to put back in her mouth when she has tremors
- Diet: consumes small quantities of high-energy soft food and high-sugar drinks frequently during the day due to difficulty swallowing hard food, to keep her energy levels up

Social History

- Lives with her husband and 2 young children
- No additional support except occasionally from her aunt
- Stopped working in 2014; her husband works as a chef
- Variable mobility; during periods of relapse, mobility limited and requires assistance to walk
- Tobacco and alcohol consumption: nil

Oral Examination

- Partially edentate (missing #12–#22, lower posterior teeth and upper left posterior teeth) (Figure 14.3.1)
- Extensive soft deposits and food debris all quadrants
- Gingivitis; most significant in the upper right quadrant
- Poorly fitting upper acrylic denture replacing the upper anterior teeth; extensive debris on the fit surface
- Erythematous area on the hard palate (Figure 14.3.2)
- Multiple retained roots: #14, #15, #23, #36 and #47
- Extensive caries with pulpal involvement: #13, #16
- Mesial caries #17

Radiological Examination

- Long cone periapical radiographs taken using a portable x-ray machine during domiciliary visit (Figure 14.3.3)
- #16: extensive mesial caries extending into the pulp
- #14, #15, #36 and #47: multiple retained roots
- #23: periapical radiolucency

A Practical Approach to Special Care in Dentistry, First Edition. Edited by Pedro Diz Dios and Navdeep Kumar.

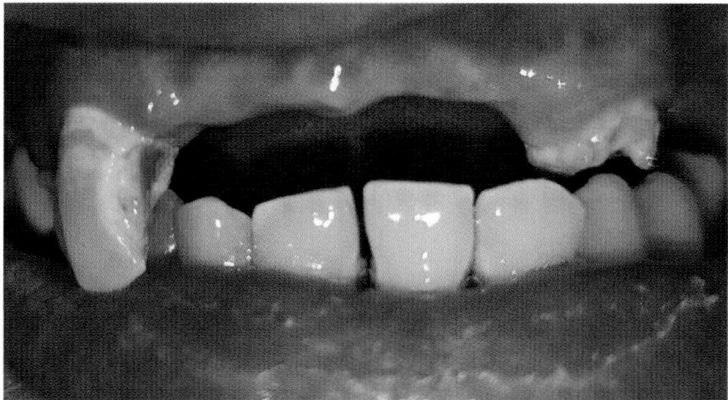

Figure 14.3.1 Partially edentate, extensive caries #13 and #23.

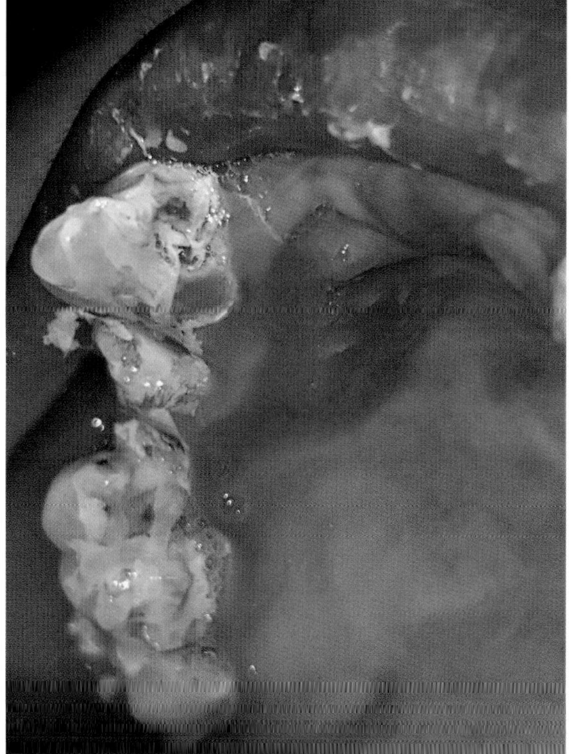

Figure 14.3.2 Upper right maxillary quadrant with extensive soft deposits and caries; erythematous localised area of the hard palate; dry lips.

Structured Learning

1) Why is domiciliary care particularly suitable for the first dental assessment of this patient?
   - Domiciliary care is offered to patients who are unable to access dental clinics due to their physical or medical condition, as is the case for this patient due to her MS relapse/exacerbation
   - Initial oral hygiene advice can be given (e.g. removing the denture at night, obtaining help when brushing her teeth, considering an electric toothbrush, using a higher fluoride toothpaste)

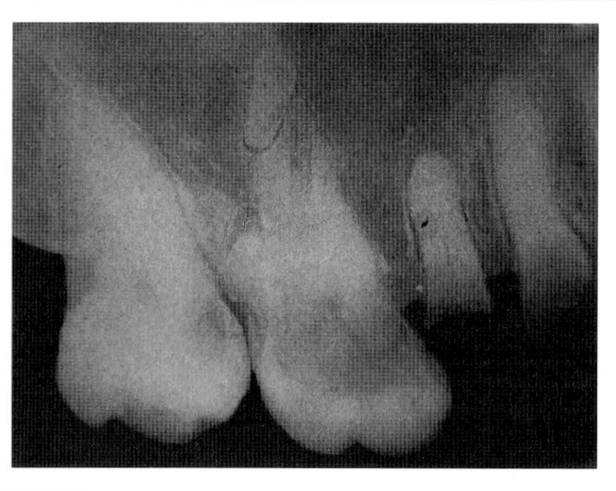

Figure 14.3.3 Long cone periapical radiograph of the upper right quadrant demonstrating retained roots and extensive caries.

   - It is also useful as the patient is symptomatic and dental screening allows a provisional diagnosis to be made
   - Radiographs can be undertaken using a mobile device in order to determine which teeth are in need of immediate treatment
   - If a clean environment can be achieved in a part of the residence, simple dental extractions can be carried out after taking radiographs, and with proper lighting and a portable suction system
   - Denture fitting and construction or simple relining of dentures can also be undertaken during domiciliary visits
   - If the patient will need more extensive treatment, a dental clinic visit can be planned with the family and transport arranged if needed
2) What factors could be contributing to the poor oral health in this patient?
   - Patients with multiple sclerosis, especially during periods of relapse, may stop brushing their teeth regularly due to fatigue, low mood and poor motivation
   - Tremors and rigidity make moving difficult and thus she may have inefficient toothbrushing techniques due to reduced dexterity and restricted access to the bathroom
   - Poor social support system – the patient has no additional carers to assist her in daily activities; unable to access dental treatment since her husband is working and she has small children to care for
   - Due to difficulty in chewing and swallowing, the patient chooses softer high-carbohydrate food/drink (for extra energy) which increases dental caries risk as well

- Xerostomia as a side-effect of medication
- Suboptimal fluoride concentration of the toothpaste
- Denture being left inside the mouth for prolonged periods and not removed at night
- Decreased sensation in the oral cavity can cause food packing and retention

3) What impact does the patient's daily dose of prednisone have on the delivery of dental treatment?
   - Prolonged glucocorticoid steroid therapy can cause multiple side-effects such as immunosuppression, delayed wound healing, decreased glucose intolerance, fluid and electrolyte imbalance, adrenocortical suppression and psychological effects (see Chapter 12.1)
4) What other factors do you need to consider in your risk assessment?
   - Social
     - Availability of escort (husband works)
     - Taking care of young children at home
     - No regular carer support
     - Reduced mobility
   - Medical
     - Currently in a relapse stage of MS when tolerance of medical/dental interventions is reduced
     - Assessing the need for steroid cover for invasive and stressful dental procedures (see Chapter 12.1)
   - Dental
     - Poor oral health
     - Cariogenic diet
     - Poorly fitting denture which is worn
     - Food pouching
     - Loss of posterior occlusal support
     - Rampant caries

5) Following discussion with the patient and her husband, an upper dental clearance with construction of a replacement full upper denture is agreed as the best way forward when the patient's MS is more stable. What would be the specific risks you would need to discuss with her?
   - A further relapse may be triggered by the planned dental extractions as it is known that stress/infections can trigger an exacerbation
   - The dental extractions are likely to require a surgical approach due to the extensive dental decay/loss of coronal structure
   - There is an aspiration risk due to dysphagia
   - Wearing a full upper denture can be difficult due to uncontrollable spasms and xerostomia, although use of denture retention pastes may help
   - Putting the denture in and out of the mouth may also be difficult due to tremors
6) What is likely to be causing the erythematous area on the hard palate and what risk factors does the patient have for its development?
   - The chronic erythematous appearance of the palate corresponds to the fit surface of her upper denture and is suggestive of denture-induced stomatitis
   - This is caused by a candidal infection and is usually asymptomatic
   - Risk factors for this patient include poor oral hygiene, xerostomia, failure to remove the denture at night, a poorly fitting acrylic denture, poor diet (possible anaemia)

General Dental Considerations

Oral Findings

- Trigeminal neuralgia. MS should be suspected when trigeminal neuralgia presents in a young patient, particularly when the symptoms are bilateral and/or there are additional neurological changes (e.g. vision disturbances, bladder dysfunction)
- Involuntary worm-like movements of the facial muscles/hemifacial spasms of the lips and tongue (Figure 14.3.4)

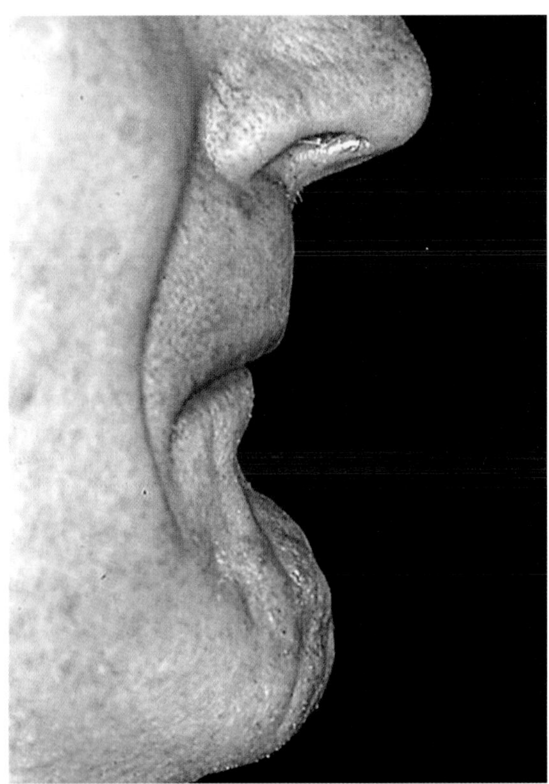

Figure 14.3.4 Multiple sclerosis presenting with sustained contracture and myokymia (involuntary worm-like movements) of the mentalis muscles.

- Facial myokimia (involuntary eyelid muscle contraction)
- Facial pain or Bell palsy
- Perioral paraesthesia/anaesthesia
- Increased risk of dental caries and periodontal disease (due to a decline in the ability to self-care)
- Difficulty in localising orofacial pain
- Tongue and facial muscle weakness
- Temporomandibular joint dysfunction
- Dysphagia in later stages
- Medication-related side-effects
  - Xerostomia (e.g. prednisone, gabapentin, baclofen, glatiramer, diazepam, amitriptyline, carbamazepine, oxybutynin)
  - Sinusitis (e.g. alemtuzumab, fingolimod, teriflunomide)
  - Orofacial pain (e.g. alemtuzumab)
  - Facial oedema (e.g. glatiramer)
  - Oral ulceration (e.g. glatiramer)
  - Dysgeusia (e.g. steroids)
  - Metallic taste (e.g. teriflunomide)

Dental Management

- Modifications in oral hygiene tools and techniques may need to be incorporated as the disease progresses
- Localising dental pain and differentiating it from facial pain may be difficult for the patient and may pose challenges in diagnosing dental disease
- Dental treatment must be adapted according to the degree of disease progression (Table 14.3.1)

Section II: Background Information and Guidelines

Definition

Multiple sclerosis is an autoimmune disease affecting the central nervous system (CNS); it is a chronic inflammatory neurodegenerative condition characterised by demyelination of nerves of the CNS producing multifocal plaques at the corticospinal tract. Although progressive, it has periods of relapse and remission. MS is the most common inflammatory neurological disease in young adults, with a peak age of onset of 30 years old.

Aetiopathogenesis

- The cause of MS is still unknown but genetic predisposition to immune dysregulation is thought to play a significant role
- Other environmental risk factors commonly associated with MS include Epstein–Barr virus (EBV), smoking, vitamin D deficiency, reduced sunlight and geographical latitude
- Although MS is generally more prevalent in countries further from the equator, such as northern Europe, North America, Australia and New Zealand, studies show that certain ethnic groups have a markedly lower prevalence of MS, despite living in countries where MS is common (e.g. Sami or Lapps of northern Scandinavia, Inuits in Canada and Maoris of New Zealand)
- MS is mediated by local inflammation from cytokines which activate macrophages and B-cells, producing destruction of the oligodendrocytes and demyelination of axons
- Nerve demyelination is predominantly caused by T-cell action against the myelin sheath
- The neurological disturbance may begin as a partial conduction blockage that changes the rate of impulse transmission along the demyelinated nerve
- In the later stages of the disease, the decreased conduction velocity along the nerve may lead to complete failure of impulse transmission
- In early stages there is resolution of local inflammation and remyelination; during a relapse, however, the nerve remains damaged and progressive loss of axons will eventually lead to brain atrophy in the advanced stages of MS

Diagnosis

- Although there are no specific diagnostic tests, a combination of clinical findings (medical history and neurological exam), magnetic resonance imaging (MRI), spinal fluid analysis and blood tests (to rule out other conditions) are commonly undertaken
- The McDonald criteria (2017) are used to confirm diagnosis, with the key requirement being evidence of neurological damage disseminated in time and space (Table 14.3.2)
- The term radiologically isolated syndrome (RIS) is used for those individuals with abnormalities on MRI of the brain and/or spinal cord consistent with lesions of MS, not explained by another diagnosis and who also have no past or current neurological symptoms or abnormalities found on neurological exam (coincidental findings); it is estimated that >50% of patients with RIS go on to develop MS within 10 years

Clinical Presentation

- There are 4 basic phenotypes of MS: clinically isolated syndrome, relapsing remitting, secondary progressive and primary progressive (Table 14.3.3)
- The term 'benign MS' has also been proposed; this is a retrospective diagnosis which is commonly given 20–30 years after disease onset; it is characterised by very

Table 14.3.1 Dental management considerations.

Risk assessment	• Stress and infections can trigger a relapse in MS • Periods of relapse may be associated with an increase in disability and reduced ability to tolerate dental interventions • Risk of falls due to poor balance and co-ordination or vision problems • Dysphagia in advanced MS may increase aspiration risk • Memory, concentration and cognition may be affected • Side-effects of pharmacological therapy (e.g. immunosuppression)
Criteria for referral	• Most patients can be seen within the primary care dental services • With progression of MS and increasing level of dependence/disability, specialist services may be required, particularly when domiciliary care is more appropriate or when there are multiple medical comorbidities
Access/position	• During periods of relapse, dental attendance may be affected • Patients with advanced MS or with those with restricted mobility require an escort to attend appointments in addition to appropriate transport • Consideration should be given to ensuring equitable access for patients who are wheelchair users; this includes ensuring safe transfer from the wheelchair to the dental chair or the use of a wheelchair recliner • Early morning appointments may be a challenge due to fatigue; inquire from the patient what time of the day is easiest to mobilise • Appointments should be kept short and procedures ideally simple as patients may tire easily • Avoid a fully supine position due to increased aspiration risk. In patients with dysphagia try a modified upright or 45° position
Communication	• Dysarthria and slurred speech may be present • Severe optic neuritis/visual problems can affect visual communication • Cognitive abilities can be affected in the advanced stages of MS and slow down effective communication • Hence patients should be given enough time to communicate their opinions on dental treatment decisions and appropriate communication aids made available (e.g. touching tools for those with visual impairment)
Consent/capacity	• Signing the consent form may require assistance/a countersignature if the patient has lost mobility of the hands due to severe tremors and spasms • If cognition is affected in the advanced stages of MS, capacity to consent must be assessed prior to planned dental intervention and reassessed on the day of treatment
Anaesthesia/sedation	• Local anaesthesia – There are no contraindications for local anaesthesia use although caution is advised if there are uncontrolled tremors/movement • Sedation – Nitrous oxide can cause further demyelination and should be avoided – Respiratory depression is not uncommon especially when intravenous sedation is undertaken; monitoring the vital signs is essential • General anaesthesia – The labile autonomic system is associated with a higher risk of hypoventilation and hypoxia with general anaesthesia
Dental treatment	• Before – Difficulty in differentiating orofacial pain and tooth pain is common – For patients on high-dose or long-term steroids, steroid cover should be considered (see Chapter 12.1) – Urinary urgency is common – ensure patient has been given the opportunity to micturate prior to the dental treatment, especially if a long procedure is planned – Patients on immunosuppressant therapy may be immunocompromised – full blood count test results should be requested and the need for antibiotic cover discussed with the physician prior to a surgical procedure

(*Continued*)

Table 14.3.1 (Continued)

	• During – Minimise the length of the planned procedure – Warn the patient when loud noises from equipment are expected to avoid startling them – Consider use of a mouth prop or bite block during prolonged procedures to increase comfort in mouth opening and decrease easy fatigability (caution if the patient has dysphagia) – Use of pillows for support of the neck and back to lessen fatigue and muscle spasms – Patients with optic neuritis and who are sensitive to light can be given dark tinted glasses when using the dental operatory light • After – Written and verbal instructions given to both the patient and escort using simple dental terms and short sentences as the patient may find it difficult to remember postoperative instructions
Drug prescription	• Consider the interaction of medication given to manage MS with any planned prescription of pain relief (e.g. in patients taking benzodiazepines, avoid opioid-based analgesics)
Education/prevention	• Rapid deterioration of oral health and progression of dental caries are commonly seen during exacerbations of MS and in late stages, due to a deterioration in the patient's ability to undertake effective oral care • Determine if the patient will need assistance from a carer/family member • Consider adapting the oral care tools in view of reduction in dexterity (electric toothbrush, wide-handled/adapted toothbrush) • Consider fluoride supplementation • Manage xerostomia and its side-effects

MS, multiple sclerosis.

Table 14.3.2 McDonald criteria for the diagnosis of multiple sclerosis (2017 update).

Clinical presentation	Additional data needed for an MS diagnosis
• Two or more relapses and either. . . objective clinical evidence of 2 or more lesions or. . . objective clinical evidence of 1 lesion together with reasonable historical evidence of a previous relapse	None
• Two or more relapses and objective clinical evidence of 1 lesion (demonstrates different dates)	Dissemination in space shown by: – One or more MRI detected lesions typical of MS or. . . – A further relapse showing damage to another part of the CNS
• One relapse and. . . objective clinical evidence of 2 or more lesions (demonstrates different parts)	Dissemination in time shown by: – Oligoclonal bands or. . . – MRI evidence of a new lesion since a previous scan or. . . – A further relapse
• One attack/relapse and. . . objective clinical evidence of 1 lesion (known as 'clinically isolated syndrome')	Dissemination in space shown by: – One or more MRI detected lesions typical of MS or. . . – A further relapse showing activity in another part of the CNS Dissemination in time shown by: – Oligoclonal bands or. . . – MRI showing new lesions since a previous scan or. . . – A further relapse
• Insidious neurological progression suggestive of multiple sclerosis (typical for primary progressive MS)	Continued progression for 1 year (from previous symptoms or by ongoing observation) plus any 2 of: 1 or more MRI detected lesions in the brain typical of MS, 2 or more MRI detected lesions in the spinal cord, oligoclonal bands in the spinal fluid

CNS, central nervous system; MRI, magnetic resonance imaging; MS, multiple sclerosis.

Table 14.3.3 Clinical subtypes of multiple sclerosis.

Clinical subtypes	Characteristics
Clinically isolated syndrome (CIS)	• First episode of neurological symptoms caused by inflammation and demyelination in the CNS • The episode, which by definition must last for at least 24 hours, is characteristic of MS but does not yet meet the criteria for a formal diagnosis (Table 14.3.2) • People who experience a CIS may or may not go on to develop MS
Relapsing–remitting MS (RRMS)	• Most common disease course (85% of MS) • Characterised by clearly defined relapses/exacerbations of new or increasing neurological symptoms • These are followed by periods of partial or complete recovery/remission when all symptoms may disappear, or some symptoms may continue and become permanent • However, there is no apparent progression of the disease during the periods of remission • RRMS can be further characterised as either *active* (with relapses and/or evidence of new MRI activity over a specified period of time) or *not active*, as well as *worsening* (a confirmed increase in disability following a relapse) or *not worsening* • Most people with RRMS are usually diagnosed in their 20s and 30s (although it can occur in childhood or later adulthood)
Secondary progressive MS (SPMS)	• Follows an initial relapsing–remitting course • Approximately 50% of those diagnosed with RRMS transition to SPMS within 10 years, and 90% transition within 25 years • Some patients with RMMS progress to SPMS with progressive worsening of neurological function (accumulation of disability) over time • SPMS can be further characterised as either *active* (with relapses and/or evidence of new MRI activity during a specified period of time) or *not active*, as well as *with progression* (evidence of disability accumulation over time, with or without relapses or new MRI activity) or *without progression*
Primary progressive MS (PPMS)	• Less common form of MS (15%) • Characterised by worsening neurological function (accumulation of disability) from the onset of symptoms, without early relapses or remissions • PPMS can be further characterised as either *active* (with an occasional relapse and/or evidence of new MRI activity over a specified period of time) or *not active*, as well as *with progression* (evidence of disability accumulation over time, with or without relapse or new MRI activity) or *without progression* • Average age of onset is approximately 10 years later in PPMS than in relapsing RRMS

CNS, central nervous; MRI, magnetic resonance imaging; MS, multiple sclerosis.

minimal disease activity, often sensory exacerbations and minimal disability

- Two of the most common symptoms are pain and spasticity that can eventually cause paralysis
- As the disease progresses, the spasticity worsens, resulting in immobility, chronic pain, fatigue and disturbed sleep
- Clinical symptoms indicative of an exacerbation of MS
  - Motor changes: urinary incontinence, ataxia, tremor, slurring and monotonous speech, jerky speech, limb weakness
  - Sensory changes: unilateral optic neuritis (i.e. visual disturbance accompanied by pain with eye movement), limb paraesthesia or anaesthesia
  - Cognitive changes: mood swings, cognitive deficits
- Specific clinical signs
  - Lhermitte phenomenon: neck flexion can bring about brief electric shock sensations in the spine, legs or arms
  - Internuclear ophthalmoplegia: almost pathognomonic of MS, characterised by change in colour vision and acuity
  - Uhthoff phenomenon: where symptoms of MS are worsened with hot weather or exercise

Management

- Although there is currently no cure for MS, treatment regimens have progressed significantly over the last 20 years

Table 14.3.4 Pharmacological treatment of multiple sclerosis.

	Action/indication	Drug
Modifying the disease course	Immunomodulators	Beta-interferon Glatiramer
	Continuous immunosuppression	Teriflunomide Fingolimod Natalizumab Ocrelizumab
	More selective immune reconstitution	Cladribine
	Less selective immune reconstitution	Alemtuzumab
Managing relapses	Anti-inflammatory	Methylprednisolone Prednisone Adrenocorticotropin
Managing symptoms	Spasticity	Baclofen Tizanidine
	Tremors	Clonazepam Primidone
	Seizures	Carbemazepine
	Depression	Citalopram Venlafaxine Amitriptyline
	Paroxysmal pain	Gabapentin Amitryptiline Pregabalin
	Bladder dysfunction	Oxybutynin Tolterodine
	Erectile dysfunction	Sildenafil

- Treatment strategies can help modify or slow the disease course, treat relapses, manage symptoms, improve function and [illegible] emotional health
- In view of this, a multidisciplinary team is required to support the patient, including the neurologist, physiotherapist, occupational therapist, speech and language therapist, and psychologist
- Pharmacological treatment focuses on 3 main areas (Table 14.3.4):
  - Modifying the disease course (e.g. ocrelizumab)
  - Managing relapses (e.g. corticosteroids)
  - Managing symptoms (e.g. baclofen)
- Complementary/alternative approaches
  - Cannabis extracts and cannabinoid oromucosal spray have been given to treat neuropathic pain, spasms and bladder overactivity
  - Exercise, stress management, acupuncture
- Surgery: tremors can be treated with neurosurgical interventions such as deep brain stimulation
- Autologous haematopoietic stem cell transplantation has gained increasing interest in recent years; it can reduce relapses but cannot repair existing damaged myelin

Prognosis

- Life expectancy of patients with MS is typically reduced by an average of 5–10 years
- Only 5% of patients experience a benign disease course with infrequent relapses
- In primary progressive MS, 10% of patients will have a gradual disease progression from diagnosis
- 30% of patients will become dependent on the use of wheelchairs

A World/Transcultural View

- There has been a reported increase in the prevalence of MS, with 2–3 million cases estimated globally, an increase of over 10% compared to 20 years ago; this may be in part due to better awareness and diagnosis of the condition

- In countries where there is limited access to medical care, there is still underdiagnosis and underreporting of the true burden of the condition
- Studies have also shown that black and ethnic minority (BAME) people with MS often reach disability levels sooner and may have a slightly different disease course to white people with MS, leading to more cognitive problems in BAME people with MS. This may be because doctors are not recognising the signs in BAME people, or that BAME people might be less likely to seek medical help for MS symptoms, and so they are only diagnosed and treated once their MS is more advanced

Recommended Reading

Cockburn, N., Pateman, K., Taing, M.W. et al. (2017). Managing the oral side-effects of medications used to treat multiple sclerosis. *Aust. Dent. J.* 62: 331–336.

Covello, F., Ruoppolo, G., Carissimo, C. et al. (2020). Multiple sclerosis: impact on oral hygiene, dysphagia, and quality of life. *Int. J. Environ. Res Public Health* 17: 3979.

Lublin, F.D., Reingold, S.C., Cohen., J.A. et al. (2016). *Multiple Sclerosis (NICE Guideline QS108).* London: NICE.

Manchery, N., Henry, J.D., and Nangle, M.R. (2020). A systematic review of oral health in people with multiple sclerosis. *Community Dent. Oral. Epidemiol.* 48: 89–100.

Thompson, A.J., Baranzini, S.E., Geurts, J. et al. (2018). Multiple sclerosis. *Lancet* 391: 1622–1636.

Yamout, B., Sahraian, M., Bohlega, S. et al. (2020). Consensus recommendations for the diagnosis and treatment of multiple sclerosis: 2019 revisions to the MENACTRIMS guidelines. *Mult. Scler. Relat. Disord.* 37: 101459.

Zhang, G.Q. and Meng, Y. (2015). Oral and craniofacial manifestations of multiple sclerosis: implications for the oral health care provider. *Eur. Rev. Med. Pharmacol Sci.* 19: 4610–4620.

14.4 Motor Neuron Disease

Section I: Clinical Scenario and Dental Considerations

Clinical Scenario

A 59-year-old woman is seen for a dental review appointment during a domiciliary visit in her private home. Her main concern is that she is finding it increasingly difficult to speak as her mouth feels dry. She also reports that food constantly gets trapped in between her upper right molar teeth and the gums in this area occasionally feel swollen/bleed.

Medical History

- Amyotrophic lateral sclerosis (ALS) diagnosed 7 years ago
- Combination of oral and percutaneous gastrostomy (PEG) feeding for the last 3 years; PEG feeding predominantly used for liquids
- Recurrent episodes of pneumonia, last hospitalisation 2 years ago
- Type 2 diabetes mellitus
- Hypertension
- Gastro-oesophageal reflux disease

Medications

- Salbutamol
- N-acetylcysteine
- Doxofylline
- Metformin
- Linagliptin
- Telmisartan
- Amlodipine
- Lansoprazole
- Escitalopram
- Calcium carbonate
- Vitamin B complex

Dental History

- Attended the dental practice regularly until 4 years ago when she requested domiciliary visits due to her reducing mobility
- Prefers dental treatment in her wheelchair which can recline by a 25° angle
- Uses a handheld toothbrush to brush her teeth independently 2–3 times daily with 1450 ppm fluoride toothpaste
- Single-tufted toothbrush used with chlorhexidine 1% gel to remove food packing
- Commercial mouthwash (not alcohol-free) almost 4 times daily to wet her mouth

Social History

- Lives with her husband and 2 adult daughters
- Company director; works from home; holding company meetings remotely
- Able to talk with the aid of a wireless microphone
- Feels increasingly anxious as her ALS progresses
- Nurse and care-giver support for all activities of daily living
- Not mobile, uses an electric wheelchair; travels if required using an adapted private car; requires a hoist for transfer
- Tobacco consumption nil; alcohol consumption 6 units a week

Oral Examination

- Xerostomia with change in consistency of saliva (frothy) (Figure 14.4.1)
- Bilateral tongue biting
- Incompetent lips/mouth breathing
- Drooling
- Full mouth rehabilitation, with porcelain fused to metal crowns and bridges on multiple teeth
- Only teeth without full coverage restorations: #17, #18, #28, #38 and #48

A Practical Approach to Special Care in Dentistry, First Edition. Edited by Pedro Diz Dios and Navdeep Kumar.

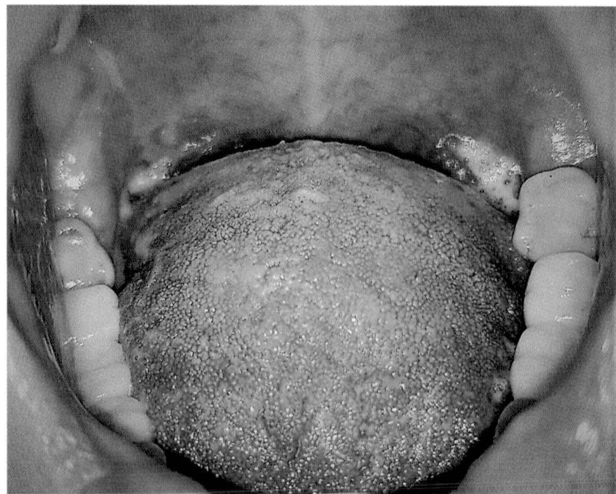

Figure 14.4.1 Xerostomia, frothy saliva, tongue biting.

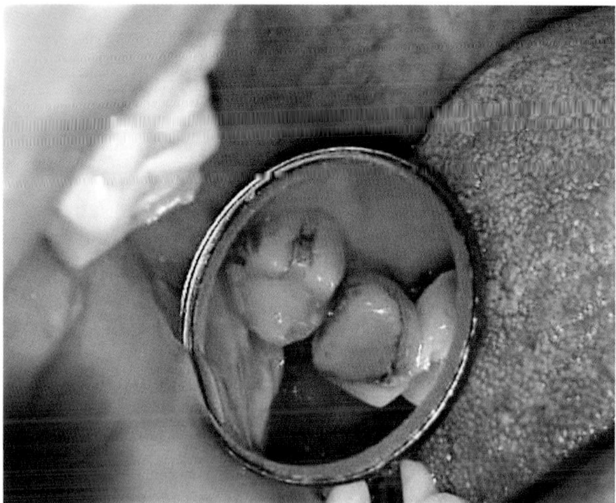

Figure 14.4.2 Heavily restored #17 and #18; food trapping interdentally.

- Extensive composite restorations in #17 and #18 with food packing interdentally (Figure 14.4.2)

Radiological Examination

- Limited to the upper right quadrant due to poor tolerance
- Long cone periapical radiograph taken bedside during domiciliary visit (Figure 14.4.3)
- Defective contact point distal to #17; #16 and #17 root filled with posts in situ

Structured Learning

1) What factors are aggravating the symptoms of xerostomia in this patient?
   - Polypharmacy (including telmisartan, amlodipine, escitalopram, lansoprazole, salbutamol, N-acetylcysteine)
   - Frequent use of alcohol-containing mouth rinse
   - Anxiety
   - Diabetes mellitus
   - Decreased fluid intake
   - Frequent suctioning of secretions
   - Mouth breathing
2) What advice would you give this patient to help manage her dry mouth?
   - Frequent sips of water throughout the day; avoid sugary drinks
   - Rinse with water after meals
   - Avoid dry or hard crunchy foods
   - Eat cool food with high liquid content
   - Avoid exacerbating factors including non essential drugs associated with xerostomia, alcohol, alcohol-containing mouthwashes, caffeine
   - Lubricate the lips frequently with petroleum jelly
   - Salivary stimulants
   - Salivary substitutes
3) Conversely, the patient reports that she also frequently experiences drooling of saliva which she finds increasingly distressing. What could be contributing to this?
   - Weakness of the muscles of the mouth and throat can cause difficulties in managing saliva/swallowing, even when the overall quantity of saliva is reduced
   - This can worsen if the head position falls forward due to weakness of the neck muscles
4) Given that the patient participates in meetings remotely and is very embarrassed about being unable to control her drooling, she asks for urgent help. What options would you discuss with her?
   - Keep the head position upright – the patient may benefit from a head support strap attached to the headrest of her electric wheelchair
   - Medications to reduce the production of saliva may help but should be used with caution given that the patient also reports a dry mouth; these can be prescribed by the neurologist/physician and include hyoscine or scopolamine patches, atropine, amitriptyline and glycopyrronium (some of them could be used only occasionally 'on request')
   - Botulinum toxin injections directly into the salivary glands can cause a temporary reduction in salivary gland production (3–6 months) and may be repeated if beneficial
   - Radiotherapy of the salivary glands causes a permanent reduction in salivary gland flow; it may be given unilaterally to start with, when drooling is severe

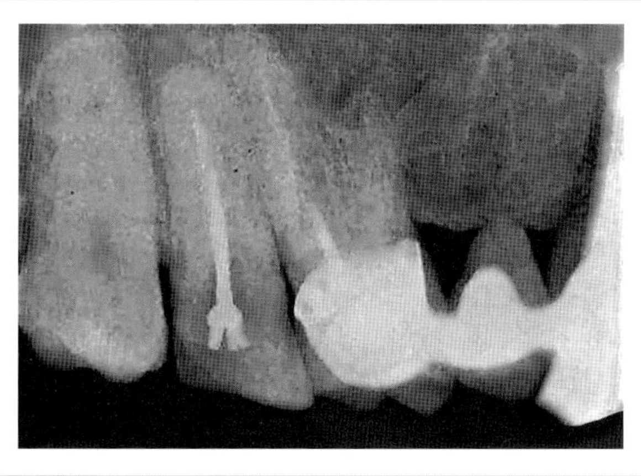

Figure 14.4.3 Long cone periapical radiograph; 1 mm space between #17 and #18; #16 and #17 root filled with posts in situ; bone resorption distal to the #15 abutment.

5) The patient asks for a permanent solution to the food packing in the upper right quadrant. What options would you discuss with her and what are their associated risks and benefits?
   - Removing part/all of the existing restoration in the #17 and replacing it with a new composite resin restoration with a better contact point with the #18
     - Risks: limited access; placement of a rubber dam will be challenging; lengthy treatment; debris generated from drilling increases the risk of aspiration; marginal leakage/further deterioration may occur
     - Benefits: avoid removal of further tooth structure; can be reviewed, replenished and replaced as required
   - Placing a porcelain crown on the #17
     - Risks: access for crown preparation; placement of gingival retraction cord and dental impressions will be limited; additional risk of aspiration related to impression material (this could be reduced with a digital intraoral scanner and fabrication of an indirect composite restoration)
     - Benefits: cast restorations usually deliver a better contact area with the adjacent teeth and protect the extensively restored tooth which is particularly vulnerable to fracture as it is root filled
   - Dental extraction of the #17
     - Risks: access to the palatal aspect of the tooth with extraction forceps may be limited; adjacent crown/bridge work may become damaged; tooth may fracture as it is root filled/heavily restored
     - Benefits: permanent solution; tooth not visible; allows easier access to the adjacent teeth for cleaning

6) The patient decides that she wants the #17 extracted. What other factors do you need to consider in your risk assessment?
   - Social
     - Complete dependence on family and carers in mobilising
     - Reduced mobility and preference to have dental treatment undertaken in her wheelchair
     - Increasing anxiety/depression
   - Medical
     - High-risk patient due to dysphagia, recurrent aspiration pneumonia and requirement for invasive ventilation
     - Increased risk of hypertensive crisis
     - Diabetes mellitus is known to be associated with increased risk of infection, impaired wound healing and risk of hypoglycaemia/hyperglycaemia in the dental setting (see Chapter 5.1)
     - Regurgitation of gastric contents due to gastro-oesophageal reflux disease
     - Stress from the dental environment can trigger an anxiety crisis (see Chapter 15.1)
   - Dental
     - Limited access for oral hygiene and dental treatment interventions
     - Easily fatigued and difficulty in keeping mouth open too long
     - Crown/root fracture risk during tooth extraction

7) In view of this patient's advanced stage of ALS and the possibility of a surgical extraction, you arrange for her to have the #17 extracted in a hospital-based oral surgery department. During attempted extraction of the tooth, the patient becomes increasingly breathless and fatigued and appears to be having difficulty breathing. What would be your concern and how would you manage this?
   - Muscle weakness associated with ALS can cause an impaired cough and increased thickness and retention of secretions
   - This is associated with a risk of aspiration which can lead to acute respiratory distress and the development of aspiration pneumonia
   - The dental extraction should be terminated
   - Suction should be used to clear the airway of any secretions/debris
   - The patient should be placed in a more upright position with the head and neck supported
   - Call the emergency services
   - Oxygen therapy can suppress respiratory drive and lead to worsening hypercapnia

General Dental Considerations

Oral Findings (Dependent on the Type of Motor Neuron Disease)

- Weakness in the tongue, mouth and throat
- Bulbar palsy leading to weak and inefficient swallow, oral-motor dysfunction, difficulty in mouth opening and dysphagia
- Self-biting due to bulbar muscle weakness
- Atrophy of tongue
- Fasciculations of the tongue (Figure 14.4.4)
- Drooling due to impaired swallowing
- Thickened mucus/saliva
- Xerostomia due to polypharmacy and mouth breathing
- Hyperactive gag reflex
- Increased dental caries if high caloric carbohydrate diet and/or xerostomia

Dental Management

- Modifications in relation to the dental management of patients with motor neuron disease (MND) dependent on the type of their disorder
- For example, for patients with ALS, consideration should be given to the fact that this form of MND is progressive and invariably fatal (Table 14.4.1)

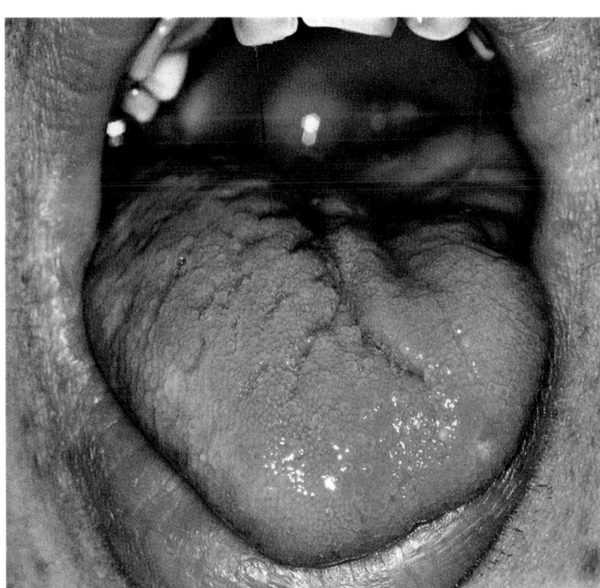

Figure 14.4.4 Fasciculations of the tongue.

Section II: Background Information and Guidelines

Definition

Motor neuron diseases are a group of clinically and pathologically heterogeneous neurological diseases characterised by progressive degeneration of motor neurons. They include both sporadic and hereditary diseases and affect the upper and/or lower motor neurons (UMN/LMN) (Table 14.4.2).

- UMNs: located in the primary motor cortex of the cerebrum (precentral gyrus), with long axons forming corticospinal and corticobulbar tracts; typically manifests as spasticity, weakness, and hyperreflexia
- LMNs: originate in the brainstem (cranial nerve motor nuclei) and spinal cord (anterior horn cells) and directly innervate skeletal muscles; typically manifests as fasciculation, atrophy, weakness, and hyporeflexia

Aetiopathogenesis

- Some MNDs are inherited, including familial amyotrophic lateral sclerosis where several gene mutations have been identified, and spinal muscular atrophy, where there is a specific gene which is abnormal/missing (Table 14.4.3)
- In sporadic or non-inherited MNDs, environmental, toxic, viral and/or genetic factors may play a role in development of the disease
- The protein TDP-43 has been found to aggregate in nervous system cells in both familial and sporadic forms of amyotrophic lateral sclerosis, causing neurodegeneration

Diagnosis

- Diagnostic tests for ALS are quite elusive and depend more on clinical history (i.e. progressive but painless muscle weakness)
- Neurological examinations such as electromyography and nerve conduction studies are used as an adjunct to detect upper and lower motor neuron dysfunction
- Additional investigations may be undertaken to exclude differential diagnoses, and may include spinal fluid analysis and occasionally nerve and muscle biopsies

Table 14.4.1 Dental management considerations.

Risk assessment	• Fatigue • Reduced mobility • Risk of aspiration during dental treatment for patients with dysphagia • Limited mouth opening/brisk gag reflex • Behavioural changes/depression • Heightened anxiety to dental treatment
Criteria for referral	• Patients in the advanced stages of the disease, where mobility and function are severely impaired, require referral to a specialist, ideally in a hospital setting
Access/position	• Avoid early morning appointments to ensure the patient has enough time to mobilise • Consider the need for a carer/escort • Determine the best time to arrange appointments when the patient is generally less fatigued • Ensure that consideration is given to the need for equipment to enable transfer, or if the patient cannot be transferred, there is access to a wheelchair recliner • For patients at risk of dysphagia, do not fully recline • Consider the need for a mouth prop and/or a finger guard • For patients who have very restricted mobility, domiciliary dental visits may be needed to assess their dental treatment needs, with simple treatments provided in the patient's home
Communication	• Patients with loss of voice function may be using speech-generating devices, microphones or writing boards • In the absence of these, determine if the patient uses a simple code for yes and no (e.g. eye blinking) and use closed questions that require a yes/no or single-word answer • Patients with a tracheostomy may be used to communicating by mouthing words; their carers may be able understand what they want to say • Face the patient directly and avoid any distractions • Allow additional time for the patient to respond
Consent/capacity	• Allow sufficient time to make a decision to consent to treatment regardless of the method they use to communicate their decision • Patients who have lost the function of their hands may be using their thumb mark prints instead to mark their signatures/ask a witness to sign on their behalf • Occasionally cognition is affected in the later stages of amyotrophic lateral sclerosis due to associated dementia; in this case a capacity assessment is required, specific to the decision; a best interest decision may be required
Anaesthesia/sedation	• Local anaesthesia – It is important to remember that patients with motor neuron disease retain the perception of pain although they may not be able to communicate it – Avoid giving inferior alveolar nerve blocks in patients with dysphagia as this may increase the risk of aspiration • Sedation – Benzodiazepines can reduce respiratory drive and airway reflexes and should be avoided – If unavoidable, sedation should be provided by an anaesthetist with appropriate respiratory support available • General anaesthesia – This should be avoided where possible as the use of general anaesthetic gases with muscle relaxants may exacerbate muscle weakness and cause respiratory depression – For those patients where a general anaesthesia cannot be avoided (e.g. profound dental anxiety, hyperactive gag reflex and/or extensive dental treatment needs which cannot be delivered with local anaesthesia), preoperative assessment and treatment with an anaesthetist must be undertaken to ensure appropriate respiratory support is in place – Total intravenous anaesthesia using propofol may be considered

(Continued)

Table 14.4.1 (Continued)

Dental treatment	• Before – Determine if an upright/semi-reclined position is required due to respiratory problems and/or dysphagia as this may hinder some dental procedures – Ensure that the patient is aware of any additional risks when reconfirming informed consent • During – Frequent breaks should be given as patients may be less tolerant to long procedures due to fatigue – Use of mouth props/bite blocks if the patient has difficulty keeping their mouth open – High-volume suction should be used to minimise aspiration risk, taking care not to induce a gag reflex – Do not use glass mirrors if there is likelihood of a gag reflex/biting on instruments – Minimise the number of dental instruments/equipment introduced in the mouth (including cotton wool rolls) – Supplemental oxygen can have a serious detrimental effect on patients with neuromuscular weakness; it should only be used in a hospital setting when recommended by the patient's neurologist/physician and often arterial blood gas monitoring is required • After – Ensure the airway is clear and that all equipment and debris has been removed
Drug prescription	• Avoid sedative medications in view of the potential for respiratory depression
Education/prevention	• If weakness of the arms and hands is present, consider the use of electric toothbrushes with a wider/longer handle and/or a 3-sided toothbrush • For patients who have difficulty keeping their mouth open and need assistance with toothbrushing, advise carers on the careful use of bite blocks, finger protectors or 2 toothbrushes stacked on top of each other • For patients with dysphagia, using a toothbrush with suction or assisting the patient with a suction device to avoid aspiration is advisable • A non-foaming fluoride toothpaste with the minimum 1450 ppm fluoride concentration is useful • Ensure dental radiographs are taken regularly to monitor for dental caries risk • Use fluoride varnish 2–4 times yearly depending on the dental caries risk of the patient • Liaise closely with the dietitian to ensure that dietary supplements do not inadvertently increase dental caries risk

Clinical Presentation

- The clinical signs of MND predominantly occur as a result of muscle weakness
- They vary in distribution and severity depending on the type of MND and whether the UMN and/or LMNs are affected (Table 14.4.2)
- Amyotrophic lateral sclerosis is the most common type of MND with typical clinical features including difficulty moving limbs, balancing and swallowing

Management

- There is currently no cure for MND
- The focus is symptomatic/supportive treatment using a multidisciplinary approach including physical, occupational, speech, respiratory and hydro therapies
- Pharmacological treatment
  - Pain control/palliative medications
  - Riluzole: a disease-modifying drug that inhibits glutamate release; first FDA-approved drug in the United States in 1995; it protects motor neurons from overproduction of glutamate which in excess is toxic to neurons
  - Edaravone: a neuroprotective drug that scavenges free radicals in the body; does not cure MND but can slow down the progression of the disease by 30–40% compared to placebo in clinical trials; FDA approved in the United States in 2017 but still not approved for prescription in Europe
- Other disease management tools
  - Ventilation assistance: non-invasive positive pressure ventilation (bilevel positive airway pressure machines – BiPAP) or invasive ventilation via a tracheostomy
  - Percutaneous gastrostomy (PEG) feeding may be required
  - Implanted baclofen pumps to reduce spasticity

Table 14.4.2 Main types of motor neuron disease

Type	UMN and/or LMN	Characteristics
• **Inherited**		
Familial amyotrophic lateral sclerosis (ALS)	UMN and LMN	• ~10% of ALS; normally follows an autosomal dominant inheritance pattern • Mutations identified in 15 genes • Approximately 40% caused by mutations in the chromosome 9 open reading frame 72/*C9orf72* gene (United States and Europe) • Worldwide, approximately 10–20% of cases are due to a mutation in the Cu/Zn superoxide dismutase-1 gene (*SOD1*) • Western Pacific ALS occurs on the islands of Guam (Guam ALS), on the Kii peninsula of Japan and in western New Guinea • Symptoms similar to sporadic ALS
Spinal muscular atrophy (SMA)	LMN	• Most common genetic cause of infant mortality • Caused by an abnormal or missing survival motor neuron gene 1 (SMN1) • Four variants have been described: – Type I (Werdnig–Hoffman disease or infantile-onset SMA) presents before 6 months of age; without treatment, many affected children die before age 1–2 years – Type II presents between 6 and 18 months of age; children unable to stand or walk unaided; respiratory difficulties common; life expectancy is reduced but most individuals live into adolescence or young adulthood – Type III (Kugelberg–Welander disease) presents between ~2 and 17 years of age; walking is usually maintained but running, rising from a chair and climbing stairs are often difficult; also associated with curvature of the spine, contractures and respiratory infections; normal lifespan with treatment – Type IV symptoms develop after 21 years of age, and are typically mild to moderate, often with leg muscle weakness
• **Sporadic/acquired**		
Sporadic amyotrophic lateral sclerosis (ALS)	UMN and LMN	• 90% of ALS; most common form of motor neuron disease • Rapidly progressive, fatal disease, commonly presenting with inability to move arms and legs, maintain balance and swallow • Can lead to inability to breathe without assistance • Fatal, commonly due to respiratory failure, usually within 3–5 years from the onset of symptoms, although ~10% survive for 10 or more years • More common in men than women, with onset between 40 and 60 years of age • A subset of ALS cases show features of frontotemporal lobar degeneration
Primary lateral sclerosis (PLS)	UMN	• Rare • Frequently affects the legs first, followed by the body, trunk, arms and hands, and, finally the bulbar muscles (muscles that control speech, swallowing and chewing) • Symptoms include weakness, muscle stiffness and spasticity, clumsiness, slowing of movement and problems with balance and speech • More common in men than women, with onset between 40 and 60 years of age • Progresses gradually over a number of years or even decades • Not typically fatal/variable progression of symptoms; some patients retain the ability to walk but others eventually require assistance/wheelchairs
Progressive muscular atrophy (PMA)	LMN	• Rare form of motor neuron disease • Features include reduced movement in the arms, legs, face, chest, throat and tongue, as well as skeletal muscle activity including speaking, walking, swallowing and breathing
Progressive bulbar palsy/ atrophy (PBP)	LMN (bulbar region)	• Commonly affects cranial nerves IX, X and XII • Presents with deterioration in swallowing, speaking, chewing • Majority of individuals eventually develop more widespread motor neurone disease/ALS

ALS, amyotrophic lateral sclerosis; LMN, lower motor neuron disease; UMN, upper motor neuron disease.

Table 14.4.3 Clinical presentation of amyotrophic lateral sclerosis

Stage of disease	Typical clinical features
Early stage	• Progressive weakening of muscles in a particular area of the body (limb weakness more common on initial onset) • Muscle spasticity • Muscle atrophy • Muscle cramping • Fasciculations • Fatigue • Frequent falling or tripping
Middle stage	• Muscle weakness and atrophy in other parts of the body • Muscle paralysis • Loss of dexterity • Dysphagia • Dyspnoea (may need non-invasive pulmonary ventilation) • Constipation • Urinary urgency • Pseudobulbar effect – crying or laughing uncontrollably or out of proportion to experienced emotion • Depression • Insomnia
Late stage	• Dysarthria, dysphonia, dysphagia, sialorrhoea • Patients with loss of voice function may be using speech-generating devices, microphones or writing boards • Hyporeflexia • Paralysis of voluntary muscles • Respiratory failure with tracheostomy and direct mechanical ventilation • Nasogastric or percutaneous gastrostomy feeding (PEG) • Frontotemporal dementia may occur in 15% of patients • Frequent episodes of bronchopneumonia or aspiration pneumonia • Ventilator-associated pneumonia

- Advance care planning
  - Advance directives in life-prolonging or -sustaining procedures
  - Focuses on respecting the autonomy and dignity of the patient in end of life care
- Areas of research
  - Stem cell therapy may protect functional motor neurons but will not replace dead motor neurons
  - Gene therapy

Prognosis

- Prognosis varies depending on the type of MND and the age of symptom onset
- Some MNDs, such as primary lateral sclerosis, are usually not fatal and progress slowly
- Spinal muscular atrophy type III/IV may be stable for long periods
- Severe forms of spinal muscular atrophy and ALS are fatal, with respiratory failure the leading cause of death

A World/Transcultural View

- Although MNDs have a relatively low prevalence across the world, they can be associated with severe disability and high fatality rates
- In terms of global prevalence, more than half of cases/associated deaths are reported in high-income regions, including North America, western Europe and Australasia
- This is likely to be related to more accurate case ascertainment and diagnosis of MND in these regions, compared with countries with low and middle income
- Availability of disease-modifying drugs varies across the world, with riluzole currently only licensed in the UK, Europe, Australia, US and Canada

Recommended Reading

Abeleira, M.T., Limeres, J., Outumuro, M. et al. (2019). Benefits of maxillary expansion for a patient with spinal muscular atrophy type 2. *Am. J. Phys. Med. Rehabil.* 98: e32–e34.

Asher, R.S. and Alfred, T. (1993). Dental management of long-term amyotrophic lateral sclerosis: case report. *Spec. Care Dentist.* 13: 241–244.

College of Dental Hygienists of Ontario (CDHO). (2018). *Advisory: Amyotrophic Lateral Sclerosis.* www.cdho.org/Advisories/CDHO_Advisory_Amyotrophic_Lateral_Sclerosis.pdf.

NICE guideline NG42. (2019). *Motor Neurone Disease: Assessment and Management*. www.nice.org.uk/guidance/ng42

Nakayama, R., Nishiyama, A., Matsuda, C. et al. (2018). Oral health status of hospitalized amyotrophic lateral sclerosis patients: a single-centre observational study. *Acta Odontol. Scand.* 76: 294–298.

Oskarsson, B., Gendron, T., and Staff, N. (2018). Amyotrophic lateral sclerosis: an update for 2018. *Mayo Clin. Proc.* 93: 1617–1628.

Tay, C.M., Howe, J., and Borromeo, G. (2014). Oral health and dental treatment needs of people with motor neurone disease. *Aus. Dent. J.* 59: 309–313.

14.5 Stroke

Section I: Clinical Scenario and Dental Considerations

Clinical Scenario

A 64-year-old female presents to your clinic accompanied by her husband. She complains of increasingly mobility from a tooth in the upper left quadrant, which is affecting her ability to eat.

Medical History

- Left-sided stroke following percutaneous coronary intervention (formerly known as angioplasty with stent) 5 years ago; 4-month stay in a rehabilitation unit; biannual reviews currently
- Coronary heart disease
- Stable angina
- Type 2 diabetes mellitus
- Mild chronic obstructive pulmonary disease – emphysema (GOLD 1)
- Pneumonia 1 year ago
- Allergy to penicillin

Medications

- Aspirin
- Clopidogrel
- Trimetazidine
- Carvedilol hydrochlorothiazide
- Losartan
- Vildagliptin/metformin

Dental History

- Regular dental attender prior to her stroke; last dental visit 5 years ago; reports refusal of other dentists to provide care after her stroke
- Now reports significant anxiety in relation to dentistry due to the length of time since her last visit
- Brushes her teeth twice daily using a manual toothbrush
- Concerned that she cannot swallow properly and hence uses a lower fluoride toothpaste so that she does not ingest too much fluoride

Social History

- Lives with her husband and adult daughter
- Worked in a corporate job before having a stroke; now receiving disability allowance
- Care-giver support daily
- Reduced mobility; requires a wheelchair for long distances; able to transfer with assistance to the dental chair
- Tobacco consumption: stopped 5 years ago after her stroke but previously smoked 20 cigarettes a day for more than 15 years
- Alcohol consumption: nil

Oral Examination

- Partially edentate (Figure 14.5.1)
- #17, #15, #41 and #48 retained root fragments (Figure 14.5.2)
- #25 grade III mobility with root caries and a cervical composite restoration
- Cervical abrasion and root caries on all the mandibular anterior teeth
- #37, #38 and #47 mesially inclined
- Flabby mucosa overlying the maxillary alveolar ridge
- Thin mandibular alveolar ridge
- Generalised plaque deposits with associated gingival inflammation, particularly in association with the lower molar teeth
- Food pouching in the right buccal sulcus
- Xerostomia and healing ulcer left lateral border of the tongue (Figure 14.5.3)
- Badly fitting upper removable acrylic partial denture (10 years old)

A Practical Approach to Special Care in Dentistry, First Edition. Edited by Pedro Diz Dios and Navdeep Kumar.

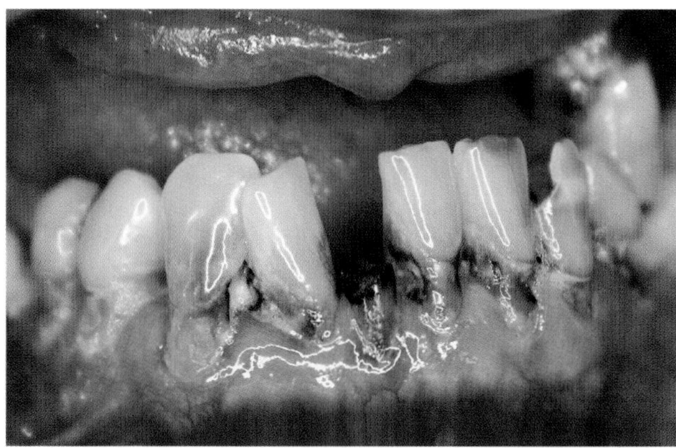

Figure 14.5.1 Partially edentate; plaque-induced gingivitis; root caries from #45 to #35; retained root #41.

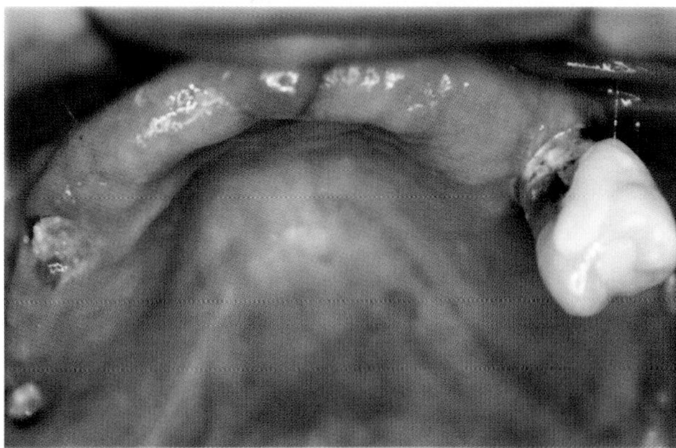

Figure 14.5.2 Retained roots #17 and #15; root caries #24.

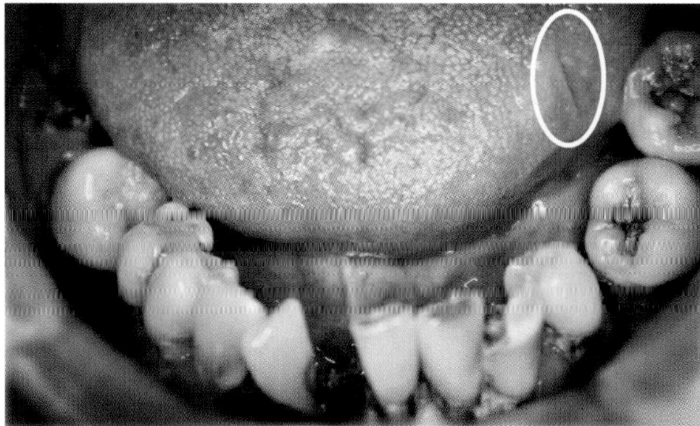

Figure 14.5.3 Xerostomia and healing ulcer left lateral border of the tongue.

Radiological Examination

- Orthopantomogram demonstrates widespread interdental decay and multiple retained roots (Figure 14.5.4)
- Cervical caries extending into the pulp of lower anterior teeth
- Moderate to severe bone loss associated with several teeth
- Significant resorption of maxillary alveolar ridge due to tooth loss

Structured Learning

1) What are the potential risk factors for stroke in this patient?
   - Age (over 55 years old)
   - Coronary heart disease
   - Diabetes mellitus
   - Emphysema
   - Former smoker
   - Job-related stress
2) What are some of the features of a left hemispheric stroke that you may see in this patient?
   - Loss of function/paralysis on the right side of the body
   - Speech/language problems
   - Dysphagia
   - Memory loss
   - Slow, cautious behaviour
3) The patient is concerned about the appearance of her broken teeth and reports that this is affecting her confidence and social interaction. What factors could have contributed to the deterioration in this patient's dentition?
   - Stroke commonly affects the patient's physical, psychological and social functioning
   - Physical factors
     - In the first few months during rehabilitation, the patient would have been highly dependent on others to brush her teeth (nursing staff, carers, family)
     - Limitations of the patient's own mobility/dexterity on discharge are likely to have negatively affected her ability to brush her teeth effectively
     - Important to determine if she was right-handed prior to her stroke; she may now have to rely on her left hand to brush her teeth which may not be as effective
     - Food pouching due to weakness of facial muscles
     - Access to dental care may be impaired due to reduced mobility
   - Psychological factors
   - Depression following a stroke can result in poor motivation to undertake self-care and access help
   - Social functioning
     - Isolation due to loss of work and inability to attend social activities can cause further post-stroke depression and make the patient less motivated to care for herself
     - Anxiety about healthcare-related procedures such as invasive dental treatment can also contribute to dental neglect

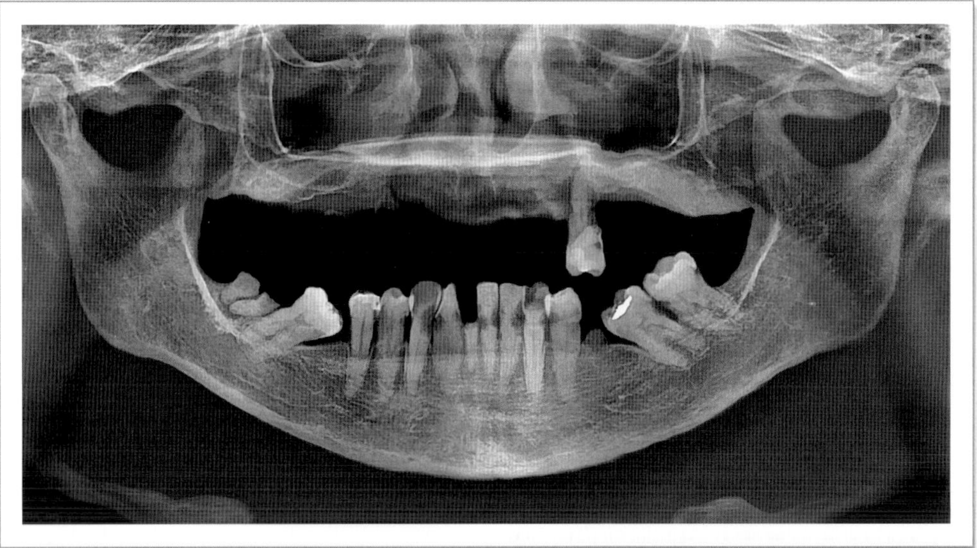

Figure 14.5.4 Orthopantomogram demonstrating extensive interdental decay in relation to multiple mandibular teeth, retained roots #17, #15, #35, #41 and #48.

4) The patient indicated that other dentists have refused to provide dental care as they considered her a high-risk patient. How can you reassure the patient that dental treatment is safe?
   - The risk of recurrence of a stroke is highest during the first 30 days after the initial event
   - Elective and invasive dental treatment is ideally deferred to 6 months after a stroke; the patient's stroke was 5 years ago; she is regularly reviewed by her physician and is also taking preventive medication
   - Patients with stable angina pectoris can be treated in the dental setting (see Chapter 8.2)
   - Dentists should be able to manage patients with mild chronic obstructive pulmonary disease (see Chapter 9.1)
5) What may also be contributing to the patient's anxiety?
   - Anxiety after stroke is common, affecting 25% of patients
   - She has not been able to access oral care for 5 years
   - It is important to have a detailed discussion regarding the best approach for anxiety management to enable delivery of dental care (see Chapter 15.1)
6) The tooth #25 is hypermobile. She wants the tooth extracted but requests that the gap is immediately filled with a denture. What factors should you discuss?
   - Explain that an immediate denture requires dental impressions
   - The tooth is likely to become dislodged in the impression material when the tray is withdrawn; in view of this, it is advisable to administer a local anaesthesia infiltration in relation to #25 to avoid pain/discomfort
   - If #25 is inadvertently removed when taking the impression, this will result in a gap for a period while the laboratory constructs a denture
   - Discuss that an alternative approach is to electively extract #25, followed by removal of the other maxillary retained roots #17, #15 and #24 at subsequent visits; once the sockets have healed, impressions can be taken at a later date for an upper denture; this approach is more likely to result in a more stable denture
   - The patient may subsequently take some time adjusting to a new denture, particularly as she has some residual weakness of the facial muscles
   - She may require assistance placing and removing the denture
7) The patient requests that #25 is removed urgently and accepts that replacement of her upper denture is best undertaken at a later stage. What factors do you need to consider in your risk assessment when planning dental treatment?
   - Social
     - Limited mobility
     - Dependence on an escort to be considered when setting up appointments
   - Medical
     - Dental treatment may elevate blood pressure and precipitate an episode of angina due to stress and anxiety (see Chapter 8.2)

- Increased bleeding risk due to dual antiplatelet therapy (see Chapter 10.5)
- Hypoglycaemia risk and potential for delayed healing related to diabetes mellitus (see Chapter 5.1)
- Emphysema and the potential for hypoxia (see Chapter 9.1)
- Anxiety (see Chapter 15.1)
- Antibiotic alternatives due to penicillin allergy (see Chapter 16.1)

- Dental
  - Poor oral health
  - Rampant dental caries
  - Poorly fitting denture
  - Food pouching persists on the right side, suggesting residual loss of function after the stroke
  - Challenges in denture construction and retention due to moderate bone loss, flabby mucosa and poor oral musculature control

8) During extraction of #25, the patient loses consciousness. What could have caused this?
   - Anxiety/vasovagal syncope
   - Hypoglycaemia: a common complication of diabetes mellitus; stress/missed meals may increase the risk
   - Orthostatic hypotension: associated with medications such as trimetazidine and carvedilol
   - Compromised airway due to dysphagia following stroke (aspiration/hypoxia)
   - Hypoxia in relation to chronic obstructive pulmonary disease
   - A further stroke/transient ischaemic attack

General Dental Considerations

Oral Findings

- Dysphagia
- Unilateral facial palsy with lack of sensation and poor muscle control of the tongue, lips and cheeks; this can cause food to accumulate on the affected side
- Reduced oral clearance increases risk of dental caries
- Poor oral hygiene
- Increased plaque accumulation, periodontal disease, halitosis
- Root caries
- Dysgeusia
- Decreased gag reflex
- Xerostomia secondary to polypharmacy (antihypertensives and antidepressants)
- Poor denture retention

Dental Management

- The appropriate adaptations in terms of dental management will be dependent on the severity of the stroke and its related impact (Tables 14.5.1 and 14.5.2)
- It is also important to consider the impact of related medical comorbidities such as diabetes and hypertension

Section II: Background Information and Guidelines

Definition

Stroke, also known as cerebrovascular accident or infarction, is an acute focal neurological condition with cerebral deficit symptoms lasting more than 24 hours which may be life threatening. There is a sudden onset of disrupted blood supply to different parts of the brain due to an infarct or haemorrhage.

It is the most common cause of acquired severe disability in adults and the most common cause of epilepsy in the elderly. It is also the second leading cause of dementia, with evidence of progressing dementia in a patient with comorbidities such as Alzheimer disease.

Aetiopathogenesis

- The primary pathophysiology of stroke is an underlying heart or blood vessel disease (Table 14.5.3)
- Genetic, demographic, medical and environmental risk factors have been described (Table 14.5.4)

Diagnosis

- Early detection for assessment using the acronym FAST
  - **F**acial weakness
  - **A**rm weakness
  - **S**peech problems
  - **T**ime to call for emergency services

- Non-contrast cranial computed tomography (CT) imaging is more sensitive for detecting an intracranial haemorrhage (Figure 14.5.5)
- Diffusion-weighted magnetic resonance imaging (DW-MRI) of the brain can be used to diagnose an ischaemic stroke and differentiate from other conditions that can be similar in presentation (e.g. seizures, migraine, hypoglycaemia, tumour, encephalitis, abscess and multiple sclerosis)

Table 14.5.1 Dental management considerations.

Risk assessment	• Recurrence of stroke is higher within the first 3–6 months • Risk of fall and difficulty in access is higher for patients with hemiparesis • Heightened anxiety • Depression • Emotional lability • Risk of aspiration if dysphagia is present • Dysarthria • Antithrombotic medication, such as antiplatelets or anticoagulants, can increase risk of bleeding • Monitor blood pressure
Criteria for referral	• Urgent dental treatment in the immediate post-stroke period (within 30 days) should be discussed with the patient's physician and provided in the hospital setting with perioperative medical management in place
Access/position	• Non ambulatory patients who are confined to their beds or those in critical care who experience acute pain may need domiciliary or in-hospital assessment • Confirm escort, transport and wheelchair requirements for patients with reduced mobility/ongoing care needs • Consider if the patient can transfer to the dental chair with or without assistance or may need a wheelchair recliner if unable to transfer • Mid or late morning appointments are ideal, when the patient is well rested and blood pressure is lower • Patients who have dysphagia and aspiration risk must be placed in a more semi reclined or upright position • Orthostatic hypotension can be experienced by patients who are taking some antihypertensive agents
Communication	• In the acute phase of stroke therapy, liaise with the physician to determine if the patient can be treated in the ambulatory setting or if a hospital setting is required • Allow adequate time to explain the proposed treatment to give the patient enough time to process the information • If dysarthria is present, the patient may require additional time/communication aids to respond
Consent/capacity	• Capacity to give consent can be temporarily or permanently impaired when there is confusion, difficulties understanding and giving opinions, or memory loss in relation to stroke • A patient may have no issues giving verbal consent but may have difficulty in signing forms due to hemiparesis or inability to write; in this case, agreement should be recorded by a witness
Anaesthesia/sedation	• Local anaesthesia – Limit local anaesthesia with epinephrine to 2–3 cartridges – Consider heightened anxiety during administration • Sedation – Oral sedation may be required to facilitate dental treatment for highly anxious patients – Consider the higher risk of aspiration for patients with dysphagia – Benzodiazepines may cause respiratory depression • General anaesthesia – This technique may be considered to facilitate treatment for patients needing extensive dental work and those who are unco-operative or with heightened anxiety
Dental treatment	• Before – Liaise with the physician to confirm if the patient is stable enough to proceed with elective dental treatment – Confirm if the patient is taking antithrombotic medication and whether any preoperative tests/adjustments are required for any planned invasive dental procedures (see Chapter 10)

(*Continued*)

Table 14.5.1 (Continued)

	• During – Extractions should be limited to no more than 3 teeth per visit for patients on antithrombotic medication and local haemostatic measures implemented (see Chapter 10) – Bleeding risk procedures (e.g. periodontal surgery or dental implants) should be limited to 1 quadrant every visit – For patients who have dysphagia and are unable to tolerate high flow of water from the handpiece for doing restorations, consider an atraumatic restorative technique (e.g. silver diamine fluoride) to arrest enamel-dentine caries – Avoid using epinephrine-soaked thread retractors – Routine use of rubber dam is recommended • After – Ensure the airway and oral cavity is free from debris – When giving postoperative instructions to the patient, consider whether there is cognitive/memory decline; involve their escort if present and provide written instructions – For patients with changes to proprioception/touch (25–85% of patients), advise regarding the increased risk of soft tissue trauma while local anaesthesia effect does not wear off
Drug prescription	• Avoid non-steroidal anti-inflammatory drugs as both non-selective (e.g. diclofenac) and selective cyclo-oxygenase-2 inhibitors (e.g. rofecoxib) can increase the risk of stroke – paracetamol is preferred for minor surgery
Education/prevention	• In the early months after a stroke, educating the family and carers is imperative in preventing deterioration of oral health • Spitting out may be difficult in the early stages of stroke due to poor oral muscular co-ordination – consider using non-foaming fluoride toothpaste and suction toothbrushes/devices; mouth rinses can be applied with a drained gauze or the toothbrush • Modify brushing techniques and toothbrushes for patients with decreased mobility in their dominant arm

Clinical Presentation

- Approximately 80% of strokes occur in the supratentorial region of the brain (cerebrum) and present with contralateral signs (hemiparesis); this is due to contralateral projection of nerve fibres across the corticospinal tract
- Initial presentation is commonly associated with a sudden onset of loss of neurological function, with symptoms including severe headache, sudden unilateral hemiparesis, numbness, visual loss or diplopia, slurred speech, ataxia and non-orthostatic vertigo
- The residual effects can be long term, affecting motor, sensory and cognitive functions
  - Motor function
    - Unilateral numbness or weakness
    - Contralateral hemiparesis (partial or complete) – face, arm, leg
    - Ataxia/frequent falling
    - Urinary incontinence and poor bowel control
    - Dysphagia
    - Sexual dysfunction
  - Sensory deficits
    - Diplopia
    - Transient monocular blindness
    - Visual field defects
    - Vertigo
    - Loss of balance
  - Cognition deficits
    - Speech and comprehension difficulties
    - Aphasia or dysphasia
    - Agnosia – inability to process sensory information
    - Mood changes – anxiety, irritability and aggression
    - Memory deficit
    - Post stroke fatigue
    - Depression
    - Recovery can be prolonged, affecting the patient's mental, psychological and social well-being

Management

- The treatment approach is determined by the type of stroke and the underlying risk factors. It consists of 3 stages: immediate treatment, prevention and rehabilitation
- Therapy immediately after a stroke

Ischaemic stroke

- Within 5 hours of symptoms, a thrombolytic drug such as recombinant tissue plasminogen activator (tPA) is given to dissolve the blood clot; this can either be given via a peripheral vein or delivered directly to the area via an endovascular procedure

  Endovascular procedures can also be used to remove the clot with a stent retriever

Table 14.5.2 Oral healthcare for patients who have had a stroke.

Level of dependence	Oral hygiene regimen
Independent	• Twice-daily toothbrushing with at least 1450 ppm fluoride toothpaste, but for patients who are at higher risk of developing caries, prescribed toothpaste of 2800 or 5000 ppm concentration is advised • Use of floss or interdental brushes before toothbrushing • Chlorhexidine 0.12% mouthwash or 1% gel used daily • Toothbrush modifications for more efficient brushing can be done such as modifying the handle or using an electric or 3-sided toothbrush • For patients with xerostomia – artificial saliva products can be used, frequent sips of water and avoiding dry food • Advise gargling and rinsing after meals to decrease food packing
Dependent on carers	• Educate caretakers on how to modify positioning during toothbrushing – Sitting on the chair with a pillow resting against the caretaker and approach toothbrushing from behind – For bed-bound patients, the bed must be close to upright to avoid aspirating fluids – A penlight and tongue depressor can be used to visualise difficult-to-clean areas such as the upper buccal and lower lingual vestibules • Patients who have difficulty spitting out or who are more prone to aspiration can use aspirating toothbrushes or a suction device during toothbrushing
With swallowing difficulties or feeding tubes	• Reducing risk of aspiration – Place the patient in an upright position when undertaking toothbrushing – Frequent suctioning of oral fluids and secretions – Using a low-foaming toothpaste (small amount) and removing excess water from the toothbrush can reduce aspiration – Careful use of a sponge stick moistened with chlorhexidine gluconate 1% gel or chlorhexidine 0.12% mouthwash can be undertaken for patients who are unable to tolerate brushing • To better clean areas of food pocketing, a gauze wrapped around the finger can be used to sweep the buccal vestibule
Denture care	• Dentures checked regularly for proper fit to be relined or replaced as needed to prevent soft tissue trauma • Dentures worn during the day and taken out during bedtime to reduce the risk of denture stomatitis and thrush • Proper denture identification to avoid losing dentures in care homes

Table 14.5.3 Main types of stroke.

Type of stroke	Characteristics
Transient ischaemic attack (TIA)	• Caused by a temporary obstruction of the blood flow to the brain, usually a blood clot • Although the symptoms are similar to those of a full stroke, they are typically temporary and disappear after a few minutes or hours • Detection of infarction on imaging can change the classification to stroke • 10–15% of people who experience a TIA have a major stroke within 3 months
Ischaemic stroke (~80%)	• There are 2 main types: thrombotic and embolic – Thrombotic stroke is due to a local thrombosis causing occlusion of vessels and decreased blood flow to the cerebral arteries – Embolic stroke is due to a detached thrombus that travels as an embolus, obstructing smaller distal arteries; may develop as a result of conditions such as atrial fibrillation
Haemorrhagic stroke (~20%)	• Often associated with a consistently elevated systolic blood pressure • There are 2 main types: intracerebral and subarachnoid – Intracerebral is the most common type of haemorrhagic stroke; associated with a focal collection of blood within the brain parenchyma or ventricular system that is not caused by trauma – Subarachnoid type is less common and is due to bleeding into the subarachnoid space (space between arachnoid membrane and pia mater of brain or spinal cord) which is not caused by trauma; presents with rapid signs of neurological dysfunction and/or headache

Table 14.5.4 Risk factors of stroke.

Type	Category	Risk factor
Non-modifiable	Race	• More frequent in people of African, Caribbean and South Asian origin
	Family history	• A positive family history of stroke is associated with an increased risk (may be related to lifestyle and genetic factors)
	Age	• The risk of stroke increases after the age of 55 years old, but it can occur at any age • It is reported as 25 times more common in individuals aged 75–85 years
	Genetics	• A large number of single-gene disorders can cause stroke but most of these are extremely rare • CADASIL (cerebral autosomal dominant arteriopathy with subcortical infarcts and leucoencephalopathy) is the most common single-gene disorder leading to ischaemic stroke
Modifiable	Lifestyle	• Smoking • Excessive alcohol consumption • Substance abuse • Poor nutrition • Lack of physical exercise • Long working hours • Stress
	Medical	• Elevated blood pressure • Dyslipidaemia • Hypercholesterolaemia • Atrial fibrillation • Arteriovenous malformations • Antiphospholipid syndrome • Diabetes mellitus/insulin resistance • Increased body mass index • Sleep-disordered breathing • Emphysema • Carotid stenosis • Chronic kidney disease • Hormonal contraception and replacement therapies • Migraine with aura
	Psychiatric	• Psychosocial stress • Depression
	Physical activity	• Neck trauma • Sexual intercourse

- Other procedures to decrease the risk of having another stroke include carotid endarterectomy, angioplasty and stents

Haemorrhagic stroke

- Medication is given to lower the intracranial pressure and blood pressure, and prevent spasms of blood vessels and seizures
- Surgical approaches include craniotomy, surgical clipping, endovascular embolisation, surgical removal of an arteriovenous malformation, if present, stereotactic radiosurgery

- Preventive approaches include smoking cessation, weight reduction and exercise, control of hypertension, atrial fibrillation and diabetes mellitus if present
- Stroke recovery and rehabilitation require a multidisciplinary team to achieve maximum function and independence; this includes a neurologist, physiotherapist, speech and language specialist, dietitian and psychologist

Prognosis

- Better prognosis is achieved with rapid assessment of presenting symptoms and early intervention

(a)

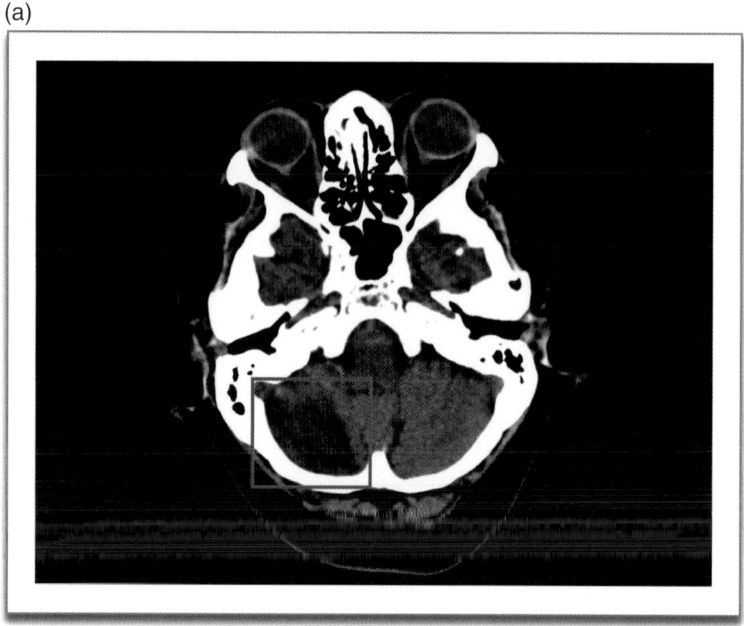

(b)

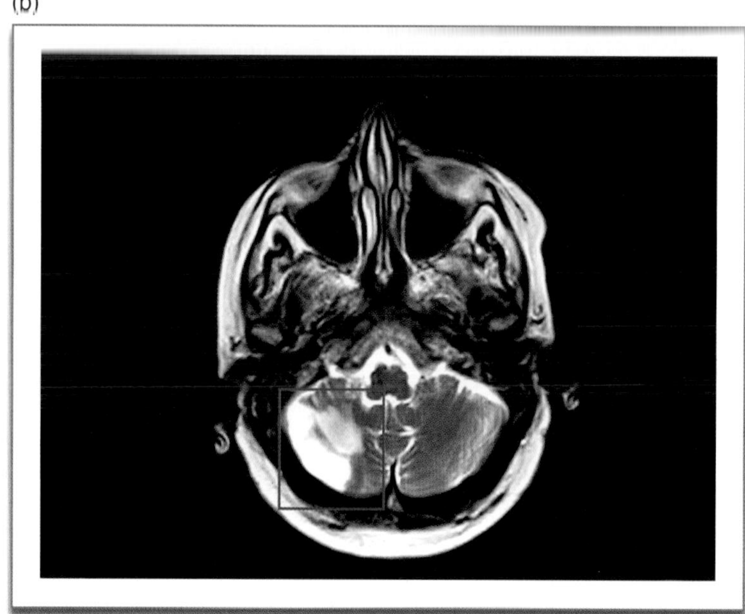

Figure 14.5.5 Acute ischaemic stroke (cerebellar infarction) confirmed by computed tomography (a) and diffusion-weighted magnetic resonance imaging (b).

- Nevertheless, it is estimated that in the first month after a stroke, there is a mortality rate of 40–50%
- On average, recovery can take place within 12–18 months
- Dysphagia associated with stroke puts the patient at a higher risk of aspiration pneumonia and its complications

A World/Transcultural View

- Stroke is the second leading cause of death and the third leading cause of disability-adjusted life-years worldwide
- Incidence is slowly declining in developed countries such as the United Kingdom where there was a 19% decrease in incidence from 1990 to 2010, mainly due to better prevention and management of the condition
- Conversely, the incidence in developing countries remains relatively high
- Although there has been a decline in overall stroke mortality rates since the 1950s, age-adjusted stroke death rates are reported to be higher in black populations within the United States

Recommended Reading

Brady, M., Furlanetto, D., Hunter, R.V. et al. (2006). Staff-led interventions for improving oral hygiene in patients following stroke. *Cochrane Database Syst. Rev.* 18: CD003864.

Bramanti, E., Arcuri, C., Cecchetti, F. et al. (2012). Dental management in dysphagia syndrome patients with previously acquired brain damages. *J. Dent. Res.* 9: 361–367.

British Society of Gerodontology. (2010). *Guidelines for the Oral Healthcare of Stroke Survivors*. www.gerodontology.com/content/uploads/2014/10/stroke_guidelines.pdf

Dickinson, H. (2012). Maintaining oral health after stroke. *Nurs. Stand.* 26: 35–39.

Fatahzadeh, M. and Glick, M. (2006). Stroke: epidemiology, classification, risk factors, complications, diagnosis, prevention, and medical and dental management. *Oral Surg. Oral Med. Oral Pathol. Oral Radiol. Endod.* 102: 180–191.

Hankey, G.J. (2017). Stroke. *Lancet* 389: 641–644.

Kim, H.T., Park, J.B., Lee, W.C. et al. (2018). Differences in the oral health status and oral hygiene practices according to the extent of post-stroke sequelae. *J. Oral Rehabil.* 45: 476–484.

Sen, S., Giamberardino, L.D., Moss, K. et al. (2018). Periodontal disease, regular dental care use, and incident ischemic stroke. *Stroke* 49: 355–362.

15

Psychiatric Disorders

15.1 Anxiety and Phobia

Section I: Clinical Scenario and Dental Considerations

Clinical Scenario

A 31-year-old female presents to the dental clinic with acute pain from her lower left third molar of 2 months' duration. The pain is triggered by cold and hot stimuli, lasts hours and is now extremely painful with associated sleep disturbance.

Medical History

- Recently diagnosed mixed anxiety-depressive disorder presented with panic attacks
- History of Bell palsy (left side) 1 year ago; linked to episode of extreme stress; 6-month recovery period
- Fatty liver (non-alcoholic fatty liver disease)
- Overweight (BMI = 26 kg/m^2)

Medications

- Sertraline
- Clonazepam (taken intermittently)

Dental History

- Dental phobia
  - Mother has dental phobia too which the patient believes is the cause of her own phobia
  - Irregular dental attender (only attends when in extreme pain); last visit 5 years ago
  - Previous dental treatment provided under general anaesthesia (multiple fillings, extractions); sedation has also been used for emergency dental treatment
  - Anxiety starts from the day before and increases with prolonged waiting time
  - History of leaving the dental practice before entering the dental surgery because of the unbearable anxiety
  - Fear of both high- and low-speed dental handpieces (sound and vibration)
  - High levels of anxiety assessed on different scales
    - Modified Dental Anxiety Scale (MDAS): 20 points
    - Revised Dental Belief Survey (R-DBS): 53 points
- Brushes twice a day but has struggled when the Bell palsy was present
- Highly cariogenic diet

Social History

- Lives with partner who often works away from home
- Two daughters (7 and 10 years old)
- Occupation: secretary, but at the moment is on medical leave (due to the mixed anxiety-depressive disorder)
- Less than 2 units of alcohol a week but when very anxious can binge drink and consume 10–12 units the day before a dental appointment to help her to sleep
- Habits: nail biting (onychophagia) and nocturnal bruxism

Oral Examination

- Hypertrophic bilateral masseters
- Scalloping/traumatic bite marks on the tongue (Figure 15.1.1)

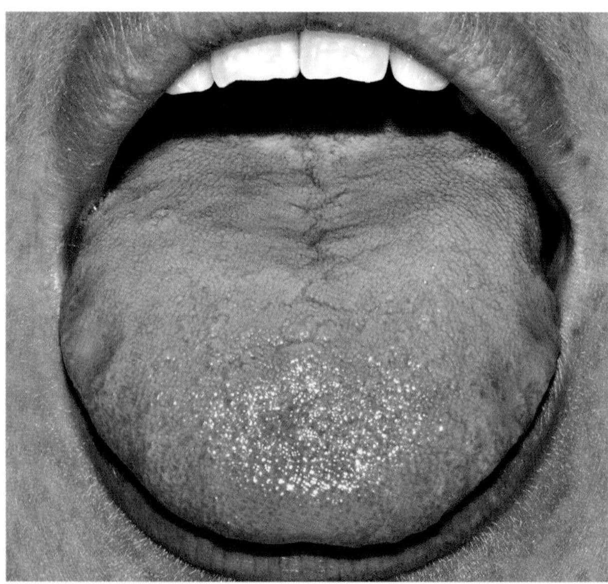

Figure 15.1.1 Scalloped tongue due to bruxism/tongue biting.

A Practical Approach to Special Care in Dentistry, First Edition. Edited by Pedro Diz Dios and Navdeep Kumar.

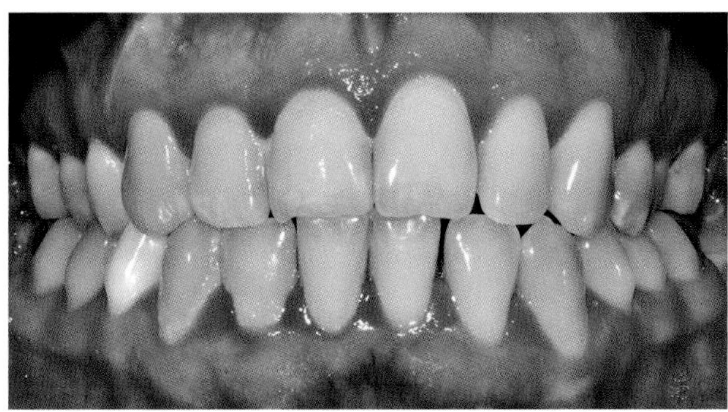

Figure 15.1.2 Poor oral health with associated gingivitis.

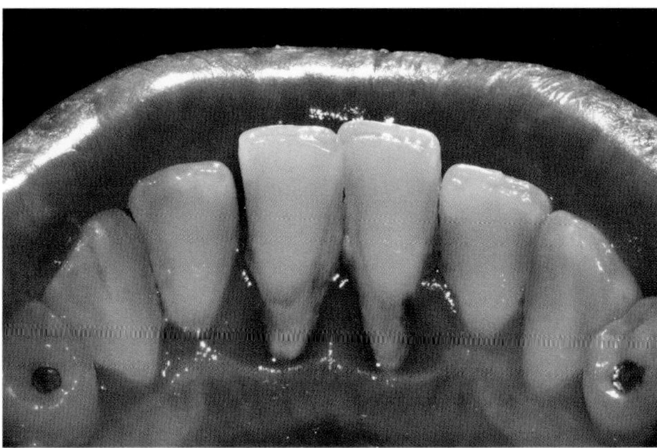

Figure 15.1.3 Lower incisors: calculus and lingual recession.

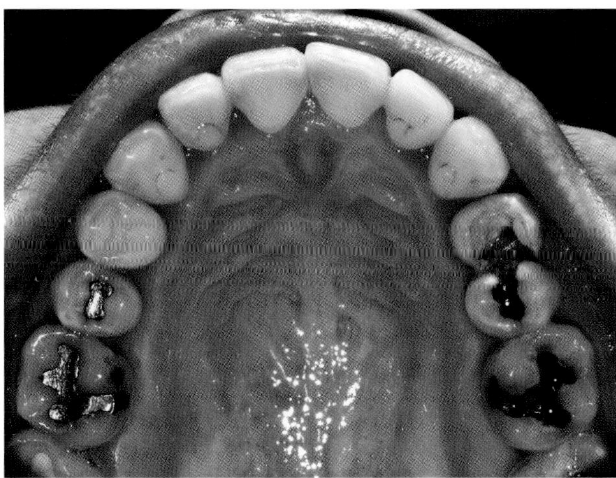

Figure 15.1.4 Multiple restorations; #25 caries; #24 disto-occlusal defective restoration.

- Presence of soft and hard deposits (Figure 15.1.2)
- Calculus and recession lingual to lower incisors (Figure 15.1.3)
- Heavily restored dentition (Figure 15.1.4)
- Caries in #17, #24 (root filled), #25 and #38
- #38 with tenderness to percussion
- Probing depth 3.5–5.5 mm in relation to the upper posterior teeth and all the lower teeth

Radiological Examination

- Long cone periapical radiographs undertaken
- #38 caries extending into dentine, no apical lesion, mesiobuccal root close to inferior dental nerve canal
- #17 cusp fracture, temporary restoration in situ
- #24 endodontic treatment, no apical lesion, occlusodistal cavity
- #25 mesial caries extending into dentine

Structured Learning

1) What aspect of this patient's behaviour is a feature of dental phobia rather than dental anxiety?
    - This patient exhibits classic avoidance behaviour
    - She only goes to the dentist when she is experiencing extreme dental pain
2) What are anxiety scales?
    - Anxiety scales are questionnaires that have been developed to assess whether a patient has a higher level of dental anxiety than an average patient (see Section II)
    - They can be helpful to identify specific triggers or just as a conversation starter
3) What do this patient's anxiety scores tell you about her degree of dental anxiety?
    - This is a highly anxious patient, with signs of dental phobia
4) The patient also reports that her mouth can feel very dry – what factors could be contributing to this?
    - Anxiety, particularly when acute, can cause sympathetic stimulation which results in a dry mouth
    - Sertraline is a selective serotonin reuptake inhibitor associated with a common side-effect of a dry mouth
    - Clonazepam is a benzodiazepine and can also cause a dry mouth
5) What factors do you need to consider in your risk assessment for the management of this patient?
    - Social
        - Availability/suitability of escort as partner works away from home and mother also has dental anxiety
        - Impact of binge drinking prior to dental visits on attendance and ability to proceed with dental treatment, especially sedation, and ability to provide informed consent
        - Panic attacks (unbearable anxiety)
        - Currently unemployed – cost of dental treatment may have an impact

- Medical
  - Consider impact of fatty liver/liver cirrhosis (see Chapter 6.1) and raised BMI on the delivery of care (see Chapter 16.4)
  - Bell palsy (rarely may recur during stressful periods)
- Dental
  - Dental phobia – only seeks dental input when she is in pain; in view of this she may not return once she is pain free
  - Presenting with acute infection in relation to apical periodontitis of #38; need to provide urgent intervention (e.g. antibiotics and/or dental extraction with sedation)
  - High caries risk: highly cariogenic diet, xerostomia, negative impact of Bell palsy on access for toothbrushing, irregular dental attender
  - Periodontal disease at an early age with spacing and recession in relation to the lower incisors; ideally needs more regular dental visits to stabilise this
  - Patient has allowed an oral examination, radiographs and photographs; hence acclimatisation for dental visits may be possible

6) The patient requests that all dental treatment, including extraction of #38, fillings and scaling, is undertaken under a general anaesthetic procedure. What are the benefits and drawbacks of this approach for this patient?
   - Benefits
     - May be an advantage if #38 requires surgical extraction
     - Multiple dental treatments required and can be completed in a single session
     - Allows to 'buy time' to do adaptation at a later stage
   - Disadvantages
     - No learning from the experience
     - Incorrectly reinforces to the patient that general anaesthesia is the normal setting for dental treatment; this may then be also assumed by daughters if they need dental treatment in the furture
     - Risks of complications higher than with local anaesthesia, especially as there are additional comorbidities to consider such as raised BMI and fatty liver disease
     - Dental treatment options may be limited due to limits of operating time (e.g. may not be possible to undertake root canal treatment on posterior teeth)
     - Increases cost (patient may need to pay for this in some countries)

General Dental Considerations

Oral Findings

- Neglect – dental fear impacts on dental health. This commonly manifests as extensive oral needs that tend to require invasive dental treatment, which further reinforces the dental fear
- Dry mouth – secondary to sympathetic stimulation or some medications prescribed for anxiety management
- Bruxism
- Lip chewing/tongue biting
- Increased gag reflex
- Atypical facial and oral pain
- Burning mouth syndrome
- Cancer phobia

Dental Management

- According to the General Dental Council (United Kingdom) all dentists have a duty to provide adequate pain and anxiety control
- Each patient will require careful assessment to ensure that the most appropriate supportive approach is implemented (Table 15.1.1)

Section II: Background Information and Guidelines

Definition

Dental anxiety or 'odontophobia' is the fifth most common cause for anxiety. It is an emotional state marked by fear of the dental environment or treatment, which is perceived as a threat. Dental phobia corresponds to an irrational and overwhelming fear of dental treatment, where the patient understands that their response is not proportional to the situation. It is characterised by avoidance behaviour. In the United Kingdom, it has been reported that 36% of patients have moderate dental anxiety, while 12% reported extreme dental fear. Both entities can be associated with stigma, which impacts on deterioration in the oral health of these individuals.

It is also important to consider if there are any additional anxieties/phobias which may impact on the provision of care, such as:

- Claustrophobia – fear of closed spaces, probably the most common phobic disorder
- Agoraphobia – fear of being in public places from which escape might be difficult or help unavailable
- Social phobia – overwhelming anxiety and excessive self-consciousness in normal social situations

Table 15.1.1 Considerations for dental management.

Risk assessment	• History of failed appointments • Patient may either appear withdrawn or talk incessantly • Unexpected movements • More likely to have associated comorbidities such as alcohol or drug dependence • Risk of vasovagal syncope
Criteria for referral	• Patients with mild anxiety can be seen by general dentists • Referral will depend on the dentist's level of competence and resource availability within the health service • The Indicator of Sedation Need (IOSN) may be used to categorise patient complexity and determine suitability for referral (Table 15.1.3) • Patients who are not able to accept dental treatment with behavioural management techniques alone may need referral for more specialised management, sedation or general anaesthesia (Table 15.1.4)
Access/position	• Suitable timing for the appointment (e.g. morning appointments may reduce stress due to less waiting time, but may also trigger insomnia/fatigue due to anxiety) • Avoid rush hour in patients with associated agoraphobia • Patients may need an escort for psychological support and to bring them to their appointment, as this reduces non-attendance of confirmed appointments (e.g. carers, support pets) • Premedication as prescribed by the physician/dentist may be required (mild benzodiazepine) the night before and/or on the day of the procedure – escort required • Relaxation techniques, meditation (e.g. use of meditation apps) or other coping strategies can start before entering the dental practice and help lower stress levels • Consider longer appointments • Consider initial acclimatisation visits in a non-dental setting • Minimise the interval between appointments
Communication	• Communication skills are key to achieve a good patient–dentist relation • Empathetic calm approach is always recommended • Allow enough time to assess the patient and talk about their concerns but do not allow this to become an avoidance strategy • Anxiety scales can help start a conversation (evidence shows that they do not increase anxiety levels) • Behavioural management techniques should be used (independent of the treatment modality) • Clear explanation of the treatment plan might help reduce anxiety
Consent/capacity	• Should not be affected, unless the patient is taking premedication to enable attendance (e.g. benzodiazepines) • Consider the impact of comorbidities such as alcohol and recreational drug use
Anaesthesia/sedation	• Local anaesthesia – Good analgesia and anaesthesia will help reduce stress levels (stress is associated with lower pain tolerance and longer lasting pain) – Computer-controlled local anaesthetic delivery (CCLAD) may be helpful – Be aware of possible unexpected movements • Sedation – Ensure an escort is available – Consider the impact of regular benzodiazepine use on the effect of dental sedation • General anaesthesia – Used as last option, as it is the most restrictive method – If there are significant dental treatment needs, it may be advantageous

(Continued)

Table 15.1.1 (Continued)

Dental treatment	• Before – Undertake a pretreatment anxiety questionnaire and review – Relaxation techniques, meditation (e.g. use of meditation apps) or other coping strategies can start before entering the dental practice and help lower stress levels – Anxiolytics (usually diazepam) might be recommended the night before and/or on the day of the procedure – Special arrangements may need to be in place before the session (e.g. for sedation: transport, escort, work arrangements) – Further investigations/assessments may be necessary if sedation or general anaesthesia is being considered • During – Preparation for medical emergencies: hyperventilation, panic attack or syncope – Use of appropriate non-pharmacological/pharmacological adjuncts to reduce anxiety • After Close follow up needs to be a priority to avoid the need for future invasive procedures
Drug prescription	• Consider interaction of benzodiazepines with azole antifungals and macrolide antibiotics (erythromycin and clarithromycin) • Benzodiazepines are potentiated with alcohol, antihistamines and barbiturates (deeper sedative effect)
Education/prevention	• Focus should be placed on the association between prevention and good oral health, as this in turn will reduce the need for invasive dental procedures • If dental treatment is carried out under general anaesthesia, the patient should be encouraged to commit to a follow-up preventive plan and a progressive acclimatisation

- Other specific phobias – commonly include those associated with heights, tunnels, driving, water, flying, insects, dogs and injuries involving blood

Aetiopathogenesis

- The aetiology of dental fear and anxiety is associated with multiple factors
- It is described as having 5 possible pathways
  1) Conditioning (personal experience)
  2) Informative (through negative connotations, dental fear environment, others' negative experiences)
  3) Vicarious (e.g. expressions of others)
  4) Verbal threat (through hearing or reading, 'word of mouth')
  5) Parental (e.g. mother's fear)
- There is some evidence that genetics may also play a role

Diagnosis

- The diagnostic criteria for anxiety/phobia are detailed in Table 15.1.2
- It is important to consider other conditions that may be contributing to changes in behaviour, including depression, obsessions, delusions, unnatural fears or hallucinations that may signify deeper diseases like schizophrenia, schizoid personality disorder, paranoias, Asperger syndrome and autism

Clinical Presentation

- Increased heart rate
- Increased respiratory rate
- Dry mouth
- Sweating
- Nausea
- Diarrhoea
- Urinary frequency
- Muscle tension
- Insomnia and sleep disturbances
- Increased pain perception
- Exaggeration of memory of pain
- Medical emergencies, such as hyperventilation or syncope

Management

- Treatment strategies are closely related to the assessment of the severity of the dental anxiety and their associated factors, including level and type of anxiety, coping strategies of the patient, presence of other psychiatric diseases and type and extent of treatment needs

Table 15.1.2 Diagnosis for specific phobias according to the main classifications.

ICD-11	DSM-V
• Fear/anxiety of 1 or more specific object(s)/situation(s) • Fear is not proportional to the danger • Avoidance of that object/situation • Persistence of symptoms for months • Results in severe distress or impairment	• Excessive anxiety/fear of an object/specific situation • The object/situation provokes immediate anxiety/fear • Active avoidance of that object/situation • The fear is disproportionate to the real danger • Lasts 6 months or more • It causes significant clinical distress and social impairment • It is not better explained by another mental disorder

ICD-11, International Classification of Diseases (2018), World Health Organization; DSM-V, Diagnostic and Statistical Manual (2013), American Psychiatric Association.

- The selection of the appropriate management technique depends on the characteristics of each individual patient, including their level of motivation, and always considering the least restrictive method
- Although an individualised approach is required, general principles include providing trust (through non-judgemental empathetic communication), realistic information (e.g. length/complexity of the procedure) and ensuring that there is high level of predictability (e.g. warning beforehand of unpleasant situations)
- A detailed pretreatment assessment should be undertaken in order to plan the most appropriate support required; common questionnaires used include:
  - Modified Dental Anxiety Scale (MDAS) (Figure 15.1.5)
    - Five questions each with a 5-category rating scale, ranging from 'not anxious' to 'extremely anxious'
    - Hence scale ranges from a minimum of 5 to a maximum of 25

CAN YOU TELL US HOW ANXIOUS YOU GET, IF AT ALL, WITH YOUR DENTAL VISIT?

PLEASE INDICATE BY INSERTING 'X' IN THE APPROPRIATE BOX

1. **If you went to your Dentist for TREATMENT TOMORROW, how would you feel?**
   Not Anxious ☐ *Slightly Anxious* ☐ *Fairly Anxious* ☐ *Very Anxious* ☐ *Extremely Anxious* ☐
2. **If you were sitting in the WAITING ROOM (waiting for treatment), how would you feel?**
   Not Anxious ☐ *Slightly Anxious* ☐ *Fairly Anxious* ☐ *Very Anxious* ☐ *Extremely Anxious* ☐
3. **If you were about to have a TOOTH DRILLED, how would you feel?**
   Not Anxious ☐ *Slightly Anxious* ☐ *Fairly Anxious* ☐ *Very Anxious* ☐ *Extremely Anxious* ☐
4. **If you were about to have your TEETH SCALED AND POLISHED, how would you feel?**
   Not Anxious ☐ *Slightly Anxious* ☐ *Fairly Anxious* ☐ *Very Anxious* ☐ *Extremely Anxious* ☐
5. **If you were about to have a LOCAL ANAESTHETIC INJECTION in your gum, above an upper back tooth, how would you feel?**
   Not Anxious ☐ *Slightly Anxious* ☐ *Fairly Anxious* ☐ *Very Anxious* ☐ *Extremely Anxious* ☐

Each item scored as follows:

Not anxious	=	1
Slightly anxious	=	2
Fairly anxious	=	3
Very anxious	=	4
Extremely anxious	=	5

Total score is a sum of all 5 items, range 5 to 25. Cut off is 19 or above which indicates a highly dentally anxious patient, possibly dentally phobic

Figure 15.1.5 The Modified Dental Anxiety Scale (MDAS).

- Simplified rating system in comparison with Corah's Dental Scale, which was an early 4-question measure of dental anxiety
- The MDAS has an extra item about the respondent's anxiety about a local anaesthetic injection

- Dental Belief Survey Revised (DBS-R)
  - The DBS-R is intended to measure 3 dimensions of the patient–dentist relationship as perceived by the patient, namely Ethics, Communication and Control
  - It is recommended for clinical use when assessing the patient's perception of the relationship to the dentist, including both trust and ethical behaviour

- Non-pharmacological approaches (most of these can be undertaken by dentists but in some cases support from a psychologist is necessary)
  - Behavioural management techniques
    - Tell–show–do (explaining every step of the process)
    - Positive reinforcement (emphasising advancements)
    - Distraction (chatting about a topic in the patient's interest, watching videos, solving mathematical problems or games)
    - Modelling
    - Enhancing control (signalling, traffic lights system)
    - Systematic desensitisation (in vivo, through pictures or videos)
    - Guided imagery (imaginal visualisation of places or colours)
  - Alternative methods
    - Aromatherapy (usually done with lavender essential oil)
    - Music therapy
    - Relaxation techniques (muscle groups)
    - Breathing techniques (diaphragmatic breathing)
    - Biofeedback
    - Acupuncture
    - Hypnotherapy
    - Cognitive behavioural therapy (undertaken by a psychologist or trained dentist)
- Pharmacological management approaches
  - A comprehensive risk assessment must be performed before deciding to undertake pharmacological management as there may be significant effects on ventilation and cardiovascular function (Table 15.1.3)
  - Indications
    - Unco-operative patients who cannot comply with dental treatment based only on behavioural management techniques (e.g. moderate or severe intellectual disabilities)
    - Challenging behaviour (e.g. autistic spectrum disorder)
    - Need for extensive dental treatment with risk of acute pain
    - Complex traumatic dental treatment
    - Medical risk factors (e.g. refractory epilepsy, movement disorders)
    - Selection of the most appropriate method of pharmacological management will require careful consideration of the indications, contraindications, benefits and limitations of each approach (Table 15.1.4)

Table 15.1.3 Continuum of depth of sedation, showing the impact on the respiratory and cardiovascular systems when increasing the sedation level.

	Level of sedation			
	Minimal Sedation (anxiolysis)	**Moderate Sedation (conscious sedation)**	**Deep Sedation**	**General Anaesthesia**
Responsiveness	Normal response to verbal stimuli	Purposeful response to verbal stimuli	Purposeful response following repeated or painful stimuli	No response to painful stimuli
Airway	Unaffected	No intervention required	Intervention may be required	Intervention required
Spontaneous ventilation	Unaffected	Adequate	May be inadequate	Inadequate
Cardiovascular function	Unaffected	Usually maintained	Usually maintained	Inadequate

Table 15.1.4 Summary of the pharmacological options for anxiety/phobia management.

	Modality		
	Inhalation	**Oral**	**Intranasal**
Indications	• Mild to moderate anxiety • Invasive dental treatments • Patients with cardiovascular risk factors • Increased gag reflex	• Mild to moderate anxiety • To increase cooperation for venepuncture[a] • Moderate to severe anxiety	• Mild to moderate anxiety • To increase cooperation for venepuncture[a] • Moderate to severe anxiety[a]
Cautions / Contra-indications	• Mouth breather • Nasal obstruction • Pulmonary diseases (e.g., COPD) • Vit B12 deficiency • Under treatment with methotrexate or bleomycin • Recent ophthalmic surgery • Middle ear disturbance/surgery • Pregnancy (1st trimester) • Current/recover drug addiction • Patients with compulsive personality • Claustrophobia • Severe personality disorders	• Under medication that interacts with benzodiazepines[b] • Renal or hepatic disease • Pregnancy • COPD • Drug consumption • Elderly • Uncontrolled hypo/ hyperthyroidism • Psychiatric illness[c]	• Nasal obstruction or abnormalities • Under medication that interacts with benzodiazepines[b] • Renal or hepatic disease • COPD • Pregnancy • Drug consumption • Elderly • Uncontrolled hypo/ hyperthyroidism • Psychiatric illness[b]
Benefits	• Easy to accept • Short latent period • Easy titration • Mild analgesia • Minimal effect on protective reflexes • Rapid recovery • No residual effect • No escort needed	• Great acceptance • Easy to administrate • Relative safety	• Easy to comply with • Good absorption • Bypasses entero-hepatic circulation • Maximum effect after 10 minutes
Limitations	• Needs partial cooperation • Needs to be used with other behavioural management techniques • Patient needs to be able to follow instructions • Cost • Occupational risks (miscarriages and infertility)	• Long time until maximum effect (~1 hour) • No titration • Unreliable drug absorption • Prolonged effect • Escort required • Monitoring equipment required	• Dosage wastage if patient sneezes • No titration • Escort required • Monitoring equipment required

(Continued)

Table 15.1.4 (Continued)

	Modality	
	Intravenous	**General Anaesthesia**
Indications	• Moderate to severe anxiety • Uncooperative patients • Uncontrolled epilepsy • Motor disturbances • Increased gag reflex	• Severe anxiety • Extreme challenging behaviour • Extensive or invasive dental treatment
Cautions / Contra-indications	• Substances/medications that interact with benzodiazepines[b] • Renal or hepatic disease • COPD • Pregnancy • Drug consumption • Elderly • Uncontrolled hypo/hyperthyroidism • Psychiatric illness[c] • Obesity • ASA III or IV (depending on the setting)	• Obesity • Complex medical history that increases the risks
Benefits	• Safest approach • Short latent period • Can be titrated • Predictable • Cannula is already inserted for reversal agent (if needed) • Amnesia • Shorter recovery than oral and intranasal techniques	• More/all procedures done per session • No need for patient cooperation • Amnesia • Rapid onset of action
Limitations	• Cooperation for venepuncture • Venepuncture complications • Escort required • Needs trained team • Monitoring equipment required	• Affects protective reflexes • Greater risks • Expensive • Waiting list • Escort required (unless inpatient) • Needs trained team

[a] When used before intravenous sedation
COPD: Chronic obstructive pulmonary disease
[b] Alcohol and some medications increase the effects of benzodiazepines (e.g., clonidine, opioids, antidepressants, antipsychotics, antihistamines, erythromycin, and antiepileptics)
[c] Patients with psychiatric illnesses (e.g., hallucinations) can react in unexpected ways to sedation

    - The 2 main options include sedation or general anaesthesia
- Sedation
    - Inhalation, oral, intranasal, intravenous
    - Consideration needs to be given to several factors, such as type of procedure, level of anxiety, medical and social history, patient's preference
    - One tool that can help to make the decision more objective and support referral pathways is the Indicator of Sedation Need (IOSN) (Table 15.1.5)
    - The risks and benefits must be carefully assessed
    - Sedation must be performed by trained health teams in primary or secondary care, dependent on the sedation techniques, the patient's ASA grading and the country's regulations
    - The least invasive sedation technique is inhalation sedation using nitrous oxide
    - For more complex cases, sedation can be achieved by benzodiazepines through different routes (usually oral, intranasal or intravenous)
    - One of the most commonly used drugs is midazolam because of its very short half-life; intravenous

Table 15.1.5 Indicator of Sedation Need (IOSN).

IOSN domain	Scores	Source
Anxiety	1–3	MDAS 5–11 (minimum anxiety) – scores 1 MDAS 12–18 (moderate anxiety) – scores 2 MDAS 19–25 (high anxiety) – scores 3
Medical history	1–4	Medical/behavioural conditions (e.g. increased gag reflex, hypertension, angina, asthma, epilepsy, Parkinson disease, arthritis, multiple sclerosis)
Treatment complexity	1–4	Expected difficulty (e.g. dental extractions with bone removal, multiple restorative treatment in all quadrants)
IOSN metric	**IOSN descriptor**	**Sedation need?**
3–4	Minimal need	No
5–6	Moderate need	No
7–9	High need	Yes
10–11	Very high need	Yes

MDAS, Modified Dental Anxiety Scale.

administration is the safest approach, as it can be titrated according to the patient's response
  - In some cases, oral or intranasal sedation is given prior to intravenous sedation to help the patient cope with the cannulation stage
  - In case of oversedation, a reversal agent (flumazenil) can be administered, although this should be avoided by careful titration
  - There are also other techniques like rectal or intramuscular sedation, but they are less commonly used
  - Sedation can also be achieved by mixing more than 1 drug, which increases the complexity of the procedure
- General anaesthesia
  - General anaesthesia is an option for the most complex cases or if there are extensive dental treatment needs
  - In patients with other phobias, high anxiety or challenging behaviour, general anaesthesia provides an opportunity to do other needed procedures (e.g. blood tests)

Prognosis

- Due to the extensive treatment modalities and variability of anxieties/phobias, the prognosis is very variable
- Predictability of the treatment is one of the most effective approaches and has shown benefits over stop signal, simple visual distraction or listening to guided imagery through headphones
- A positive effect on tension and anxiety has also been seen when high levels of attention to distraction techniques are achieved
- Impact of listening to music or observing a picture poster seems to be limited
- Videos appear to achieve this better than audio distraction
- Low long-term success rates have been seen in people treated with hypnosis
- There is also evidence showing success over time with psychological interventions
- The use of sedatives does not allow the patient to 'learn' from the experience
- Therefore, a pharmacological approach should not be considered as an option to reduce anxiety in the long term, but as an adjunct in the treatment/used in the acute phase of treatment

A World/Transcultural View

- Anxiety disorders are highly prevalent worldwide and are associated with significant disability and economic impact
- The incidence of dental anxiety is reported to be within relatively similar ranges (10–42%) across the world, with most countries reporting incidences close to 20% of the population
- The settings and professionals that can administrate each type of sedation vary depending on the country

Recommended Reading

American Dental Association (ADA) (2016). *Guidelines for the Use of Sedation and General Anaesthesia by Dentists*. Chicago: ADA.

Asl, A.N., Shokravi, M., Jamali, Z., and Shirazi, S. (2017). Barriers and drawbacks of the assessment of dental fear, dental anxiety and dental phobia in children: a critical literature review. *J. Clin. Pediatr. Dent.* 41: 399–423.

Bellini, M., Maltoni, O., Gatto, M.R. et al. (2008). Dental phobia in dentistry patients. *Minerva Stomatol.* 57: 485–495.

Carter, A.E., Carter, G., Boschen, M. et al. (2014). Pathways of fear and anxiety in dentistry: a review. *World J. Clin. Cases* 2: 642–653.

Coulthard, P., Bridgman, C.M., Gough, L. et al. (2011). Estimating the need for dental sedation. 1. The Indicator of Sedation Need (IOSN) – a novel assessment tool. *Br. Dent. J.* 211: E10.

Kisely, S., Sawyer, E., Siskind, D., and Lalloo, R. (2016). The oral health of people with anxiety and depressive disorders – a systematic review and meta-analysis. *J. Affect. Disord.* 200: 119–132.

Kogan, C.S., Stein, D.J., Maj, M. et al. (2016). The classification of anxiety and fear-related disorders in the ICD-11. *Depress. Anxiety* 33: 1141–1154.

The Dental Faculties of the Royal College of Surgeons of England and the Royal College of Anaesthetists. (2020). *Standards for Conscious Sedation in the provision of Dental Care and Accreditation (The Report of the Intercollegiate Advisory Committee on Sedation in Dentistry)*. www.rcseng.ac.uk/dental-faculties/fds/publications-guidelines/standards-for-conscious-sedation-in-the-provision-of-dental-care-and-accreditation/

15.2 Depression

Section I: Clinical Scenario and Dental Considerations

Clinical Scenario

A 47-year-old female attends your dental clinic asking for replacement of her lost teeth. The appearance of her mouth is contributing to her low self-esteem. She no longer smiles and avoids leaving the house. She appears unkempt and is extremely thin.

Medical History
- Depression, diagnosed 22 years ago
- Asthma (controlled)
- Underweight (BMI = 16.3 kg/m^2)

Medications
- Fluoxetine
- Fluticasone/salmeterol
- Salbutamol

Dental History
- Irregular dental attender; last visit was 4 years ago
- Reports consuming chocolates, pastries and soft drinks several times a day but does not have regular meals
- Brushes her teeth intermittently; often forgets

Social History
- Single, lives alone, no next of kin
- No contact telephone number
- Occasional informal jobs helping her neighbours
- Receives disability pension due to depression
- Tobacco: cigarettes 2–4/week
- Alcohol: 14 units per week (binge drinking)
- Other drugs: cocaine base paste (cocaine, tobacco, cannabis mix) with tobacco in a pipe once a week (5 years); previously used to consume cannabis

Oral Examination
- Vertical dimension loss
- Palatine torus
- Dry tongue/mouth
- Generalised soft and hard deposits
- Generalised periodontitis
- Partially edentate (Figure 15.2.1)
- Retained roots: #17, #24, #27 and #41(Figure 15.2.2)
- Extensive caries: #15, #23, #34, #32, #31, #43 and #44 (Figure 15.2.3)

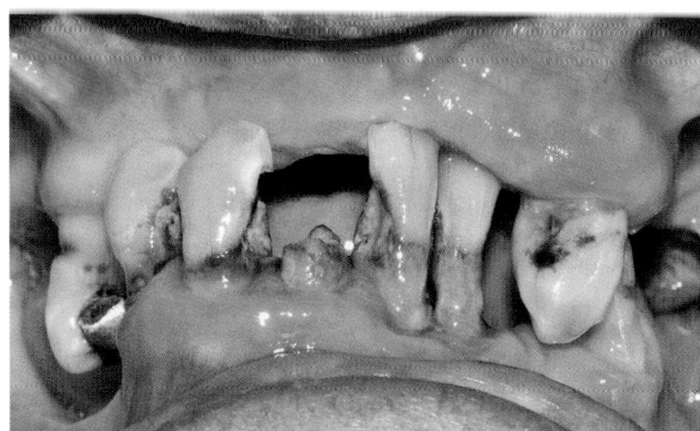

Figure 15.2.1 Partially edentate, deep overbite, multiple carious teeth.

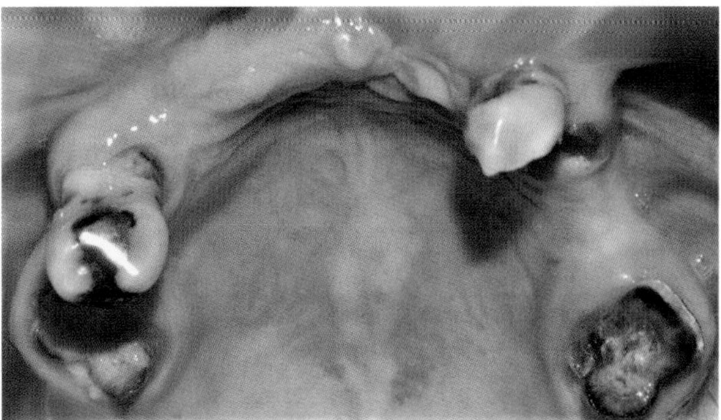

Figure 15.2.2 Maxillary dentition: retained roots #17, #24 and #27; palatine torus.

A Practical Approach to Special Care in Dentistry, First Edition. Edited by Pedro Diz Dios and Navdeep Kumar.

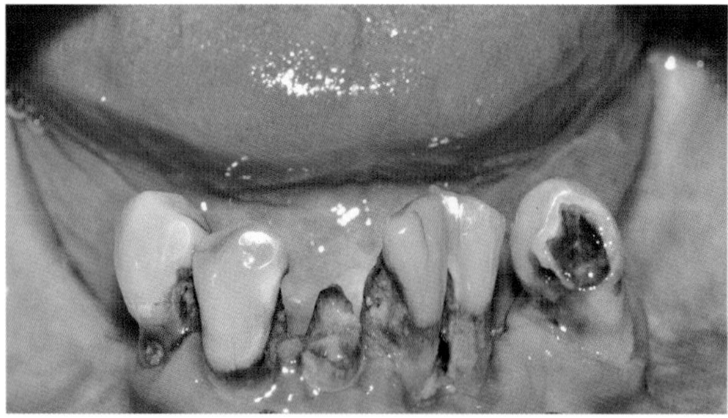

Figure 15.2.3 Mandibular dentition: retained root #41; caries in #34, #32, #31, #43 and #44.

Radiological Examination

- Full-mouth periapical radiographs undertaken (Figure 15.2.4)
- #17, #24 and #27: retained roots with apical lesions
- #41: retained root
- #23: deep distal caries with pulpal involvement, mesial caries
- #31 and #32: extensive cervical caries; extensive horizontal bone loss
- Further dental caries: #15 deep cervical caries, #34 buccal and distal caries, #43 deep mesial caries, #44 mesial caries, #42 missing; generalised bone loss (~60–80%)

Structured Learning

1) What could be the connection between the patient's depression and her low body mass index (BMI)?
   - Depression and eating disorders have a bidirectional relationship
   - An additional diagnosis of anorexia nervosa should be considered
   - This will have a further impact on the social, medical and dental risk factors when planning care
2) What factors have contributed to the poor dental status of this patient?
   - Self-neglect
   - Irregular dental attender
   - Cariogenic diet
   - Fluoxetine can cause a dry mouth and hence increase the dental caries risk further
   - Cocaine use can also result in a dry mouth
   - Binge drinking can lead to further oral neglect
   - Asthma medication oral side-effects (see Chapter 9.2)
3) The patient is convinced that improving her dental appearance will help her find a job and hence cure her depression. Is she correct?
   - Loss of teeth and unattractive smile can have an impact on the patient's psychological state, increasing low self-esteem, withdrawal and isolation

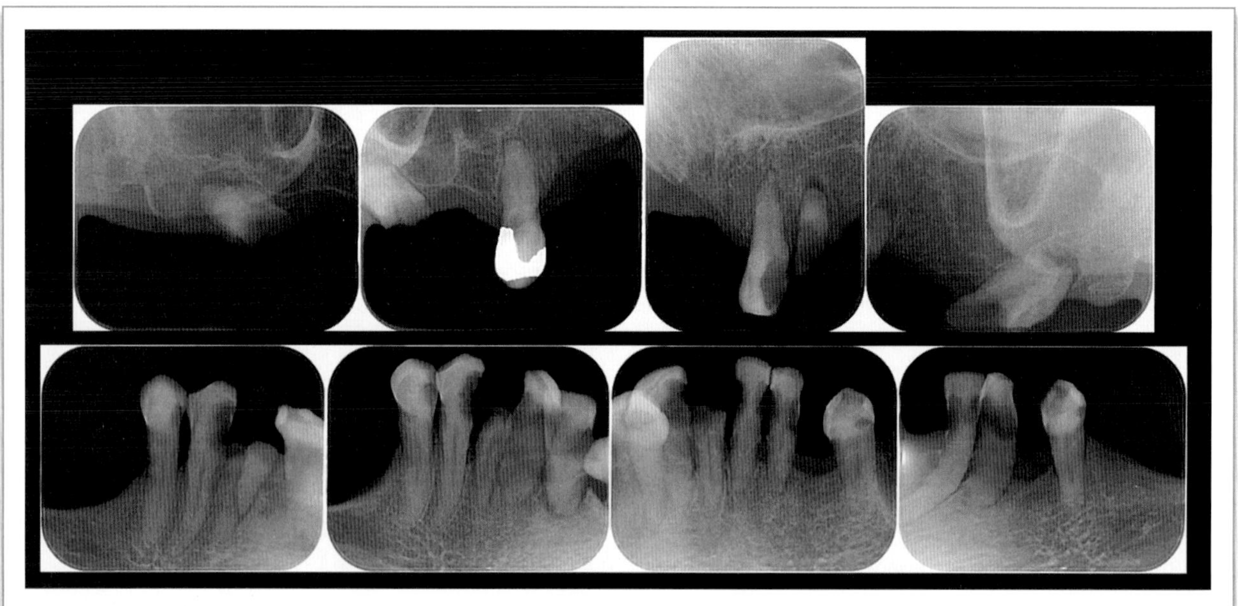

Figure 15.2.4 Full-mouth periapical radiographs demonstrating multiple retained roots and carious teeth.

- Although improving the appearance of the teeth may be a positive action, it will not cure her depression
- The patient's expectations need to be realistic

4) What factors do you need to consider in your risk assessment for the management of this patient?
   - Social
     - Irregular attender, poor compliance and tolerance
     - Associated habits (see Chapters 15.4 and 15.5)
     - No telephone contact number
     - No escort or next of kin
     - Financial constraints (irregular income)
   - Medical
     - Asthma (consider patient's triggers) (see Chapter 9.2)
     - Low BMI; poor diet (risk of deficiencies/anaemia/delayed healing)
     - Potential increased bleeding risk (side-effect from fluoxetine)
   - Dental
     - Deep overbite
     - Reduced denture retention (mandibular ridge resorbed posteriorly; palatine torus; dry mouth)
     - Poor dental status
     - Managing expectations
5) The patient wants dental treatment to commence immediately. What would you need to ensure in relation to her depression?
   - Ideally, a course of dental treatment should be scheduled when the patient is actively accessing support for their depression
   - This will increase the likelihood of a successful dental treatment outcome
   - Some simple dental procedures (e.g. retained root extractions) can be provided to stimulate the patient and help change attitudes and habits
6) Given that the prognosis of her remaining teeth is poor, you advise a dental clearance followed by provision of complete denture. What would be the challenges in relation to construction of a denture?
   - Construction of an immediate denture is not advisable due to the loss of multiple teeth and gross caries in the remaining teeth
   - Healing after the dental extractions may be delayed
   - Multiple visits required to construct the denture
   - Retention may be reduced in relation to xerostomia and the presence of a palatine torus
7) The patient fails to attend the dental appointment booked to commence dental extractions. What would you do?
   - This may be a safeguarding concern, particularly if the patient reports suicidal ideation
   - As the patient has no next of kin/family or telephone number, contact the doctor to register your concern

General Dental Considerations

Oral Findings

- Oral neglect
- Xerostomia
- Caries
- Periodontal disease (including necrotising ulcerative gingivitis/periodontitis in severe cases of depression)
- Bruxism and attrition
- Sialadenitis
- Cheilitis
- Dysphagia
- Facial dyskinesia caused by antidepressants
- Oral lichen planus
- Recurrent aphthous stomatitis
- Atypical facial pain
- Burning mouth syndrome
- Temporomandibular pain dysfunction syndrome
- People with depression are 20–30% more likely to be edentulous
- Depression is closely linked to unhealthy habits (tobacco, alcohol and drug consumption, and poor eating habits); oral manifestations linked to these, including the risk of oral cancer, need to be considered

Dental Management

- Referral for psychological diagnosis and support should be considered in a patient where depression is suspected
- If there is immediate concern regarding the patient's well-being (e.g. suicidal ideation), emergency services should be contacted
- A sympathetic, non-judgemental approach is essential when planning and providing care
- Goals are difficult to maintain in the long term and recurrences are frequent. Treatment goals may need to be reassessed depending on the patient's level of engagement and compliance (Table 15.2.1)

Section II: Background Information and Guidelines

Definition

Depression is a common mental disorder affecting 320 million people worldwide. It is characterised by persistent sadness and a lack of interest or pleasure in previously rewarding or enjoyable activities (WHO). It can lead to a variety of emotional and physical problems, and can dramatically affect a person's ability to function and live a

Table 15.2.1 Considerations for dental management.

Risk assessment	• The patient may appear withdrawn, difficult or aggressive • Safeguarding concerns if there is associated self-harm ideation
Criteria for referral	• Dentists should be able to manage the vast majority of patients with mild depression • Uncontrolled depression (e.g. suicidal ideation) requires referral • Institutionalised patients may require a home visit
Access/position	• Avoid early morning appointments if there is associated sleep disturbance • Failed appointments should be followed up with a phone call to ensure that the patient is not at risk
Communication	• Empathetic and non-patronising approach • Identifying a specific goal in conjunction with the medical team (social/medical) is the key to motivating the patient (e.g. improving appearance and ability to eat)
Consent/capacity	• Depression can cause problems with attention and memory – it is important to ensure that the patient understands and can remember what is being discussed
Anaesthesia/sedation	• Local anaesthesia – Potential interaction of antidepressants and epinephrine (no clinical evidence); common measures should be undertaken such as avoid intravascular injection, use of aspirating syringe, not exceeding 0.05 mg of epinephrine • Sedation Best avoided in patients on or within 21 days of MAOIs (risk of coma) and SSRIs (potentiation) • General anaesthesia – Best avoided in patients on MAOIs (risk of respiratory depression and coma) – Caution in patients on amitriptyline (sedative)
Dental treatment	• Before – Adapt the planned treatment in relation to patient's mood and ability to continue that day • During – Continued empathetic communication • After – TCAs and MAOIs can cause postural hypotension; the dental chair should be slowly brought upright if the patient has been reclined during treatment – Close follow-up needs to be a priority to avoid the need for future invasive procedures
Drug prescription	• Paracetamol inhibits metabolism of TCAs • MAOIs interact with opioids • Erythromycin can be potentiated by SSRIs • Issue minimum effective quantity of medication, ideally to be administered by the escort
Education/prevention	• Focus should be placed on the association between prevention and the maintenance of a healthy dentition/smile • A strict preventive programme is recommended in major depression as it is usually associated with multiple risk factors (e.g. lack of interest in oral hygiene, cariogenic diet, decreased salivary flow)

MAOI, monoamine oxidase inhibitor; SSRI, selective serotonin reuptake inhibitor; TCA, tricyclic antidepressant.

rewarding life. The lifetime risk of developing depression is 10% in the general population, affecting more women than men (2:1). It is a major global cause of disability, and is the most common disorder contributing to suicide.

Aetiopathogenesis

Depression is the result of complex interactions between multiple factors.

- Genetics
  - Depression is known to run in families, suggesting that genetic factors contribute to the risk of developing this disease
  - However, research into the genetics of depression is in its early stages
  - Studies suggest that variations in many genes, each with a small effect, combine to increase the risk of developing depression
- Biological
  - Changes in the hypothalamus (which regulates serotonin, dopamine and noradrenaline) are common in people with depression and have implications for circadian rhythms, food intake and libido
  - Higher risk of depression in women has been associated with hormonal changes (e.g. menstrual cycle changes, pregnancy, menopause)
  - Consequence of drug treatments (e.g. ibuprofen, corticosteroids, benzodiazepines, levodopa, oral contraceptives) or withdrawal of psychoactive drugs
  - More common in patients with viral infections (e.g. viral hepatitis, mononucleosis, HIV/AIDS), Parkinson disease, myocardial infarction, malignant diseases, arthritis, endocrinopathies, diabetes, cancer, brain injury, dementia
  - A bidirectional relation between cardiovascular disease and depression has been established
- Social
  - Significant life events (e.g. unemployment, trauma, grief)
  - Not exercising, being under- or overweight and having fewer social relationships can also increase the risk of experiencing depressive symptoms
- Psychological
  - Other mental health conditions such as schizophrenia
  - Psychological impact of chronic conditions
- Duration, timing or presumed aetiology differentiates several types of depressive disorders:
  - Disruptive mood dysregulation disorder
  - Major depressive disorder (classic presentation)
  - Persistent depressive disorder (dysthymia)
  - Premenstrual dysphoric disorder
  - Substance/medication-induced depressive disorder
  - Depressive disorder due to another medical condition
  - Other specified depressive disorder
  - Unspecified depressive disorder

Table 15.2.2 Major depressive disorder diagnostic criteria according to the American Psychiatric Association.

Diagnostic criteria	Assessment for diagnosis
A. Symptoms – Depressed mood: feels sad, empty, hopeless, appears tearful Evident reduced interest or pleasure in all (or almost all) activities. – Significant weight loss (without diet) or weight gain (more than 5% of body weight in a month), or appetite change – Insomnia or hypersomnia – Psychomotor agitation or retardation – Loss of energy – Feelings of worthlessness or excessive guilt – Concentration problems or indecisiveness – Recurrent thoughts of death, suicidal ideation or a suicide attempt B. The symptoms affect areas of functioning or cause clinically significant distress C. Not attributable to the effects of a substance or to another medical condition D. It is not better explained by other psychotic disorders E. There has never been a manic or hypomanic episode	• Needs at least 5 symptoms of criterion A during the same 2-week period • At least 1 of the symptoms is either depressed mood or loss of interest or pleasure • All of the symptoms present every day or nearly every day (exception suicidal ideation)

Source: Modified from American Psychiatric Association, Diagnostic and Statistical Manual of Mental Disorders (DSM-5®), American Psychiatric Pub, 2013.

Diagnosis

- Depressive disorders are defined by their characteristic features:
  - Depressive mood (e.g. sad, irritable, empty)
  - Loss of pleasure or interest (anhedonia), which can be accompanied by other symptoms such as cognitive, neurovegetative or behavioural changes
- Diagnosis is undertaken on clinical assessment, following psychiatric guidelines such as the DSM-5 (Table 15.2.2)
- Severity of depression (from mild to severe) tends to be assessed on the clinical evaluation of the number and severity of symptoms and their impact in the daily life
- The presence of anhedonia is associated with severe depression, in contrast to somatic symptoms being related to moderate depression. There are also tools that have been designed to assess severity of the illness, such as the Hamilton Depression Rating Scale (HAMD)

Clinical Presentation

- Symptoms of depression may be psychological, social, cognitive and/or somatic (Table 15.2.3)
- Men tend to present with irritable mood, exhaustion, sleeping pattern alterations and loss of interest in their hobbies, while women are more likely to have feelings of sadness, worthlessness and guilt

Management

- Community prevention programmes
  - Examples include school-based programmes for children, interventions for parents of children with behavioural problems, exercise programmes for the elderly
- Psychological support
  - Individual counselling or group approaches
  - Techniques consist of talking therapies such as behavioural activation, cognitive behavioural therapy and interpersonal psychotherapy
  - In cases of severe depression, the treatment focus must be prevention of suicide
- Antidepressant medication (Table 15.2.4)
  - Antidepressants are not recommended for the initial treatment of mild depression, because the risk–benefit ratio is poor
  - Antidepressant are indicated where mild depression persists or is associated with psychosocial and medical problems, as well as in moderate to severe depression
  - In severe cases, where augmentation of antidepressants is needed, antipsychotics, lithium or other antidepressants may be considered
- Diet and exercise
  - A healthy diet and regular exercise may be as effective as antidepressants in reducing symptoms of depression
- Complementary therapies
  - Herbal therapy (*Hypericum perforatum* – St John's wort) has been used in cases of mild depression
  - Mindfulness, aromatherapy, acupuncture, massage, meditation and yoga may also improve emotional well-being
- Electroconvulsive therapy
  - Based on the concept of inducing a seizure in a controlled environment (under general anaesthesia)
  - It is a controversial treatment, indicated in cases of severe depression when a quick response is needed or when other techniques have proved unsuccessful
  - Amnesia is the most common side-effect
- Transcranial direct current stimulation (tDCS)
  - Involves using a small battery-operated machine to pass a low current through the brain to stimulate activity
  - Although there are no major safety concerns, there is limited evidence regarding the effectiveness of this technique

Table 15.2.3 Symptoms of depression.

Psychological	Social	Cognitive	Somatic
• Low/irritable mood • Feeling of emptiness/hopelessness • Low self-esteem • Feeling guilty • Pessimism • Self-harm • Suicidal thoughts/attempts	• Lack of motivation • Social isolation • Loss of interest in hobbies • Avoiding contact with loved ones	• Problems concentrating • Difficulty when learning new things • Difficulty in making decisions • Problems at work	• Fatigue • Moving/speaking slower • Changes in appetite/weight • Unexplained pains • Changes in sleep patterns • Anxiety • Loss of libido • Constipation • Menstrual cycle changes

Table 15.2.4 Most common types of antidepressant drugs.

Type of antidepressant	Mode of action	Systemic side-effects	Oral side-effects	Examples
Monoamine oxidase inhibitors (MAOIs)	• Inhibit MAO-A, an enzyme that breaks down norepinephrine and serotonin • First type of antidepressants used • Not commonly prescribed now due to side-effects • Interaction with opioids	• Hypotension • Anorexia • Nausea • Diarrhoea • Constipation • Insomnia • Sexual dysfunction • Weight gain • Tremor • Food and drug interactions (risk of hypertensive crises)	• Dry mouth • Stomatitis • Oral ulcers	• Moclobemide • Phenelzine • Isoniazid • Tranylcypromine • Selegiline • Isocarboxazid
Tricyclic antidepressants (TCAs)	• Block reuptake of norepinephrine and serotonin • Most effective but slow onset (4 weeks for full effect) • Greatest risk of overdose (excluding lofepramine)	• Sedation (especially amitriptyline) • Constipation • Bladder problems • Sexual dysfunction • Blurred vision • Dizziness • Weight gain • Drowsiness • Tardive dyskinesia (amoxapine) • Photosensitive rashes (trimipramine)	• Dry mouth • Dysgeusia • Sialadenitis • Stomatitis • Gingivitis • Caries • Cheilitis • Dysphagia • Oral ulcers • Facial oedema	• Amitriptyline • Imipramine • Nortriptyline • Dolesupin • Doxepin • Lomipramine • Lofepramine • Protriptyline • Amoxapine • Trimipramine • Clomipramine • Desipramine
Selective serotonin reuptake inhibitors (SSRIs)	• Block reuptake of serotonin • First line of treatment • Fewer adverse effects • Do not interact with alcohol • Affect metabolism of benzodiazepines, erythromycin	• Headaches • Dizziness • GI problems • Arrhythmias (terfenadine) • Agitation • Anorexia • Nausea • Diarrhoea • Anxiety • Sexual dysfunction • Visual disturbances • Insomnia	• Dry mouth • Dysgeusia • Sialadenitis • Stomatitis • Gingivitis • Caries • Glossitis • Bruxism • Dysphagia • Gingival hyperplasia[a]	• Fluoxetine • Sertraline • Citalopram • Escitalopram • Fluvoxamine • Paroxetine • Terfenadine • Vilazodone
Serotonin and norepinephrine reuptake inhibitors (SNRIs)	• Block reuptake of norepinephrine and serotonin • Slow onset (4–6 weeks for full effect) • Higher risk of death due to overdose	• Headaches • Dizziness • Sweating • Fatigue • Insomnia • Constipation • Weight gain • Sexual dysfunction • Hypertension	• Dry mouth • Dysgeusia • Stomatitis • Candidiasis • Glossitis • Bruxism • Dysphagia • Halitosis • Oral ulcers	• Venlafaxine • Desvenlafaxine • Levomilnacipran • Duloxetine

(Continued)

Table 15.2.4 (Continued)

Type of antidepressant	Mode of action	Systemic side-effects	Oral side-effects	Examples
Noradrenergic and specific serotonergic antidepressants (NASSAs)	• Block reuptake of norepinephrine and serotonin • No significant drug interactions • Commonly used in elderly • Fewer side-effects than SSRI (specific receptors targeted) • Sometimes classified as tetracyclic antidepressant	• Sedation • Headaches • Anxiety • Insomnia • Fatigue • Diarrhoea • Constipation • Arthralgia • Myalgia • Weight increase • Orthostatic hypotension • Bone marrow depression	• Dry mouth	• Mirtazapine • Esmirtazapine • Setiptiline

Other types of antidepressant drugs include selective norepinephrine reuptake inhibitors (NRIs), serotonin antagonist and reuptake inhibitors (SARIs), norepinephrine and dopamine reuptake inhibitors (NDRIs), tetracyclic antidepressants, melatonergic agonist and serotonin antagonist, multimodal serotonergic antidepressants.
GI, gastrointestinal; [a]Sertraline.

- Repetitive transcranial magnetic stimulation (rTMS)
  - TMS uses electromagnetic coils to deliver pulses of magnetic energy to specific parts of the brain
  - This stimulates the brain and may help to reduce depression and anxiety
  - There is evidence that this is a relatively safe and effective technique but it is not widely available

Prognosis

- Depending on the type of depression, it is possible to recover from depression with the correct support in place
- Success rates are higher in younger patients and may approach 80–90%
- Pharmacological treatment is given on average for 2 years, although some patients may require it for a lifetime
- After one episode of depression, the risk of another is 50%
- With each additional episode, this risk rises, increasing to 70% after a second episode and 90% after the third
- Moderate to severe depression can significantly affect the person's ability to function in terms of daily living
- Depression plays a role in more than half of all suicide attempts, whereas the lifetime risk of suicide among patients with untreated depressive disorder is nearly 20%
- Despite depression being more commonly diagnosed in women, suicide is 4 times more likely in men (men are less likely to admit signs of severe depression and doctors are less likely to recognise it in them)
- Smoking, drugs and alcohol use are more common in depression and are associated with health risks
- Serotonin toxicity (serotonin syndrome) is a potentially life-threatening condition resulting from excess serotonin in the central nervous system; it can appear as a result of taking high doses of medication, due to the summative effect of different antidepressants, or as a result of interaction between antidepressants and other drugs

A World/Transcultural View

- Depression is the most common disease worldwide
- Most people will exhibit depressive symptoms at some point in their life and hence the burden of depression and other mental health conditions is on the rise globally
- Although there are known effective treatments for depression, fewer than half of those affected in the world (in many countries, fewer than 10%) receive such treatments
- Barriers to effective care include a lack of resources, lack of trained healthcare providers and social stigma associated with mental disorders
- Another barrier to effective care is inaccurate assessment – in countries of all income levels, people who are depressed are often not correctly diagnosed, and others who do not have the disorder are too often misdiagnosed and prescribed antidepressants

Recommended Reading

Cademartori, M.G., Gastal, M.T., Nascimento, G.G. et al. (2018). Is depression associated with oral health outcomes in adults and elders? A systematic review and meta-analysis. *Clin. Oral Invest.* 22: 2685–2702.

Friedlander, A.H., Friedlander, I.K., Yagiela, J.A., and Eth, S. (1993). Dental management of the child and adolescent with major depression. *ASDC J. Dent. Child.* 60: 125–131.

Friedlander, A.H., Kawakami, K.K., Ganzell, S., and Fitten, L.J. (1993). Dental management of the geriatric patient with major depression. *Spec. Care Dentist.* 13: 249–253.

Friedlander, A.H. and Mahler, M.E. (2001). Major depressive disorder. Psychopathology, medical management and dental implications. *J. Am. Dent. Assoc.* 132: 629–638.

Friedlander, A.H. and Norman, D.C. (2002). Late-life depression: psychopathology, medical interventions, and dental implications. *Oral Surg. Oral Med. Oral Pathol. Oral Radiol. Endod.* 94: 404–412.

Fukuhara, S., Asai, K., Kakeno, A. et al. (2021). Association of education and depressive symptoms with tooth loss. *J. Dent. Res.* 100: 361–368.

Malhi, G.S. and Mann, J.J. (2018). Depression. *Lancet* 392: 2299–2312.

National Institute for Health and Care Excellence (NICE). (2009). *Depression in Adults: Recognition and Management. NICE Clinical Guideline [CG90].* www.nice.org.uk/guidance/cg90

15.3 Schizophrenia

Section I: Clinical Scenario and Dental Considerations

Clinical Scenario

A 53-year-old male presents for an emergency dental appointment complaining that a crown in the upper right quadrant (#14) became the day before when he was eating. There is no associated pain or swelling. The patient has brought the crown with him and wants it recemented. He attends with his wife.

Medical History
- Schizophrenia
  - Diagnosed when 19 years old; first episode associated with an incident of severe stress
  - Followed by hospital admission for 1 month during which he received 3 electroshock therapy sessions
  - Under treatment with psychiatrist; several inpatient admissions over the years
  - In the past managed with pipotiazine injections twice a month for 11 years, but discontinued due to the development of severe tardive dyskinesia
- Tardive dyskinesia predominantly of the hands and face (persistent movement of the mandible)
- Depression
- Hypertension
- Hypercholesterolaemia
- Gastro-oesophageal reflux disease
- Nasal obstruction due to polyps
- Possible mild cognitive deterioration (reported by wife)

Medications
- Quetiapine
- Trihexyphenidyl
- Fluoxetine
- Hydrochlorothiazide
- Losartan
- Atorvastatin
- Metoclopramide

Dental History
- Irregular attender; only attends if there are dental problems; last visit was a month ago to a mobile clinic close to his home after his anterior bridge came off – he had this recemented
- Prior to this, no dental treatment for the last 5 years
- He states that he does not trust dentists because every time he visits, they are always trying to take his teeth out
- Brushes once a day (only in the morning)
- Uses a mouthwash intermittently as he has a bad taste in his mouth
- Highly cariogenic diet, including high-sugar carbonated drinks 4–6 times/day

Social History
- Lives in the countryside with his wife, 2 daughters and 3 grandchildren
- ‘Disappears’ occasionally and has been found in shelters (reported by wife)
- Currently unemployed; has difficulty keeping jobs due to paranoid thoughts; previously worked as a security guard
- Receiving disability pension
- Relies on his wife to accompany him to his appointments as he reports that he has extreme exhaustion
- Tobacco consumption: 20–30 cigarettes daily for 30 years
- Alcohol consumption: sporadic; binge-drinking episodes weekly with 15–20 units consumed
- Cocaine use: 2 recent episodes associated with suicide attempts

Oral Examination
- Incompetent lips with gingival show
- Mouth breather
- Xerostomia (Figure 15.3.1)
- Bilateral tongue and cheek biting (clenches teeth together when stressed)
- Fissured tongue
- Generalised periodontal disease
- Gingival recession

A Practical Approach to Special Care in Dentistry, First Edition. Edited by Pedro Diz Dios and Navdeep Kumar.

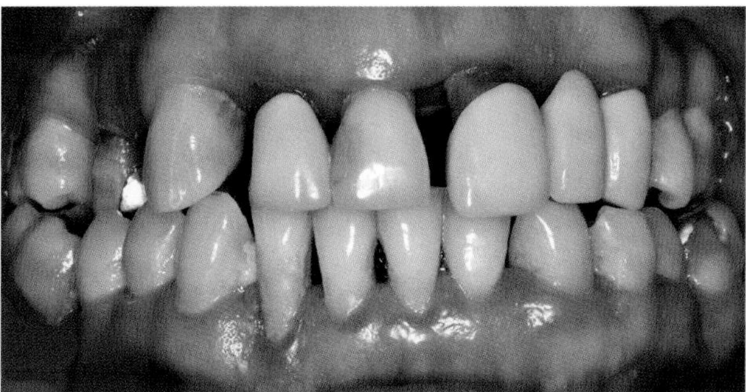

Figure 15.3.1 Anterior dentition – gingival recession, xerostomia.

- #14: retained and carious root (Figure 15.3.2)
- #12: grade II mobility
- Bridge upper left quadrant: grade I mobility, gingival recession
- #46: pus exudate from buccal sinus

Radiological Examination

- Orthopantomogram undertaken (Figure 15.3.3)
- #14: short retained root, no endodontic treatment, radiolucent periapical area
- #15: endodontic treatment (short in length)
- #12 and #21: endodontic treatment
- #46: perio-endo lesion with advanced bone loss
- Generalised bone loss (~60–70%) and subgingival calculus present

Structured Learning

1) How may this patient's schizophrenia have affected his dental attendance?
   - Low dental care utilisation is more common
   - This may be related to factors such as heightened anxiety, lack of interest in self-care, amotivational state/extreme exhaustion, unemployment (limited financial means)

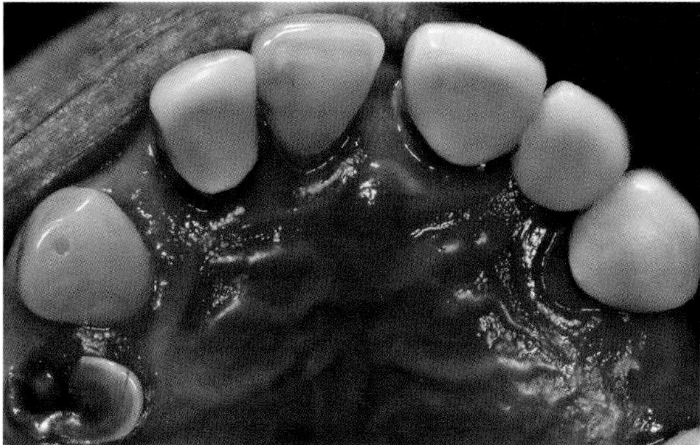

Figure 15.3.2 Maxillary dentition – retained root #14, extensive subgingival caries.

2) What information would you need in order to carry out an appropriate risk assessment for the management of this patient?
   - Further detail on the management of his mental illness and compliance with treatment
   - Presence of any comorbidities/confirmation of the details with his medical practitioner
   - Social history/availability of escort (wife normally looks after the grandchildren)
3) What characteristics of this specific patient are likely to have had a negative impact on his oral health?
   - Compliance issues in daily life (reported by wife)
   - Lack of perceived need
   - Attitudinal and possibly cognitive difficulties
   - Underlying depression (see Chapter 15.2)
   - Motor problems due to tardive dyskinesia
   - Long-term tobacco consumption
   - Mouth breather
   - Dry mouth (related to mouth breathing and polypharmacy)
   - Poor oral health habits and diet
   - Gastro-oesophageal reflux disease
4) The tooth #14 retained root has subgingival caries. The core has fractured and is inside the detached crown. The bad taste in his mouth originates from the #46 draining buccal sinus. The #14 and #46 require extraction. What are the challenges when discussing this with the patient?
   - Mistrust due to problems with inference of people's intentions (particularly with dentists)
   - Anxiety and phobia
   - Cognition and potential attention defects
   - Delusions/disorganised thought processes
   - Irregular attender – may not return if he feels you are not providing the treatment he wants (tooth replacement)
5) After a lengthy discussion, the patient agrees to have the #14 and #46 extracted as long as the gaps are filled immediately. What are some of the gap replacement options and associated risks?
   - Removable prosthesis (immediate/post-immediate denture): cost, compliance, reduced retention due to xerostomia and dyskinetic movements, loss of denture, poor aesthetics (high smile line, gaps)
   - Fixed prosthesis: cost, periodontal disease, poor support from potential abutment teeth, multiple gaps, maintenance
   - Dental implants: cost, periodontal disease, smoking, clenching, compliance, maintenance
6) What factors do you need to consider in your risk assessment for the management of this patient?

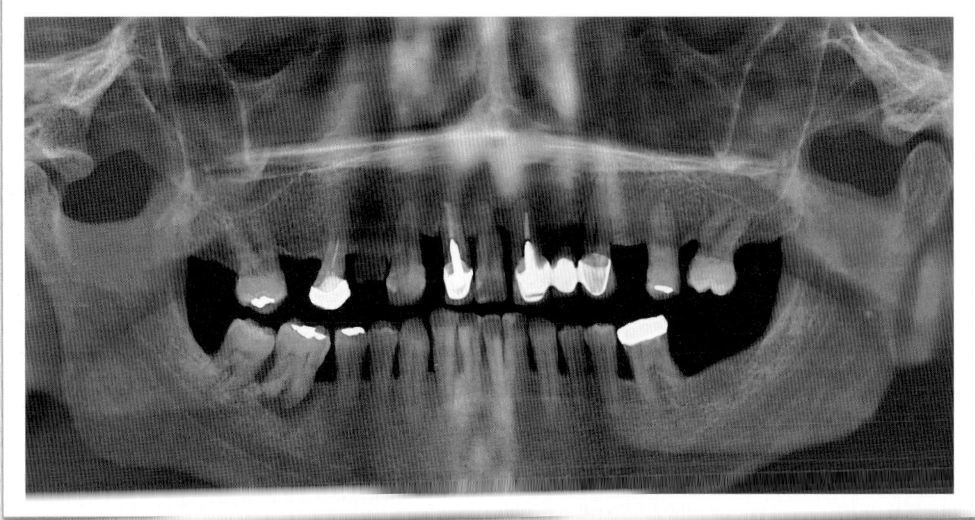

Figure 15.3.3 Orthopantomogram showing generalised bone loss, #46 perio-endo lesion, retained root #14.

- Social
  - Availability/suitability of wife as an escort
  - Impact of binge drinking prior to dental visits on attendance and ability to proceed with dental treatment, especially sedation, and capacity to provide informed consent
  - Limited financial means
- Medical
  - Side-effects of medication, most notably tardive dyskinesia
  - Depression (see Chapter 15.2)
  - Hypertension (see Chapter 8.1)
  - Potential airway obstruction due to nasal polyps
  - Possible mild cognitive deterioration (reported by wife)
- Dental
  - Lack of perceived need for dental care, poor attendance
  - High caries risk: highly cariogenic diet, xerostomia, suboptimal oral hygiene habits, irregular dental attender
  - Access to the mouth impaired by persistent movements of the mandible
  - Gastro-oesophageal reflux disease is associated with an increased risk of dental erosion
  - Capacity and compliance for dental treatment are likely to be impaired

General Dental Considerations

Oral Findings

- Severity of schizophrenia is negatively related to oral health, with more severe symptoms associated with more caries, periodontal disease and prosthetic unmet needs
- Presence of negative symptoms has been linked to self-neglect
- Patients treated with atypical antipsychotics may have better oral health when compared to individuals treated with typical neuroleptics
- Oral findings associated with schizophrenia include:
  - Poor oral hygiene (limited compliance, tardive dyskinesia)
  - Caries
  - Periodontal disease
  - Heavily stained teeth/prostheses (associated with tobacco consumption) (Figure 15.3.4)
  - Dry mouth (as a side-effect of neuroleptic medication)
  - Hypersalivation (as a side-effect of haloperidol and clozapine)
  - Attrition (in cases of tardive dyskinesia)
  - Candidosis (as a consequence of dry mouth)
  - Oral pigmentation (as a side-effect of neuroleptic medication)
  - Dysphagia and speech difficulties (due to muscle rigidity or spams)

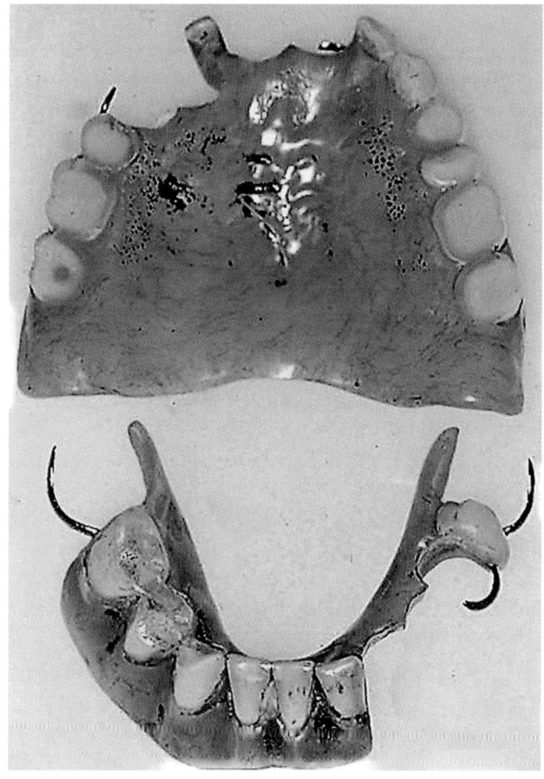

Figure 15.3.4 Dental prosthesis heavily stained due to compulsive smoking and severe tooth wear due to dental attrition (after only 1 year of use).

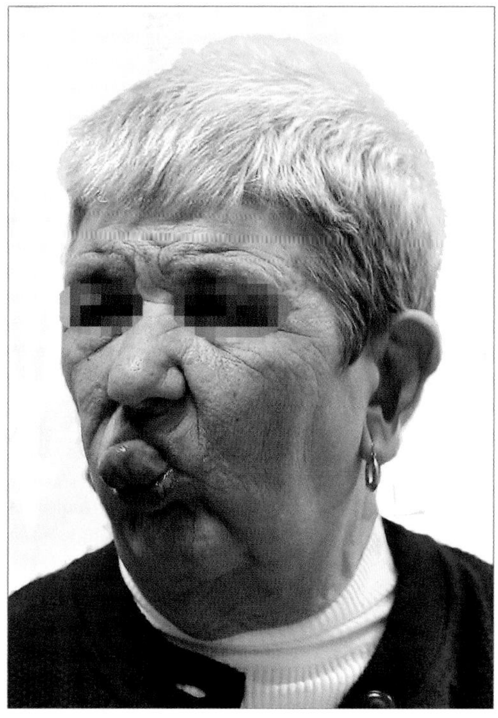

Figure 15.3.5 Tardive oral dyskinesia.

- Orofacial dystonia/tardive dyskinesia (as a side-effect of neuroleptic medication, e.g. phenothiazines) (Figure 15.3.5)
- Parafunctional habits (e.g. nail or lip biting, bruxism)
- Delusional oral symptoms
- Self-mutilation
- A palatal rugae randomly distributed pattern has been described
- Oral cancer risk (associated with tobacco consumption)

Dental Management

- Each patient will require careful assessment to ensure that the most appropriate supportive approach is implemented (Table 15.3.1)

Section II: Background Information and Guidelines

Definition

Schizophrenia is considered a chronic, severe and heterogeneous mental disorder, characterised by distortions in thinking, perception, emotions, language, sense of self and behaviour (WHO). It has an important impact on daily life, leading to one-third of patients being severely disabled by the condition. Lifetime prevalence is close to 1% but it may vary according to race and country. Reported differences in distribution between males and females depend on the definition and diagnostic criteria used. Wider concepts, such as those that include mood symptoms, allow more women to be included, with a similar risk for both sexes emerging.

Aetiopathogenesis

- Schizophrenia appears to be the result of an imbalance related to dopamine and glutamate, with dopamine overactivity in the mesolimbic pathway of the brain
- Brain structure abnormalities in variable regions of the brain have also been described; these can affect the prefrontal and temporal cortex, grey matter volume, white matter connectivity and cellular architecture
- Some studies also propose that the condition is due to a neurodevelopmental disorder in the foetus, in which inappropriate neuron connections have been formed
- Risk factors
  - Genetic: implicated in only 10% of cases

Table 15.3.1 Considerations for dental management.

Risk assessment	• Behaviour may appear bizarre, unpredictable or inappropriate • Self-neglect, loss of drive, lack of coping strategies, leading to difficulty achieving compliance • Lack of perceived need for medical/dental care • Loss of facial expression, monotonous voice and disordered speech are common, making communication and assessment of patient motivation difficult • Higher incidence of unhealthy habits, including higher consumption of tobacco, alcohol and/or drugs • Extrapyramidal symptoms related to neuroleptic drugs may be present, making dental management challenging • Gag reflex impairment and dysphagia have also been described; may be related to tardive orofacial dyskinesia, anticholinergics, neuroleptic-induced dystonia or inherent swallowing abnormalities/tongue thrust • Phenothiazines can cause dose-related impaired temperature regulation and are also occasionally associated with obstructive jaundice, leucopenia or electrocardiogram (ECG) changes
Criteria for referral	• Most patients with schizophrenia should be seen in primary care • The patient should be referred if they have significant medical issues or there is a concern regarding their behaviour where treatment in the same hospital setting as their psychiatry care would be advantageous
Access/position	• Access to dental care may be limited: financial issues (unemployment levels higher); frequent inpatient stays • Timing: determine patterns in patient compliance (e.g. sleep pattern alterations and risk of drug or alcohol abuse) • Elective dental treatment may need to be postponed in the case of an acute episode • Short appointments are recommended
Communication	• Challenging to obtain a full medical history, as patients have difficulty separating non-relevant information from important details; they may also avoid talking about their mental illness • Open, non-judgemental approach required (especially when asking about schizophrenia diagnosis) • Avoidance of whispering as this can induce paranoid thoughts • Anticipation/explanation of next steps during treatment can help reduce anxiety
Consent/capacity	• Variable – may be unaltered if the schizophrenia is under control • However, cognitive changes including verbal memory impairments, social cognition difficulties and attention deficits and paranoia may affect the decision-making process
Anaesthesia/sedation	• Local anaesthesia – Consider avoidance of vasoconstrictor: interaction with phenothiazines causing epinephrine reversal, hence vasodilation instead of vasoconstriction; haloperidol and droperidol can also block vasoconstriction with epinephrine • Sedation – Best avoided – Risk of hallucinations due to interaction between some neuroleptics and sedatives • General anaesthesia – May be the only management option if urgent/emergency treatment is required – Best avoided due to risk of severe hypotension, especially with intravenous barbiturates

(*Continued*)

Table 15.3.1 (Continued)

Dental treatment	• Before – Importance of clear, confirmed medical history – Confirm compliance with schizophrenia treatment – Consider possible side-effects of medication, such as tardive dyskinesia and agranulocytosis – Treatment should be modified based on reassessment of the patient on the day of the appointment • During – Focus on stress and anxiety reduction – Consider semi-reclined position to avoid aspiration (involuntary movement disorders of the mouth/dysphagia) – To reduce the risk of injury to the patient and foreign body inhalation, consider consented clinical holding due to movement disorder (tardive dyskinesia) – Monitor closely (sudden unexpected behaviour) • After – Careful repositioning after dental treatment is indicated in patients with orthostatic hypotension due to haloperidol and phenothiazines
Drug prescription	• Risk of seizures with tramadol
Education/prevention	• Due to the higher risk of caries and periodontal disease, close oral hygiene support is required • Promotion of healthy habits is also very important but hard to achieve • Dietary advice to reduce consumption of sweet/acidic food/drink is essential • High-concentration fluoride toothpaste and chlorhexidine mouthwash should be considered • Management of dry mouth is required • Cessation advice for tobacco, alcohol and drug use

- Physiological: pregnancy, birth and perinatal complications (e.g. hypoxia) and paternal age
- Environmental: cannabis consumption, migration, urbanicity, seasonality
- Race: people of Afro-Caribbean heritage and some minority groups appear to have a higher risk
- Other: acute episodes may be precipitated by cannabis consumption, stress or traumatic situations

Diagnosis

- There is no pathognomonic sign or symptom of schizophrenia, as symptoms can be variable and must be interpreted in the context of impact on daily life (e.g. social and occupational functions)
- Furthermore, there are no biological markers or psychometric tests to diagnose this disorder
- Hence diagnosis can be challenging and must be done by an experienced psychiatrist, with average diagnosis time from onset around 1 year
- Diagnostic criteria usually used are those defined by the DSM-V or ICD-11 (Table 15.3.2)

Clinical Presentation

- The traditional pattern of schizophrenia consists of the following (Table 15.3.3):
  - Most individuals show a slow development with different signs and symptoms, with 50% of them manifesting depressive symptoms
    Prodromal period can last from a few days to several months and precedes a first episode of psychosis
  - Acute episode with presence of positive symptoms, accompanied by agitation and distress
  - Negative symptoms may be the first sign of the disorder (prodromal symptoms), but usually appear after the acute episode symptoms lessen or disappear (residual phases)
  - Negative symptoms might persist for years, are responsible for considerable morbidity, and are associated with worse prognosis
- Peak age for a first psychotic episode varies between women and men, with males presenting earlier (early to mid-20s) and females manifesting in their late 20s
- A late-onset presentation can appear in women over age 40, with predominance of psychotic symptoms

Table 15.3.2 Diagnostic criteria according to the American Psychiatric Association.

1 Presence of at least 2 of the following active-phase manifestations[a] (with at least 1 of them being one of the first 3):
- Delusions
- Hallucinations
- Disorganised speech
- Catatonic or grossly disorganised behaviour
- Negative symptoms

2 Level of functioning in at least 1 major area (e.g. work, interpersonal relations or self-care) is clearly lower than before the commencement of the disturbance

3 Signs of disturbance continue manifesting for a period of 6 months or more

During this time, presence of at least 1 month of active-phase symptoms (or less if treated successfully)

It may include periods of prodromal or residual symptoms, during which signs of the disturbance may be manifested by negative symptoms or by 2 or more active-phase symptoms in an attenuated form

4 Differential diagnosis with schizoaffective disorder and depressive or bipolar disorders has been made

5 It is not attributable to other causes like drug abuse, medication side effects or another medical condition

6 In case of autism spectrum disorder or a communication disorder of childhood onset, prominent delusions or hallucinations are present beside other required symptoms of schizophrenia

[a] Each manifestation must be present for a significant part of time during at least a 1 month period (or less if successfully treated).
Source: Modified from American Psychiatric Association, Diagnostic and Statistical Manual of Mental Disorders (DSM-5®), American Psychiatric Pub, 2013.

Table 15.3.3 Clinical presentation of schizophrenia.

Positive symptoms	Negative symptoms	Other common features
• Hallucinations • Delusions • Altered thoughts	• Flat facial expression • Avolition (loss of self-initiated purposeful activities) • Anhedonia (decreased ability to experience pleasure) • Asociality (apparent lack of interest in social interactions) • Alogia (diminished speech output)	• Dysphoric mood (depression, anxiety, anger) • Alterations in sleep pattern • Inappropriate affect (e.g. person laughing for no apparent reason) • Absence of eating • Somatic concerns • Anxiety and phobias • Abnormal sensory processing • Problems with inference of people's intentions • Anosognosia (absence of insight into their disorder) • Tardive dyskinesia (uncontrollable movements in the mouth and/or other body parts)

- Females tend to manifest symptoms that are affect laden, can usually maintain social functioning better and are less likely to manifest negative symptoms and disorganisation

Management
- Most patients need daily living support, as they often remain chronically ill with either exacerbations and remissions, or a progressive course of the disorder
- Treatment modalities include psychotherapy, cognitive behavioural therapy, supportive therapy (in community psychiatric services) and pharmacological treatment with antipsychotics (typical or atypical) (Table 15.3.4)
- Older (typical) antipsychotics (e.g. phenothiazines) tend to have extrapyramidal side-effects such as drug-induced movement disorders (dystonia, parkinsonism, restlessness, stiffness, tardive dyskinesia and tremors) and are usually less effective on negative symptoms
- Newer antipsychotics (atypical) do not usually cause movement disorders but are associated with increased risk of obesity and diabetes
- In cases of catatonia or absence of medication response, electroconvulsive therapy might be used
- Hospital admission might be necessary in cases of potential risk to self or others; approximately 10% of patients remain hospitalised long term

Table 15.3.4 Antipsychotic medications and their characteristics.

Type of medication	Examples	Characteristics
Phenothiazines	• Chlorpromazine • Promazine • Methotrimeprazine	– Pronounced sedative effects – Moderate antimuscarinic and extrapyramidal effects – Chlorpromazine is the most commonly used for anxiety or hyperactivity associated with schizophrenia
	• Pericyazine • Pipotiazine • Thioridazine	– Moderate sedative and antimuscarinic effect – Low extrapyramidal effects – Thioridazine is cardiotoxic
	• Fluphenazine • Perphenazine • Prochlorperazine • Trifluoperazine • Thioproperazine • Acetophenazine • Mesoridazine	– Indicated when sedation is not needed – Marked extrapyramidal effects – Can worsen depression
Butyrophenones	• Haloperidol • Benperidol • Droperidol	– Mainly used for violent patients
Thioxanthines	• Flupentixol • Zuclopentixol	– Common extrapyramidal effects
Diphenylbutylpiperidines	• Fluspirilene • Pimozide	– Risk of sudden death
Atypical antipsychotics	• Clozapine • Olanzapine • Quetiapine • Amilsulpride • Risperidone • Sertindole • Zotepine • Aripiprazole	– Increasingly used as first-line management option – Cause long QT syndrome – Clozapine is indicated in resistant cases – Clozapine can cause agranulocytosis and has antimuscarinic effects – Aripiprazole is contraindicated in patients with dementia

Prognosis

- Variable and unpredictable
- Estimated that in 20% of cases the outcome is favourable
- However, people with schizophrenia can die 20 years earlier than the rest of the population and receive less health promotion and physical healthcare
- The presence of anosognosia (unawareness or insight to their disorder) predicts poor treatment adherence, high relapse rates and poor course of the disorder
- Poor compliance with healthy behaviours along with other factors, such as polypharmacy, harmful habits and poor diet, impact on systemic health
- Substance use disorders are very common in people with schizophrenia, with more than 50% consuming tobacco regularly
- Anxiety, obsessive-compulsive and panic disorders are also common
- Suicide ideation is very high in people with schizophrenia, as is suicide attempt (around 20%), with 5–6% individuals dying by suicide
- Suicide risk remains high for the whole lifespan, but is particularly increased in young males with substance use, people with depressive symptoms and in particular periods (e.g. after psychotic episodes and hospital discharges)

A World/Transcultural View

- Schizophrenia is linked to strong social stigma, limited public understanding, fear and disability; in view of this, patients might not be willing to admit the disease, making diagnosis and true prevalence figures challenging
- Although reported prevalence and incidence rates vary across the world, and at local and neighbourhood levels, this may be due to variations in resources, diagnosis and support by specialised mental health services
- Nevertheless, developing countries have lower reported prevalence rates
- Schizophrenia prevalence is also reported as higher in migrants, in penal institutions and areas of social deprivation

Recommended Reading

Agarwal, D., Kumar, A., Manjunath, B.C. et al. (2019). Effectiveness of oral health education on oral hygiene status among schizophrenic patients: a randomized controlled study. *Spec. Care Dentist.* 39: 255–261.

Friedlander, A.H. and Marder, S.R. (2002). The psychopathology, medical management and dental implications of schizophrenia. *J. Am. Dent. Assoc.* 133: 603–610; quiz 624-5.

National Institute for Health and Clinical Excellence (NICE). (2014). *Psychosis and Schizophrenia in Adults: Schizophrenia Prevention and Management [CG178].* www.nice.org.uk/guidance/cg178/evidence/full-guideline-490503565

National Institute for Health and Clinical Excellence (NICE). (2010). *Psychosis and Schizophrenia in Children and Young People: Recognition and Management [CG155].* www.nice.org.uk/guidance/cg155/resources/psychosis-and-schizophrenia-in-children-and-young-people-recognition-and-management-pdf-35109632980933

Wey, M.C., Loh, S., Doss, J.G. et al. (2016). The oral health of people with chronic schizophrenia: a neglected public health burden. *Aust. N.Z. J. Psychiatry.* 50: 685–694.

Yaltirik, M., Kocaelli, H., and Yargic, I. (2004). Schizophrenia and dental management: review of the literature. *Quintessence Int.* 35: 317–320.

Yang, M., Chen, P., He, M. et al. (2018). Poor oral health in patients with schizophrenia: a systematic review and meta-analysis. *Schizophr. Res.* 201: 3–9.

15.4 Recreational Drug Use

Section I: Clinical Scenario and Dental Considerations

Clinical Scenario

A 38-year-old female presents to you requesting replacement of her upper denture as the current denture fractured 6 months ago and now keeps falling out. She does not want any other treatment and appears agitated, anxious and unkempt.

Medical History

- Borderline personality disorder associated with depression and psychosis
  - Diagnosed at age 16
  - Several inpatient stays in psychiatric hospital due to suicide attempts and drug overdose
  - Last hospitalisation: 10 months ago, inpatient for a month
- Hypertension
- Fatty liver
- Anaemia
- Asthma
- History of obesity: gastric sleeve surgery 10 years ago; BMI reduced from 39 kg/m^2 to 23 kg/m^2

Medications

- Sertraline
- Propranolol
- Salbutamol (as required; not taken regularly)
- Methadone

Dental History

- Irregular dental attender; last visit was 2 years ago
- Mild–moderate dental anxiety due to negative childhood experience (clinical holding used to deliver treatment)
- Brushes teeth irregularly when she remembers
- Highly cariogenic diet

Social History

- Disability pension since she was 24 years of age
- Lives with partner who suffers from depression and drug use disorder
- Has 2 children who live with her parents; loss of custody due to drug abuse
- Used to work in sex commerce but currently not working
- History of childhood family violence/sexual abuse from male sibling
- Tobacco: 2 to 3 cigarettes/day
- Alcohol: binge drinking approximately twice a month; up to 40 units daily
- Recreational drugs: regular consumption of cocaine (snorted) and cocaine base paste (smoked), and recently began injecting heroin

Oral Examination

- Missing teeth: #16, #12, #25, #26, #36, #34 and #46 (Figure 15.4.1)
- Gap replacement with an upper partial acrylic denture which is fractured (Figure 15.4.2)
- Palatine torus
- Xerostomia
- Soft and hard deposits
- Generalised gingival inflammation
- Lingual gingival recession on the mandibular anterior teeth
- Multiple defective restorations: #15, #11, #21, #23, #27 and #44
- Temporary filling: #45
- Caries: #13, #24, #33, #35 and #43
- Retained roots: #14 and #22

Radiological Examination

- Orthopantomography undertaken (Figure 15.4.3)
- #14 and #22: retained roots with apical lesions

A Practical Approach to Special Care in Dentistry, First Edition. Edited by Pedro Diz Dios and Navdeep Kumar.

(a)

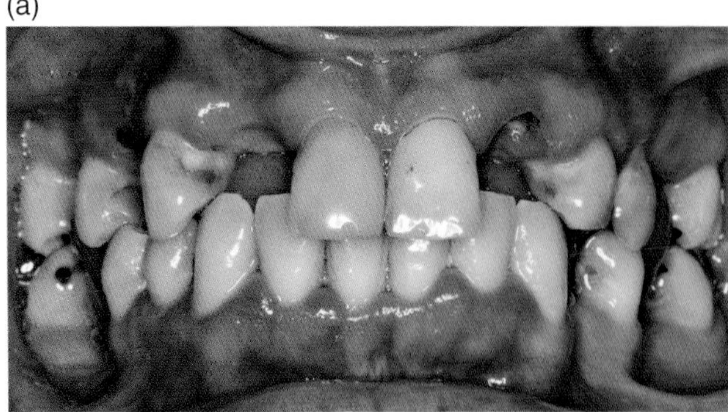

(b)

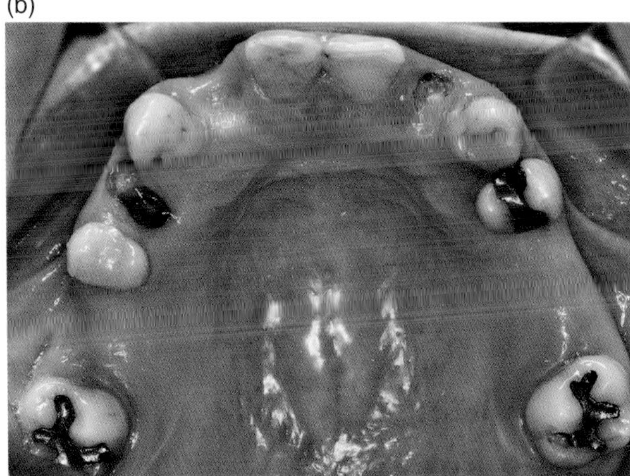

Figure 15.4.1 (a) Anterior dentition demonstrating gaps in the lateral incisor regions. (b) Missing maxillary teeth (#16, #12, #25 and #26), palatine torus and xerostomia.

(a)

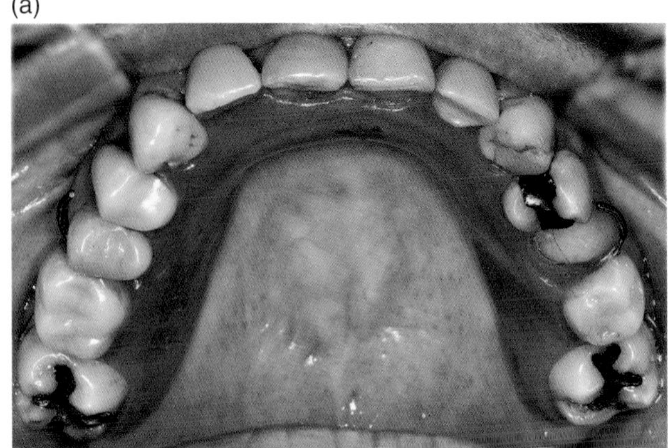

(b)

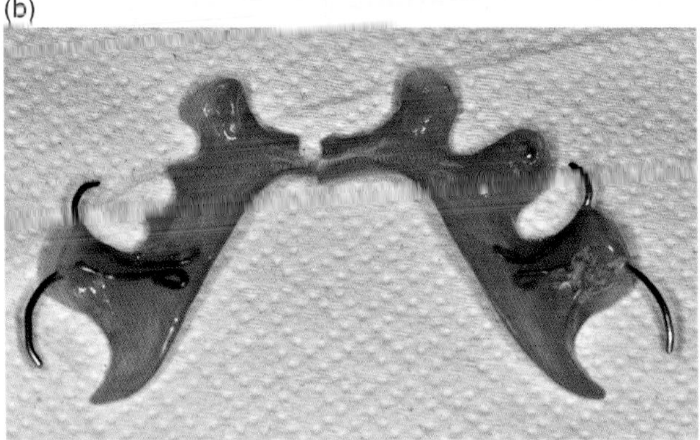

Figure 15.4.2 (a) Upper partial denture in situ. (b) Fractured upper partial acrylic denture.

- Multiple carious teeth: #13 extensive distal caries, #24 extensive palatal caries, #35 mesial caries, #33 distal caries and #44 distal caries
- #23: endodontic treatment
- #15: deep restoration; no apical involvement
- #45: deep restoration with possible pulpal involvement
- Generalised bone loss (~20–30%)

Structured Learning

1) What characteristics of this patient are likely to be linked to the use of recreational drugs?
   - Self-neglect
   - Agitated state
   - Close association with other psychiatric illness (e.g. depression), social issues and dangerous behaviours (e.g. previous sex worker, heavy alcohol consumption)
2) What additional information about the recreational drug use would you need in order to carry out appropriate risk assessment for the management of this patient?
   - Most recent recreational drug use consumption, i.e. is the patient still under the influence of these drugs when she presents for treatment?
   - Further detail regarding the type, frequency, quantity and modality of drug consumption
   - Confirm if she is receiving active support and treatment for her recreational drug use (identify physician/specialist involved in her care)
   - Social history (including other risk behaviours, dependants, suitable escort)
   - Presence of other comorbidities, including blood-borne viruses, cardiac valve damage/infective endocarditis (intravenous drug use; more commonly involving the tricuspid valve), liver injury (viruses, alcohol, drugs)
3) What characteristics of this patient's borderline personality disorder may impact on dental management?
   - This disorder is a mental illness characterised by severe mood instability, impulsive behaviour and lack of emotion control
   - The patient has associated features of paranoia and depression (see Chapter 15.2)

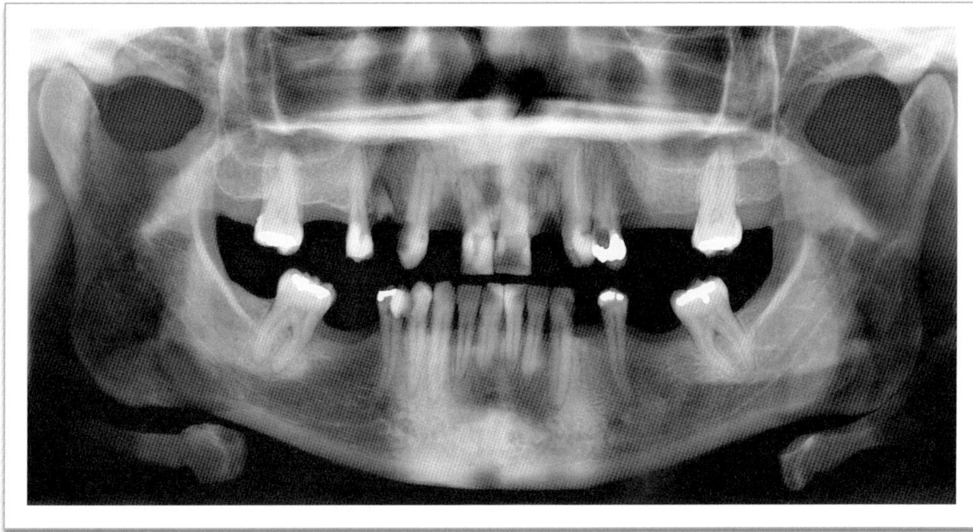

Figure 15.4.3 Orthopantomogram demonstrating multiple carious teeth and generalised bone loss.

- Features of this disorder may be misinterpreted as signs of recreational drug use
- It is likely to be associated with a negative impact on her interpersonal relationship and self-identity, with further impairment of her personal life

4) Despite the presence of retained roots, carious lesions and periodontal disease, the patient insists that she only wants her denture replaced and does not want to return for multiple appointments. What are your options?
   - Refuse to proceed as you do not want to leave untreated dental disease – risk is that the patient is lost to care and will never return
   - Temporarily repair the existing denture on the same day using a cold cure acrylic material; gain patient's confidence and arrange a review to follow up denture when you can rediscuss the untreated oral disease – risk is that the repair is unstable; the patient will not return and/or may lose confidence
   - Take impressions for an immediate denture and use a copy technique if the current denture fits reasonably well (duplicate horseshoe design to avoid palatine torus); gain patient's confidence and attempt acclimatisation to care when the patient returns for this to be fitted. If the patient gains confidence and sees the benefit of dental care, stabilise the remaining dentition and construct a definitive replacement denture
5) Following replacement of the upper denture, the patient agrees to proceed with extractions and fillings as required. What factors do you need to consider in your risk assessment for the management of this patient?
   - Social
     - Difficulties finding suitable escort (i.e. the partner of this patient also uses recreational drugs and suffers from depression)
     - Additional unhealthy habits (tobacco, alcohol, poor diet)
     - Recreational drug use likely to be uncontrolled as she has recently also started using intravenous heroin
     - Currently unemployed – cost of dental treatment may have an impact
     - Capacity/consent impaired by recreational drug use and alcohol excess – if the patient is unable to comply with abstaining for 12 hours, you will not be able to obtain informed consent
     - Likely to have issues with trust due to physical/sexual abuse when younger; may prefer a female dentist
   - Medical
     - Fatty liver, likely to be linked to excess alcohol consumption; depending on the extent, may result in impaired liver function (see Chapter 6.1)
     - Iron deficiency and anaemia are common after bariatric surgery (see Chapter 16.4)
     - Increased risk of hypertensive crisis and orthostatic hypotension (see Chapter 8.1)
     - Asthma – risk of an acute presentation increased by general anxiety (see Chapter 9.2)
     - Eating disorder (history of excess weight) – still consuming excess sweet foods
     - Intravenous drug use (more recently using heroin) – associated with the risk of infective endocarditis and parenterally transmitted infections (e.g. HBV, HCV, HIV)
   - Dental
     - Dental anxiety – may further impact on compliance and attendance

    - High caries risk: highly cariogenic diet, poor oral hygiene habits, hyposalivation (secondary to cocaine/heroin use, methadone treatment and other psychoactive drugs), possible sugar content in methadone
    - Increased risk of tooth surface loss due to attrition/bruxism, secondary recreational drug use, erosion from dietary acids and reflux secondary to gastric surgery
    - Caution with epinephrine-containing local anaesthesia as cocaine use is associated with a risk of arrhythmias, hypertension and cardiac failure

6) What preoperative investigations would you consider for this patient?
    - Full blood count: risk of anaemia (related to malnutrition)
    - Coagulation profile due to the liver disease and additional risk of thrombocytopenia (linked to heroin use)
7) The patient asks for medication to help control her dental anxiety. Why would you have concerns regarding providing this?
    - The patient may be attempting to access further opioid/benzodiazepine medication to supplement her recreational drug use
    - Risk of interaction between prescribed medications and recreational drugs
    - Methadone can interact with benzodiazepines and cause severe respiratory depression

General Dental Considerations

Oral Findings

- Dental neglect
- Caries and periodontal disease
- Bruxism
- Dental erosion
- Wide array of oral changes associated with specific drugs
- Medications used to treat drug use disorder can also cause oral manifestations, for example, dry mouth (e.g. lofexidine) and increased dental caries risk (e.g. non-sugar-free methadone)
- Oral findings secondary to comorbidities such as malnutrition, psychiatric conditions, hepatitis B/C, HIV/AIDS or tuberculosis may also be observed

Dental Management

- Although dental professionals should ask patients routinely about recreational drug use, it is known that most do not do this
- This may be due to a lack of understanding of the oral signs of drug consumption, as well as the implications of recreational drug use on dental treatment (e.g. co-operation, capacity, medical comorbidities) (Table 15.4.1)
- Treatment goals and priorities should be continually reassessed depending on how the patient presents on the day of treatment

Table 15.4.1 Considerations for dental management.

Risk assessment	• Feelings of shame may lead to inaccurate information regarding true levels of recreational drug use • Low motivation and negative attitudes towards oral health • Variable compliance, capacity and engagement • Social and financial challenges as drug abuse is strongly correlated with unemployment and homelessness • Presence of systemic comorbidities (e.g. psychiatric comorbidities, malnutrition) • Intravenous drug use is associated with the risk of transmission of viral infections (HIV, HBV, HCV) and infective endocarditis (which will require antibiotic prophylaxis) • Hypersensitivity to stress and pain • Patients may request opioid analgesics for an oral complaint, even when there is no objective evidence of the disorder • Risk of interaction between prescribed medications and recreational drugs
Criteria for referral	• Most patients who recreationally misuse drugs can be seen in primary care • Refer the patient when they have significant secondary medical issues or serious behavioural problems

(Continued)

Table 15.4.1 (Continued)

Access/position	• Access issues due to higher incidence of financial constraints • An escort is ideal, although a suitable person may be challenging to identify • Consider whether the patient is actively using recreational drugs or not • At least 12 hours should be left between the last consumption of drug and the dental appointment • Also advise against the use of alcohol within 12 hours of the appointment • Morning appointments may be more appropriate as this time is less likely to be associated with drug consumption • Attendance might be erratic and contacting the patient in between appointments can be difficult
Communication	• May be affected by recent use of a recreational drug • Depending on the drug used, speech may be slow and unclear or fast and erratic
Consent/capacity	• Impaired if the patient is under the influence of the drugs • May be further impaired if alcohol is also used and/or there are concurrent psychiatric conditions
Anaesthesia/sedation	• Local anaesthesia – Ideally given 12 hours after the last use of a recreational drug; where this is not achievable, local anaesthesia may be given at least 6 hours after the last dose of cocaine – Avoid/limit the use of epinephrine vasoconstrictor due to risk of arrhythmias, hypertension and cardiac failure (associated with cocaine, ecstasy, amphetamines, cannabis use) – Avoid ester anaesthetics in intravenous cocaine users (possible allergy to benzoic acid) – Recreational drug users are associated with resistance to local anaestheic drugs • Sedation – Ideally, the patient should not use recreational drugs for at least 48 hours; if this is not possible, a hospital/specialist sedation environment is preferred – Opioids such as heroin can cause significant respiratory depression with benzodiazepines (e.g. midazolam); this is also observed with methadone – Cocaine adversely affects respiratory/cardiovascular control with sedation – Cannabis makes oxygen saturation levels unpredictable during sedation – Central nervous system depressants for related mental health conditions can act synergistically with benzodiazepines – Tolerance may have developed in these patients similar to recreational drug users – Veins are often unusable in intravenous drug users – Opioids are contraindicated – Risk of relapse to drug abuse postoperatively should be considered • General anaesthesia – If there are significant dental treatment needs, this may be advantageous Isoflurane or sevoflurane are preferred – Steroid cover may be necessary in opiate users (opioid-induced adrenal insufficiency) – Barbiturates should be avoided in amphetamine users – Halothane can precipitate arrhythmias (cocaine users) – Ketamine and suxamethonium should be avoided (cocaine users) – Hyperthermia might occur in cocaine users – Resistance to general anaesthesia can also occur (especially in amphetamine users) – Risk of relapse to drug abuse postoperatively should be considered

(Continued)

Table 15.4.1 (Continued)

Dental treatment	• Before – Consider blood tests: full blood count (anaemia related to malnutrition), coagulation profile (alcohol- and drug-induced liver injury) – Confirm timing of the last recreational drug use – Reassess the planned treatment at each visit depending on the patient's capacity/compliance • During – Monitor carefully and adapt treatment depending on the patient's ability to cope with treatment • After – Close follow-up needs to be a priority to avoid the need for future invasive procedures – Safe discharge into the care of an escort
Drug prescription	• Issue minimum effective quantity of medication, ideally to be administered by the escort • Medication metabolism can be impaired in liver damage • In patients addicted to opioids, these should be avoided unless expert consultation is sought • Opioids are contraindicated in amphetamine users • Avoid prescription of benzodiazepines or tricyclic antidepressants in patients taking methadone • Consider potential for addiction in the prescription of pain relief drugs (non-steroidal anti-inflammatory drugs are safer)
Education/prevention	• Drug abuse is commonly associated with a cariogenic diet, xerostomia and poor hygiene • Use of high-fluoride toothpaste or other supplements is helpful • Management of dry mouth may be necessary • Smoking, alcohol and recreational drug consumption cessation advice should be given • Signposting for assistance as required

Section II: Background Information and Guidelines

Definition

'Recreational drugs' are defined as substances used without medical justification for psychoactive effects, often in the belief that occasional use of such a substance is not habit forming or addictive. Drug use is a worldwide problem that affects 275 million people, of which 31 million suffer from drug use disorders. An estimate of 5.6% of the global burden of diseases is related to drug abuse. Drug use is increasing by approximately 3 million new users each year. The most common drug of consumption is cannabis, followed by cocaine-related substances and opioids. In 2015, approximately 450 000 people died as consequence of drug use. Intravenous drug users (10.6 million worldwide) face the greatest health risks, as half of them suffer from hepatitis C and 1 in 8 have acquired HIV.

Aetiopathogenesis

- Recreational drug use is a consequence of the confluence of several biological, psychological, economic and social circumstances, with presence of risk factors and absence of protective factors (Table 15.4.2)

Table 15.4.2 Protective and risk factors related to substance consumption.

Protective factors	Risk factors
Family involvement	Childhood trauma (abuse and neglect)
Coping strategies	Poor school environment
Emotional regulation	Sensation seeking
Physical safety	Peer drug use and substance availability
Social inclusion	Low income
Safe environment	Mental health problems
	Being in prison

- Different drugs have a variety of modes of action, but they all affect the brain reward system and can lead to long-term dependence
- They can be classified according to their primary effect
  - Stimulants: amphetamines, methamphetamine, cocaine, khat, synthetic cathinones, nicotine
  - Depressants: benzodiazepines, gamma-hydroxybutyrate, kava, alcohol
  - Dissociatives: methoxetamine, ketamine, nitrous oxide
  - Empathogens: 3,4-methylenedioxymethamphetamine (MDMA/ecstasy), para-methoxyamphetamine (4-MA/PMA), medrophedrone, ethylone

- Opioids: buprenorphine, codeine, fentanyl, heroin, methadone, naltrexone, opium, oxycodone
- Psychedelics: lysergic acid diethylamide (LSD), psilocybin (magic mushrooms), N-benzyl-ortho-methoxy derivatives of psychedelic phenethylamines (NBOMes), ayahuasca
- Cannabinoids: synthetic, medicinal or traditional cannabis, butane hash oil

- Of concern, there are numerous new psychoactive substances whose side-effects are not fully known. This group includes synthetic cannabinoids, new phenethylamines, tryptamines, piperazines, new cathinones (mephedrone or 'meow meow' and methylone) and novel benzodiazepines

Diagnosis

- Substance use disorder is diagnosed when a person continues to use a drug despite important problems arising from its use
- It presents with cognitive, behavioural and psychological features and can be classified according to the DSM-5 criteria

Clinical Features

- Lack of control of drug consumption, inability to quit and spending a great amount of time in activities related to drug consumption (obtaining, consuming and recovering from it)
- Impact on social life is characteristic, with damage to work and family life
- Personality changes
- Lack of sense of danger and impulse control
- Psychological problems (e.g. depression and anxiety)
- Poor personal hygiene and self-neglect
- Tolerance and withdrawal symptoms are especially noticeable with opioids, sedatives, hypnotics and anxiolytics, and less evident with amphetamines, cocaine and cannabis
- Physiological signs of drug consumption include tachycardia (amphetamines), hyperpyrexia (ecstasy), bruxism, psychosis and maxillofacial injuries
- Specific side-effects are dependent on the type of recreational drug used (Table 15.4.3)
- Presence of drug-associated diseases (HIV, hepatitis B/C, infective endocarditis) due to intravenous drug use
- Withdrawal symptoms can include sweating, anxiety, appetite changes, muscle twitching, sleep alteration, tachycardia, increased respiratory rate and hypertension

Management

- Brain changes may persist despite detoxification, especially when drug use disorders are severe
- The combination of craving, withdrawal symptoms and environmental circumstances (e.g. risk factors that precipitated consumption in the first place) makes it difficult to stop drug use and to remain abstinent
- Multiple unsuccessful efforts to stop drug consumption are common, with only 1 in 6 people with drug use disorders receiving treatment
- Treatment options can be delivered within the inpatient, residential, day-patient and outpatient services
- The approach will vary depending on the type of drug: pharmacological therapy is the primary option for opioid misuse while psychosocial interventions are the main treatment for cannabis and stimulant misuse
- Pharmacological treatments have 3 main phases
  - *Maintenance*: this stage is also known as substitution or harm reduction. The main aim is to provide stability; this is achieved through different targets, such as reduction of craving, prevention of withdrawal symptoms, elimination of hazards of injectable drugs and removal of the preoccupation with obtaining illegal drugs. A substitution regimen (methadone or buprenorphine) can be prescribed at high doses to prevent withdrawal symptoms in cases of opioid abuse
  - *Detoxification*: need to be supported by relapse prevention strategies and psychological support because of high relapse rate. Withdrawal symptoms may be managed with medications such as lofexidine or clonidine
  - *Abstinence*: period when a person has stopped taking drugs. In some cases of opioid addiction, naltrexone (opioid antagonist) can be prescribed to help maintain abstinence as it competitively displaces opioid agonists, blocking their positive reward effect
- Psychological interventions include:
  - Brief interventions for self-help (e.g. Narcotics or Cocaine Anonymous)
  - Formal psychological therapy (e.g. cognitive behavioural therapy)
  - Other approaches, such as contingency management focus on positive reinforcement to motivate patient to achieve reduction of drug use or to maintain abstinence.
- There should be testing for hepatitis B/C, tuberculosis and HIV
- Immunisation to hepatitis B should be offered

Table 15.4.3 Recreational drugs, mode of action, examples and oral implications.

Type of drug	Mode of consumption/ mode of action	Side-effects		Oral findings
OPIOIDS (NARCOTICS)				
Heroin Oxycodone Opium Fentanyl Buprenorphine Codeine Tramadol Naloxone Methadone	• Orally, smoked, sniffed, injected (SC/IV) • Mimic enkephalins and endorphins • Activate reward system • Increase dopamine production • Pain relief • Euphoric effect • Naloxone is an opioid antagonist	Arrhythmias Cognitive problems Confusion Constipation Depression Drowsiness Flushed skin Hypertension Immune system changes Infective endocarditis	Irritability Loss of weight Lung abscess/fibrosis Myoclonus Nausea Orthostatic hypotension Pupil constriction Respiratory depression Sedation Thrombocytopenia	Oral neglect Cervical caries Untreated caries Dental erosion Attrition Periodontal disease ANUG Mucosal atrophy Oral epithelial dysplasia Sialadenitis Sialosis Dry mouth Taste alteration Burning mouth syndrome
		Withdrawal symptoms: Abdominal pain Insomnia Lacrimation Muscle spasm Nausea and vomiting	 Pupil dilation Rhinorrhoea Sweating Tremor	
COCAINE				
C. hydrochloride Crack C. base paste **Slang names:** C, coke, nose candy, snow, white lady, toot, charlie, blow, white dust, stardust	• Orally, smoked, snorted, injected • Potentiation of catecholamines • Blockage of dopamine reabsorption • Potent addictive euphoric effect	Cluster headaches Dilated pupils High temperature Hypertension	Loss of appetite Sudden death Tachycardia Vasoconstriction	Caries Bruxism Dental erosion Periodontal disease ANUG Ulceration and necrosis of nasal septum/palate Ankyloglossia in babies of cocaine-using mothers Dry mouth
		Chronic toxicity: Angina Anxiety Coronary spams Depression Impotence Myocardial infarction Paranoia	 Psychosis Respiratory arrest Seizures Sleep disorders Sphenoidal sinusitis Haemorrhagic stroke Ventricular arrhythmias	
		Withdrawal symptoms: Bradycardia Depression	 Fatigue Psychosis	

(Continued)

Table 15.4.3 (Continued)

Type of drug	Mode of consumption/ mode of action	Side-effects		Oral findings
AMPHETAMINES Speed Ice/crystal meth Base **Slang names:** fast, up, uppers, louee, goey, whiz, tik	• Orally, smoked, snorted, injected • Stimulation of alpha- and beta-adrenergic receptors • Similar effect to cocaine • Euphoriant effect • Used to avoid fatigue • Used to lose weight	Anorexia Anxiety Mood swings Nausea	Psychosis Respiratory failure Sleeplessness	Rampant caries ('meth mouth') Attrition Bruxism Periodontal disease Orolingual dyskinesia Trismus Dry mouth
		Acute toxicity: Aggression Arrhythmias Collapse Dilated pupils Dry mouth Hallucinations	Hyperpyrexia Hypertension Seizures Tachycardia Tachypnoea	
		Chronic toxicity: Cardiovascular problems Haemorrhagic stroke Hyperactivity Loss of weight	Mood disorders Repetitive movements Restlessness Tremors	
LSD (lysergic acid diethylamide) **Slang names:** acid, trips, tabs, microdots, lucy	• Orally • Activation of serotonin receptors • Potent hallucinogen • Long-lasting unpredictable effect • Not addictive	Delusions Dilated pupils Flashbacks Hallucinations Hyperpyrexia Hypertension Loss of appetite	Mood changes Panic Paranoia Sleeplessness Synaesthesia Tachycardia Tremors	Dry mouth
CANNABIS Marijuana (herb) Hashish (oil) Joint (cigarette) Bong (pipe) **Slang names:** yarndi, pot, weed, hash, dope, gunja, joint, stick, chronic, cone, choof, mull, 420, dabs, dabbing, BHO	• Smoked, eaten (mixed with food) • Tetrahydrocannabinol binds to brain receptors • Most common illicit drug used • Can trigger schizophrenia • When smoked, has 50–70% more carcinogenics than tobacco	Anxiety Co-ordination loss Depression Distorted perception Immune system changes Impaired memory Impaired thinking	Lung cancer Myocardial infarction Neurodevelopment alterations in babies of cannabis-using mothers Respiratory diseases	Cariogenic diet (munchies) Gingival hyperplasia Periodontal disease Candidiasis Erythroplakia Leucoplakia Cannabis stomatitis (inflammation, leuco-oedema and hyperkeratosis) Dry mouth Oral cancer

(Continued)

Table 15.4.3 (Continued)

Type of drug	Mode of consumption/ mode of action	Side-effects		Oral findings
MDMA (3,4-methylenedioxy-methamphetamine) **Slang name:** ecstasy	• Orally • Synthetic drug • Similar to amphetamines • Affects dopamine-containing neurons • Potent hallucinogen • Stimulant effect • Euphoriant effect • No dependence • No withdrawal symptoms	Anxiety Appetite suppression Arrhythmia Ataxia Brain damage Hepatic failure Hypertension Hyperthermia Hyponatraemia Malignant hypertension Muscle tension Myocardial infarction Nausea Paranoia	Parkinsonism Renal failure Seizures Sleep problems Sweating Tachycardia Vision alteration **Chronic toxicity:** Anxiety Cognitive impairment Depression	Bruxism Attrition Erosions Mucosal ulceration Periodontitis TMJ dysfunction Paraesthesia Dry mouth

ANUG, acute necrotising ulcerative gingivitis; IV, intravenous; SC, subcutaneous; TMJ, temporomandibular joint.

Prognosis

- Recreational drug use is linked to multiple health problems and other health risk behaviours such as alcohol dependence
- Deaths can be directly or indirectly associated with drug use
- Deaths directly related to drug use tend to be a consequence of opioid overdose (76% of deaths), especially heroin, the most widely used opiate
- Heroin drug users have a higher mortality risk (12 times higher than the general population)
- Indirect deaths are mostly attributable to HIV and hepatitis C acquired through intravenous drug use

A World/Transcultural View

- Recreational drug use is common around the world and affects both young and older people
- The variety of drugs available and their markets are expanding due to high-level manufacture of cocaine and opium and online drug trafficking
- Prescription drug abuse is also increasing (e.g. fentanyl and tramadol) and in addition, new substances are continuously being synthesised
- Drug use disorders are associated with social impairment, several health risks and crime
- There are regional variations in the pattern of drug use due to local availability. For example, cocaine base paste is predominantly consumed in South America. Afghanistan remains the world's largest illicit opium producer with over 70% of global production. Methamphetamine manufacturing is mainly concentrated in East and South-East Asia. The use of novel psychoactive substances is largely a European/North American/Oceania phenomenon

Recommended Reading

Abed, H. and Hassona, Y. (2019). Oral healthcare management in heroin and methadone users. *Br. Dent. J.* 226: 563–567.

Baghaie, H., Kisely, S., Forbes, M. et al. (2017). A systematic review and meta-analysis of the association between poor oral health and substance abuse. *Addiction* 112: 765–777.

Hasan, A. and Sharma, V. (2019). Substance abuse and conscious sedation: theoretical and practical considerations. *Br. Dent. J.* 227: 923–927.

Maripuri, S., Sadi, H., Nevius, A. et al. (2020). Using evidence-based dentistry in the clinical management of methadone maintenance therapy patients. *J. Evid. Based Dent. Pract.* 20: 101399.

Rommel, N., Rohleder, N.H., Wagenpfeil, S. et al. (2016). The impact of the new scene drug "crystal meth" on oral health: a case–control study. *Clin. Oral Invest.* 20: 469–475.

Stanciu, C.N., Glass, M., Muzyka, B.C., and Glass, O.M. (2017). "Meth mouth": an interdisciplinary review of a dental and psychiatric condition. *J. Addict. Med.* 11: 250–255.

United Nations Office on Drug and Crime (UNODC). (2018). *World Drug Report*. www.unodc.org/wdr2018

15.5 Alcoholism

Section I: Clinical Scenario and Dental Considerations

Clinical Scenario

A 42-year-old male presents to you requesting dental implants to help him improve his appearance and find a job. He reports being unable to wear his dentures as his mouth is too sore and dry. He appears emaciated and unkempt.

Medical History

- Alcoholism/alcohol use disorder (AUD)
- Anaemia
- Mixed anxiety-depressive disorder, under treatment with psychologist
- Insomnia
- History of fall from stairs (2 years ago): right clavicle and humerus fracture, treated with surgery and physiotherapy; residual physical disability (50%)
- Allergy to metamizole

Medications

- Clonazepam
- Diazepam

Dental History

- Last dental visit 2 years ago when the previous dentures were made; no follow-up visits
- No dental anxiety
- Brushes teeth once a day
- Diet – often forgets to eat; sucks mints to mask the smell of alcohol

Social History

- Divorced, has 4 daughters and 3 sons, but estranged and lives alone
- No regular contact telephone number
- Used to work as a painter but had to stop after the fall, now does occasional ad hoc jobs
- Tobacco consumption: 25–30 cigarettes/day
- Alcohol intake: reports an average of 30 units/week but when he feels lonely admits to binge drinking in excess of 80 units/week

Oral Examination

- Angular cheilitis
- Dry lips/mouth
- Fissured tongue (Figure 15.5.1)
- Partially edentate with multiple missing teeth and lack of posterior occlusal support: #16, #14, #21, #22, #24,

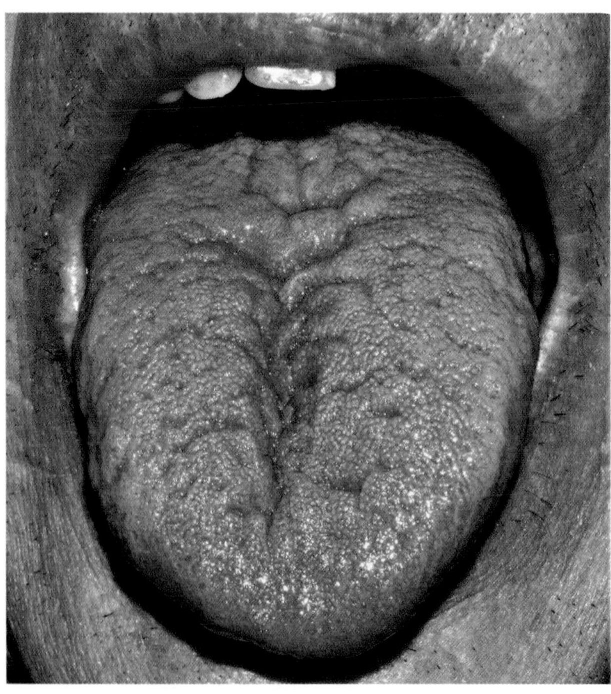

Figure 15.5.1 Angular cheilitis, dry lips/mouth, fissured tongue.

A Practical Approach to Special Care in Dentistry, First Edition. Edited by Pedro Diz Dios and Navdeep Kumar.

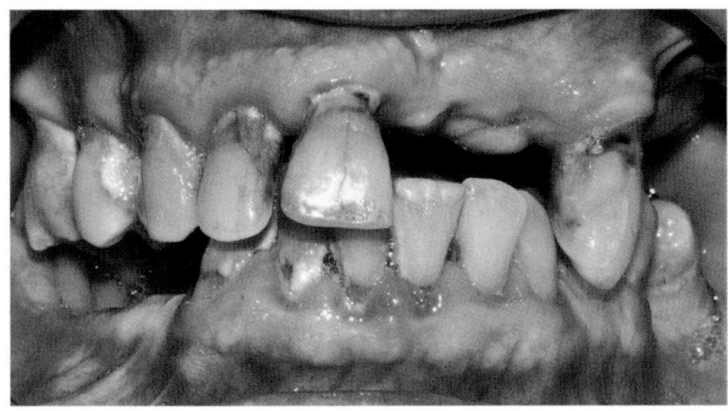

Figure 15.5.2 Partially edentate, xerostomia, gingival recession, poor oral hygiene.

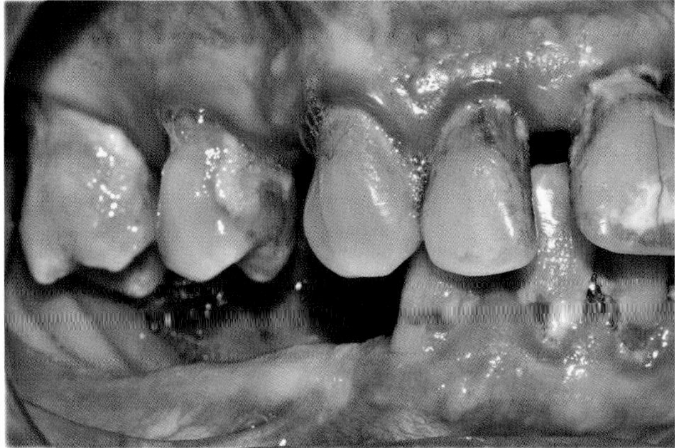

Figure 15.5.3 Lack of posterior occlusal support on the right side.

#25, #26, #27, #36, #44, #45, #46 and #47 (Figures 15.5.2 and 15.5.3)
- Caries: #12, #11, #23, #41, #42 and #43
- Mobility: #15, #12 and #42 (grade I); #11, #31 and #41 (grade II); #17 (grade III)
- Extensive soft and hard deposits and staining all quadrants
- Generalised gingival recession
- Generalised periodontal disease

Radiological Examination
- Full-mouth long cone periapical radiographs undertaken (Figure 15.5.4)
- Pneumatisation of the maxillary sinus
- Generalised horizontal alveolar bone loss
- #17: severe bone loss (~80%), close proximity to maxillary sinus
- #16: covered retained root
- #12: cervical mesial caries
- #11: cervical caries (mesial to distal); bone loss (~60%)
- #31 and #41: bone loss (~60%)

Structured Learning

1) What are the possible contributing factors resulting in xerostomia in this patient?
    - Alcohol use (diuretic)

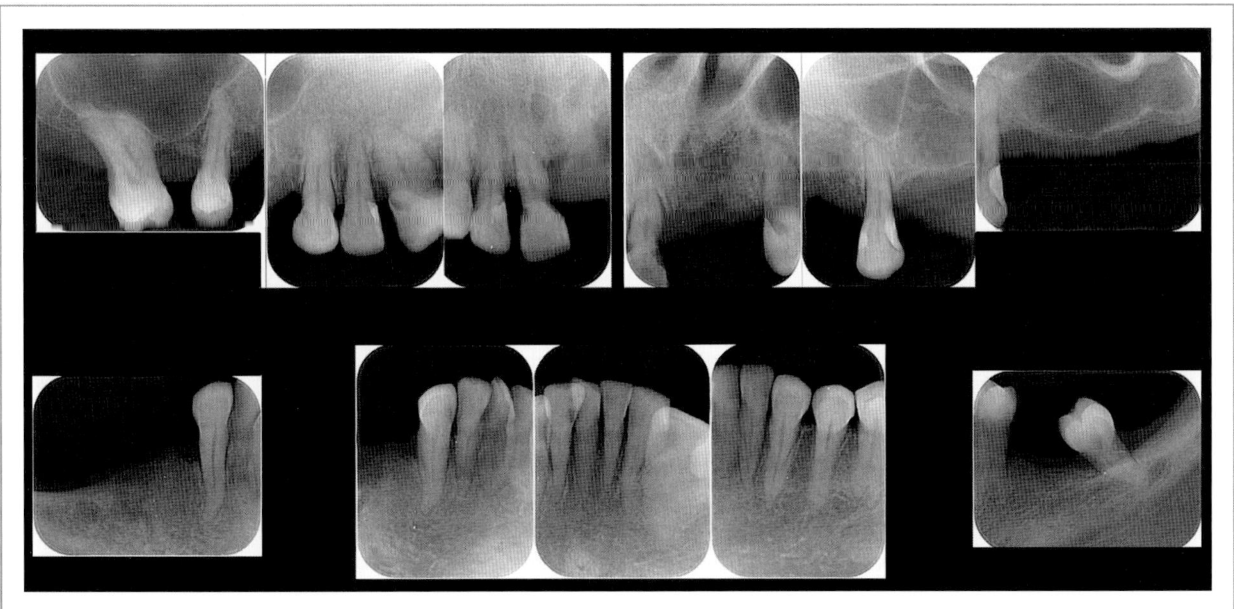

Figure 15.5.4 Full-mouth periapical radiographs.

- Anxiety/depression
- Side-effect of clonazepam/diazepam
- Tobacco use – some evidence that long-term smoking is associated with reduced salivary flow rates
- Dehydration due to inadequate fluid intake

2) What other oral features in this patient may be related to his alcohol use disorder?
   - Generalised oral neglect and partially dentate, widespread dental decay and periodontal disease
   - Angular cheilitis (anaemia)
   - Sore mouth (anaemia)
3) Following discussion of the oral findings, the patient agrees to have #17 removed as it is increasingly painful and moves when he tries to eat. What factors do you need to consider in your risk assessment for the management of this patient?
   - Social
     - Currently unemployed – cost of dental treatment may have an impact
     - Capacity/consent impaired by alcohol excess and daily benzodiazepines (diazepam and clonazepam)
     - Attendance may be erratic due to alcohol use disorder, depression, insomnia
     - Unable to contact the patient by telephone
     - Tobacco consumption
     - Lack of a suitable escort
   - Medical
     - Alcohol-related liver disease may be associated with nausea, weight loss, anorexia, jaundice, confusion, peripheral oedema and increased bleeding (see Chapter 6.1)
     - Impaired liver function will also require caution when prescribing drugs (antibiotics/painkillers) which are commonly metabolised in the liver
     - Additional alcohol-related comorbidities may be present (e.g. peptic ulceration)
     - Emaciation, lack of regular meals and possible bleeding from a peptic ulcer commonly associated with iron deficiency (anaemia)
     - Caution with non-steroidal anti-inflammatory drugs due to increased likelihood of peptic ulceration and reported allergy to metamizole
   - Dental
     - High caries risk: sucks mints daily, poor oral hygiene habits, xerostomia
     - High dental treatment needs
     - Delayed healing (alcohol excess, malnutrition)
     - Related psychiatric conditions, such as depression, will impact on the ability to tolerate dental treatment
     - Oral cancer risk – higher due to alcohol excess, tobacco use and malnutrition
4) You advise the patient to avoid alcohol prior to his appointment. How might this impact on his presentation?
   - Patients who are trying to stop their drinking can present with withdrawal symptoms including tremors, hallucinations and mood alterations
   - This can impact on their ability to consent for and cope with dental treatment
   - It may be preferable to schedule an appointment at a time of day when the patient does not usually drink alcohol
5) The patient asks you for sedation as he is anxious regarding the dental extraction. What would be your concerns?
   - Lack of escort for the appointment and to support the patient at home
   - Not recommended as complicated by tolerance to benzodiazepines (patient takes diazepam/lorazepam daily) or, conversely, they may have prolonged duration if there is significant liver damage
6) Following extraction of #17, the patient returns asking you again for dental implants. What specific risks would you discuss?
   - Cost of dental implant placement (unemployed)
   - Difficulty in achieving compliance with stages of implant placement
   - Poor quality of bone (osteoporosis linked to heavy drinking) and pneumatisation of maxillary sinuses
   - Increased bleeding risk during placement (pancytopenia, liver cirrhosis)
   - Infection at the implant site (active periodontal disease in other sites of the mouth, impaired immunity, malnutrition)
   - Failure/peri-implantitis (smoking, self-neglect, active periodontal disease, suboptimal maintenance, possible bruxism)

General Dental Considerations

Oral Findings

- Neglect may lead to advanced caries and periodontal disease
- This may be exacerbated by underlying anxiety and depression, which can also contribute to attrition, dry mouth and burning mouth syndrome (see Chapters 15.1 and 15.2)
- Excessive alcohol consumption is one of the main risk factors causing violent behaviour – this can result in trauma to the face and teeth
- Alcohol is a risk factor for oral cancer
- Other orofacial features include a smell of alcohol on the breath, telangiectasias, rhinophyma (enlargement of the

nose with dilation of follicles and redness and prominent vascularity of the skin, also known as 'grog blossom')
- Oral manifestations may also occur as a result of concomitant diseases (Table 15.5.1)

Dental Management

- Dental treatment will be mainly conditioned by behavioral disturbances, severity of liver injury and presence of comorbidities (Table 15.5.2)

Section II: Background Information and Guidelines

Definition

Alcohol is the most common drug of abuse and alcoholism is considered the most extreme form of alcohol abuse. It can also be referred as 'alcohol use disorder' (AUD). AUD has been defined as a chronic relapsing brain disturbance characterised by an impaired ability to stop or control alcohol use despite adverse social, occupational or health consequences. Around 240 million people worldwide are alcohol dependent.

Aetiopathogenesis

- The aetiology of AUD is still not well established but is generally considered to be due to a complex relationship between genetic and environmental factors
- Triggers include stress or anxiety reduction, grief, socialisation and a traumatic event/unresolved trauma
- Alcohol consumption increases the release of the neurotransmitter dopamine through its interactions with other neurotransmitter systems (glutamate, gamma-aminobutyric acid [GABA], corticotropin-releasing factor, serotonin) and the effect on the endogenous opioid system, including endorphins and enkephalins
- Alcohol addiction is based on the concept of neuroadaptation and reward. GABA is associated with impulsivity control and dopamine with feelings of happiness and euphoria. The more alcohol that is consumed, the more accustomed the person is to the electrochemical imbalance. As a consequence, when people with AUD are deprived of alcohol, a state of hyperexcitability presents, manifesting as negative withdrawal symptoms
- Risk factors for AUD include bachelors over 40 years old, housewives, commercial travellers, entertainers, armed forces personnel, miners, construction workers, lawyers and healthcare professionals

Diagnosis

- Healthcare providers, including dentists, have an important role in identifying harmful drinking
- One of the screening tools used is the Alcohol Use Disorders Identification Test (AUDIT) (Table 15.5.3)
- Patients identified as at risk should be referred to specialist services where other factors will be assessed, such as dependence, with Severity of Alcohol Dependence Questionnaire (SADQ), Leeds Dependence Questionnaire (LDQ) or Alcohol Problems Questionnaire (APQ)
- In the WHO classification, chronic alcoholism is described as alcohol dependence (ICD-11, 2018), while the DSM-5 uses the term AUD
- Blood tests: gamma-glutamyl transpeptidase increased, full blood count (macrocytosis without anaemia), blood alcohol levels raised

Clinical Features

- Long-term drinking can manifest as damage to multiple systems (Table 15.5.1)
- The toxic effect of alcohol on most organs can be observed at doses above 1–2 drinks/day, with cellular toxicity caused by accumulation of acetaldehyde and changes in the oxidation–reduction state of the cells
- The clinical presentation can be described as acute, chronic and withdrawal related (Table 15.5.4)
- Alcohol can interact with other drugs such as warfarin, paracetamol/acetoaminophen and central nervous system-active agents such as benzodiazepines
- Individuals with AUD can be categorised into 5 main groups, with 50% of those affected being relatively young in age, contrary to the traditional misconception (Table 15.5.5)

Management

- Alcohol dependence treatment is a long process that involves not only the patient but also their close contacts
- The treatment options depend on the extent of the drinking and the proposed goal
- Usually treatment is done in 3 stages: detoxification, rehabilitation and maintenance
- Medication can be used to enable the process (Table 15.5.6)
- Behavioural therapies: counselling sessions, cognitive behavioural therapy, 12-Step facilitation therapy, family therapy, motivational enhancement therapy, self-help groups (e.g. Alcoholics Anonymous)

Table 15.5.1 Alcoholism-related comorbidities and orofacial manifestations.

System	Alcohol-related changes	Orofacial manifestations
Liver	Raised liver enzymes (e.g. GGT) Raised bilirubin and albumin Fatty liver disease (steatosis) Alcohol-induced hepatitis and cirrhosis	• Jaundice • Bleeding (reduced clotting factors II, VII, IX and X) • Sialosis • Foetor hepaticus in end-stage decompensated disease
Gastro-oesophageal	Gastritis Gastric ulcers Gastro-oesophageal reflux Vomiting Mallory–Weiss syndrome (gastro-oesophageal laceration/haemorrhage)	• Dental erosion • Effects of anaemia (e.g. ulcers, angular cheilitis, glossitis, paraesthesia, dysgeusia)
Intestinal	Malnutrition Malabsorption of glucose, zinc, vitamins (B1, B9, B12, A, D, E and K)	• Effects of anaemia (as above) • Sialosis (may be due to malnutrition)
Haematological	Bone marrow suppression leading to pancytopenia and immune defects Macrocytosis	• Effects of anaemia (as above) • Infections (leucopenia) • Bleeding (thrombocytopenia)
Cardiac	Hypertension Coronary artery disease Cardiomyopathy Arrhythmias	• Side-effect of medications (see Chapters 8.1, 8.2, 8.3 and 8.4)
Central nervous system	Atrophy of the cerebellum Reticular system stimulation Progressive neurological syndrome Peripheral neuropathy Wernicke encephalopathy (amnesia, capacity affected) Korsakoff psychosis Dementia	• Generalised neglect • Nocturnal bruxism • Temporomandibular joint disorder • Oral dystonia
Pancreas	Acute pancreatitis Pancreatic cancer	• Poor oral health • Possible link between periodontal disease and pancreatic cancer
Bone	Secondary osteoporosis	• Osteoporotic jawbones (see Chapter 7.1) • Risk of medication-related osteonecrosis of the jaw (see Chapter 16.2)

GGT, gamma-glutamyl transferase.

Prognosis

- Mortality due to alcohol excess is greater than that caused by diseases such as diabetes and HIV
- It is mainly associated with road traffic accidents and secondary systemic disease, predominantly liver cirrhosis
- Every year, about 3 million deaths are the consequence of alcohol misuse (5.3% of worldwide deaths)
- Most of the alcohol-related deaths in the United Kingdom are currently men (66%)
- AUD is also associated with a significant social impact, including higher rates of divorce, domestic violence, unemployment, loss of personal possessions, homelessness and dangerous behaviours

A World/Transcultural View

- Guidelines for maximum alcohol intake vary across the world; in the United Kingdom, the maximum consumption for men and women is 14 units of alcohol a week – the equivalent of 6 pints of average-strength beer or 7 glasses of wine
- Alcohol consumption varies depending on several factors, including cultural norms, economic wealth of the country and religion

Table 15.5.2 Considerations for dental management.

Risk assessment	• Unpredictable behaviour – disinhibited and may become violent • Variable compliance • May lose control of body functions (e.g. urinating) • Risk of trauma (due to inco-ordination) • Amnesia is also common • Alcohol-related liver cirrhosis will delay the metabolism of many drugs, and also result in a bleeding tendency (see Chapter 6.1) • Consider presence of other medical comorbidities (Table 15.5.1) and malnutrition • Suppression of protective reflexes such as the cough reflex may result in risk of inhalation of fluids/debris
Criteria for referral	• Most patients with alcohol misuse should be seen in primary care • Referring the patient is appropriate if the patient has significant secondary medical issues, severe behavioral disturbances or suspected oral cancer
Access/position	• Schedule appointment time that is not associated with drinking hours (e.g. morning instead of afternoon) • Presence of an escort recommended (to help with attendance, follow-up appointments, postoperative instructions)
Communication	• Communication with the general medical practitioner/physician is particularly important if the patient has secondary medical conditions (e.g. liver disease) • Contacting the patient to schedule subsequent appointments may be challenging (patient may be under the influence of alcohol, in temporary/changing accommodation, homeless) • If the patient presents under the influence of alcohol, slurred speech may impact on the clarity of communication
Consent/capacity	• Impaired if the patient attends under the influence of alcohol • Dementia and neurological damage could be present in late-stage chronic alcohol excess (Wernicke encephalopathy, Korsakoff psychosis)
Anaesthesia/sedation	• Local anaesthesia – Analgesia may be difficult to achieve due to tolerance (limited efficacy and duration) – Consider possible liver impairment (prilocaine and articaine recommended) • Sedation – Not recommended as benzodiazepines are potentiated by alcohol consumption – Interactions are not predictable as sedatives increase central nervous system depression – Consider possible liver impairment when selecting drugs and calculating dosages – Consider availability of a suitable escort • General anaesthesia – Best avoided – If used, careful consideration given to the risks versus benefits – Tolerance might be an issue – Excessive effect from drugs in liver impairment – Higher aspiration risk (aspiration lung abscess)
Dental treatment	• Before – Consider preoperative blood tests: full blood count (anaemia, pancytopenia), coagulation screen (bleeding risk related to liver injury) – Plan for any additional support in relation to comorbidities – Confirm timing of the last alcohol consumption – Reassess the planned treatment at each visit depending on the patient's capacity/compliance

(Continued)

Table 15.5.2 (Continued)

	• During – Local haemostatic measures to control increased bleeding risk • After – Safe discharge into the care of an escort – Wound healing may be impaired; alcoholism implicated in the development of osteomyelitis after jaw fractures – Close follow-up is a priority to avoid the need for future invasive procedures
Drug prescription	• Consider the hepatotoxic effect of paracetamol (dose adjustment and minimising the dose/duration) • Most non-steroidal anti-inflammatory drugs can increase the risk of gastric erosions and intestinal bleeding and should be avoided • Consider possible impairment of liver function and its implication on the metabolism of drugs • Opioids enhance sedation and should be avoided • Interaction between antibiotics and alcohol such as metronidazole (disulfiram effect) and cephalosporins • Avoid alcohol-containing preparations (e.g. mouth rinses) • Issue minimum effective quantity of medication, ideally to be administered by the escort
Education/prevention	• Motivation to improve better oral health is challenging • Education on association of alcoholism with dental trauma and oral cancer • Alcohol and tobacco cessation advice • Brief interventions (short, evidence-based, structured conversations about alcohol consumption) are appropriate in a primary care setting

Table 15.5.3 Alcohol Use Disorders Identification Test (AUDIT), created by the World Health Organization (WHO/MSD/MSB/01.6a).

1) How often do you have a drink containing alcohol?
2) How many drinks containing alcohol do you have on a typical day when you are drinking?
3) How often do you have 6 or more drinks on one occasion?
4) How often during the last year have you found that you were not able to stop drinking once you had started?
5) How often during the last year have you failed to do what was normally expected from you because of drinking?
6) How often during the last year have you needed a first drink in the morning to get yourself going after a heavy drinking session?
7) How often during the last year have you had a feeling of guilt or remorse after drinking?
8) How often during the last year have you been unable to remember what happened the night before because you had been drinking?
9) Have you or someone else been injured as a result of your drinking?
10) Has a relative or friend or a doctor or another health worker been concerned about your drinking or suggested you cut down?

Source: Babor, T.F., et al. AUDIT: The Alcohol Use Disorders Identification Test. Guidelines for Use in Primary Care. Geneva: World Health Organization.

- Alcohol use disorders are a worldwide issue, with the highest alcohol consumption in the European regions, the Americas and the western Pacific region
- Alcohol represents the third leading preventable cause of death in the United States; the first is tobacco, and the second is poor diet and physical inactivity
- More than 200 health conditions have been linked to excessive alcohol drinking, increasing the burden on health economies across the globe

Table 15.5.4 Clinical presentation of alcohol consumption.

Effects of chronic consumption	Acute effects of alcohol	Signs of withdrawal[a]
Alcohol-smelling breath Self-neglect Anxiety Tremor Sleep disturbances	Impaired judgement Lack of concentration Loss of inhibitions Slurred speech Altered co-ordination Ataxia	Sweating Shaking Tremor Sleep disturbances Hallucinations

[a] Withdrawal symptoms tend to be worst in the first 48 hours and improve gradually for up to 3–7 days.

Table 15.5.5 Classification of alcoholics according to demographics.

Subtype	AUD	Characteristic of the subtype
Young adult	32%	– Compulsive behaviours around alcohol associated with addiction begin when they are around 20 years old – Due to few drinking occasions during an average week, they tend to binge drink
Young antisocial	21%	– Average age of this group is 26 years old – Antisocial personality disorder, which leads them to an early start on drinking (average age of 15), with AUD by age 18 – Increased risk of polydrug abuse
Functional	19%	– Usually middle aged – Superficial appearance of stability, with higher income, education and relationships – Drinking is sparse with binge drinking
Intermediate familial	19%	– Individuals in families struggling with AUD (around half have a close family member affected) – Drinking starts around age 17 due to family stress and addiction symptoms appear by their early 30s
Chronic severe	9%	– Usually men, with high divorce rate and likelihood of polydrug abuse

AUD, alcohol use disorder.

Table 15.5.6 Medication commonly used in alcohol dependence.

Medication	Characteristics
Acamprosate	– Controls gamma-aminobutyric acid (GABA) levels – Used after abstinence is achieved to prevent alcohol craving and relapse – Treatment course can last for up to 6 months
Disulfiram	– Used to achieve abstinence – Discourages drinking by causing unpleasant physical reactions to alcohol, such as dizziness, nausea, vomiting and chest pain – Treatment course includes an initial follow-up every 2 weeks for the first 2 months, and then monthly for the following 4 months
Naltrexone	– Blocks the opioid receptors, hence stopping the effects of alcohol – Helps to prevent relapse or reduce alcohol consumption – Treatment course can last up to 6 months
Nalmefene	– Blocks opioid receptors in the brain, reducing cravings for alcohol – Helps to prevent relapse or reduce alcohol consumption

Recommended Reading

Friedlander, A.H., Marder, S.R., Pisegna, J.R., and Yagiela, J.A. (2003). Alcohol abuse and dependence: psychopathology, medical management and dental implications. *J. Am. Dent. Assoc.* 134: 731–740.

Kwasnicki, A., Longman, L., and Wilkinson, G. (2008). The significance of alcohol misuse in the dental patient. *Dent. Update* 35: 7–8, 10–12, 15–16.

Manicone, P.F., Tarli, C., Mirijello, A. et al. (2017). Dental health in patients affected by alcohol use disorders: a cross-sectional study. *Eur. Rev. Med. Pharmacol. Sci.* 21: 5021–5027.

National Institute for Health and Care Excellence (NICE). (2011). *Alcohol-Use Disorders: Diagnosis, Assessment and Management of Harmful Drinking (High Risk Drinking) and Alcohol Dependence [CG115]*. www.nice.org.uk/guidance/cg115

Plessas, A. and Nasser, M. (2019). Can we deliver effective alcohol-related brief advice in general dental practice? *Evid. Based Dent.* 20: 77–78.

Roked, Z., Moore, S., and Shepherd, J. (2015). Feasibility of alcohol misuse screening and treatment in the dental setting. *Lancet* 385: S84.

World Health Organization. (2018). *Global Status Report on Alcohol and Health*. Geneva: WHO.

16

Other Special Considerations

16.1 Allergies

Section I: Clinical Scenario and Dental Considerations

Clinical Scenario

A 20-year-old man with cerebral palsy presents for an urgent dental appointment accompanied by his mother. She reports that her son had a severe seizure that morning and hit his face against a cupboard adjacent to his bed. She is concerned that this could have damaged his teeth

Medical History
- Cerebral palsy (hypotonic paraparesis)
- Spina bifida
- Epilepsy (daily seizures)
- Aortic valve insufficiency
- Dorsal-lumbar scoliosis
- Allergy to bananas

Medications
- Sodium valproate
- Topiramate
- Diazepam

Dental History
- Fair oral hygiene; toothbrushing twice daily by his care-giver
- Patient underwent dental treatment under general anaesthesia 4 years earlier
- Since then, he has had yearly check-ups
- Although the patient is co-operative, he has moderate dental anxiety resulting in an increase of his involuntary movements

Social History
- Lives with his parents; attends a day care centre
- Completely dependent for daily life activities
- Wheelchair user
- Non-verbal; his mother interprets his non-verbal language and is able to determine when he is in pain

Oral Examination
- Not compliant for a full oral examination
- Oral hygiene fair
- Trauma to the inside of the lower lip observed: 2 cm linear cut
- #32 grade II mobility but not extruded

Radiological Examination
- Not compliant for radiographs

Structured Learning

1) What additional questions should you ask regarding the reported trauma to the face?
   - The patient is a vulnerable young adult as he is unable to look after himself and is dependent on others; as a result, he is unable to protect himself against significant harm or exploitation
   - In view of this, it is important to establish further details of the reported cause of the traumatic event and make further assessments to ensure that there are no other indicators of the patient being at risk, due to either neglect (left unsupervised) or physical abuse (confirm whether there are any other signs/history of trauma)
   - If concerned, it is important to raise a safeguarding alert (it is important to take clinical photographs)
2) In the case of this patient, you determine that the facial/dental injuries are consistent with the explanation given and the mother has already requested a raised bed rail is fitted on the bed. Following discussion with the patient and his mother, it is agreed that you need to anaesthetise the area of trauma to investigate further. Topical anaesthetic (20% benzocaine) is applied prior to administration of a local anaesthetic injection (2% lidocaine with 1:80 000 epinephrine). A sudden increase in the

A Practical Approach to Special Care in Dentistry, First Edition. Edited by Pedro Diz Dios and Navdeep Kumar.

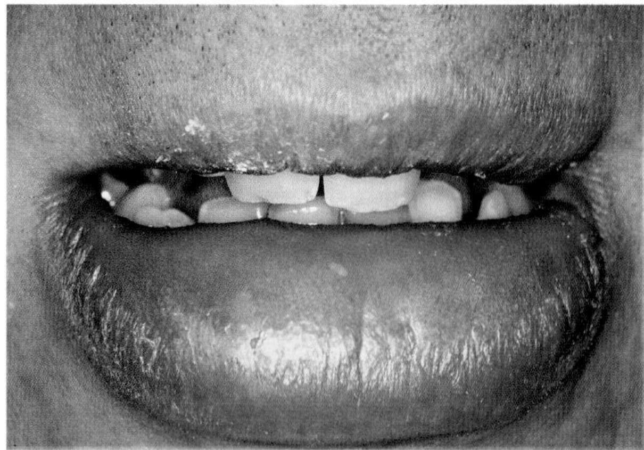

Figure 16.1.1 Sudden lip swelling during dental treatment may become a medical emergency.

volume of the lower lip is observed (Figure 16.1.1). What differential diagnoses would you consider for this presentation?
- Allergic reaction
- Hereditary angio-oedema
- Haematoma due to intravascular injection
- Subcutaneous/submucosa emphysema related to the use of compressed air is another cause of facial/lip swelling but would not apply in this case

3) What would be your immediate concern?
   - This rapid presentation of lip swelling should be treated as an emergency situation as it can be life-threatening, with features of a type I allergic reaction
   - It is important to assess if there are breathing difficulties, abdominal pain, dizziness and/or an urticarial rash
4) What factors are important for this patient when handling this emergency situation?
   - Social
     - Non-verbal communication – challenging to confirm with the patient how he is feeling; hence it is essential for his mother to be present to reassure the patient and interpret his non-verbal communication
     - Wheelchair user – unable to transfer without a hoist
   - Medical
     - Scoliosis may impair breathing further
     - Increased risk of epileptic seizure as the result of the stress generated by this incident
     - Acute complications of aortic regurgitation (uncommon)
   - Dental
     - Emergency management should be the priority with emergency empirical treatment implemented for a type I allergic reaction/angio-oedema event
     - The mobile #32 may be a risk to the airway if it becomes extruded
     - Avoid the use of any potential allergens (e.g. latex, benzocaine)
5) What drugs may be prescribed to treat this episode?
   - If the condition is limited to the lips, with no systemic involvement:
     - Monitor closely; if the lip swelling abates, refer to the patient's physician for allergy testing
     - If there is local support from a physician, H_1 antihistamines (e.g. diphenhydramine, chlorpheniramine and hydroxyzine) and/or corticosteroids (e.g. prednisone and methylprednisolone) may be prescribed at the same visit
   - If there are signs of systemic involvement/respiratory distress:
     - Request emergency medical assistance
     - Oxygen in facemask
     - Subcutaneous epinephrine
     - Inhaled salbutamol
     - If there is on-site medical assistance and the patient stabilises, antihistamines and corticosteroids may also be given
6) The lip swelling abates and you refer the patient to his physician to arrange allergy testing. It is confirmed that the patient is allergic to latex. What factors in this patient's medical history increase his risk of latex allergy?
   - Spina bifida (failure of fusion of the neural tube during embryonic development); may be related to repeated exposure to latex, higher incidence of atopy and possible genetic predisposition
   - Allergy to bananas; cross-reactivity to latex is known
7) What precautions should be adopted for the next dental visit?
   - Liaise with the physician to confirm if they wish to prescribe prophylaxis with antihistamines and corticosteroids to enable dental treatment
   - Schedule the patient for the first appointment of the day
   - Ensure a latex-free environment (i.e. use latex-free gloves, remove any instrumentation, equipment and accessories that contain latex, confirm that the dental local anaesthetic used is latex free)

- Ensure the surgery is labelled as a 'latex-free zone' to avoid contamination/staff entering without permission
- All team members to be aware of the implications of the allergy and trained in emergency management

General Dental Considerations

Oral Findings

- Type I allergy
  - Labial or lingual oedema
  - Perioral urticaria
  - Glottic oedema (anaphylactic shock)
- Type II allergy
  - Signs of anaemia (mucosal pallor, depapillated tongue)
  - Haemorrhagic lesions (petechiae, ecchymosis, haematomas)
  - Necrotic ulcers
- Type III allergy
  - Haemorrhagic ulcerative stomatitis
  - Localised haemorrhagic necrotic vasculitis
  - Erythema multiforme (Stevens–Johnson syndrome)
- Type IV allergy
  - Fixed drug eruption
  - Lichenoid reactions
  - Allergic stomatitis induced by drugs or prosthetic material
  - Granulomatous cheilitis
  - Non-specific findings such as burning mouth, pain, flaking and xerostomia (Figure 16.1.2)

Dental Management

- In recent years, the number of allergic reactions related to the dental clinic environment has increased significantly (Table 16.1.1)
- For the dental team, the most common triggers for allergic reactions are latex, acrylate and formaldehyde
- For dental patients, it is also important to consider contact allergy to certain metals and resins, as well as hypersensitivity reactions to commonly used drugs
- Before proposing a dental procedure for a patient with presumed allergies, the allergy diagnosis should be confirmed; the allergen panels selected for analysing hypersensitivity to dental materials vary between countries
- Once the responsible allergen(s) have been identified, these should be avoided, the requirement for drug prophylaxis should be assessed, and preparations should be in place to manage emergency situations (Tables 16.1.2 and 16.1.3)

Section II: Background Information and Guidelines

Definition

Allergy is a hypersensitivity reaction of the immune system during which the system identifies certain substances as harmful which are in fact safe for most of the population. These substances are known as allergens. The most common allergic diseases are allergic rhinitis (hay fever), allergic asthma, urticaria, atopic dermatitis, allergic contact dermatitis and food allergies.

Allergies are the most typical cause of chronic disease in industrialised countries. Worldwide, the rate of sensitisation to 1 or more common allergens is estimated at approximately 40%, with certain underlying conditions known to be more commonly associated with the development of allergies (Table 16.1.4).

Aetiopathogenesis

- There are 4 main types of allergic reaction which are mediated in different ways; the risk of developing these

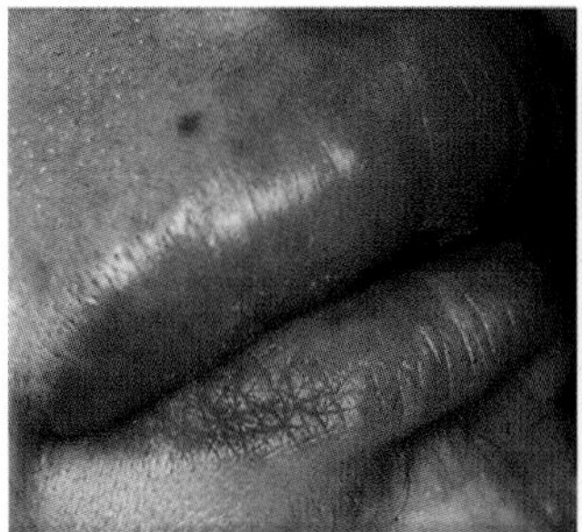
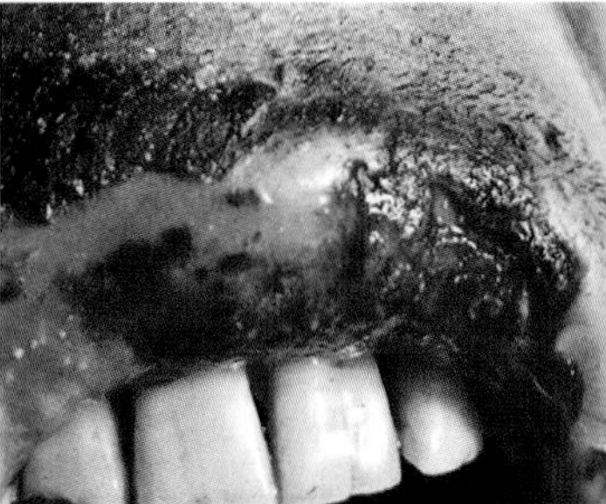
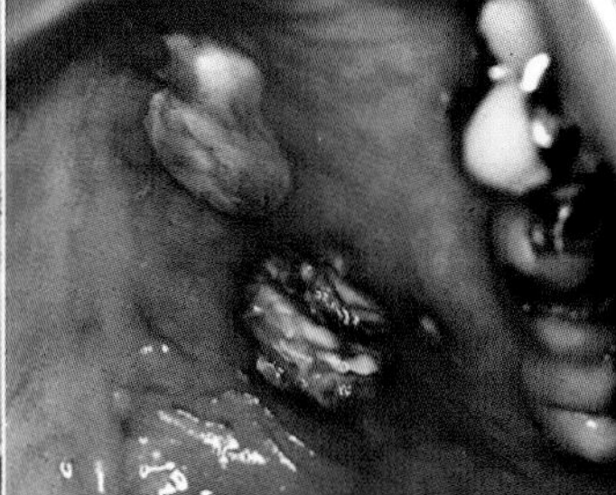
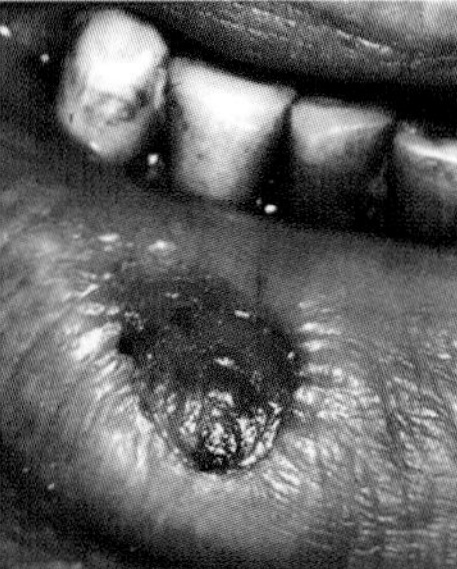

Figure 16.1.2 Oral manifestations of allergic reactions (types I–IV).

Table 16.1.1 Allergens with particular relevance to dentistry.

Allergen	Clinical presentation	Characteristics
Metals	Type IV or type I	– Nickel and cobalt are the most allergenic metals – Mercury amalgam and, to a lesser extent, copper, zinc and tin may also cause reactions – Gold has reported cross-hypersensitivity with mercury – Less common reactions may occur to palladium, titanium and other metals
Acrylic resins	Type IV or type I	– The most common is methyl methacrylate (MMA), with a 1% prevalence of contact allergy in the general population – Can also occur with other methacrylates such as 2-hydroxyethyl methacrylate (HEMA), ethylene glycol dimethacrylate (EGDMA) and triethylene glycol dimethacrylate (TEG-DMA)
Latex	Type I or type IV	– Allergic dermatitis should be differentiated from irritant dermatitis – The allergen can also act through inhalation – There are known risk groups such as health professionals, atopic patients and those with spina bifida or myelomeningocoele – Certain fruits such as kiwi, banana, avocado, pineapple and chestnuts can have cross-reactivity with latex antigens (latex-fruit syndrome) – Examples of dental equipment that may contain latex include anaesthetic cartridges, amalgam carriers, aspirators, rubber dam, endodontic rubber stops, polishing cups, temporary crown/matrices, mixing bowls, Bunsen burner tubing, medical syringes, cannulas, anaesthetic masks – It has been suggested that gutta-percha may have the potential to exhibit cross-allergenicity with latex; however, there is no reliable scientific evidence to confirm this
Local anaesthetics	Type I or type IV	– It is important to note that adverse effects experienced after administration of local anaesthetics may be mistaken for allergic reactions, but often there is another explanation for the symptoms (e.g. psychogenic, intravascular administration) – Allergies are infrequent with ester anaesthetics (benzocaine, tetracaine, procaine and dibucaine) and very rare with amide anaesthetics (lidocaine, mepivacaine, bupivacaine or prilocaine) – Reported allergies may also be linked to the preservatives added to the anaesthetic (methylparaben and sulfites) – The allergy test for local anaesthetics is typically performed with a mixture of 3 ester derivatives of para-aminobenzoic acid; if a patient is positive, the allergist may still recommend an amide group anaesthetic, with single-use cartridges and avoidance of vasoconstrictors
Antibiotics	Type I or type IV	– Antibiotics are responsible for 60% of allergic drug reactions – The diagnosis is confirmed with a controlled exposure test – The most common allergens are penicillins (followed far behind by cephalosporins and quinolones) – The true rates of cross-reactivity from penicillins to cephalosporins appear to be low – Allergy to macrolides is extremely unusual and rarely involves all antibiotics in the group – Hypersensitivity to clindamycin has declined in recent years – Ciprofloxacin causes the most cases of allergy to quinolones
Non-steroidal anti-inflammatory drugs (NSAIDs)	Type I or type IV	– Aspirin is the most common allergen (10% of individuals with asthma have aspirin allergy); 1 in every 5 cases has a cross-sensitivity to other NSAIDS – Allergy to COX-1 inhibitors or paracetamol may occur; the recommendation is to use selective COX-2 inhibitors

(Continued)

Table 16.1.1 (Continued)

Allergen	Clinical presentation	Characteristics
Mouthwashes/gels	Type I and type IV	– Anaphylaxis (type IV) to chlorhexidine mouthwash has been increasingly reported throughout the world, including 2 incidents in the United Kingdom where chlorhexidine-containing mouthwash had been used to wash alveolar sockets following recent tooth extraction – Dentists should be aware of this potential adverse reaction and avoid its use for the irrigation of dry sockets (evidence of benefit limited)

Table 16.1.2 Basic series of allergens for analysing hypersensitivity to dental materials and oral hygiene products (testing allergens authorised by the International Contact Dermatitis Research Group).

1,4-Butanediol dimethacrylate	Epoxy resin
1,6-Hexanediol diacrylate	Ethylene glycol dimethacrylate
2,2-Bis(4-(2-methacryl-oxyethoxy)phenyl)propane (BIS-EMA)	Eugenol
2,2′-Dihydroxy-4-methoxybenzophenone	Formaldehyde
2-Hydroxyethyl methacrylate	Glutaraldehyde
4-Tolyldiethanolamine	Gold sodium thiosulfate dihydrate
Aluminium chloride hexahydrate	Hexylresorcinol
Benzalkonium chloride	Menthol
Benzoylpyridine	Mercury
Bisphenol A dimethacrylate (BIS-MA)	Methyl methacrylate (MMA)
Bisphenol A-glycidyl methacrylate (BIS-GMA)	Methyl hydroquinone
Bornanedione	N,N-Dimethyl-4-toluidine
Carvone	N-Ethyl-p-toluenesulfonamide
Chlorhexidine	Nickel sulfate hexahydrate
Cobalt chloride hexahydrate	Palladium chloride
Colophonium	Phenylmercuric acetate
Copper sulfate pentahydrate	Potassium dichromate
Dimethylaminoethyl methacrylate	Sodium tetrachloropalladate hydrate
Drometrizole	Tetrahydrofurfuryl methacrylate
	Tin
	Triethylene glycol dimethacrylate
	Urethane dimethacrylate

is increased in relation to certain predisposing diseases and risk factors

- Type I (anaphylactic)
  - Immediate (minutes)
  - Requires prior sensitisation in which B-cells produce antibodies (IgE)
  - In a new exposure, mast cells and basophils are activated, releasing inflammatory mediators
  - Examples of typical allergens include transfusions (e.g. in patients with IgA deficiency), drug reactions (e.g. penicillin, muscle relaxants), food allergies (e.g. nuts, shellfish, eggs, soy), insect venom (e.g. bee, wasp) and inhaled/environmental agents (e.g. dust mites, animal dander, pollen, latex)
- Type II (cytotoxic)
  - Onset can be delayed by minutes or hours
  - Caused by antigens that bind to antibodies (IgG and IgM)
  - Antigen–antibody complexes stimulate macrophages and K-cells (phagocytosis) and activate the complement cascade
  - Examples include autoimmune haemolytic anaemia, Graves disease, Goodpasture syndrome, hyperacute transplant reaction, pernicious anaemia, bullous pemphigoid, pemphigus vulgaris
- Type III (mediated by immune complexes)
  - Occurs 3–10 hours after contact with the allergen
  - The mechanism of action is similar to that of type II, but the antigen–antibody complexes are located in vessels and tissues

Table 16.1.3 Considerations for dental management.

Risk assessment	• The medical record, including history of any allergies, will assist in identifying any previous allergic events, in addition to predisposing diseases/risk factors (Table 16.1.4) • The reaction can be mild (e.g. urticaria) to potentially fatal (e.g. anaphylaxis)
Criteria for referral	• For all patients with a history of allergy, it is essential to obtain an allergy report and consult with the physician/allergist before starting dental treatment • Most patients can be seen in a primary care setting as long as adequate precautions are in place • Patients with a history of severe allergy episodes or angio-oedema are best seen within a hospital setting, particularly when prophylactic medication is recommended by the physician/allergist
Access/appointment	• Appointments for patients with latex allergy should be scheduled for first thing in the morning, when the number of latex particles suspended in the air in the dental office is at a minimum
Communication	• The medical history should include detailed information regarding allergies and should be checked at each visit • It is important that all members of the dental team are aware of the patient's allergies and what precautions are required
Consent/capacity	• The consent should reflect the patient's allergy history, specifying the identified allergens and risk factors (e.g. predisposing diseases) • The prophylaxis measures adopted need to be described • Warn of the possibility of cross-reactions and potential complications
Anaesthesia/sedation	• Local anaesthesia – Confirm the patient's history of allergy to local anaesthetics (numerous reported adverse reactions are psychogenic, vasovagal or attributable to intravascular injections) – In the allergy report on anaesthetic allergens, confirm the safe alternatives that are usually listed – Use single-use cartridges (to avoid methylparabens) – Use anaesthetics without vasoconstrictor (to avoid sulfites) • Sedation – There are no reports of allergic reactions to nitrous oxide – Hypersensitivity reactions to benzodiazepines are extremely uncommon • General anaesthesia – There are no documented cases of inhaled anaesthetics causing anaphylaxis in the perioperative setting – Allergic reactions in the operating room are caused, in order of decreasing frequency, by muscle relaxants, latex and antibiotics – Malignant hyperthermia is not an allergy but rather an autosomal dominant inherited disorder primarily triggered by volatile anaesthetics and the muscle relaxant succinylcholine
Dental treatment	• Before – For patients with latex allergy: ○ Prepare a latex-free dental clinic/operating room ○ Confirm with the physician whether drug prophylaxis needs to be arranged ○ Diphenhydramine (1 mg/kg of weight/6 h IV or orally), ranitidine (1 mg/kg of weight/8 h IV), and methylprednisolone (1 mg/kg of weight/6 h IV or orally) ○ Prophylaxis is typically commenced 12–24 hours prior to the procedure and maintain the antihistamines and corticosteroids for 1 week – For patients with allergies to metals, resins or other dental materials: ○ Refer the patient to the allergist for allergy tests for suspicious intraoral lesions ○ When hypersensitivity to a dental material included in a restoration or prosthesis is confirmed, this material should be removed and replaced, although it has been noted that the original lesion does not always resolve – For patients with hereditary angio-oedema (although strictly speaking this is not an allergic disease): ○ Typical support is recommended by the physician to reduce bradykinin-induced swelling ○ Recombinant human C1 inhibitor (1000 U starting 24 h before the procedure), stanozolol (2 mg/8–12 h from 5 days before the operation to 3 days after the operation) and tranexamic acid (1000 mg/8 h from 5 days before the operation to 3 days after the operation)

(Continued)

Table 16.1.3 (Continued)

	• During – Have a protocol prepared to manage allergic reactions and especially anaphylactic shock – For patients with allergies to metals, resins or other dental materials, avoid the allergen and potential cross-reactions – For patients with hereditary angio-oedema, minimise invasive dental procedures and oral trauma • After – For patients with allergies to metals, resins or other dental materials, the oral manifestations of allergies are occasionally non-specific (e.g. peri-implantitis and implant failure in patients with titanium allergy) – For patients with hereditary angio-oedema, a 24-hour postprocedural follow-up is mandatory
Drug prescription	• Confirm the hypersensitivity with specific diagnostic tests • Avoid using any drug responsible for a reported/confirmed allergy, including any pharmacologically related drugs • In the case of an antibiotic, the recommendation is to avoid all antibiotics belonging to that group • About 80% of patients with an allergy to an NSAID also have an allergy to other NSAIDs (multiple reactivity) • In general, cross-reactivity between COX-1 inhibitors, paracetamol and selective COX-2 inhibitors is unusual
Education/prevention	• Carefully record history of drug allergies (especially antibiotics, non-steroidal anti-inflammatory drugs and local anaesthetics), allergy to dental materials or oral hygiene products • Avoid exposure to the identified allergens and to those that might cause cross-reactions with the allergens • For patients allergic to tropical fruit, avoid materials with latex (latex-fruit syndrome) • Drug prophylaxis should be administered under medical supervision

COX, cyclo-oxygenase; IV, intravenous; NSAID, non-steroidal anti-inflammatory drug.

Table 16.1.4 Conditions that promote sensitisation and the development of allergies.

Predisposing diseases	Risk factors
Chronic rhinitis	Allergen composition (e.g. preservatives)
Asthma	Degree of exposure (e.g. doses and rate of exposure)
Atopic dermatitis	Entry/administration route (worse for parenteral)
Chronic urticaria	Adulthood
Sjögren syndrome	Female sex
Mastocytosis	
HIV infection/AIDS	
Hereditary angio-oedema (C1 inhibitor abnormality)	

- Examples include polyarteritis nodosa, poststreptococcal glomerulonephritis, systemic lupus erythematosus, serum sickness

- Type IV (late or cell mediated)
  - The reaction time is 48–72 hours (although it can be delayed by weeks)
  - Mediated by T-cells, which causes the release of cytokines
  - These inflammatory mediators activate macrophages and neutrophils, which end up generating a cell infiltrate
  - Examples include acute/chronic transplant rejection, contact dermatitis (e.g. nickel, latex, cosmetics), drug reactions

Diagnosis

- A full medical history, including allergy history, should be taken to ensure that the appropriate tests are undertaken for any suspected allergens
- Skin tests
  - Prick test: a drop of the allergen extract is placed on the front side of the forearm, and the skin is punctured

with a lancet through the drop (e.g. to study hypersensitivity to local anaesthetics)
  - Intradermal test: the allergen extract is injected directly into the dermis (e.g. to study hypersensitivity to local anaesthetics)
  - Patch test: the allergen is diluted and placed in contact with the skin by means of special dressings or polyethylene patches (e.g. to study hypersensitivity to dental materials) (Figure 16.1.3)
- Blood test
  - Serological techniques such as specific antibody measurements (IgE) (e.g. to study hypersensitivity to latex)
  - Cell techniques such as the histamine release test in response to certain allergens
- Drug provocation tests or controlled exposure
  - The tests consist of administering, under medical supervision, progressive doses of the allergen, generally orally (e.g. to study hypersensitivity to drugs)

Clinical Presentation (Type I Reaction)

- The clinical manifestations of these diseases can range from mild (e.g. urticaria) to potentially fatal (e.g. anaphylaxis) (Figure 16.1.4)
- Localised reactions
  - Skin: urticaria, eczema or angio-oedema
  - Eye: conjunctivitis
  - Nasopharyngeal: rhinorrhoea or rhinitis
  - Sinuses: sinusitis
  - Airways: asthma or angio-oedema
  - Gastrointestinal tract: abdominal pain or gastroenteritis
- Severe generalised reactions
  - Anaphylaxis: sudden onset and rapid progression of symptoms including respiratory distress (bronchospasm, laryngeal oedema), circulatory problems (hypotension), disorientation, restlessness, discomfort and/or dizziness, erythema, pruritus, edema and/or exanthema, syncope
  - Generalised toxicoderma (e.g. toxic epidermal necrolysis)

Treatment

- Avoidance of exposure to the causal agent
- Antihistamines
  - Classic or first-generation (e.g. hydroxyzine and diphenhydramine)
  - Second-generation (e.g. cetirizine and ebastine), with fewer adverse effects
- Beta-2-adrenergic agonist bronchodilators
  - Short-acting (e.g. salbutamol and terfenadine)
  - Long-acting (e.g. salmeterol and formoterol), which are commonly combined with corticosteroids
- Corticosteroids (see Chapter 12.1)
  - To minimise their adverse effects, commonly administered as low-dose, low-potency corticosteroids, for only the necessary duration and preferably locally (topical or inhaled)
  - Other drugs occasionally used include theophylline, anticholinergics, immunosuppressants, monoclonal IgE antibodies, antileukotrienes and, in cases of acute emergency, adrenaline
- Emergency management of anaphylaxis
  - Acute phase:
    - Oxygen via facemask (10 L/min)
    - Epinephrine (1:1000/0.5 mL subcutaneous)
    - Salbutamol (400 μg inhaled)
  - Stabilised patient:
    - Antihistamines (e.g. diphenhydramine 50 mg intramuscular or intravenous)

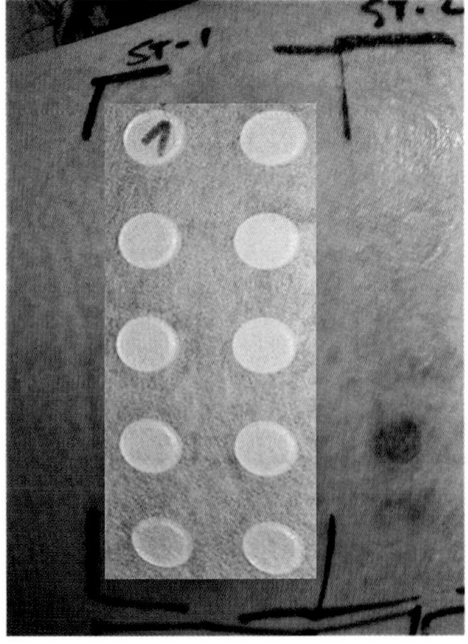

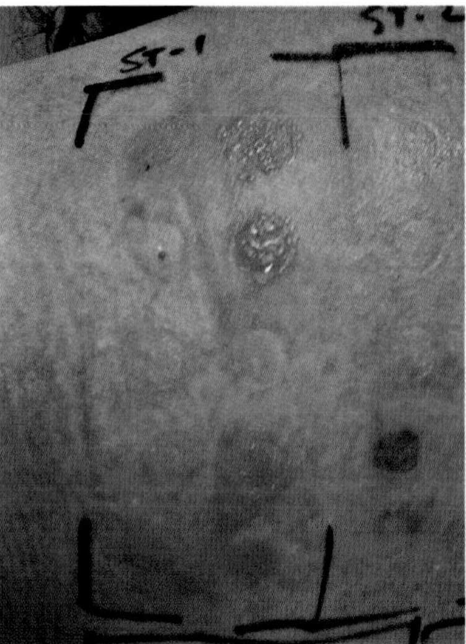

Figure 16.1.3 Patch test to study hypersensitivity to dental materials.

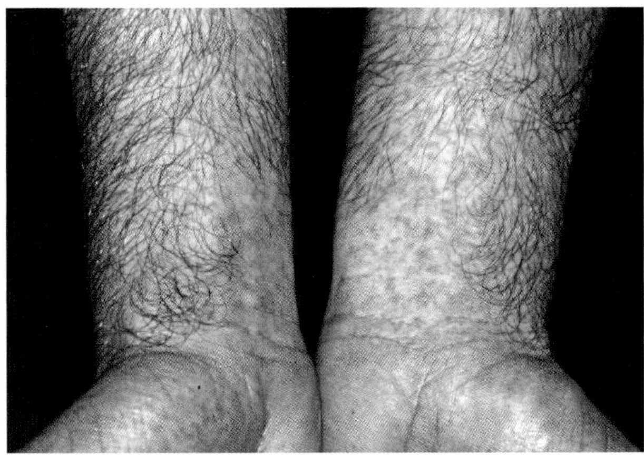

Figure 16.1.4 Hypersensitivity reaction to amoxicillin-clavulanate in an HIV-infected patient.

  - Corticosteroids (e.g. methylprednisolone 40 mg intramuscular or intravenous)
  - Transfer to hospital

Prognosis

- Immunotherapy has been shown to alter the natural history of allergic asthma and can even be curative
- The prognosis for chronic urticaria is good, although patients can experience recurrent flare-ups for long periods
- Hypersensitivity pneumonitis has a better prognosis in young patients and those with less than 2 years of exposure; when the disease progresses to pulmonary fibrosis, its prognosis is severe
- The mortality associated with anaphylaxis varies between 0.5% and 1%

A World/Transcultural View

- There are significant geographical differences in the prevalence of certain allergic diseases
- For example, in the United States, Canada, Chile, Brazil and Australia, it is estimated that more than 10% of the population has clinical asthma, while in Russia, Siberia, China and Mongolia, this rate is less than 2.5%
- Gold sensitisation rates vary worldwide between 0.78% and 30.7%
- Chronic urticaria affects 1.4% of the Asian population, 0.5% of the European population and 0.1% of the American population
- The rate of penicillin allergy among hospitalised patients varies from 6% in The Netherlands to 19% in Canada, although there is a significant lack of data from low- to medium-income countries
- Countries with scarce resources do not always have certain diagnostic tests, such as inhaled nitric oxide quantification, which is applied to assess the progress of patients with asthma and rhinitis
- To diagnose latex allergies, it is important to have reliable recombinant allergens, given that several European countries and the United States no longer market the allergen extracts to perform prick tests or the latex gloves with talc for the bronchial sensitivity tests

Recommended Reading

Comino-Garayoa, R., Cortés-Breton Brinkmann, J., Peláez, J. et al. (2020). Allergies to titanium dental implants: what do we really know about them? A scoping review. *Biology* 9: 404.

Maher, N.G., de Looze, J., and Hoffman, G.R. (2014). Anaphylaxis: an update for dental practitioners. *Aust. Dent. J.* 59: 142–148. quiz 273.

Minciullo, P.L., Paolino, G., Vacca, M. et al. (2016). Unmet diagnostic needs in contact oral mucosal allergies. *Clin. Mol. Allergy.* 14: 10.

National Institute for Health and Care Excellence. (2011). *Anaphylaxis: Assessment and Referral after Emergency Treatment [CG134]*. www.nice.org.uk/guidance/cg134

Olms, C., Yahiaoui-Doktor, M., and Remmerbach, T.W. (2019). Contact allergies to dental materials. *Swiss Dent. J.* 129: 571–579.

Peroni, D., Pasini, M., Iurato, C. et al. (2019). Allergic manifestations to local anaesthetic agents for dental anaesthesia in children: a review and proposal of a new algorithm. *Eur. J. Paediatr. Dent.* 20: 48–52.

Ramsey, A. and Brodine, A.H. (2019). Allergy topics for dental practitioners. *Gen. Dent.* 67: 38–45.

Syed, M., Chopra, R., and Sachdev, V. (2015). Allergic reactions to dental materials – a systematic review. *J. Clin. Diagn. Res.* 9: ZE04–ZE09.

16.2 Antiresorptive and Antiangiogenic Drugs

Section I: Clinical Scenario and Dental Considerations

Clinical Scenario

A 73-year-old man presents to the dental clinic with an ulcer on the right side of the tongue which is particularly painful when speaking and eating. He feels that it may be related to an adjacent rough area on the lower jaw which he first became aware of approximately 2 months ago.

Medical History

- Prostate cancer diagnosed 8 years earlier
  - Intermediate-risk, Gleason score of 7
  - Bone metastases recently confirmed
  - Previous treatment has included various combinations of androgen-deprivation agents (bicalutamide), gonadotropin-releasing hormone superagonist (goserelin) and cytostatic drugs (leuprorelin)
- Arterial hypertension (with target organ impairment)

Medications

- Denosumab (for the last 2 years, every 6 months, last given 2 months ago)
- Prednisone (5–10 mg for the last 5 years)
- Docetaxel (antineoplastic agent)
- Calcium
- Vitamin D
- Candesartan/hydrochlorothiazide

Dental History

- Irregular dental visit attender
- Stopped going due to ongoing treatment and side-effects related to his oncological disease
- Often feels tired and forgets to brush his teeth

Social History

- Widowed, lives alone
- Son lives nearby and is next of kin
- Care-giver support daily
- Reduced mobility; relies on a walking aid and can only manage short distances

Oral Examination

- Poor oral hygiene with multiple soft and hard deposits all quadrants
- Chronic periodontal disease in relation to all the remaining teeth
- An area > 1 cm of bony exposure in the region of the right mandibular alveolar crest, painful on probing; no purulent discharge (Figure 16.2.1)
- An ulcer > 1 cm in the right lateral border of the tongue adjacent to the exposed area of bone
- Extensive caries in #44
- Partially edentate with missing posterior teeth: #14–17, #24–26, #35–37 and #45–47
- Overlying trauma from a poorly fitting lower partial denture

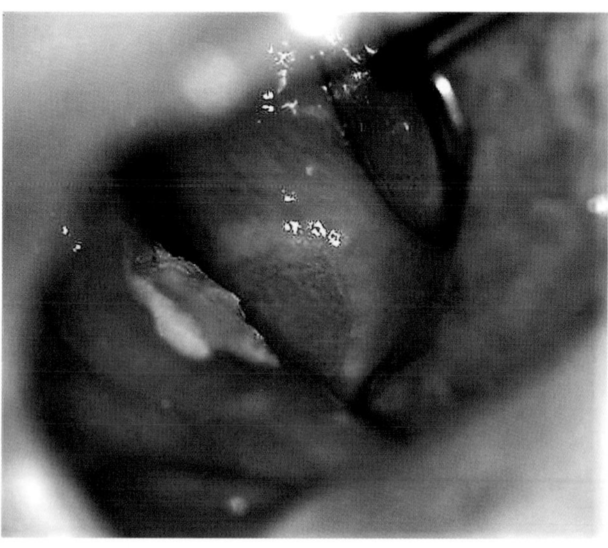

Figure 16.2.1 An area > 1 cm of exposed bone on the right lingual surface of the mandible, and adjacent traumatic tongue ulceration.

A Practical Approach to Special Care in Dentistry, First Edition. Edited by Pedro Diz Dios and Navdeep Kumar.

Radiological Examination

- An orthopantomogram was undertaken and demonstrated scarce and irregular bone trabeculation in the region of the exposed bone area and adjoining areas
- Computed tomography confirmed the presence of a sequestrum in the lower right mandibular region

Structured Learning

1) What is your provisional diagnosis for the exposed area of bone?
   - Whilst it is important to exclude bone metastasis secondary to prostate cancer, the appearance of bone coupled with the patient's history of taking an antiangiogenic drug suggests that the area of exposed bone is due to medication-related osteonecrosis of the jaw (MRONJ)
   - This patient has associated pain on probing, suggestive of infection; hence this would be described as Stage 2 MRONJ
2) What MRONJ risk factors does this patient have?
   - Related to the antiresorptive drug: denosumab (high-potency drug)
   - Related to other drugs: chemotherapy and corticosteroids
   - Patient-related: older age
   - Local factors: poorly fitting lower partial denture causing trauma to the mandibular crestal ridge, poor oral health/existing periodontal disease
3) What are the treatment options for managing this lesion?
   - Antimicrobial treatment with a 0.12–0.2% chlorhexidine mouthwash (twice per day)
   - Antibiotics, e.g. doxycycline (200 mg/day) from 7 days prior to the surgery until 3 weeks after the procedure (or an alternative antibiotic regime)
   - Removal of sequestrum
   - Reduce trauma to the tongue (gently smooth the exposed bone)
   - Pain relief for the tongue ulcer (anaesthetic gel/anti-inflammatory mouthwash)
   - Reduce trauma from the denture (avoid wearing it, adapt by adjusting it so that there is no contact, and/or replace with once the area has stabilised)
4) What factors are considered important in assessing the risk of managing this patient?
   - Social
     - Reduced mobility
     - Requires escort/support for attending appointments
   - Medical
     - Poor prognosis (metastasised prostate cancer)
     - Risk of acute adrenal insufficiency/crisis due to systemic steroids (see Chapter 12.1)
     - Local and distant infection risk, delayed wound healing and bleeding tendency due to adverse effects of the antineoplastic agent (see Chapter 12.2)
     - Risk of a hypertensive crisis (see Chapter 8.1)
     - Risk of complications due to hypertension-related target organ involvement (see Chapter 8.1)
   - Dental
     - Poor oral hygiene
     - Periodontal disease
     - Lack of posterior occlusal support and hence increased risk of continued denture-associated trauma may trigger further MRONJ
     - Extensive caries in #44: dental extraction can trigger further MRONJ; preferable to undertake endodontic treatment and seal the root surface; this also maintains support for the denture as an overdenture abutment
5) Would you advise the patient to discontinue denosumab in view of the MRONJ?
   - There is insufficient evidence to support or refute the discontinuation of bone-modifying agents such as denosumab
   - Administration of denosumab may be deferred at the discretion of the treating physician, in conjunction with the patient and with input from the dentist regarding the oral findings
   - However, careful consideration should be given to the risks of discontinuation as the systemic complications in relation to the bony metastases in this patient are significant
   - As denosumab has a shorter half-life than bisphosphonates, it has been suggested that if an oral surgical procedure is planned, this should be conducted no sooner than 1 month after the last injection and when there are at least 6 weeks until the next injection to allow for adequate healing (although there is some controversy on this matter)
6) What circumstances would justify referring the patient to a hospital-based maxillofacial surgery department?
   - Medical comorbidities and frailty related to cancer diagnosis and the arterial hypertension (close liaison with the physician/oncologist required)
   - Significant haematological abnormalities due to the antineoplastic chemotherapy
   - If the sequestrum is large (greater than 3 cm) and/or if primary closure appears impossible
7) What antibiotics are indicated during the perioperative period?
   - Maxillofacial/oral surgeons mostly prefer penicillin-based antibiotics plus beta-lactamase inhibitor or metronidazole for MRONJ surgery
   - Based on empirical experience, doxycycline has also shown satisfactory results

General Dental Considerations

Oral Findings: Medication-Related Osteonecrosis of the Jaw (MRONJ)

- MRONJ is an adverse effect of antiresorptive and antiangiogenic drugs and can appear spontaneously, although it is generally triggered by a dental procedure that involves bone manipulation (Figure 16.2.2)
- Signs and symptoms include delayed healing following a dental extraction or other oral surgical procedure, as well as pain, soft tissue infection and swelling, numbness, paraesthesia and exposed bone
- Patients might also complain of pain or altered sensation in the absence of exposed bone
- MRONJ can be spontaneous and also present as an incidental finding in the absence of any symptoms, appearing either as areas of radiopacity or radiolucency in the jaw bones

Dental Management

- For patients who are administered antiresorptive or antiangiogenic agents, the recommendation is to implement a protocol that includes preventive and procedural measures, mainly applicable when performing surgical procedures in the dentoalveolar area (Table 16.2.1)
- A risk assessment is required to ensure a specific informed consent is undertaken before any invasive dental procedure (Table 16.2.2)

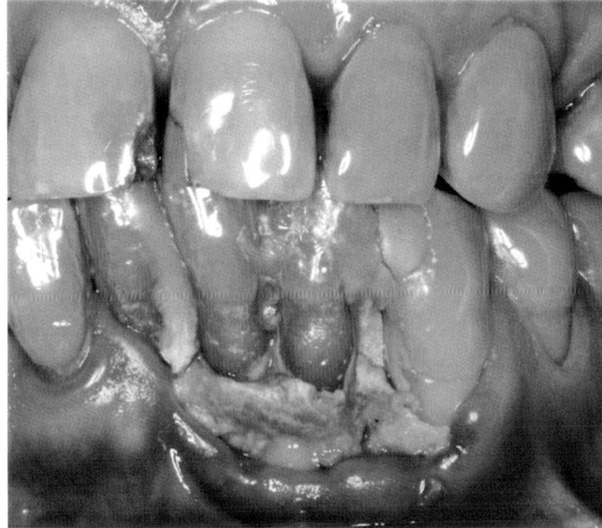

Figure 16.2.2 Spontaneous bone exposure following periodontal treatment, suggestive of medication-related osteonecrosis of the jaw.

Table 16.2.1 Recommended clinical protocol before starting antiresorptive treatment.

• Collect information on the drug product, dosage, envisaged treatment duration and concomitant administration of other drugs
• Provide verbal and written information to the patient about the risk of medication-related osteonecrosis of the jaw (informed consent)
• Extract the non-restorable teeth
• Perform restorative and prosthodontic treatment for the teeth with good prognoses
• Diagnose and treat periodontal disease
• Assess the risk of caries and periodontal disease
• Teach the patient oral hygiene techniques and implement an individual maintenance protocol
• For patients with cancer, close liaison with the oncologist is required to ensure adequate healing in relation to the timing of cancer therapy

Section II: Background Information and Guidelines

Definition

Medication-related osteonecrosis of the jaw is a rare side-effect of antiresorptive and antiangiogenic drugs (Table 16.2.3). It is defined as exposed bone or bone that can be probed through an intraoral or extraoral fistula in the maxillofacial region, that has persisted for more than 8 weeks in patients with a history of treatment with antiresorptive or antiangiogenic drugs but no history of radiation therapy to the jaw and no obvious metastatic jaw disease.

The incidence of MRONJ increases with the duration of antiresorptive or antiangiogenic therapy, with notable differences observed with respect to drug type and potency, route of administration and underlying disease. MRONJ can develop in approximately 7% of patients with cancer who take high-potency bisphosphonates or high-dose denosumab and about 0.001–0.01% of those with osteoporosis using low-potency oral bisphosphonates or low-dosage denosumab.

More recently, novel targeted chemotherapy drugs have been implicated in MRONJ (see Chapter 12.2) and the risk may be compounded further if given in conjunction with bisphosphonates or denosumab (Table 16.2.4).

Aetiopathogenesis

- The aetiopathogenesis of MRONJ has not been fully determined and is likely to be multifactorial, with both genetic and immunological components
- Several genes (e.g. *CP2C8*) have been investigated as having either an increased or decreased association with

Table 16.2.2 Risk assessment of medication-related osteonecrosis of the jaw (MRONJ) and recommended clinical protocol during antiresorptive treatment.

	Clinical situation	Recommended clinical protocol
Low risk	• Patients presenting prior to commencement of antiresorptive treatment • Patients who have been administered low-dose antiresorptive agents for less than 5 years, with no additional risk factors	– Restorative treatment does not require specific precautions – Endodontic treatment is preferable to extraction and periapical surgery (apicectomy is not recommended) – Basic periodontal treatment (non-surgical) is not considered to be a procedure associated with risk – Although surgical procedures (including extraction, periodontal surgery and dental implants) are not contraindicated, it is imperative to have specific informed consent – Peri-implantitis has been associated with the onset of MRONJ – Assess the prophylactic administration of antibiotics in each case depending on the individual patient-related comorbidities
Moderate Risk	• Patients who have been administered low-dose antiresorptive agents for less than 5 years, with additional risk factors • Patients who have been administered low-dose antiresorptive agents for 5 or more years	– Surgical procedures (including extraction, periodontal surgery and dental implants placement) are not contraindicated. It is imperative to have specific informed consent. The prescribing physician should assess the temporary interruption of administering the drug at least during the 2 previous months (drug holiday[a]) provided the systemic conditions allow for it, although this measure remains controversial – It has been proposed that in order to reduce the bacterial load prior to invasive surgery, perioperative administration (preventive therapy) of antiseptics (e.g. 0.12–0.2% chlorhexidine rinses every 8 h) and antibiotics (e.g. amoxicillin 500–750 mg/8 h, penicillin V, amoxicillin/clavulanic acid or metronidazole) at therapeutic doses may be of benefit; however, the evidence regarding this approach is limited – Dental extractions should be planned sequentially by tooth or by sextant, waiting for each extraction site to heal before continuing with the next – Dental extractions should be performed in the least traumatic manner possible (resorting to odontosection if necessary), with bone regularisation and primary alveolar closure – Healing after surgery should be closely monitored – Oral antiresorptive agents for the management of osteoporosis does not constitute a contraindication for the placement of dental implants. The consent document needs to inform the patient of the risk of MRONJ and failure of the implants. The recommendation is to perform a primary closure of the surgical site – The long-term prognosis of implants and the risk of developing MRONJ in patients who take low-dose antiresorptive agents subcutaneously or intravenously remains unknown
High risk	• Patients who will take or have taken high-dose antiresorptive agents	– Therapeutic surgical procedures should be avoided in this patient group unless there are uncontrollable infections with conservative approaches; in this case, the same precautions should be adopted as for patients with moderate risk – Elective surgical treatments (dental implants) are contraindicated

[a] In patients treated with denosumab, the surgical procedure should be conducted no less than 1 month after the last injection and when there are at least 6 weeks until the next one.

Table 16.2.3 Drugs implicated in the development of medication-related osteonecrosis of the jaw (MRONJ).

	Active ingredient	Mechanism of action	Primary indications	Posology (dose/frequency)
Bisphosphonates (relative potency)	• Etidronate (×1)	Non-nitrogen BPs (minimal risk of MRONJ) Inhibit ATP-utilising enzymes and induce osteoclast apoptosis	Paget disease	300–700 mg/day (PO)
	• Clodronate (×10)		Malignant hypercalcaemia Osteolysis secondary to malignant tumours	1600–3200 mg/day (PO)
	• Tiludronate (×50)		Paget disease	400 mg/day (PO)
	• Alendronate (×1000)	Nitrogen BPs FPPS inhibition	Prevention and treatment of osteoporosis Paget disease	OP: 10 mg/day or 70 mg/week (PO) Prev OP: 5 mg/day or 35 mg/week (PO) Paget disease: 40 mg/day (PO)
	• Ibandronate (×1000)		Prevention and treatment of postmenopausal osteoporosis in women	150 mg/month (PO) 3 mg/3 months (IV)
	• Risedronate (×1000)		Prevention and treatment of postmenopausal osteoporosis in women Paget disease	OP: 5 mg/day or 35 mg/week or 150 mg/month (PO) Paget disease: 30 mg/day (PO)
	• Pamidronate (×5000)		Hypercalcaemia produced by malignant tumours Bone metastasis, predominantly lytic, in breast cancer and multiple myeloma	90 mg/3 weeks (IV)
	• Zoledronate (×10 000)		Prevention and treatment of postmenopausal osteoporosis in women Hypercalcaemia produced by malignant tumours Multiple myeloma and bone metastases of solid tumours	OP: 5 mg/year (IV) Prev OP: 5 mg/2 years (IV) Bone metastases: 4 mg/3 weeks (IV)
Biological antiresorptives	• Denosumab	Anti-RANKL	Osteoporosis in postmenopausal women Bone loss associated with hormone suppression in men with prostate cancer Prevention of skeletal events in adults with advanced neoplasia with bone involvement Treatment of unresectable giant cell bone tumour	OP: 60 mg/6 months (SC) Bone metastases: 120 mg/month (SC)

(*Continued*)

Table 16.2.3 (Continued)

	Active ingredient	Mechanism of action	Primary indications	Posology (dose/frequency)
Antiangiogenics	• Bevacizumab	Anti-VEGF	Cervical cancer Metastatic colorectal cancer, renal carcinoma, non-small cell lung cancer Glioblastoma	5–10 mg/kg/2 weeks (IV)
	• Aflibercept		Macular degeneration Diabetic macular oedema/retinopathy	2 mg/4 weeks (IVI)
	• Pazopanib		Renal cell carcinoma Soft tissue sarcoma	800 mg/day (PO)
	• Cabozantinib		Thyroid cancer Renal cell carcinoma Hepatocellular carcinoma	60–140 mg/day (PO)
	• Sunitinib	Anti-TKI	Renal cell carcinoma Gastrointestinal stromal tumour Pancreatic cancer	37.5–50 mg/day (PO)
	• Axitinib		Renal cell carcinoma	5 mg/twice a day (PO)
	• Dasatinib		Leukaemia	100 mg/day (PO)
	• Imatinib		Leukaemia Myelodysplastic disease	400–600 mg/day (PO)
	• Erlotinib		Non-small cell lung cancer Pancreatic cancer	100–150 mg/day (PO)
	• Sorafenib		Renal cell carcinoma Thyroid cancer Hepatocellular carcinoma	400 mg/twice a day (PO)

ATP, adenosine triphosphate; FPPS, farnesyl pyrophosphate synthase; IV, intravenous; IVI, intravitreal; OP, osteoporosis; PO, oral (per os); Prev, prevention; RANKL, receptor activator of nuclear factor kappa-B ligand; SC, subcutaneous; TKI, protein tyrosine kinase inhibitors; VEGF, vascular endothelial.

Table 16.2.4 Other drugs considered to be implicated in the development of medication-related osteonecrosis of the jaw (MRONJ).

	Active ingredient	Mechanism of action	Primary indications	Posology (dose/frequency)
Biological immunomodulators	• Infliximab	Anti-TNF-alpha	Crohn's disease, ulcerative colitis Rheumatoid arthritis, ankylosing spondylitis, psoriatic arthritis	3 mg/kg at 0, 2 and 6 weeks (IV)
	• Adalimumab	Anti-TNF-alpha	Crohn's disease, ulcerative colitis Rheumatoid arthritis, ankylosing spondylitis, juvenile idiopathic arthritis, psoriatic arthritis Hidradenitis suppurativa Uveitis	40–160 mg/2 weeks (SC)
	• Rituximab	Anti-CD20	Non-Hodgkin lymphoma, leukaemia Rheumatoid arthritis Granulomatosis with polyangiitis	375 mg/m^2/week (IV)
Other immunomodulators	• Methotrexate	ATIC inhibition	Autoimmune disorders (e.g. rheumatoid arthritis) Solid tumours Haematological malignancies	7.5–25 mg/day or week (PO, IV, IM, SC)
	• Temsirolimus	Anti-mTOR	Advanced breast cancer, kidney cancer, neuroendocrine tumours Leukaemia	25 mg/week (IV)
	• Everolimus	Anti-mTOR	Breast cancer, kidney cancer, neuroendocrine tumours Tuberous sclerosis complex Prevention of transplant rejection	0.75–1 mg/twice daily (PO) Prev TR: 10 mg/day (PO)
Other drugs	• Ipilimumab	Anti-CTLA-4	Advanced melanoma	3 mg/kg/3 weeks (IV)
	• Azacitidine	DNMT inhibition	Myelodysplastic syndromes and leukaemia	75–100 mg/m^2/day (IV, SC)

ATIC, 5-aminoimidazole-4-carboxamide ribonucleotide formyltransferase; BPs, bisphosphonates; CD20, B-lymphocyte antigen CD20; CTLA-4, cytotoxic T-lymphocyte antigen 4; DNMT, DNA methyltransferase; IM, intramuscular; IV, intravenous; mTOR, mammalian target of rapamycin; PO, oral (per os); Prev TR, prevention of transplant rejection; SC, subcutaneous; TNF-alpha, tumour necrosis factor-alpha.

Table 16.2.5 Main risk factors for medication-related osteonecrosis of the jaw.

• Related to the patient	Older age Tobacco users
• Related to the antiresorptive/antiangiogenic drug	Cumulative dose Relative potency Treatment duration Therapeutic indication (higher risk for cancer vs osteoporosis)
• Related to other drugs	Other antiresorptive or antiangiogenic drugs Chemotherapy Erythropoietin Glucocorticoids (long-term)
• Comorbidity related	Anaemia Diabetes mellitus Cardiovascular disease Chronic kidney disease Systemic inflammatory disease
• Related to local factors	Site (more frequent in the mandible vs maxilla) Invasive dental procedures (e.g. dental extractions) Chronic infections (e.g. periodontal disease) Mucosal trauma (e.g. dentures)

MRONJ but evidence for a single causative gene is not clear

- Possible contributing factors for the development of MRONJ include bone turnover suppression, angiogenesis inhibition, toxic effects on soft tissue, inflammation and infection
- Risk factors include the underlying medical condition for which the patient is being treated, the cumulative drug dose (also linked to the drug treatment duration), concurrent treatment with systemic glucocorticoids, dentoalveolar surgery, mucosal trauma, mandible more likely than maxilla to develop MRONJ (Table 16.2.5)

Diagnosis

- The diagnosis is based on clinical findings and a history of medication known to be associated with the development of MRONJ
- Additional tests
  - Orthopantomography (limited use in early-stage MRONJ) (Figure 16.2.3)
  - Computed tomography: very useful for early diagnosis, defining the true extent of the lesions(s) and confirming the staging (Figure 16.2.4)
  - Magnetic resonance: useful for assessing the involvement of the medullary bone and soft tissue

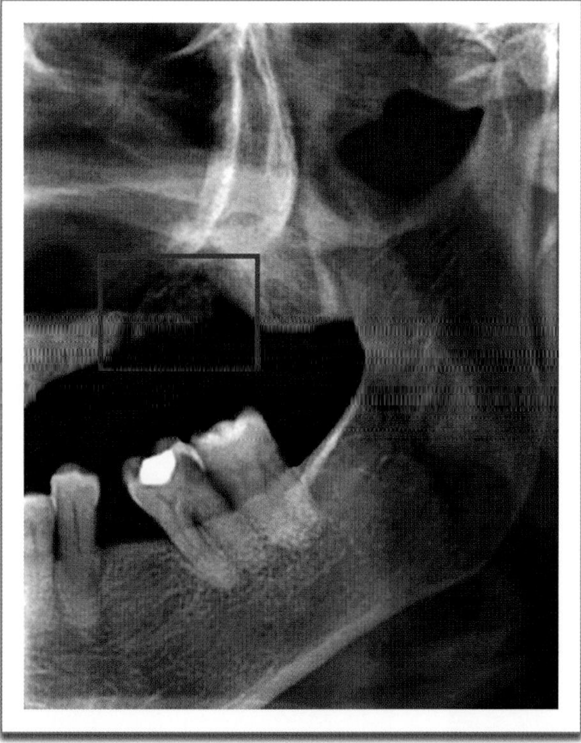

Figure 16.2.3 Detail of an orthopantomogram showing bone sequestration in the upper left quadrant maxillary tuberosity region.

- Microbiological cultures and antibiogram
- Histological study: biopsy is required if the origin of the lesion is suspected to be related to the condition that initiated the use of antiresorptive agents (e.g. for patients with a history of multiple myeloma)

Clinical Presentation

- Clinically, 4 stages have been described, ranging from non-specific findings with no evidence of bone necrosis (Stage 0) to extensive lesions with exposed necrotic bone or extraoral fistula, which progress with pain and infection (Stage 4) (Table 16.2.6)

Management

- There is no consensus regarding the effectiveness of treatment strategies for management of MRONJ as the evidence base remains poor
- Management approaches are currently determined by the clinical stage
- A conservative approach is generally preferred, i.e. administration of antibacterial agents, elimination of infectious oral foci and local trauma
- There is some evidence that a more extensive surgical approach is beneficial in selected cases (including wider resection, mucoperiosteal and mylohyoid flaps)
- Evidence regarding adjuvant approaches is very limited (e.g. drug holidays, supplemental hyperbaric oxygen, teriparatides, autologous platelet concentrate therapy and low-level laser therapies)

Prognosis

- To date, there are no biomarkers with a substantial level of evidence to establish the risk of an individual developing MRONJ or the prognosis of the condition if they develop it
- The clinical determinants include:
  - The stage at the time of diagnosis
  - The location of the lesions (mandibular MRONJ has a poorer prognosis than maxillary MRONJ)
  - It has been suggested that surgery improves the prognosis compared with a strictly drug management approach
  - Relapses appear to be more frequent among patients with diabetes

A World/Transcultural View

- Antiresorptive and antiangiogenic drugs are predominantly indicated in breast cancer and prostate cancer patients to prevent/treat bone metastasis. The incidence of breast cancer varies widely, ranging from 27 cases/100 000 persons in

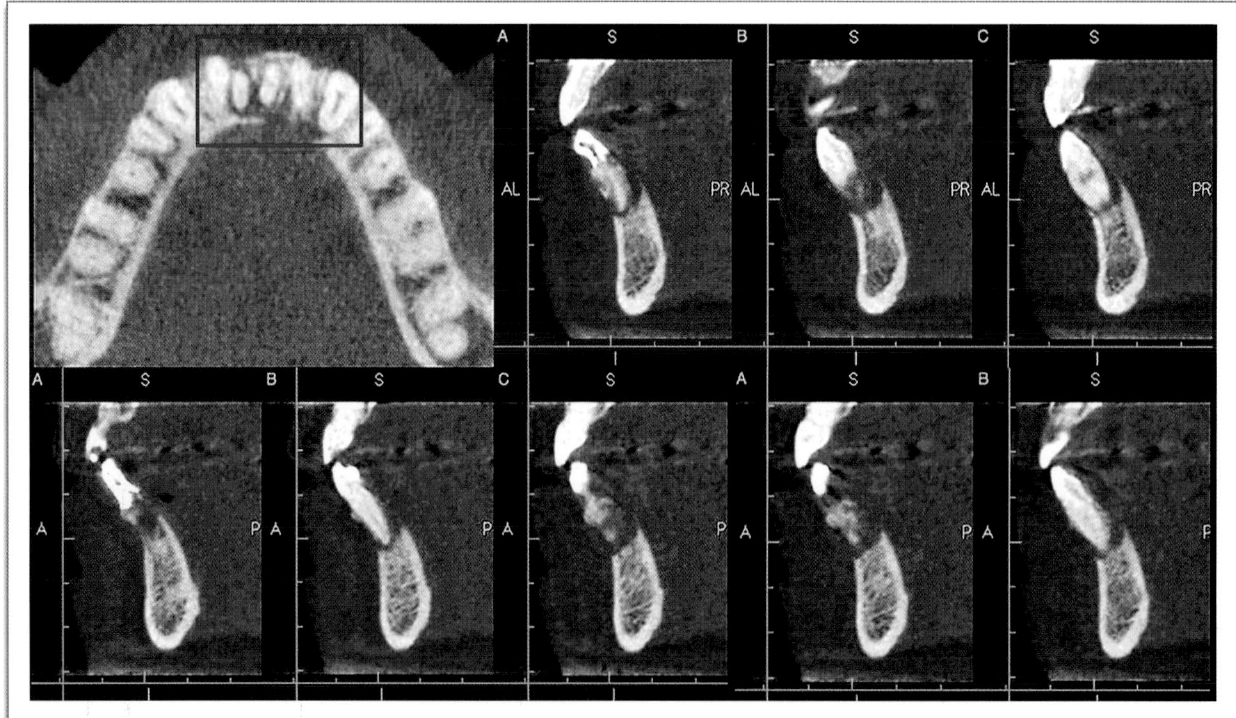

Figure 16.2.4 Cone beam computed tomography demonstrating the extent of medication-related osteonecrosis of the jaw in the anterior region of the mandible.

Table 16.2.6 Staging and management of medication-related osteonecrosis of the jaw (MRONJ).

Clinical stage	Clinical presentation	Management
Stage 0	• No clinical evidence of necrotic bone but non-specific clinical findings, radiographic changes and symptoms	Systemic management, including use of pain medication and antibiotics
Stage 1	• Exposed and necrotic bone or fistula that probes to bone in patients who are asymptomatic and have no evidence of infection	Systemic management, including use of pain medication and antibiotics Removal of sequestrum[a] Clinical follow-up on a quarterly basis Patient education Review of indications for continued antiresorptive/antiangiogenic therapy
Stage 2	• Exposed and necrotic bone or fistula that probes to bone associated with infection as evidenced by pain and erythema in the region of exposed bone with or without purulent drainage	Pain control Oral antibacterial mouth rinse Oral antibiotics Debridement to relieve soft tissue irritation and infection control Removal of sequestrum[a]
Stage 3	• Exposed and necrotic bone or fistula that probes to bone in patients with pain, infection and at least 1 of the following: – Osteolysis extending beyond the alveolar bone – Pathological fracture – Extraoral fistula – Oroantral or oronasal communication	Pain control Oral antibacterial mouthrinse Oral antibiotics Debridement or resection for longer term palliation of infection and pain Removal of sequestrum[a]

[a] Removal of bone sequestration is recommended in all stages.

Central-East Asia and Africa to 85–94 cases/100 000 persons in Australia, North America and Western Europe. Prostate cancer incidence rates are also consistently highest in North America and Oceania and lowest in Asia
- Osteoporosis, another common indication for bisphosphonates, is estimated to affect 200 million women worldwide. Osteoporosis is most common in whites, followed by Asians and African Americans
- These epidemiological differences justify a great variability in the antiresorptive and antiangiogenic prescription rate worldwide
- Moreover, a susceptibility factor to MRONJ might be particularly prevalent in the population of a well-defined geographical region

Recommended Reading

Eguia, A., Bagan, L., and Cardona, F. (2020). Review and update on drugs related to the development of osteonecrosis of the jaw. *Med. Oral Patol. Oral Cir. Bucal.* 25: e71–e83.

Di Fede, O., Panzarella, V., Mauceri, R. et al. (2018). The dental management of patients at risk of medication-related osteonecrosis of the jaw: new paradigm of primary prevention. *Biomed. Res. Int.* 2018: 2684924.

Jayaraj, R., Kumarasamy, C., Ramalingam, S., and Devi, A. (2018). Systematic review and meta-analysis of risk-reductive dental strategies for medication related osteonecrosis of the jaw among cancer patients: approaches and strategies. *Oral Oncol.* 86: 312–313.

Khan, A.A., Morrison, A., Kendler, D.L. et al. (2017). International Task Force on Osteonecrosis of the Jaw. Case-based review of osteonecrosis of the jaw (ONJ) and application of the international recommendations for management from the International Task Force on ONJ. *J. Clin. Densitom.* 20: 8–24.

Nicolatou-Galitis, O., Schiødt, M., Mendes, R.A. et al. (2019). Medication-related osteonecrosis of the jaw: definition and best practice for prevention, diagnosis, and treatment. *Oral Surg. Oral Med. Oral Pathol. Oral Radiol.* 127: 117–135.

Ruggiero, S.L., Dodson, T.B., Fantasia, J. et al. (2014). American Association of Oral and Maxillofacial Surgeons position paper on medication-related osteonecrosis of the jaw – 2014 update. *J. Oral Maxillofac. Surg.* 72: 1938–1956.

Scottish Dental Clinical Effectiveness Programme (SDCEP) (2017). *Oral Health Management of Patients at Risk of Medication-Related Osteonecrosis of the Jaw.* www.guidelinecentral.com/summaries/oral-health-management-of-patients-at-risk-of-medication-related-osteonecrosis-of-the-jaw/#section-society

Yarom, N., Shapiro, C.L., Peterson, D.E. et al. (2019). Medication-related osteonecrosis of the jaw: MASCC/ISOO/ASCO Clinical Practice Guideline. *J. Clin. Oncol.* 37: 2270–2290.

UK Chemotherapy Board. (2019). *Medication-Related Osteonecrosis of the Jaw: Guidance for the Oncology Multi-Disciplinary Team.* www.ukchemotherapyboard.org/osteonecrosis

16.3 Pregnancy and Breastfeeding

Section I: Clinical Scenario and Dental Considerations

Clinical Scenario

A 24-year-old pregnant patient attends her routine dental check-up complaining that her gums feel swollen, with associated sensitivity and bleeding when brushing her teeth.

Medical History
- Pregnant – 10 weeks at presentation
  - Nausea/morning sickness since the fifth week
  - Subclinical hypothyroidism
- Migraines
- History of vertebral fractures due to car accident (2 years earlier); episode of peripheral dizziness 4 weeks earlier attributed to residual cervical spine damage

Medications
- Folic acid
- Levothyroxine
- Potassium iodide
- Doxylamine/pyridoxine

Dental History
- Dental anxiety related to unpleasant experience as a child when a filling was placed without local anaesthesia
- Two years earlier, the patient underwent oral rehabilitation with fixed prosthesis with conscious sedation
- History of orthodontic treatment (from 10 to 16 years old)
- Wears an occlusal splint nocte
- Brushing teeth twice daily but has been using a soft brush as the gums feel sore
- Diet: consuming ginger ale regularly during the day to manage her nausea; unable to tolerate full meals; snacks on small amounts of food throughout the day

Social History
- Married
- Works as an accountant
- Travels to appointments using her own car
- Nil tobacco/alcohol consumption

Oral Examination
- Poor oral hygiene
- Swollen/inflamed gingivae which bleed easily on contact (Figure 16.3.1)
- Fully dentate
- Left temporomandibular joint click on opening

Structured Learning

1) Apart from the poor oral hygiene, what could have caused the change in gingival appearance?
   - Pregnancy gingivitis, also known as gingivitis gravidarum, may present in the first trimester of pregnancy

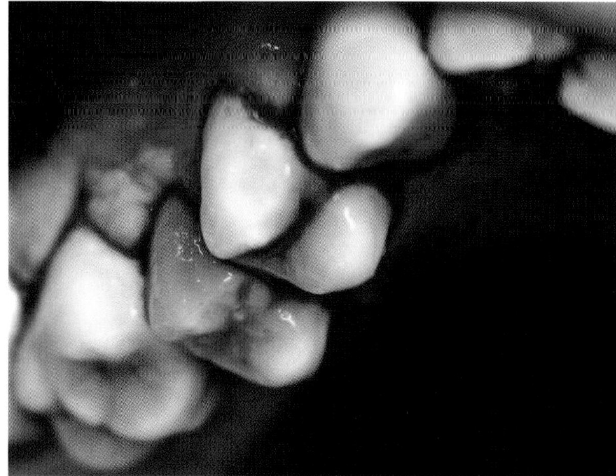

Figure 16.3.1 Gingival hyperplasia and bleeding gums.

A Practical Approach to Special Care in Dentistry, First Edition. Edited by Pedro Diz Dios and Navdeep Kumar.

- This form of gingivitis results from increased levels of progesterone and oestrogen causing an exaggerated gingival inflammatory reaction to local irritants

2) What factors are considered important in assessing the risk of managing this patient?
   - Social
     - Drives to appointments (not suitable if dental sedation is considered)
   - Medical
     - Still in the first trimester of pregnancy when elective dental treatment should be avoided
     - There can be an increased tendency to nausea and sickness
     - Selective drugs prescription
     - Risk of peripheral dizziness when reclined in the dental chair (car accident sequela)
   - Dental
     - Using a soft toothbrush which is likely to be ineffective at removing oral deposits
     - Gingival recession can occur if the gingival inflammation persists
     - Vomiting related to pregnancy increases the risk of dental erosion
     - Cariogenic dietary habits
     - Potential for anaemia and related oral manifestations due to poor oral intake
     - Dental anxiety may reduce compliance for treatment
     - Only strictly necessary radiographs should be undertaken
3) When is it most appropriate to schedule her dental appointments for periodontal treatment?
   - The patient is taking an antiemetic (doxylamine/pyridoxine) because of her hyperemesis gravidarum; it is preferable to wait a few weeks to see if she progresses favourably once the second trimester of pregnancy is under way, particularly as she is also anxious about dental treatment
   - Elective dental procedures are also usually safer in the second trimester
   - Avoid scheduling the patient when she usually feels the most tired (generally early in the morning)
4) Following oral hygiene advice, the patient returns for periodontal treatment when she is 14 weeks pregnant. In order to assess her level of anxiety, you ask her to complete a Modified Dental Anxiety Scale questionnaire (see Chapter 15.1). Her score is 20 which means that she is extremely anxious. She requests dental sedation. What sedation technique do you choose?
   - Close liaison with the patient's physician is required before providing sedation
   - One option which the physician could assist with is diphenhydramine, although consideration would need to be given to the fact she is already taking doxylamine, an antihistamine with sedative activity
   - Avoid benzodiazepines, since they are not recommended in pregnancy or hypothyroidism
   - Nitrous oxide may be employed with strict restrictions and a hospital setting may be preferable (the sessions should not exceed 30 minutes, and the oxygen concentration should not be lower than 50%)
5) What considerations are there regarding the patient's position in the chair?
   - Place the backrest of the chair in the semi-reclined position to promote respiration and prevent gastro-oesophageal reflux
   - Remember the patient's history of peripheral dizziness and vertebral fractures
   - Supine hypotensive syndrome occurs starting in the second trimester
6) What factors may increase the risk of bleeding as the result of the periodontal treatment?
   - The interproximal papillae in pregnancy gingivitis are oedematous and bleed easily but this can be controlled with local measures
   - Hypothyroidism can cause vascular endothelial disorders but not in its subclinical form
7) Unfortunately, the patient subsequently presents with a periodontal abscess in relation to #14. What antibiotics should be avoided in pregnancy?
   - Do not prescribe metronidazole in the first trimester of pregnancy
   - Clarithromycin is contraindicated throughout pregnancy and during breastfeeding
   - Quinolones and tetracyclines should also be avoided during pregnancy

General Dental Considerations

Oral Findings

- Pregnancy
  - Gingivitis: due to an increase in capillary patency, gingivitis affects the marginal gum and interdental papilla and preferentially occurs in patients with pre-existing gingivitis (Figure 16.3.2)
  - Periodontal disease: pregnancy does not cause periodontal disease but can worsen it in patients with pre-existing periodontitis
  - Gingival hyperplasia and bleeding gums: result from an increase in capillary patency
  - Pyogenic granuloma (gravidarum): due to an increase in angiogenesis caused by oestrogens, sometimes com-

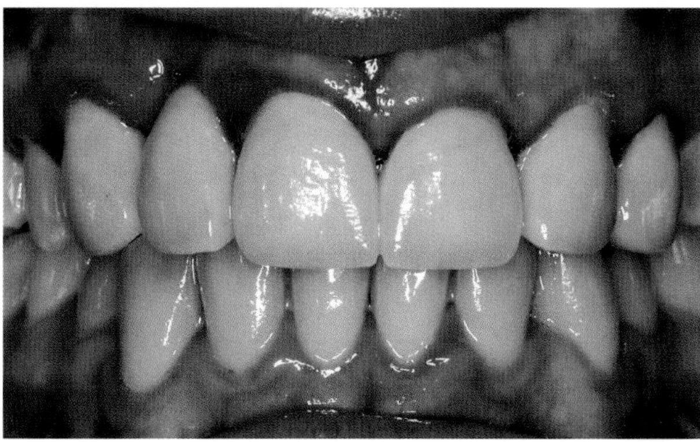

Figure 16.3.2 Pregnancy-related mild gingivitis.

bined with local irritative factors; more common in the first pregnancy and in the first and second trimesters; usually resolves spontaneously following childbirth (Figure 16.3.3)
  - Qualitative changes in the saliva: these changes decrease sodium and pH levels and increase potassium, protein and oestrogen levels
  - Tooth mobility: due to changes in the lamina dura, which generally resolve spontaneously after childbirth
  - Enamel erosion: the increase in gonadotropin levels causes morning sickness, especially during the first trimester
  - Risk of caries: the saliva concentration of *Streptococcus mutans* increases during the second and third trimesters; accompanied by a decrease in pH and calcium concentrations of saliva in the third trimester, this may increase dental caries risk
- Breastfeeding
  - A role has been suggested for breastfeeding in preventing primary dentition malocclusion

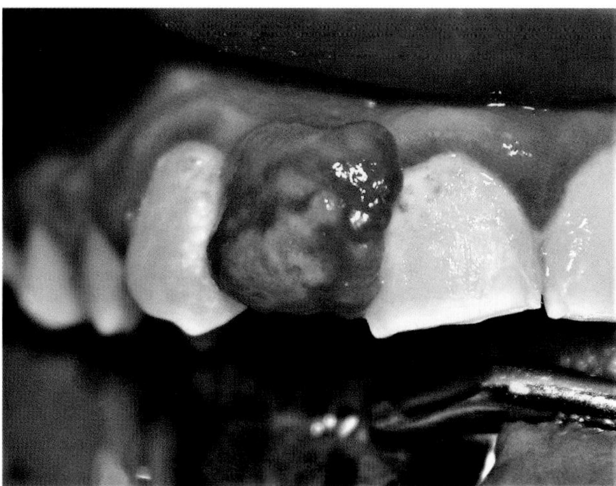

Figure 16.3.3 Pyogenic granuloma (gravidarum).

  - Breastfeeding is considered a protective factor for childhood caries under 1 year of age
  - Conversely, breastfeeding beyond 1 year has been associated with an increased caries risk

Dental Management

- Patients who are pregnant should continue to attend their dental practice for regular care
- They should be reassured that dental treatment is safe and can be adapted in relation to their trimester, with avoidance of all potentially teratogenic drugs (Tables 16.3.1 and 16.3.2)
- Pregnancy is also considered an ideal time for establishing educational and preventive programmes, given that during this period women are more receptive to adopting health practices for their own well-being and that of their babies

Section II: Background Information and Guidelines

Definition

Pregnancy is a dynamic physiological condition, with associated temporary changes in cardiovascular, haematological, respiratory, gastrointestinal, genitourinary and endocrine systems (Table 16.3.3). These physiological changes can represent challenges for the mother's general and oral health, and healthcare should be adapted appropriately. Nevertheless, myths and beliefs exist regarding the relationship of medical and dental interventions with complications during pregnancy such as spontaneous miscarriage, teratogenicity and low birth weight. These often create barriers for pregnant women, dentists and other healthcare practitioners.

A World/Transcultural View

- Numerous barriers have been identified in accessing dental treatment during pregnancy, barriers that are subject to geographical variations and include a mix of factors such as the lack of perceived importance of oral health, financial barriers, employment issues, social support, lack of information, barriers for healthcare practitioners and the incorrect beliefs regarding the safety of dental treatment
- It has been suggested that the oral health of pregnant women who live in rural settings is substantially poorer than that of pregnant women living in cities, with greater reluctance among those living in rural areas to visit oral health services due to their concerns about the safety of dental care during pregnancy

Table 16.3.1 Considerations for dental management.

Risk assessment	• Dental treatment during pregnancy is generally safe but can be affected by systemic abnormalities caused by the physiological changes of pregnancy: – Nausea and vomiting due to the effects of sex hormones (hypersensitive gag reflex) – Dyspnoea due to diaphragm compression – Hypotension due to peripheral vasodilation – Gastro-oesophageal reflux due to increased intragastric pressure – Anaemia due to haemodilution and iron deficiency – Increased renal clearance (might require a dosage adjustment of renal metabolism drugs) • Additional risk of hypertension (pre-eclampsia) and gestational diabetes • Bleeding tendency in patients receiving anticoagulants or antiplatelets to treat hypercoagulability
Criteria for referral	• A medical consultation is required prior to dental treatment for patients with high-risk pregnancies, gestational diabetes, pre-eclampsia or other comorbidities
Access/position	• Avoid dental procedures in the first trimester: – Greater risk of teratogenesis – Can result in falsely attributing a spontaneous miscarriage to these procedures (the prevalence of spontaneous miscarriages during this trimester reaches 20%) – If an emergency procedure is essential, avoid scheduling the appointments for the early morning (hyperemesis gravidarum) • The ideal period for undertaking dental treatment is between weeks 14 and 20 of pregnancy • In the third trimester: – A semi-reclined position should be used to promote respiration and prevent gastro-oesophageal reflux – In addition, the patient should be placed in left lateral decubitus, with the right hip raised 10–15 cm to prevent hypotension due to inferior vena cava compression
Communication	• Anxiety and depression disorders are fairly common during pregnancy and can affect compliance with oral hygiene instructions and increase the stress level during dental clinic visits
Consent/capacity	• Consent should reflect the dental treatment needs and justify the timing of sessions • Indicate that only strictly necessary radiographs will be performed • The patient should be advised that under no circumstance will contraindicated drugs be prescribed during pregnancy and breastfeeding
Anaesthesia/sedation	• Local anaesthesia – Lidocaine and prilocaine are considered safe anaesthetics – If an anaesthetic with vasoconstrictor is required, adrenaline may be employed, but it is preferable to avoid using felypressin • Sedation – Avoid the use of diazepam and midazolam – Nitrous oxide may be employed in the second and third trimesters under strict precautions, with a maximum session duration of 30 minutes; the oxygen concentration should not be <50% • General anaesthesia – It is preferable to postpone it until after delivery

(*Continued*)

Table 16.3.1 (Continued)

Dental treatment	• Throughout the pregnancy – Only necessary radiographs should be performed (not routinely) – The use of lead aprons, collimators and high-speed radiographic film helps reduce foetal exposure – Avoid placing and removing amalgams because mercury can pass through the placental barrier and is secreted in breast milk • First trimester – Periodontal prophylaxis – Only emergency treatments • Second trimester – Periodontal prophylaxis – Scaling and root planing, if necessary – Elective dental procedures are safe • Third trimester – Periodontal prophylaxis – Scaling and root planing, if necessary – Elective dental procedures should be avoided during the second half of the third trimester
Drug prescription	• It is advisable to consult supplementary sources before prescribing drugs to a pregnant or breastfeeding mother (e.g. British National Formulary/Drugs and Lactation Database LactMed; available at www.ncbi.nlm.nih.gov/books/NBK501922) • If medication is prescribed to a breastfeeding mother, it should be taken immediately after breastfeeding (pumping the milk ahead of time and keeping it refrigerated could also be considered) • See Table 16.3.2 for examples of modifications required
Education/prevention	• Dental care during pregnancy is not only safe but recommended • However, there is a lack of knowledge among healthcare practitioners and their patients regarding poor oral hygiene and its impact on pregnancy • A relationship has been reported between periodontal disease and an increased risk of premature childbirth, low birth weight and pre-eclampsia. Periodontal care during pregnancy can reduce this risk (although this association has not been definitively confirmed) • Early prenatal clinical and educational interventions are effective in reducing the transmission of *Streptococcus mutans* from mother to child, delaying colonisation and the onset of caries in young children • Oral hygiene should be encouraged, providing instructions on plaque control and diet advice • Patients should be informed of the oral changes that appear during pregnancy and how to prevent them (e.g. to prevent enamel erosion, rinse the mouth with a solution of sodium bicarbonate after each episode of vomiting)

Table 16.3.2 Drugs prescribed during pregnancy and breastfeeding.[a]

Antibiotics			**Analgesics**[a]			**Sedatives**		
	Pregnancy	Breastfeeding		Pregnancy	Breastfeeding		Pregnancy	Breastfeeding
• Penicillin V	+	+	• Paracetamol	+	+	• Hydroxyzine	–	–
• Amoxicillin	+	+	• Metamizole	–	–	• Diphenhydramine	+	+
• Amoxicillin-clavulanate	+	+	• Ibuprofen	- TT	+	• Doxylamine	+	+
• Clindamycin	+	+	• Diclofenac	- TT	–	• Diazepam	–	–
• Metronidazole	- FT	+	• Naproxen	- TT	–	• Midazolam	–	–
• Azithromycin	+	+	• Dexketoprofen	–	–	• Lorazepam	–	–
• Clarithromycin	–	–	• Codeine	–	–	• Alprazolam	–	–
			• Tramadol	–	–			

+, safe; –, avoid; - FT, avoid in the first trimester; TT, avoid in the third trimester.
[a] Some non-steroidal anti-inflammatory drugs can cause teratogenesis when given during the first trimester and delay/prolong labour or prematurely close the ductus arteriosus during the third trimester; prescribing corticosteroids and oral antifungals is not recommended.

Table 16.3.3 Systemic disorders during pregnancy.

System	**Disorders**
Cardiovascular	• Increase in systolic volume and tachycardia, which cause an increase in cardiac output • Functional heart murmurs (disappear shortly after childbirth) • Supine hypotension (second and third trimesters) • Risk of deep vein thrombosis
Haematological	• Increase in the number of erythrocytes and leucocytes • Physiological anaemia • Increase in coagulation factors V, VII, VIII, X and XII (hypercoagulability) • Risk of thromboembolism • Increase in fibrinolytic activity (reactive)
Respiratory	• Dyspnoea • Hyperventilation, due to reduced residual functional capacity • Moderate hypoxaemia • Snoring • Increased chest circumference and widening of the intercostal spaces, due to foetal compression • Rhinitis, which predisposes patients to nasal haemorrhaging and upper respiratory tract infections
Gastrointestinal	• Heartburn, prolonged gastric emptying and reflux, due to increased intragastric pressure and hypotonia of the lower oesophageal sphincter • Nausea and vomiting (maximum prevalence at 8–12 weeks)
Hepatic	• Hepatic dysfunction, which predisposes to pre-eclampsia • Obstructive cholestasis • Fatty liver
Renal and genitourinary	• Increased renal perfusion • Increased urine excretion of renal metabolism drugs (dosage adjustments might be required) • Oedema due to protein loss • Risk of urinary tract infection • Ureteral dilation and risk of pyelonephritis
Endocrine	• Increased levels of sex hormones, thyroxine, steroids and insulin • Risk of gestational diabetes

- The availability of dental services that are culturally appropriate for pregnant women of indigenous communities varies significantly among countries
- In some low-income African countries, significant dental treatment needs have been detected among pregnant women. Accordingly, it has been suggested that routine dental check-ups should be performed, preferably during the first trimester of pregnancy, and that oral hygiene guidelines should be provided in maternal health clinics

Recommended Reading

Donaldson, M. and Goodchild, J.H. (2012). Pregnancy, breast-feeding and drugs used in dentistry. *J. Am. Dent. Assoc.* 143: 858–871.

Kurien, S., Kattimani, V.S., Sriram, R. et al. (2013). Management of pregnant patient in dentistry. *J. Int. Oral Health* 5: 88–97.

Paglia, L. and Colombo, S. (2019). Perinatal oral health: focus on the mother. *Eur. J. Paediatr. Dent.* 20: 209–213.

Peres, K.G., Chaffee, B.W., Feldens, C.A. et al. (2018). Breastfeeding and oral health: evidence and methodological challenges. *J. Dent. Res.* 97: 251–258.

Robinson, B.J. and Boyce, R.A. (2014). Why is dental treatment of the gravid patient regarded with caution? When is the appropriate time for care – be it emergent or routine – in the gravid patient? *J. N. J. Dent. Assoc.* 85: 11–14.

Stern, A. and Elmore, J. (2016). Medication for gravid and nursing dental patients. *Dent. Clin. North Am.* 60: 523–531.

Suresh, L. and Radfar, L. (2004). Pregnancy and lactation. *Oral Surg. Oral Med. Oral Pathol. Oral Radiol. Endod.* 97: 672–682.

Vitale, S.G., Privitera, S., Gulino, F.A. et al. (2016). Dental management in pregnancy: recent trends. *Clin. Exp. Obstet. Gynecol.* 43: 638–642.

16.4 Bariatric Patients

Section I: Clinical Scenario and Dental Considerations

Clinical Scenario

A 55-year-old female presents to your dental clinic complaining of pain in an upper left first molar tooth.

Medical History

- Raised body mass index (BMI = 46.9 kg/m^2)
- Hypertension
- Ischaemic heart disease – stable angina
- Hypercholesterolaemia
- Type 2 diabetes mellitus
- Asthma, well controlled and on follow-up
- Sleep apnoea: continuous positive airway pressure (CPAP) device used at night
- Gastro-oesophageal reflux disease
- Osteoarthritis
- Major depressive disorder

Medications

- Amlodipine
- Atenolol
- Aspirin
- Glyceryl trinitrate (inhaler)
- Atorvastatin
- Metformin
- Corticosteroid (inhaler)
- Salbutamol (inhaler)
- Lansoprazole
- Sertraline

Dental History

- Irregular attender, previous visit over 5 years ago
- Dental anxiety associated with injections and drilling sensation/sounds; avoids fillings and prefers dental extractions
- No history of dental sedation or general anaesthesia for dental treatment
- Brushes twice a day with fluoridated toothpaste but unable to reach upper posterior teeth
- Snacks on cakes and biscuits between meals with 10 sweetened beverages daily

Social History

- Divorced and lives alone; rarely leaves her home
- Two sons who are married and live separately
- Requires hospital transport to attend appointments
- Mobility: although able to stand for short periods, using a bariatric wheelchair to attend hospital appointments
- Tobacco and alcohol consumption: nil

Oral Examination

- Limited visualisation of the posterior teeth due to extensive adipose tissue
- Partially edentulous with lack of posterior occlusal support
- Soft deposits and food debris
- Generalised gingival inflammation
- Food packing between #26 and #27
- #26: distal caries; tender on palpation; grade I mobility
- Generalised tooth surface loss with combined signs of erosion and attrition, particularly on #11, #12 and all lower anterior teeth

Radiological Examination

- Patient unable to tolerate intraoral radiographs due to limited space/access in the mouth
- Difficulty with orthopantomogram due to tissue mass around shoulders obstructing movement of emission tube and cartridge frame (wider machine required; accessed in another clinic) (Figures 16.4.1)
- Orthopantomogram confirms distal caries in #26 and generalised bone loss (10–30%) (Figure 16.4.2)

A Practical Approach to Special Care in Dentistry, First Edition. Edited by Pedro Diz Dios and Navdeep Kumar.

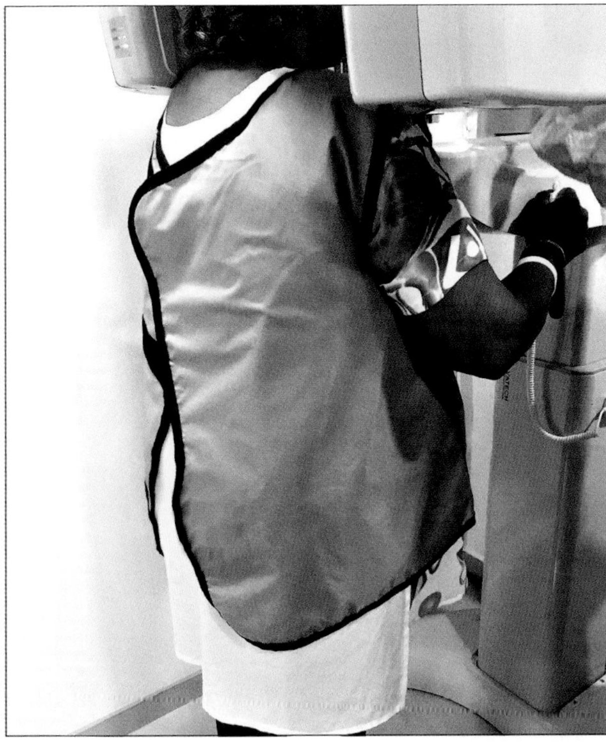

Figure 16.4.1 Shoulder obstruction during attempt to undertake an orthopantomogram.

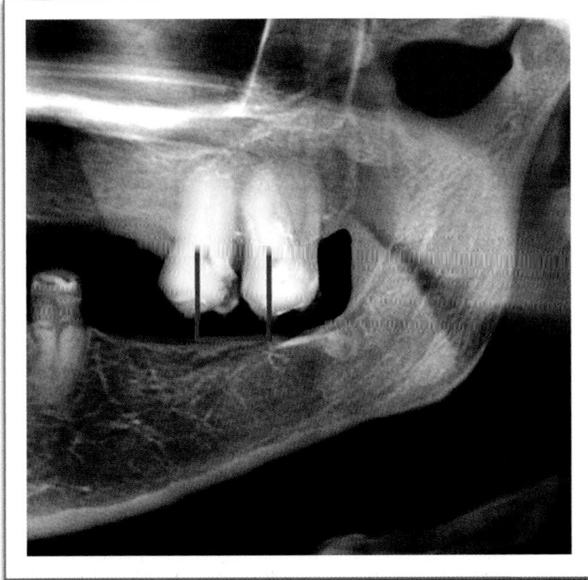

Figure 16.4.2 Orthopantomogram demonstrating caries on the distal aspect of #26.

Structured Learning

1) What does the raised BMI of this patient indicate?
   - This patient has a BMI of 46.9 kg/m^2, which is classified as morbidly obese
   - She has an 'extremely high risk' of cardiovascular diseases, stroke, diabetes and also weight-related diseases
2) The patient asks that you only recline her slightly in the dental chair as lying flat makes her feel breathless. What could be contributing to this feeling?
   - Obesity can be associated with compressive effects of the excess abdominal weight which prevents the lungs from inflating fully, particularly when lying down; patients should be seen in a semi-upright position
   - Other factors which may exacerbate her shortness of breath include her underlying dental anxiety, asthma, pulmonary hypertension and ischaemic heart disease
3) The dental chair fails to move upright at the end of your examination (Figure 16.4.3). What is the most likely reason for this?
   - Most standard dental chairs have a safe working limit (SWL) in the region of 140 kg/22 stone
   - The dental chair will not reposition as the maximum weight limit has been exceeded
4) The patient bursts into tears. She is embarrassed and apologises that her weight is the likely reason the dental chair does not move. How would you respond?
   - Apologise and reassure the patient that she is not at fault
   - Explain it is a legal-ethical duty of service providers to make 'reasonable adjustments' to enable equitable access to dental care regardless of any disability
   - Advise her that it is possible for her to access dental care with suitable and safe facilities, practices and equipment – inform her that you will attempt to make these available for her next visit (e.g. access to a bariatric dental chair/bench and platform; SWL 203 kg/32 stone) (Figures 16.4.4 and 16.4.5)
   - Reassure her that the staff will have specific training on bariatric handling and transfer to optimise safety
5) The patient consents to extraction of the carious #26. What other factors do you need to consider in your risk assessment?
   - Social
     - Identifying a suitable escort; essential if sedation is being considered to manage her dental anxiety
   - Medical
     - Airway compromise/respiratory distress due to obesity
     - Increased risk of hypertensive crisis and orthostatic hypotension (see Chapter 8.1)
     - Acute presentation of angina-related chest pain (see Chapter 8.2)

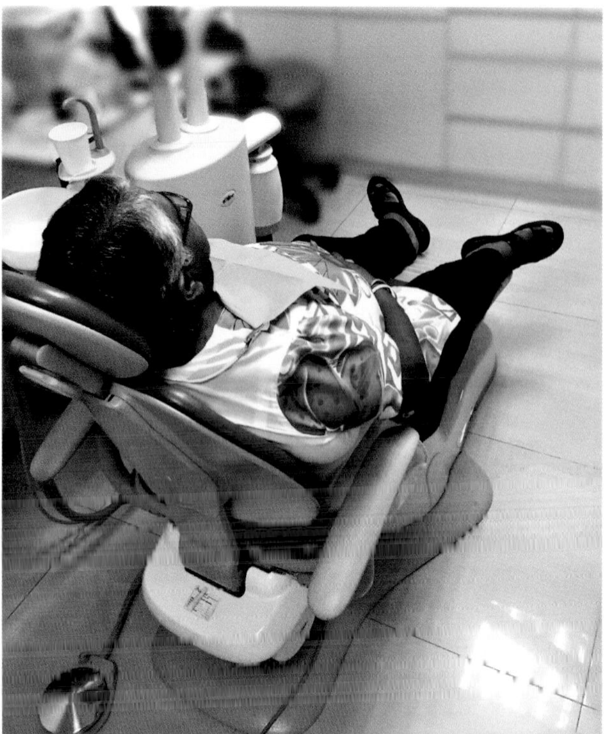

Figure 16.4.3 Dental chair unable to reposition.

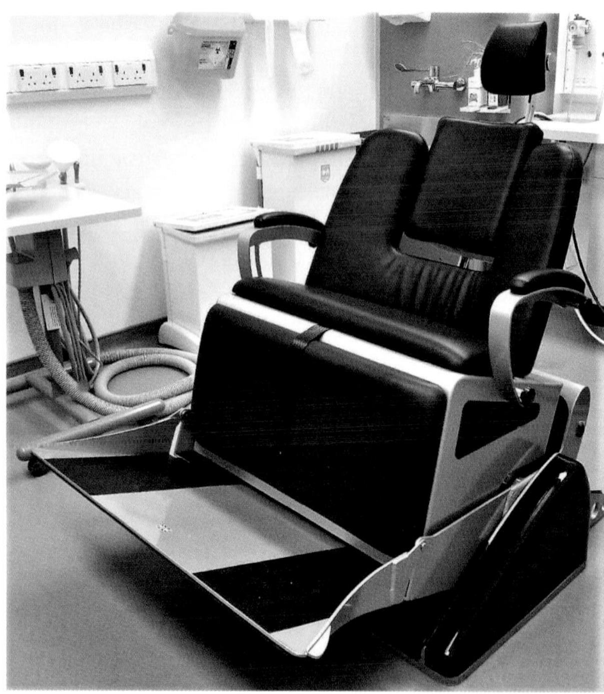

Figure 16.4.4 Bariatric bench.

- Hypoglycaemia, infection risk and delayed wound healing due to diabetes (see Chapter 5.2)
- High risk of thromboembolic events (see Chapter 14.5)

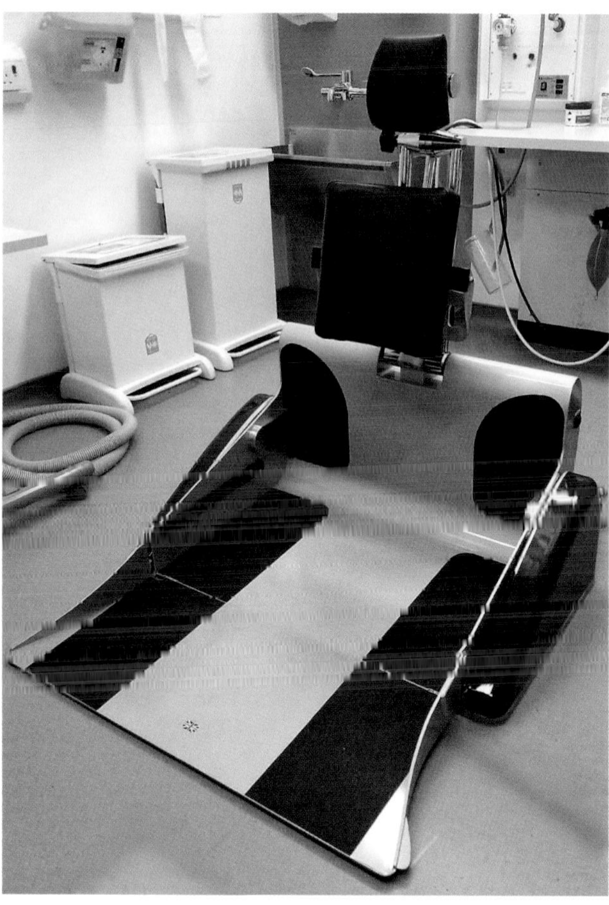

Figure 16.4.5 Wheelchair platform.

- Risk of an acute asthma attack (see Chapter 9.2)
- Stress from the dental environment can trigger an anxiety crisis (see Chapter 15.1)
- Polypharmacy

• Dental
  - Dental anxiety may reduce compliance for dental treatment
  - Unable to recline the dental chair
  - It may not be possible to place the forceps on #26 in the correct position due to the buccal adipose tissue
  - Limited access for further radiographs, operative dentistry/instrumentation and oral hygiene practices due to increased adipose tissue
  - Tooth surface loss likely to be secondary to gastro-oesophageal reflux disease and bruxism
  - Poor oral hygiene (increased incidence of dry socket)

6) The patient asks for sedation due to her dental anxiety. What factors should you consider?
   • The abundant adipose tissues act as a 'reservoir' for the sedatives, attenuating the active drug concentra-

tion in plasma; therefore, the sedative available to the central nervous system is reduced
- The effect of sedation agents is often prolonged; this is due to the fat-soluble molecular structure of benzodiazepines and propofol
- Concomitantly, available plasma sedative to the liver or kidneys is also reduced, slowing down elimination rate and recovery
- Furthermore, benzodiazepines (e.g. midazolam) cause respiratory depression
- The patient also has multiple medical comorbidities
- If sedation is being considered, this should be undertaken in a hospital environment with the support of an anaesthetist; a presedation assessment will be required to assess the airway and impact of the concurrent medical condition
- Propofol, ketamine and nitrous oxide have a less airway-depressive effect and may be preferred to benzodiazepines
- Titration induction is essential
- Prolonged recovery is likely; access to an inpatient bed is advisable

General Dental Considerations

Oral Findings

- Increased adipose tissue deposition in perioral tissues, floor of mouth and the tongue affects accessibility and visibility, especially to posterior tooth surfaces
- Sleep apnoea due to increased tissue mass around the oral facial region and the pharynx
- Bruxism – associated with sleep apnoea
- Dental erosion more frequent; linked to gastric reflux/vomiting (side-effects of bariatric surgery) and poor dietary choices
- Dentine hypersensitivity can occur in relation to frequent consumption of acidic beverages; exacerbated by presence of gastric reflux
- Xerostomia may be observed in patients taking appetite suppressants or in those who have undergone bariatric surgery
- A correlation has been found between obesity and periodontal disease; it has been suggested that this is related to the fact that obese individuals have an increased local inflammatory response, as well as possibly an altered oral microflora
- Increased dental caries risk, particularly in children, is likely to be linked to an unhealthy diet, high in sugary drinks and snacks
- Poor wound healing may be observed in patients following bariatric surgery

Dental Management

- Dental management considerations depend on the severity of the obesity and any related comorbidities (Table 16.4.1)
- Careful assessment of the airway is required before considering whether to recline the patient (Table 16.4.2)

Section II: Background Information and Guidelines

Definition

Bariatrics is the branch of medicine that deals with the causes, prevention and treatment of obesity. It focuses on preventing worsening of both health and quality of life. The BMI is commonly used as a measure of obesity and is calculated by dividing a person's weight in kilograms by their height in metres (squared). Obesity is a global epidemic. Over 1.9 billion adults 18 years and older were overweight in 2016 (approximately 39% of the world's population); of these, over 650 million were obese as defined using the World Health Organization classification of weight (Table 16.4.3).

Aetiopathogenesis

- Weight gain results due to a surplus of caloric intake (overeating and physical underactivity)
- It is influenced by a complex variety of factors (Table 16.4.4)

Diagnosis

- BMI is the most validated measure of obesity using the World Health Organization definition (Table 16.4.4), although easy to measure, it is a poor predictor of body fat and lean mass
- Waist circumference, waist-to-hip ratio, skinfold thickness
- Bioelectric impedance
- Underwater weighing (hydrodensitometry)
- Computed tomography and magnetic resonance imaging

Clinical Presentation

- Characterised by excessive generalised deposition and storage of fat
- Exercise intolerance
- Development of medical comorbidities, including:
  - Coronary heart disease/cardiovascular disease (congestive heart failure)

Table 16.4.1 General dental management considerations.

Risk assessment	• Accessibility • Airway management • Multiple comorbidities, including sleep apnoea, diabetes mellitus, ischaemic heart disease and osteoarthritis, may impact on the delivery of dental care • May have an immune dysfunction leading to delayed wound healing • Coagulation abnormalities may occur (e.g. due to non-alcoholic fatty liver disease)
Criteria for referral	• Dentists should be able to treat the vast majority of bariatric patients in primary care provided the service has the appropriate equipment and access requirements • However, if there are significant medical comorbidities/ASA III, they should be referred to a hospital-based dental service for any invasive dental treatment/sedation
Access/position	• An accurate weight/body mass index (BMI) is essential when considering whether specialised equipment/facilities are required • The safe working limit (SWL) for a standard dental chair is typically 140 kg/22 stone – if the patient exceeds this, a bariatric dental chair (SWL 203 kg/32 stone), wheelchair recliner (SWL 500 kg/79 stone) or bariatric wheelchair (318 kg/50 stone) may be needed • Waiting rooms should have a suitable high-weightbearing chair which should be armless • Toilet facilities should have suitable SWL or specialist bariatric surround • In certain situations, heavy-weightbearing hoists for wheelchair transfer, bariatric-suitable ambulance, bariatric suitable wheelchair, physical access through the door frame or even domiciliary care may be considered • A higher SWL operating table may be required for general anaesthesia (e.g. [illegible] kg/[illegible] stone) • If there are mobility issues and/or fatigue in association with sleep apnoea, avoid early morning appointments
Communication	• Whilst conversations about obesity can be difficult, healthcare workers, including dentists, should still engage patients regarding weight-related health issues and refer to the primary care doctor as required • Avoiding these essential topics will undermine the importance of weight management in oral health • Anxiety and depression may be associated with overeating; these can negatively impact on effective communication (see Chapters 15.1 and 15.2)
Consent/capacity	• Mental capacity is generally not impaired • Depression and anxiety may result in lack of engagement or understanding • Consider the impact of any related alcoholism or syndrome-associated learning disabilities related to obesity (e.g. Prader–Willi syndrome)
Anaesthesia/sedation	• Local anaesthesia – Intraoral anatomical landmarks may be obscured by adipose tissue – Gow-Gates technique, or intraligamental infiltration, may be alternatives to inferior alveolar nerve block • Sedation – Presedation airway assessment should be undertaken using tools such as the L.E.M.O.N law (Table 16.4.2) and Mallampati classification – Patients with a compromised airway and/or BMI of 40 kg/m^2 or more (ASA III) are at risk of significant respiratory depression and should be seen in a hospital setting with the support of an anaesthetist – Nitrous oxide is the sedation agent of choice as it causes minimal depression, and concurrently provides oxygen; a larger nasal hood may be required to enable better adaptation to the facial tissues – Intravenous cannulation may be challenging as veins tend to be less visible – Increased adiposity is known to prolong the recovery and reduce peak sedative effect of benzodiazepines and propofol – Avoid administering opioids and benzodiazepines concurrently as the sedative effects of these drugs can be synergistic • General anaesthesia – Intubation and airway management can be challenging, due to constriction of airways and reduced neck mobility – Consider medical comorbidities and management of medical emergencies – inpatient beds may be required

(*Continued*)

Table 16.4.1 (Continued)

Dental treatment	• Before – A light meal prior to the dental appointment will reduce risk of hypoglycaemia (if diabetic) and also limits excessive gastric reflux – An adequately sized blood pressure cuff should be available – Ensure manual handling training and a risk assessment have been undertaken – Intraoral radiography may be challenging due to restricted access in relation to increased oral adipose tissues – Orthopantomograms may not be possible if the machine is unable to accommodate the patient's size; an alternative technique in these situations is the lateral oblique radiograph • During – Consider placing the patient in a semi-supine (Fowler's position 45–60°) or upright position to optimise airway and breathing – Avoid prolonged procedures as these may cause fatigue and exacerbate pressure ulcers/soreness for the patient; it may also lead to musculoskeletal issues for the operator if they are unable to work in an ideal position – Operators who are petite may find it beneficial to use a stool for extra reach – Soft tissue retractors may help to improve intraoral access – Placement of sectional matrix systems may be challenging due to encroaching buccal tissues – ensure a variety of bands are available, including circumferential designs – Emergency management: wider blood pressure cuffs, longer intramuscular needles (to get through fat layer) may be needed; may be unable to place the patient into supine/recovery position or physically move patient (do not attempt as this may cause injury to the operator); airway management and resuscitation are more challenging, with additional difficulty with identification of landmarks for chest compressions; urgent assistance is required and the resuscitator should rotate with a colleague to avoid fatigue • After – Factor in additional time for patient transfer, operator positioning and intraoral access – Arrange earlier review after invasive dental treatment as healing may be impaired
Drug prescription	• Non-steroidal anti-inflammatory drugs may exacerbate gastric reflux, particularly in patients who have undergone bariatric surgery • Avoid opioids as they can cause respiratory depression • Paracetamol is the painkiller of choice • Azoles, macrolides and benzodiazepines employ the CYP3A4 enzyme complex for elimination via the liver, which is shared by various appetite suppressants (e.g. tesofensine, lorcaserin, sibutramine); caution should be exercised when prescribing these
Education/prevention	• Dietary advice to manage caloric intake is essential and should be undertaken in collaboration with a dietitian where possible; discuss sugar substitutes such as xylitol • Remineralisation products, such as amorphous calcium phosphate, may help with dental erosion secondary to reflux • A mandibular advancement device may be beneficial for patients with sleep apnoea (referral to sleep medicine experts is sometimes warranted) • Consider salivary substitutes for patients with xerostomia secondary to appetite suppressants

Table 16.4.2 Airway assessment (L.E.M.O.N tool).

L.E.M.O.N evaluation criteria	Points
L = Look externally	
Facial trauma	1
Large incisors	1
Beard or moustache	1
Large tongue	1
E = Evaluate the 3-3-2 rule	
Incisor distance under 3 finger breadths	1
Hyoid–mental distance under 3 finger breadths	1
Thyroid-to-mouth distance under 2 finger breadths	1
M = Mallampati class III or IV	1
Class I: Soft palate, uvula, fauces, pillars visible	
Class II: Soft palate, major part of uvula, fauces visible	
Class III: Soft palate, base of uvula visible	
Class IV: Only hard palate visible	
O = Obstruction	1
Presence of pathology like epiglottitis, retropharyngeal abscess, peritonsillar abscess, trauma or a foreign body in the upper airway cause difficulty for intubation and laryngoscopy	
N = Reduced neck mobility	1
Reduced range of motion in the neck can be due to arthritis, cervical spondylosis and obesity. This affects intubation. A healthy atlanto-occipital joint movement ranges around 35°	
Total	10

The presence of each condition or pathology scores 1 point; no points are allocated with its absence; a higher score is associated with increasing difficulty of airway management.

Table 16.4.3 World Health Organization classification of weight by body mass index (BMI).

Classification	BMI (in kg/m^2)
Underweight	<18.5
Normal	18.5–24.9
Overweight	25.0–29.9
Obese	30.0–39.9
Morbidly obese	>40

- Type 2 diabetes mellitus
- Musculoskeletal disorders (e.g. osteoarthritis)
- Obstructive sleep apnoea (OSA); a STOP-Bang questionnaire is used to assess the risk of OSA (Table 16.4.5)
- Obesity hypoventilation syndrome – chronic hypoventilation due to excess weight preventing full expansion of the lungs
- Stroke
- Gout, gallstones
- Various cancers, including endometrial, breast, colon and liver
- About 10% of obese people have Pickwickian syndrome – a combination of apnoea, episodic somnolence and cor pulmonale

Management

- The primary goal of treatment is weight loss via lifestyle changes
  - Supported by dietitians and nutritionists
  - Supported by physical therapists or specialised trainers
- Appetite suppressants and other medications can also be used
  - Many suppressants are available but are used for a limited duration (months) due to tachyphylaxis and potential side-effects
  - Diethylpropion and phentermine are norepinephrine-releasing agents, approved for short-term use of around 3 months, phentermine is not recommended for people with uncontrolled hypertension or heart disease
  - Lorcaserin (a serotonin receptor agonist not available in the United States) and orlistat (a pancreatic and gastric lipase inhibitor) are recommended for patients with cardiovascular disease
- Bariatric surgery is indicated for people with a BMI above 40 kg/m^2
  - There are 4 main categories: gastric bypass, adjustable gastric band, gastric sleeve and duodenal switch
  - Associated with risk due to medical comorbidities associated with obesity
  - Approximately 10% are reportedly unsuccessful

Prognosis

- Persons with BMI >40 kg/m^2 have a life expectancy reduced by an average of 10 years
- Persons with BMI 30–39.9 kg/m^2 have a reduced life expectancy of around 3 years
- Seeking bariatric treatment may improve longevity by 10 years and also improve quality of life

A World/Transcultural View

- The obesity epidemic is not restricted to industrialised societies
- In developing countries, it is estimated that over 115 million people have obesity-related problems
- Ethnicity influences the age of onset and the rapidity of weight gain

Table 16.4.4 Factors influencing the risk of obesity.

Factors	Risks
Lifestyle	Overeating, dietary choices (high in simple carbohydrates/fat)
	Sedentary lifestyle
	Alcoholism
Psychological	Binge-eating disorder (compulsive overeating)
	Eating excessively in response to emotions such as sadness, stress, anger or depression
Medications	Antidepressants
	Anticonvulsants (e.g. carbamazepine, sodium valproate)
	Antidiabetic medication (e.g. insulin, sulfonylureas, thiazolidinediones)
	Certain hormones (e.g. oral contraceptives, corticosteroids)
	Some antihypertensives and antihistamines
Diseases	Hypothyroidism
	Insulin resistance
	Polycystic ovary disease
	Cushing syndrome
Genetic predisposition	May be related to defects in hormones such as leptin which signal the brain to eat less
	Genetic conditions (e.g. Prader–Willi syndrome)
	More likely for a child to develop obesity if both parents are obese (also linked to lifestyle)
Childhood weight	Being overweight during older childhood is highly predictive of adult obesity, especially if one or both parents are also obese
Hormones	Women tend to gain weight especially during certain events such as pregnancy and menopause
	However, with the availability of lower-dose oestrogen pills, weight gain has not been as great a risk
Socioeconomic issues	Lack of money to purchase healthy foods or lack of safe places to walk/exercise

Table 16.4.5 STOP-Bang questionnaire for sleep apnoea.

	Yes	No
Snoring *Do you snore loudly?*		
Tiredness *Do you often feel tired, fatigued or sleepy during the daytime?*		
Observed Apnoea *Has anyone observed that you stop breathing or choke or gasp during your sleep?*		
High Blood **P**ressure *Do you have or are you being treated for high blood pressure?*		
BMI *Is your body mass index more than 35 kg/m²?*		
Age *Are you older than 50 years old?*		
Neck Circumference[a] *Is your neck circumference greater than 40 cm or 15.75 in.?*		
Gender *Are you male?*		
Score 1 point for each positive response		
Risk of sleep apnoea (total of scores):		
Low risk = 0–2		
Intermediate risk = 3–4		
High risk ≥5, or		
Yes to 2 or more of 4 STOP questions + male gender, or		
Yes to 2 or more of 4 STOP questions + BMI >35 kg/m², or		
Yes to 2 or more of 4 STOP questions + neck circumference		

[a] Usually measured at the level of the Adam's apple; alternative measurement via shirt collar: 43 cm (17 in.) or larger for males or 41 cm (16 in.) or larger for females. *Source:* Adapted from: www.stopbang.ca/osa/screening.php

Table 16.4.6 Ethnicity-specific obesity indices.

Country or ethnic group	Overweight (BMI)	Obese (BMI)	Waist circumference cut-off for abdominal obesity
International standards European descent United States African descent[a]	≥25 kg/m²	≥30 kg/m²	Male ≥94 cm Female ≥80 cm
China Japan	≥24 kg/m²	≥28 kg/m²	Male ≥90 cm Female ≥80 cm
South Asia South-East Asia	≥22–24 kg/m²[b]	≥27 kg/m²	Male ≥90 cm Female ≥80 cm

BMI, body mass index.
[a] International standards apply for people of African descent until more specific instructions are available.
[b] Range of BMI index cut-off (e.g. Singapore ~22, India ~23, Indonesia ~24).

- People of African descent reportedly have lower body fat and higher lean muscle mass than Caucasians of the same BMI
- Asians have 3–5% higher total body fat than their Caucasian counterparts
- In view of these differences, ethnicity-specific obesity indices have been proposed within countries to stratify obesity-related risks (Table 16.4.6)

- Access to social or medical support, including bariatric surgery, is very variable across the world
- Furthermore, legislation and policies to protect people with obesity from discrimination, such as the Equality Act 2010 in the United Kingdom, are not universal

Recommended Reading

Abed, H. and Reilly, D. (2018). Bariatric dentistry: managing the plus-size patient. *J. Ir. Dent. Assoc.* 62: 333–335.

Barbosa, C.S., Barbério, G.S., Marques, V.R. et al. (2009). Dental manifestations in bariatric patients: review of literature. *J. Appl. Oral Sci.* 17 (Suppl): 1–4.

Blüher, M. (2019). Obesity: global epidemiology and pathogenesis. *Nat. Rev. Endocrinol.* 15: 288–298.

Khan, M.S., Alasqah, M., Alammar, L.M., and Alkhaibari, Y. (2020). Obesity and periodontal disease: a review. *J. Family Med. Prim. Care.* 9: 2650–2653.

Marshall, A., Loescher, A., and Marshman, Z. (2016). A scoping review of the implications of adult obesity in the delivery and acceptance of dental care. *Br. Dent. J.* 221: 251–255.

Suvan, J., D'Aiuto, F., Moles, D.R. et al. (2011). Association between overweight/obesity and periodontitis in adults. A systematic review. *Obes. Rev.* 12: e381–e404.

World Health Organization. (2020). *Fact Sheet: Obesity and Overweight*. www.who.int/news-room/fact-sheets/detail/obesity-and-overweight

16.5 Homelessness

Section I: Clinical Scenario and Dental Considerations

Clinical Scenario

You are contacted by the local community services regarding a 64-year-old man temporarily residing in one of their lodgings. The man is complaining of persistent pain in the region of left maxillary sinus, with discharge from his nose.

Medical History

- Mild chronic obstructive pulmonary disease (Gold I score)
- Mild asthma
- Latent tuberculosis
- Chronic sinusitis and allergic rhinitis
- Chronic hepatitis C, on 6-monthly follow-up without active treatment; recent serum viral load undetectable
- Gastro-oesophageal reflux disease
- Benign prostate hypertrophy

Medications

- Salbutamol (inhaler, as required)
- Fluticasone (inhaler)
- Omeprazole
- Variety of traditional Chinese tonics and herbs taken daily when accessible

Dental History

- Brushes once a day with a hard-bristled toothbrush; no toothpaste
- Irregular dental attender; visits only when symptoms arise
- Prison dental service only provided dental extractions
- History of delayed healing after dental extractions, with surgical repair of an oral antral fistula on the left side 2 years ago

Social History

- Separated from wife for 20 years; no contact with daughter for over 10 years; no other close family (distant relationship with siblings)
- Ex-offender, released from prison 1 month ago after a 5-year period of imprisonment
- Homeless; recently moved to temporary lodging by the local community services
- Unemployed
- Previous injecting drug user and a heavy ex-smoker (stopped 1 year ago)
- Alcohol consumption: 30 units a week

Oral Examination

- Mouth breather
- Edentulous upper jaw with frictional keratosis and traumatised ridge from lower teeth
- No oroantral communication observed on the left side
- Lower teeth grade I-II mobility with very poor periodontal health
- Generalised tooth surface loss

Radiological Examination

- Orthopantomogram undertaken (Figure 16.5.1)
- Metal mesh on left orbital floor
- Edentulous upper ridge with pneumatisation of the nasal sinuses
- 20–50% bone loss around teeth #33, #34, #35, #43, #44 and #45

Structured Learning

1) The patient is unable to recall the reason why the metal mesh on left orbital floor was placed. What factors could be responsible for his lack of recall?
   - Excess alcohol consumption can affect the ability to recall past events; this can be temporary or permanent, i.e. Wernicke encephalopathy (see Chapter 15.5)

A Practical Approach to Special Care in Dentistry, First Edition. Edited by Pedro Diz Dios and Navdeep Kumar.

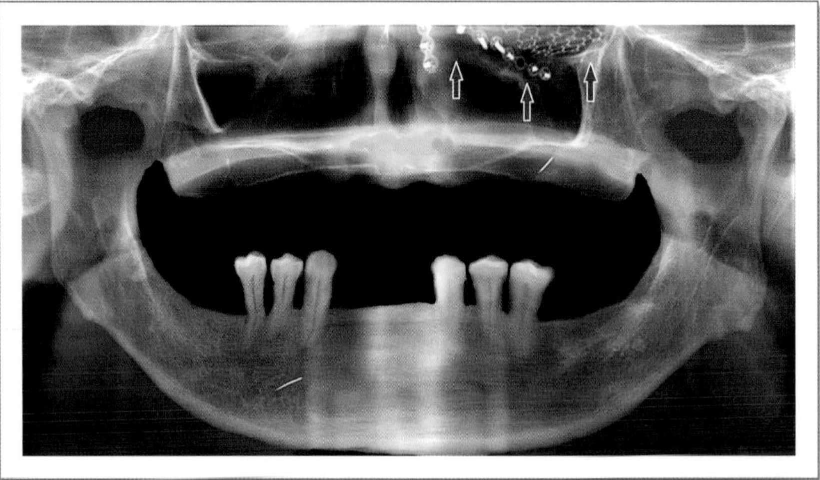

Figure 16.5.1 Orthopantomogram demonstrating metal mesh on the left orbital floor and bone loss in relation to the lower canines and premolar teeth.

- The patient has a history of recreational drug use which may impact on his ability to recall previous events
- Social stigmatisation may make the patient reluctant to divulge the details of a past event which may be related to abuse, assault or trauma due to incapacitation (drugs/alcohol)

2) Following liaison with the patient's social and medical team, you confirm that the patient had an orbital blowout fracture 6 years ago due to blunt trauma related to an assault. Titanium mesh, together with a bone graft, was used for reconstruction of an orbital floor fracture. What could be a possible explanation of this patient's symptoms?
   - As there are no maxillary teeth, and no observed oro-antral communication, a dental cause is unlikely
   - Chronic sinusitis and allergic rhinitis may be contributing to his symptoms
   - Infection of the mesh is a plausible cause of the nasal discharge
   - Although this complication is generally uncommon (~2%), the patient's medical comorbidities considerably increase the risk of infection
   - Shortly after the orbital reconstruction surgery, the patient was imprisoned, hence was lost to surgical follow-up
3) The nasal discharge appears purulent. What are important considerations when prescribing antibiotics and pain relief for this patient while you arrange a surgical review?
   - Avoid drugs that are metabolised in the liver due to the history of hepatitis C and continued excess alcohol consumption (see Chapter 4.3)
   - The analgesics of choice are paracetamol and COX-2 inhibitor; however, consider the hepatotoxic effect of paracetamol (dose adjustment and minimising the dose/duration)
   - The antibiotics of choice are amoxicillin and penicillin V
   - Clindamycin and metronidazole may be prescribed at reduced doses
   - Quinolones are a fairly safe option and do not require dose adjustment
   - In view of the high alcohol intake, avoid non-steroidal anti-inflammatory drugs as they can increase the risk of gastric erosions and intestinal bleeding
   - Do not prescribe metronidazole (disulfiram effect)/cephalosporins due to the interaction between these antibiotics and alcohol (see Chapter 15.5)
   - Opioids enhance sedation and should be avoided, particularly as the patient has a history of recreational drug use and prescribing opioids can trigger a relapse
4) What factors may make this patient more likely to mouth breath?
   - Chronic rhinitis/asthma
   - Chronic sinusitis
   - History of trauma to the facial structures may have also caused a compromised nasal airway (e.g. deviated septum)
   - Chronic obstructive pulmonary disease
5) What factors could be contributing to this patient's poor oral health?
   - Poor oral hygiene habits, including not using fluoride toothpaste
   - Poor awareness regarding the importance of oral care
   - Lack of motivation

- Poor access to dental services (previous prison dental service only provided dental extractions; homeless)
- Comorbidities including asthma and gastro-oesophageal reflux disease

6) The patient returns to you asking for removal of all his remaining teeth and a set of dentures to improve his appearance. He feels that his improved dental appearance will help him find employment. What factors do you need to consider in your risk assessment for the management of this patient?
   - Social
     - Vulnerable adult
     - Currently homeless/unemployed – cost of dental treatment may have an impact
     - Capacity/consent impaired by alcohol excess
     - Attendance may be erratic due to alcohol excess, lack of permanent housing, cost of transport
     - Unable to reliably contact the patient
     - Lack of family support/suitable escort (need to liaise with social services)
     - Ex-offender with a history of violence – ensure a chaperone is present as per the local lone worker policy
     - Unrealistic expectations that a new set of dentures will enable him to find employment
   - Medical
     - Alcohol-related liver disease/comorbidities (see Chapter 6.1)
     - Caution when prescribing drugs due to increased likelihood of impaired liver function/side-effects and interaction with alcohol
     - Malnutrition, lack of regular meals commonly associated with iron deficiency (anaemia)
     - Impaired respiratory function in relation to tuberculosis and chronic obstructive pulmonary disease/asthma (see Chapters 4.1 and 9.2)
     - Reactivation of latent tuberculosis
     - Asthma is associated with an increased risk of other atopic reactions, including drug allergies (e.g. penicillin)
     - Ibuprofen and aspirin are associated with a risk of precipitating asthmatic attacks (see Chapter 9.2)
   - Dental
     - Poor oral hygiene habits and poor oral health
     - Increased risk of xerostomia (mouth breather, alcohol excess)
     - Tooth surface loss in relation to use of a hard toothbrush, gastro-oesophageal reflux disease (increased due to alcohol excess)
     - Requirement to attend multiple appointments for dental extraction and subsequently for denture construction
     - Delayed healing (alcohol excess, malnutrition)
     - Steroid inhaler use is associated with an increased risk of oral candidiasis
     - Oral cancer risk – higher due to alcohol excess, tobacco use and malnutrition

General Dental Considerations

Oral Findings

- Homelessness has a significant negative impact on the condition of a patient's mouth and teeth, with poor oral health being a common finding
- Approximately 90% of people who are homeless may report oral symptoms, with the most common complaints being bleeding gums, dental cavities and dental abscesses, often with associated pain
- Higher levels of tooth decay and periodontal disease are common due to limited dietary choices and poor access to oral hygiene practices/health prevention
- Higher levels of tooth loss are present (either due to trauma or being removed either by an emergency dentist or the homeless individual themselves)
- Tobacco-related lesions such as staining of the teeth and oral mucosa, and smoker's keratosis of the palate
- Increased risk of oral cancer from smoking and alcoholism

Dental Management

- Being homeless creates social, behavioural and health-related barriers in accessing dental care; in view of this, consideration should be given to adapting services to support the delivery of dental care (Table 16.5.1)
- Dental management will be conditioned by the high prevalence of medical conditions, mental health problems and substance abuse (Table 16.5.2)
- Minimally invasive/preventive approaches, such as the use of silver diamine fluoride, may be of benefit (Figure 16.5.2)

Section II: Background Information and Guidelines

Definition

Although there is no international consensus on how homelessness is defined, it is generally considered to include people without a reliable shelter. Other than not having a permanent home, it entails an additional element of social disadvantage with an element of poor access to resources and a way of life that is not by choice.

Table 16.5.1 Barriers and enablers of oral healthcare in homelessness.

Themes	Barriers	Enablers
Social/community-related challenges	• Unemployment • Poverty • Lack of fixed address/poor accommodation • Turbulent lifestyle and history • Limited social contact and community support; lack of suitable escort • Seldom contactable – typically do not have a fixed address, contact number or close point of contact • Exposure to crimes, violence, accidents and substance abuse; related to higher risk of trauma • Erroneous belief that there are dedicated welfare dental services for homeless people • Information on dental services and welfare benefits have to be made accessible in the context of homelessness • Prejudices and stigmatisation leading to unwillingness to accept homeless patients for dental care • Language/cultural barriers (e.g. refugees)	• Improve experience and training of the dental team in managing socially excluded communities • Holistic approach for psychosocial, physical, social and dental well-being by ensuring close liaison between dental, social and medical services • Increase flexibility in relation to organisational structures: – Enable access if fixed patient address – Common hours between shelters and dental clinics and/or booking a block of appointments for shelter services rather than single slots – Provide after-work hours services – Remove financial penalties for failed appointments Screening services to triage emergency, one-off treatment and those who wish to access routine dental services – Provide/signpost to mobile dental services (removes the cost of travel, improves access) • Primary and secondary care dental services for people who are homeless should be integrated and liaise closely • Increase awareness of eligible beneficial schemes • Ensure access to translator as required • Raise safeguarding concerns as appropriate – some may be victims of physical, psychological or sexual abuse
Behavioural	• Embarrassment • Mistrust/dislike • Perception of discrimination and provision of lower standard of care • Dental anxiety • Symptomatic visits (e.g. for management of acute dental infection) worsen experience • Lower perceived need for dentistry • Lack of awareness of oral hygiene	• Enhance ethos of compassion and empathy • Consider the use of additional non-pharmacological and pharmacological approaches to manage dental anxiety (see Chapter 15.1) • Educate regarding the importance of oral hygiene and regular preventive measures to avoid repeated episodes of pain/infection
Health related	• Health neglect and poor health-seeking behaviours • Limited healthcare provision • Malnutrition leading to poor healing/recovery • Communicable diseases are not uncommon, including tuberculosis, hepatitis B and C, and other blood-borne infections such as HIV • Mental health problems including depression, anxiety, psychotic illnesses • Substance abuse, alcoholism and smoking	• Liaise closely with the homeless team who are providing medical services for this cohort of patients • Confirm the medical complexity and support required • Support the smoking, alcohol and recreational cessation advice • Signpost patients to medical care as required

Table 16.5.2 General dental management considerations.

Risk assessment	• These can be social, behavioural and health related (Table 16.5.1)
Criteria for referral	• Dentists based in primary care should be able to treat the vast majority of individuals who are homeless using the enablers outlined in Table 16.5.1 • If there are significant medical comorbidities or behavioural problems, referral to a secondary care setting with appropriate medical support may be required
Access/position	• Ensure the patient has access/has been given an option to receive support from social services • Employ a flexible approach • Mobile clinics improve accessibility
Communication	• Empathetic approach required • Translators may be required for immigrants or refugees • Liaise closely with relevant medical teams as required
Consent/capacity	• Mental capacity is generally not impaired unless affected by recreational drug use and/or alcoholism • Mental health and psychiatric illnesses are not uncommon and may impact on capacity
Anaesthesia/sedation	• Local anaesthesia – Consider impact of dental anxiety and medical comorbidities • Sedation – Injecting drug users/previous users may be tolerant to sedatives, have poor access to suitable veins and/or may be susceptible to relapse and further drug use – Respiratory tract conditions such as chronic obstructive pulmonary disease or tuberculosis are common, and can affect airway and breathing – Liver conditions from alcoholism and hepatitis can affect use of drugs like propofol • General anaesthesia – Consider medical comorbidities in the risk assessment – Overnight admission may be required if no suitable escort and/or accommodation in place for discharge
Dental treatment	• Before – Liaise with the homelessness, medical and social care teams to ensure appropriate adaptations and support are in place – Consider the increased likelihood of ectoparasites on the patient's body and clothing (e.g. bedbugs, lice, fleas, mites and ticks); may require additional drapes and disposable head covers – Consider the need for additional support in relation to dental anxiety (see Chapter 15.1) • During – Ensure an empathetic and supportive approach is maintained throughout the treatment episode – Silver diamine fluoride is effective in preventing and arresting dental caries, especially if there are multiple cavities to be stabilised (Figure 16.5.2); may be beneficial for patients who are irregular attenders • After – Arrange close follow-up in view of the increased risk of poor surgical healing expected due to tobacco use, alcoholism, malnutrition and other health issues
Drug prescription	• Adaptations may be required in relation to associated health issues • Caution with use of azole antifungals and macrolide antibiotics for those with liver conditions (see Chapter 6.1) • Caution should be exercised in relation to individuals with substance dependency who may request additional sedatives, opioid painkillers and other controlled drugs (see Chapter 15.4)
Education/prevention	• Support the patient by providing smoking and/or alcohol cessation advice • Provide oral care tools (toothpaste/toothbrush) to enable oral hygiene practices

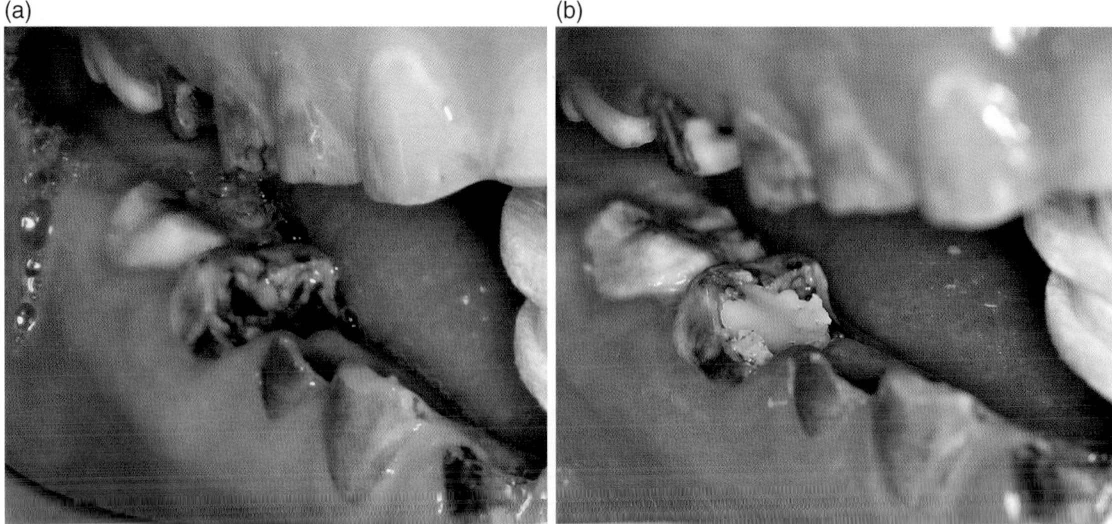

Figure 16.5.2 (a,b) Silver diamine fluoride may be beneficial for patients who are irregular attenders.

The person would seldom be able to attain a minimum standard of living, as compared to a nomadic person who is considered to have an option of choice, has access to resources, is part of a community and is sustainable in this way of life.

Aetiopathogenesis

- More prevalent in men (up to 80% of adults over 55 years of age), where isolation and difficulty of finding employment were cited as the main reasons
- Many factors contribute to homelessness worldwide, including natural hazards and political, economic, social or community circumstances (Table 16.5.3)
- People who are homeless may be grouped as follows:
  - Primary homeless are people living on the streets (Figure 16.5.3)
  - Secondary homeless are people moving between temporary shelters, including houses of friends/family and emergency accommodations (e.g. charities, shelters)

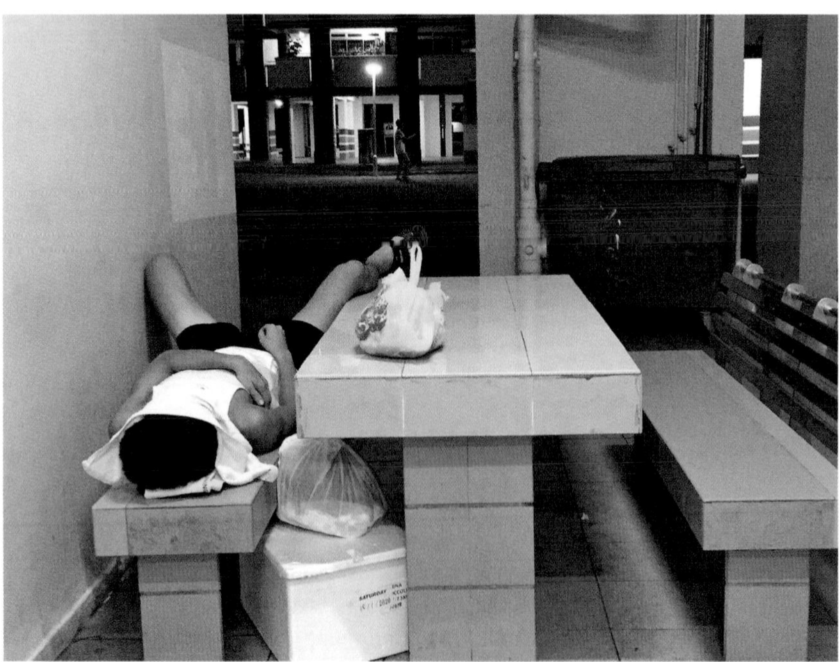

Figure 16.5.3 Homeless man sleeps in a public space.

Table 16.5.3 Factors contributing to homelessness.

- International/national
  - Natural disasters
  - Wars/refugees
  - Internally displaced persons
- Economic/political
  - Urban migration (e.g. developing cities where the supply of affordable accommodation does not match demand)
  - Poverty and unemployment
  - Asylum seekers
- Social/community
  - Includes people who are displaced from their families or communities due to crime, violence and addiction (e.g. alcohol, drugs, gambling)
  - Fugitives
- Others
  - By choice or culture (e.g. nomadic, such as Inuit, indigenous tribes and seafarers)

  - Tertiary homeless are people living in private boarding houses without a private bathroom and/or security of tenure, and marginal caravan park residents

Clinical Presentation

- Homelessness is associated with marginalisation, minority status, socio-economic disadvantage, poverty, poor physical health, limited social support, psychological distress and the failure to thrive
- It is commonly associated with multiple medical problems (e.g. substance abuse, mental health issues, infectious diseases, cardiovascular conditions, gastrointestinal disorders) (Table 16.5.4)

Management

- Healthcare for homeless people remains a challenge due to poorer nutrition, exposure to elements of weather, higher exposure to violence, inability to access social support

Table 16.5.4 Prevalent medical conditions associated with homelessness.

Categories	Details of types of conditions
Abuse	• Physical • Psychological • Sexual
Dependency	• Alcoholism • Tobacco use • Injecting drug use • Volatile substance abuse
Exposure	• Hypothermia • Tropical diseases (e.g. malaria, cholera) • Sanitation-related diseases (e.g. ascariasis)
Mental health issues	• Depression • Anxiety • Major psychiatric illness (e.g. schizophrenia)
Infectious diseases	• Lower respiratory infections (e.g. tuberculosis) • Upper respiratory viral infections • Sexually transmitted diseases (e.g. HIV infection) • Viral hepatitis • Ectoparasites (diseases they may carry in brackets) – Arthropods: ticks (e.g. Lyme disease), mites (e.g. scabies) – Insects: fleas (e.g. plague), bedbugs, lice (e.g. epidemic typhus)
Cardiovascular diseases	• Hypertension • Vascular disease
Nutrition	• Malnutrition • Dehydration
Gastrointestinal disorders	• Vomiting • Gastritis • Diarrhoea
Oral diseases	• Orofacial pain • Dental caries • Periodontal disease

- A multidisciplinary approach between social and healthcare services is essential
- Prevention of homelessness requires large-scale collaboration between government agencies, social and welfare organisations and the public, with 3 important areas of focus:
  - Provision of suitable accommodation
  - Food, training and employment
  - Enhanced access to support services, including mental health services, clothing, addiction support groups (i.e. gambling, smoking, drug use)

Prognosis

- The health and functional problems in a homeless adult are on a par with someone chronologically older in that same population
- Younger homeless adults (under 50 years old) are reportedly more prone to psychotic symptoms and substance abuse
- Life expectancy is approximately 30 years less than the rest of the population, with age-adjusted death rates 4 times higher
- Drug and alcohol abuse account for one-third of all deaths

A World/Transcultural View

- In 2005, approximately 100 million people worldwide were homeless
- This figure is thought to be increasing steadily and although it is difficult to measure, it may be as high as 1 billion people
- There remains tremendous social stigma around homelessness in both developing and developed countries
- Homelessness is poorly studied or understood in developing countries, where homeless people are very likely to suffer adverse health outcomes

Recommended Reading

Ahmadyar, M. (2018). Care for the homeless: dental services for the homeless. *Br. Dent. J.* 225: 1048.

Bonin, E., Brehove, T., Carlson, C. et al. (2010). *Adapting Your Practice: General Recommendations for the Care of Homeless Patients.* Nashville: Health Care for the Homeless Clinicians' Network, National Health Care for the Homeless Council, Inc.

Bramley, G. (2017). *Homelessness projections: Core homelessness in Great Britain.* London: Crisis. www.crisis.org.uk/media/237582/crisis_homelessness_projections_2017.pdf

Csikar, J., Vinall-Collier, K., Richemond, J.M. et al. (2019). Identifying the barriers and facilitators for homeless people to achieve good oral health. *Community Dent. Health* 36: 137–142.

King, T.B. and Gibson, G. (2003). Oral health needs and access to dental care of homeless adults in the United States: a review. *Spec. Care Dentist.* 23: 143–147.

Paisi, M., Kay, E., Plessas, A. et al. (2019). Barriers and enablers to accessing dental services for people experiencing homelessness: a systematic review. *Community Dent. Oral Epidemiol.* 47: 103–111.

Stormon, N., Sowa, P.M., Anderson, J., and Ford, P.J. (2021). Facilitating access to dental care for people experiencing homelessness. *J.D.R. Clin. Trans. Res.* 6: 420–429.

16.6 End of Life

Section I: Clinical Scenario and Dental Considerations

Clinical Scenario

You are contacted by the palliative care physician responsible for the care of an 80-year-old woman who is currently residing in a hospice. The physician is concerned that the patient has a mobile lower incisor which poses an aspiration risk and asks that you undertake an urgent domiciliary visit.

Medical History

- Severe multi-infarct (vascular) dementia – fluctuating consciousness between stupor and hypersomnia; unable to mobilise
- Aspiration pneumonia, hospitalised following 2 episodes over the past 3 months
- Thromboembolic stroke, right middle cerebral artery stroke 3 years ago
- Ischaemic heart disease
- Severe dysphagia – nasogastric tube in place for 2 years; nil-by-mouth
- Double incontinence
- History of laryngeal carcinoma 25 years ago treated with conventional radiotherapy (70 Gy in 33 fractions)
- Methicillin-resistant *Staphylococcus aureus* (MRSA) positive
- Hypertension (target organ damage)

Medications

- Clopidogrel
- Timolol maleate (eye drops)
- Vitamin B, vitamin D and calcium supplements
- Omeprazole

Dental History

- Has not received oral hygiene assistance at the long-term care facility over the past year
- Last visit to a dentist over 5 years ago

Social History

- Husband is the main care-giver and next of kin
- Patient resident in a hospice and confined to the bed
- Hospital transport with capacity to allow for a trolley bed required for essential hospital visits

Oral Examination

- Limited co-operation for examination
- Mouth breathing/xerostomia (Figure 16.6.1)
- Persistent bruxism and clenching
- #14: grade III mobility
- Coating on tooth surfaces and palate

Radiological Examination

- Not possible

Structured Learning

1) What could be causing the coating on the palate?
    - The coating consists of a dehydrated mix of secretions from minor salivary glands in the palate and exfoliated epidermal or mucosal tissues
    - These can coat the oral mucosal surfaces and the occlusal surfaces of teeth
    - Contributing factors include:
        - Xerostomia (mouth breathing)
        - Poor hydration
        - Reduced oral cleansing due to reduced oromuscular function
        - Lack of oral care provision in the hospice
2) What is the significant risk associated with the palatal debris?
    - Microbial colonisation can occur
    - The debris can dislodge and obstruct the airway
    - Despite placement of the nasogastric tube to aid feeding, the patient remains at risk of aspiration of fragments of the debris, increasing the likelihood of aspiration pneumonia

A Practical Approach to Special Care in Dentistry, First Edition. Edited by Pedro Diz Dios and Navdeep Kumar.

(a)

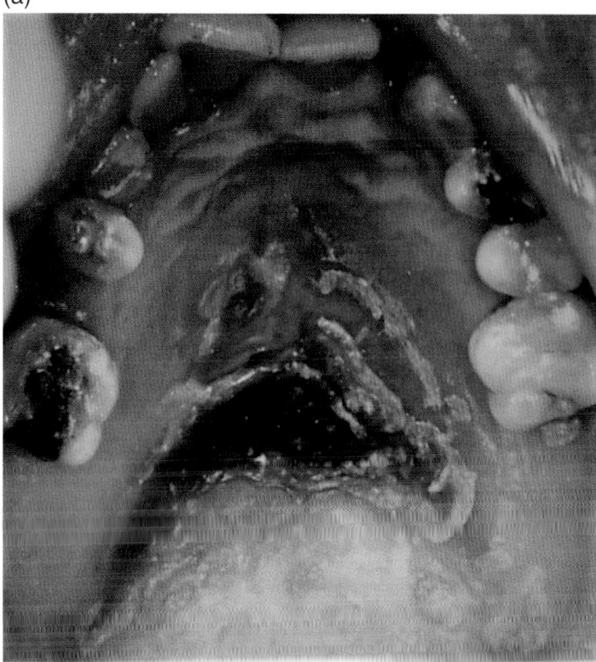

(b)

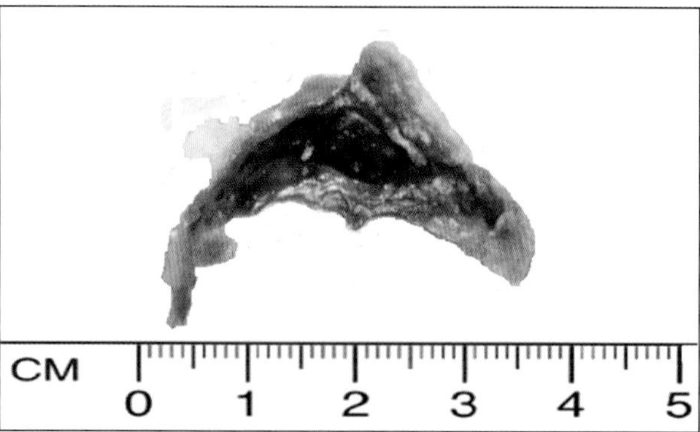

Figure 16.6.1 (a,b) Xerostomia with collection of debris/secretions on the palate and teeth (removed coating/debris from the palate).

3) What factors would have contributed to the inability to obtain radiographs?
   - Avaliability of a portable X-ray device
   - Limited co-operation (dementia)
   - Limited access (stroke)
   - Bruxism/clenching
   - Possibility of displacing #14
4) What other factors do you need to consider in your risk assessment when planning to extract #14?
   - Social
     - Non-ambulatory
     - Fully dependent
   - Medical
     - Multiple comorbidities, ASA IV (severe systemic disease that is a constant threat to life)
     - Dementia resulting in limited co-operation and capacity
     - Significant dysphagia/aspiration risk; related pneumonia risk
     - Dental treatment may elevate blood pressure and precipitate an episode of angina due to stress and anxiety (see Chapter 8.2)
     - Increased bleeding risk due to antiplatelet therapy and hypertension (not clinically significant; see Chapter 10.5)
     - MRSA positive
     - Double incontinence (require facilities to change pads as required)
   - Dental
     - Risk of aspiration of the mobile tooth
     - Neglected oral health/poor oral hygiene
     - Chronic complications of radiotherapy, including osteoradionecrosis of the bone
     - Inability to open mouth
     - Limited co-operation
5) The decision is made to extract the hypermobile #14 urgently at the hospice with sedation provided via the nasogastric tube and close monitoring by the palliative care physician. Why is this particularly appropriate given the patient's MRSA status?
   - Arranging to see the patient in her hospice room avoids transport, thereby minimising further environmental contamination/exposure of additional persons to MRSA
6) What additional precautions would you take given that the patient is MRSA positive?
   - Standard recommendations for disease control and prevention are generally adequate for preventing the transmission of MRSA and include:
     - Minimise the number of dental staff attending to essential members only
     - Use of personal protective equipment is essential and should be donned before entering the patient's room
     - Strict hand hygiene protocols should be in place
     - Appropriate handling of contaminated equipment, materials and surfaces is essential
     - Safe handling of sharps and safe injection practices should be observed
7) Three weeks later, you are contacted by the hospice again as the patient has developed a painful swelling on the side of her face. The concern is that this may be due to a dental abscess. What would be your approach?
   - Confirm that the patient has received pain control and antibiotics have been prescribed given the likelihood of infection
   - Confirm if the patient is still MRSA positive

- Discuss whether further sedation can be administered by the physician to allow improved access to the mouth to visualise the teeth/deliver urgent dental treatment
- Domiciliary care:
  - Portable handheld/wireless x-ray radiation devices can be useful to obtain intraoral radiographs
  - Undertake required dental treatment if this can be provided safely in the hospice setting (e.g. simple dental extraction of a mobile tooth where the tooth can be fully visualised/the airway protected)
- Transfer to hospital-based dental service, ensuring that appropriate facilities/equipment are available to accommodate the patient presenting supine on a trolley and their MRSA-positive status if this is confirmed:
  - Obtain radiographs as required (e.g. extraoral lateral oblique radiograph or an orthopantomogram using a horizontal panoramic unit) (Figure 16.6.2)
  - Provide dental care with medical support given the ASA IV status of the patient

General Dental Considerations

Oral Findings

- Dental plaque and remnant food debris are often not actively cleansed in those with reduced oromuscular sensitivity (e.g. stroke or dementia), resulting in rampant caries and severe gum disease
- Other common findings are orofacial pain, dysphagia, salivary gland dysfunction (drooling or dry mouth), oromucosal infections (e.g. candidiasis), taste changes and accumulation of dry secretions
- With age-related deterioration of dentition and/or edentulism, the lack of stable occlusion can worsen dysphagia
- Those undergoing palliative cancer treatment may experience mucositis/stomatitis
- Deviation from routine behaviour may be an expression of dental pain (e.g. bruxism, lip biting and rejection of toothbrushing)

Dental Management

- Although dental diseases are seldom life-threatening, pain and infection can significantly affect a patient's quality of life
- The dental team should ensure that any planned intervention is focused on preserving dignity, quality of life and comfort for the remaining duration of the patient's life (Table 16.6.1; Figure 16.6.3)
- Domiciliary care with a portable dental unit may be required if there are significant risks/discomfort associated with transferring the patient to the dental surgery (Figure 16.6.4)
- A multidisciplinary input is valuable to understand the optimal outcome for the end-of-life patient

(a)

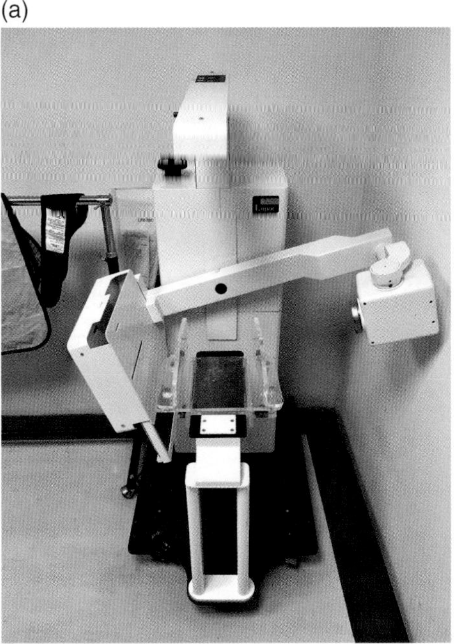

(b)

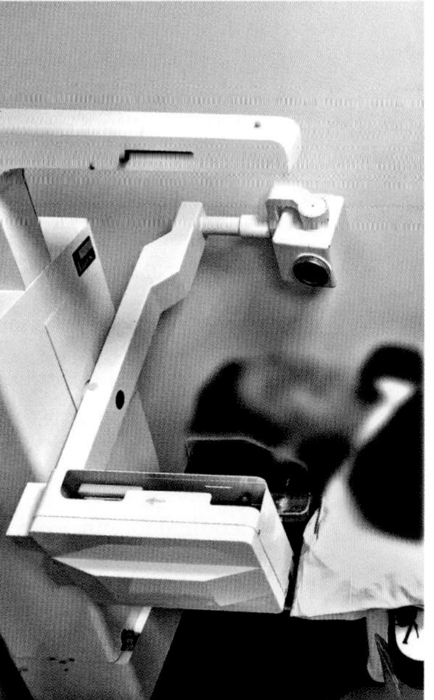

Figure 16.6.2 (a,b) Supine panoramic radiography device. *Source:* Courtesy of Kaohsiung Medical University.

Table 16.6.1 Dental management considerations.

Risk assessment	• ASA III, IV or V due to medical complexities such as chronic diseases and cancer • Often older patients with features of geriatric syndrome/frailty • Polypharmacy • Commonly reduced mobility/non-ambulatory • Fall risk • Dysphagia, malnutrition • Altered mental state and consciousness level (Glasgow Coma Scale) • Care-resistant behaviours may be expected particularly if the patient is in a state of confusion or delirium is present
Criteria for referral	• Domiciliary care or referral to services which provide this may be required for patients who are not ambulatory • Referral to a hospital-based dental service is required if invasive/complex dental intervention is required • For patients who are admitted for medical care, hospital-based teams are more appropriate to manage urgent oral/dental concerns
Access/position	• Frailty is common, with patients requiring support/aids for walking if they are ambulatory • Physical assistance may be required for transfer • Wheelchairs or trolley beds may be required for non-ambulatory patients; premises should be suitably adapted/equipped to enable care to be provided • Domiciliary care at the patient's home or hospice may be needed • It may be more appropriate to see the patient in a semi-reclined position/supine if they cannot be elevated • Short sessions should be planned
Communication	• Communication with the multidisciplinary team, including palliative care consultant, is essential to determine the risks and how best to proceed • The patient may have impaired communication as a result of their medical complexities and sedative medication • Patients who are admitted may be mechanically ventilated and hence unable to communicate verbally
Consent/capacity	• Mental capacity may be reduced due to a reduced consciousness level; this is exacerbated if opioids are used for pain control • It is important to determine if there is an advance directive, a lasting power of attorney (LPA) or court-appointed deputy • If the patient is assessed as lacking capacity for a proposed intervention, a best interest decision is needed to proceed; this should involve consultation with the next of kin, carers, an LPA/deputy if one is required, and physicians involved in the care of the patient, including the palliative care team
Anaesthesia/sedation	• Local anaesthesia – Adequate local anaesthesia should still be provided, even if the patient is in a minimally conscious state – Consideration should be given to the medical complexities when determining the agent/dose • Sedation – Antipsychotic medications can be synergistic with sedative drugs – Referral to a specialist centre is warranted if the patient is ASA III and above. • General anaesthesia – Should be generally avoided due to high ASA status – If required for other medical reasons, it may be possible to deliver urgent dental treatment in the same session

(Continued)

Table 16.6.1 (Continued)

Dental treatment	• Before – Dentistry should be kept simple in line with the palliative philosophy of healthcare – The focus is on pain and infection control in order to improve quality of the person's remaining life – Treatment plans should be simple, safe and serviceable – Minimally invasive dentistry is preferable, with asymptomatic diseased teeth stabilised rather than definitive treatment provided – Hypermobile teeth pose a risk to the airway in patients with reduced consciousness/dysphagia and should be planned for extraction – Close liaison with the multidisciplinary team is required if any dental intervention is required to determine the risks and benefits in the context of the patient's overall prognosis • During – Keep dental treatment simple and appointments short – Use high-volume suction to prevent aspiration – Arrest caries with 38% silver diamine fluoride or sodium fluoride varnish. Fillings are sometimes possible but present a greater risk • After – Ensure the oral cavity is clear of all debris – If there is any bleeding, ensure that this is controlled as it poses an additional aspiration risk – Consider the need for pain relief in the context of existing pain medication prescribed by the palliative care team
Drug prescription	• Consider the impact of polypharmacy and drug interactions • Concomitant liver and renal conditions may require adaptation of drug dosages
Education	• Encourage daily oral hygiene to remove dry secretions and accumulated debris • Reinforce that patients on tube feeding/nil by mouth should still receive oral hygiene measures • Non-foaming toothpaste and access to suction are beneficial for those with dysphagia • Sponge sticks can be used to remove dry secretions

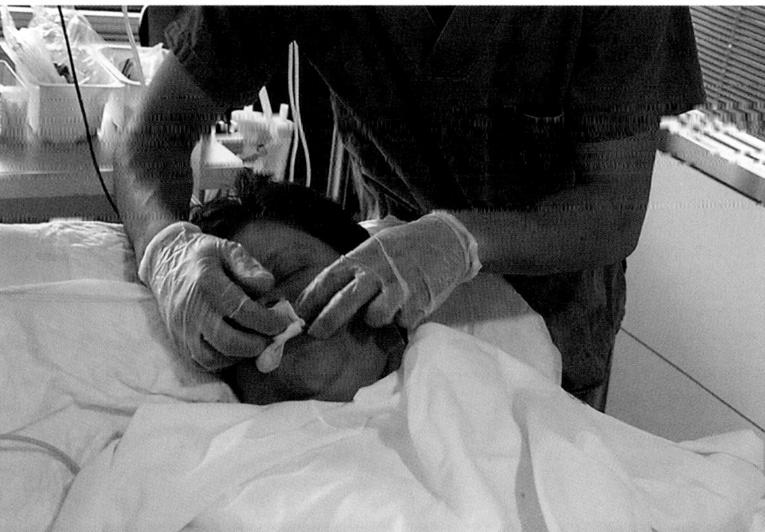

Figure 16.6.3 Using damp gauze wrapped round a gloved finger to gently moisten and cleanse coated areas.

Section II: Background Information and Guidelines

Definition

End-of-life care falls under a broad umbrella termed 'palliative care'. Palliative care is provided to any patient with a life-threatening illness and who experiences a reduced quality of life because of the disease symptoms or treatment. That illness can be at any stage, and the resulting life expectancy can be for any duration. Comparatively, end-of-life care typically indicates a life expectancy of under 6 months and progresses to terminal care when the patient is only expected to live for days to hours.

The philosophy that underpins end-of-life care is that the sanctity of life is preserved in terms of its quality and dignity, rather than simply by longevity of a life. Hence, the emphasis is on relief of symptoms, pain and distress (Figure 16.6.5). An estimated 40 million people worldwide are in need of palliative care each year, with the numbers increasing as people live longer with increasingly debilitating conditions.

Aetiopathogenesis

- Common chronic illnesses that give rise to the need for end-of-life or palliative care include cancer, cardiovascular disease, chronic respiratory diseases, AIDS and diabetes
- Frailty is associated with an age-related decline in physiological reserve and organ function and can also require palliative care

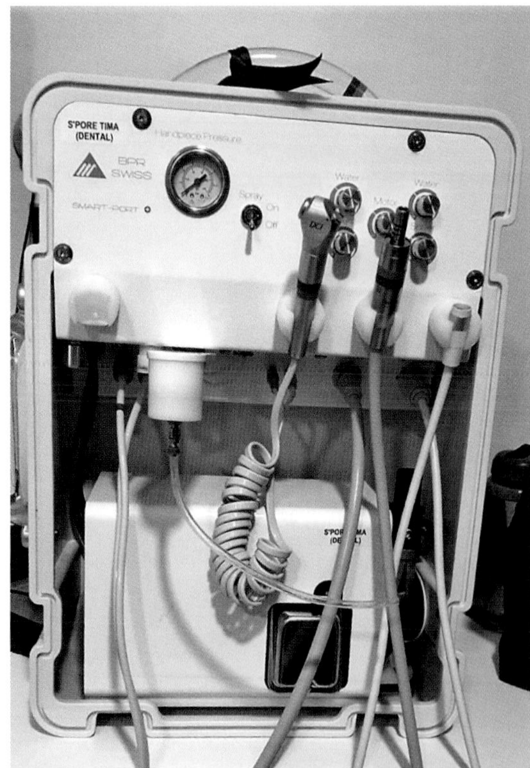

Figure 16.6.4 Portable dental unit.

Clinical Presentation

- Patients present with a combination of physical, cognitive and functional impairments
- Common features include frequent falls, incontinence, pressure ulcers, pneumonia, ascending urinary tract infection, delirium, antibiotic resistance
- Many end-of-life patients will be non-ambulatory and confined to bed as they are physically too weak to transfer; as a result, they will be unable to undertake activities of daily living safely or independently
- MRSA carriage is more common in patients who are receiving palliative care; it commonly colonises saliva and dental plaque, with the potential to spread via respiratory droplets and body fluids; if it is not adequately treated in the immunocompromised patient, it can result in multiorgan failure or 'toxic shock syndrome'
- Aspiration of oral fluids can occur asymptomatically in patients with dysphagia; this can cause 'silent aspiration' and lead to aspiration pneumonia
- Patients may experience a wide range of consciousness, confusion (e.g. delirium), parasomnias, minimally conscious states and vegetative states
- Consciousness level can be assessed by the Glasgow Coma Scale (Appendix D)
- Approximately 30% of end-of-life patients have anxiety or depression, which can in some instances lead to suicide

Management

- End-of-life planning
  - Advanced care planning (advanced medical directive) involves making plans for the person's future healthcare, particularly when one loses the ability to make decisions
  - Advanced estate planning, sometimes termed a 'will', is used to perpetuate family values and protect assets
- Psychological support
  - It can be difficult for the patient to accept the fact that they are not expected to live for more than 6 months
  - Healthcare professionals should be tactful and respectful when discussing difficult topics such as treatment side-effects and prognosis
  - Meaningful conversations with partners and family will help the patient with closure and also the loved ones during bereavement
  - An 'emotional will' is sometimes helpful for a dying person to express their feelings to family or friends,

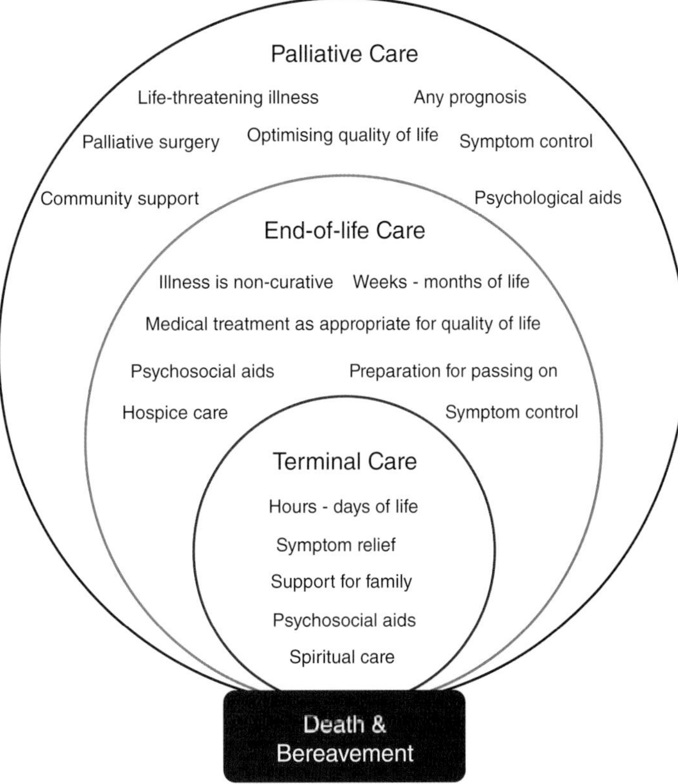

Figure 16.6.5 Phases of care when approaching death.

particularly when there is difficulty in direct interactions; this can be voice recorded, videoed or written
  - Counselling services and local spiritual support groups can be helpful
- Pain control
  - Approximately 70–80% of people with AIDS, cancer and/or severe cardiac or pulmonary disease will experience moderate to severe pain at the end of their lives
  - Pain control, using narcotics and antidepressants, is often required
  - The World Health Organization (WHO) 3-step analgesic ladder is a guide for effective pain management, although it was designed for the control of cancer pain (Appendix E)

Prognosis

- End-of-life care is often provided in long-term care facilities such as hospices
- The emphasis is on quality of life and relief of symptoms/pain, not curative treatment
- Respecting the dignity of the patient and family is a key concept
- Death is inevitable

A World/Transcultural View

- Worldwide, only around 14% of individuals who need palliative care receive it
- Discussions about death and dying are still difficult in many cultures, creating barriers for optimal communication about patient care
- There is evidence to support that physicians differ in their practice influenced by their own cultural beliefs and depending on the class or cultural origins of the patient
- When an early diagnosis can be made, patients and families are increasingly involved in decision making in many countries
- Different cultures have different views on nutrition and hydration at the end of life
- In the developing world, additional barriers to accessing end-of-life care include inability to afford care and lack of training or awareness

Recommended Reading

Chen, X., Chen, H., Douglas, C. et al. (2013). Dental treatment intensity in frail older adults in the last year of life. *J. Am. Dent. Assoc.* 144: 1234–1242.

Delgado, M.B., Burns, L., Quinn, C. et al. (2018). Oral care of palliative care patients – carers' and relatives' experiences. A qualitative study. *Br. Dent. J.* 224: 881–886.

Fitzgerald, R. and Gallagher, J. (2018). Oral health in end-of-life patients: a rapid review. *Spec. Care Dentist.* 38: 291–298.

Venkatasalu, M.R., Murang, Z.R., Ramasamy, D.T.R., and Dhaliwal, J.S. (2020). Oral health problems among palliative and terminally ill patients: an integrated systematic review. *BMC Oral Health.* 20: 79.

Wiseman, M. (2017). Palliative care dentistry: focusing on quality of life. *Compend. Contin. Educ. Dent.* 38: 529–534.

World Health Organization. (2018). *Integrating Palliative Care into Health Care: WHO Guides for Planners, Implementers and Managers.* www.who.int/palliativecare/en

Appendix A

Case Mix Model

Case mix is a tool developed by the British Dental Association to help dentists gauge the complexity of patients (updated version 2019).

CRITERIA	0	A	B	C
Ability to communicate	0	2	4	8
Ability to co-operate	0	3	6	12
Medical status	0	2	6	12
Oral risk factors	0	3	6	12
Access to oral care	0	2	4	8
Legal and ethical barriers to care	0	2	4	8

Total score interpretation: 0, standard patient; 1-9, some complexity; 10-19, moderate complexity; 20-29, severe complexity; ≥ 30, extreme complexity. Maximum score interpretation: of the 6 scoring criteria, only the most complex criteria is used - for example, a patient requiring a general anaesthesia would be described as a 'C' category patient. Available at: https://bda.org/dentists/governance-and-representation/craft-committees/salaried-primary-care-dentists/Documents/Case%20mix%202019.pdf

A Practical Approach to Special Care in Dentistry, First Edition. Edited by Pedro Diz Dios and Navdeep Kumar.

Appendix B

Common Oral Manifestations of Systemic Diseases

Oral manifestation	Associated conditions	
White lesions	Infections	Candidosis
		Epstein–Barr virus (hairy leucoplakia)
		Measles (Koplik spots)
	Mucocutaneous diseases	Lichen planus
		Lupus erythematosus
	Developmental	Darier disease
		Dyskeratosis congenita
Red/purple lesions	Infections	Candidosis
		Deep mycosis
		Herpesvirus-8 (Kaposi sarcoma)
	Mucocutaneous diseases	Lichen planus
		Lupus erythematosus
	Granulomatous diseases	Granulomatosis with polyangiitis
	Blood extravasation and vascular defects	Congenital coagulation disorders (e.g. von Willebrand disease)
		Acquired coagulation disorders (e.g. liver disease, antithrombotic drugs)
		Congenital vascular defects (e.g. Rendu–Osler syndrome)
		Acquired vascular defects (e.g. senile purpura)
		Thrombocytopenia
		Functional platelet disorders
	Haematological disorders	Megaloblastic anaemia
		Lymphoproliferative disease
	Chemotherapy	Mucositis
	Drug allergies	
Pigmented lesions	Drug-induced	Antibiotics (black tongue)
		Corticosteroids (black tongue)
		Antidepressants (black tongue)
		Methyldopa (black tongue)
		Proton pump inhibitors (black tongue)
		Iron (brown)
		Antimalarials (yellow)
		Minocycline (grey)
		Cytotoxics (brown)
		Oral contraceptives (brown)
		Anticonvulsants (brown)

(*Continued*)

A Practical Approach to Special Care in Dentistry, First Edition. Edited by Pedro Diz Dios and Navdeep Kumar.

(Continued)

Oral manifestation	Associated conditions	
		Phenothiazines (brown) Gold (purplish) Heavy metals (black)
	Endocrinopathies	Addison disease (black)
Swellings	Hereditary conditions	Hereditary angio-oedema
	Granulomatous diseases	Crohn's disease Sarcoidosis Tuberculosis Melkersson–Rosenthal syndrome Granulomatosis with polyangiitis
	Endocrinopathies and deposits	Acromegaly Amyloidosis Myxoedema Nephrotic syndrome Cushing syndrome
	Drug induced	Hydantoins Calcium channel blockers Cyclosporine
	Malignant neoplasms	Lymphomas Leukaemia Metastatic oral neoplasms
Blisters	Infections	Coxsackie Enterovirus Herpesviruses
	Mucocutaneous diseases	Dermatitis herpetiformis Epidermolysis bullosa Erythema multiforme Lichen planus Linear IgA disease Pemphigoid Pemphigus
	Others	Drugs Amyloidosis Paraneoplastic disorders
Ulcers and erosions	Infections	Deep mycosis Herpesviruses Cytomegalovirus HIV infection Gram-negative bacteria Necrotising ulcerative gingivitis Tuberculosis Non-tuberculous mycobacteria Syphilis

(Continued)

(Continued)

Oral manifestation	Associated conditions	
	Mucocutaneous diseases	Dermatitis herpetiformis
		Epidermolysis bullosa
		Erythema multiforme
		Lichen planus
		Linear IgA disease
		Pemphigoid
		Pemphigus
		Lupus erythematosus
		Graft-versus-host disease
		Felty syndrome
		Reiter syndrome
		Behçet disease
	Gastrointestinal diseases	Coeliac disease
		Crohn's disease
		Ulcerative colitis
	Haematological disorders	Anaemia
		Iron deficiency
		Neutropenia
		Leukaemia
		Myelodysplasia
		Multiple myeloma
		Plasminogen deficiency
	Drug induced	Non-steroidal anti-inflammatory drugs
		Anticonvulsants
		Antiretrovirals
		Hypoglycaemic agents
		Antiresorptives/antiangiogenics
		Antihypertensives
		Antianginal drugs
		Cytotoxics
		Immunosuppressive agents

Appendix C

American Society of Anesthesiologists (ASA) Physical Status Classification System

The purpose of the system is to assess and communicate a patient's pre-anaesthesia medical comorbidities. The classification system alone does not predict the perioperative risks, but used with other factors (e.g. type of surgery), it can be helpful in predicting perioperative risks.

ASA classification	Definition
ASA I	A normal healthy patient
ASA II	A patient with mild systemic disease
ASA III	A patient with severe systemic disease
ASA IV	A patient with severe systemic disease that is a constant threat to life
ASA V	A moribund patient who is not expected to survive without the operation
ASA VI	A declared brain-dead patient whose organs are being removed for donor purposes

Simplified from: www.asahq.org/standards-and-guidelines/asa-physical-status-classification-system

A Practical Approach to Special Care in Dentistry, First Edition. Edited by Pedro Diz Dios and Navdeep Kumar.

Appendix D

Glasgow Coma Scale (GCS)

Criterion	Observation	Score
Eye Opening Response	Spontaneous open with blinking	4
	To verbal stimuli, command, speech	3
	To pain only (not applied to face)	2
	No response	1
	Non testable	NT
Verbal Response	Oriented	5
	Confused conversation, but able to answer questions	4
	Inappropriate words	3
	Incomprehensible sounds	2
	No response	1
	Non testable	NT
Motor Response (pressure on finger tip, trapezius or supraorbital notch)	Obeys commands for movement	6
	Purposeful movement to painful stimulus	5
	Withdraws in response to pain	4
	Flexion in response to pain (decorticate posturing)	3
	Extension response in response to pain (decerebrate posturing)	2
	No response	1
	Non testable	NT

The total score is calculated by adding up the scores from the different categories shown above and ranges from a minimum total score of 3 (totally unresponsive) to a maximum of 15 (fully alert), with the level of brain injury broadly categorised as follows:
- Minor, GCS ≥ 13
- Moderate, GCS 9 – 12
- Severe, GCS ≤ 8

Of note, there are modifications to the score for intubated patients and paediatric patients, as their responses may not adequately grade their level of consciousness.
Adapted from: www.glasgowcomascale.org/downloads/GCS-Assessment-Aid-English.pdf?v=3

A Practical Approach to Special Care in Dentistry, First Edition. Edited by Pedro Diz Dios and Navdeep Kumar.

Appendix E

WHO Three-step Ladder for Pain Relief

Steps			Examples
1	Non-opioid +/- Adjuvant drugs	If pain persists or increases, go to step 2	Aspirin Paracetamol
2	Opioid for mild to moderate pain +/- Non-opioid +/- Adjuvant drugs	If pain persists or increases, go to step 3	Codeine Hydrocodone
3	Opioids for moderate to severe pain +/- Non-opioid +/- Adjuvant drugs	Free from pain	Morphine Hydromorphone Methadone Fentanyl (patches) Levorphanol

Adapted from: Anekar, A.A. and Cascella, M. (2021). *WHO Analgesic Ladder*. Treasure Island, FL: StatPearls Publishing.

A Practical Approach to Special Care in Dentistry, First Edition. Edited by Pedro Diz Dios and Navdeep Kumar.

Appendix F

Medical Conditions Associated with Increased Bleeding Risk

Medical condition	Increased bleeding due to...
Chronic renal failure	• Associated platelet dysfunction
Liver disease (e.g. caused by alcohol abuse, chronic viral hepatitis, autoimmune hepatitis, primary biliary cirrhosis)	• Reduced production of coagulation factors • Reduction in platelet number and function due to splenomegaly • Alcohol excess resulting in direct bone marrow toxicity and reduced platelet numbers
Haematological malignancy or myelodysplastic disorder	• Impaired coagulation or platelet function (even in remission)
Recent or current chemotherapy	• Pancytopenia including reduced platelet numbers
Advanced heart failure	• Resulting liver failure
Inherited bleeding disorders (e.g. haemophilia, von Willebrand disease)	• Defective or reduced levels of coagulation factors
Idiopathic thrombocytopenic purpura	• Reduced platelet numbers

A Practical Approach to Special Care in Dentistry, First Edition. Edited by Pedro Diz Dios and Navdeep Kumar.

Appendix G

Classes of Drugs Associated with Increased Bleeding Risk

Drug class	Effect
Anticoagulant or antiplatelet drugs	• Patients on dual, multiple or combined antiplatelet or anticoagulant therapies have higher risk of bleeding complications than those on single therapy
Non-steroidal anti-inflammatory drugs	• Impair platelet function to various extents
Cytotoxic drugs or drugs associated with bone marrow suppression (e.g. chemotherapy – cancer; immunosuppressants – cancer, autoimmune disorders)	• Reduce platelet numbers and/or impair liver function, affecting coagulation factor production
Corticosteroids	• Inhibit thromboxane A2, thus decreasing platelet function • Exert effects on vessel wall, interfering with initial haemostatic interactions between vessel wall, platelets and clotting factors • Immunosuppression increases infection risk, and therefore increases fibrinolysis
Selective serotonin reuptake inhibitors	• Potential platelet aggregation impairment. Although unlikely to be clinically significant in isolation, may increase bleeding time in combination with other antiplatelet drugs
Carbamazepine	• Affects liver function and bone marrow production of platelets • Patients most at risk are those recently started on the drug, or following dose adjustment
Alpha-tocopherol (vitamin E)	• Inhibits platelet adhesion to the adhesive proteins collagen, fibrinogen and fibronectin
Alcohol	• Liver disease resulting in coagulopathy • Thrombocytopenia through folate deficiency or direct suppression of bone marrow • Potentiates bleeding time prolongation of aspirin and other non-steroidal anti-inflammatory drugs
Herbal medications (e.g. garlic, *Ginkgo biloba*, ginseng, fish oil, glucosamine, St John's wort)	• Inhibit platelet adhesion and aggregation, or contain coumarins

A Practical Approach to Special Care in Dentistry, First Edition. Edited by Pedro Diz Dios and Navdeep Kumar.

Appendix H

Bleeding Risk Associated with Dental Procedures

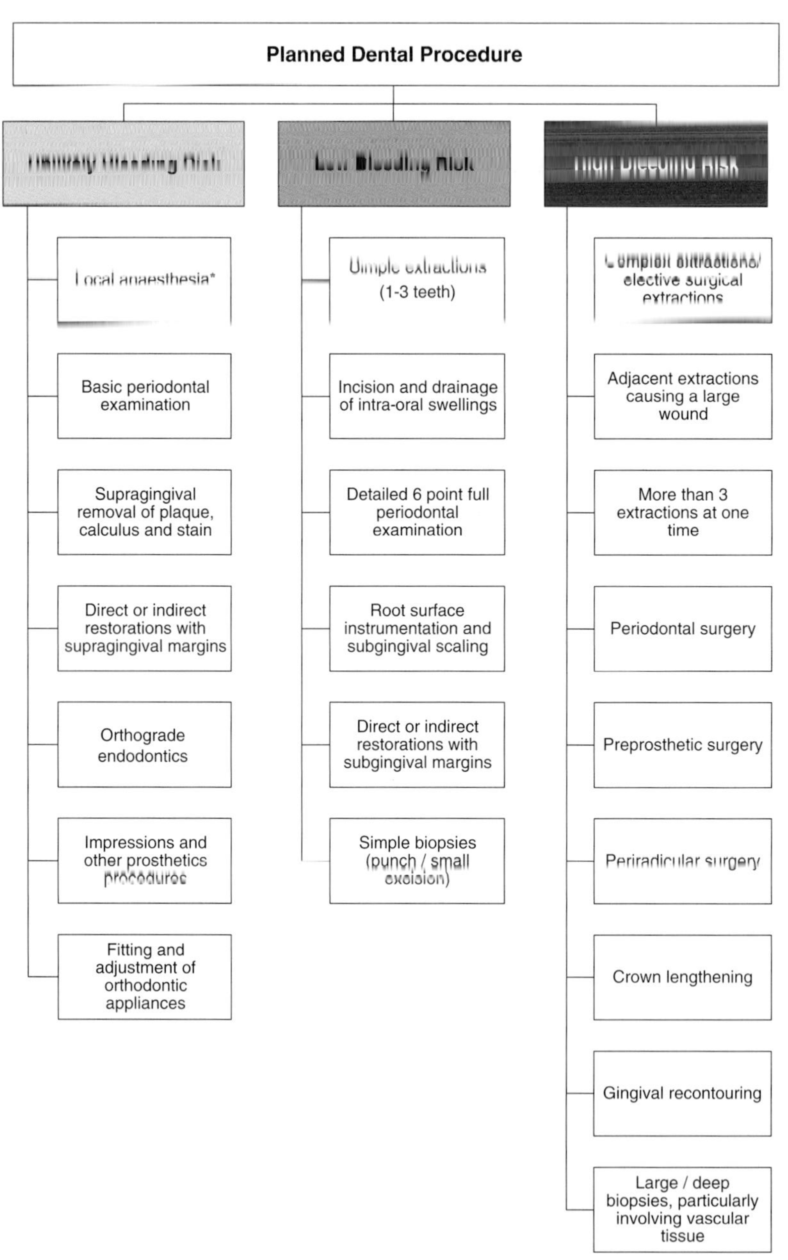

* As with all patients (whether anticoagulated or not) , avoid regional nerve blocks where possible and use an aspirating syringe and local anaesthesia containing a vasoconstrictor unless contraindicated; request an INR for patients taking warfarin if they have an unstable INR.
Adapted from: https://www.sdcep.org.uk/wp-content/uploads/2015/09/SDCEP-Anticoagulants-Guidance.pdf

A Practical Approach to Special Care in Dentistry, First Edition. Edited by Pedro Diz Dios and Navdeep Kumar.

Appendix I

Topical Haemostatic Agents for Invasive Dental Procedures

Topical agent	Characteristics
Tranexamic acid (5% mouthwash and 8% gel)	• Synthetic analogue of the amino acid lysine • Acts as an antifibrinolytic by reversibly binding 4–5 lysine receptor sites on plasminogen • This reduces conversion of plasminogen to plasmin, preventing fibrin degradation and preserving the framework of fibrin's matrix structure • It also directly inhibits the activity of plasmin with weak potency • It has approximately 8 times the antifibrinolytic activity of an older analogue, aminocaproic acid
Gelatin sponge	• Medical device which is a water-insoluble, non-elastic, porous, pliable product prepared from purified pork skin gelatin granules and water • Primary haemostatic properties related to physical absorption of blood and body fluids • Also acts as a scaffolding to help stabilise the clot • Resorbs and does not need to be removed • May cause swelling and hence should not be overpacked
Oxidised regenerated cellulose	• Resorbable oxidised cellulose material in a sterile fabric meshwork derived from plant-based alpha-cellulose • Swells on contact with blood to increase pressure in socket to enhance haemostasis • Lowers the pH of the surrounding tissue, causing red cell lysis and dark discolouration • Caustic and should ideally be removed as it may delay healing and interfere with osteogenesis
Microfibrillar collagen	• Derived from bovine skin • Provides a matrix for clot formation and strengthening, as well as enhancement of platelet aggregation, degranulation and release of clotting factors • If left in place, absorbed in 8–10 weeks • Ideally should be removed as may cause swelling/an allergic reaction
Topical thrombin	• Protein substance produced through a conversion reaction in which prothrombin of bovine origin is activated by tissue thromboplastin in the presence of calcium chloride • Converts fibrinogen to fibrin • Should not be used with collagen and cellulose products due to inactivation from pH alterations • Potential for formation of antibodies to bovine thrombin that cross-react with human coagulation factors • Human thrombin, isolated from pooled donor plasma, developed to minimise this risk but availability is limited and cost high; also potential for the transmission of blood-borne pathogens • Recombinant human thrombin (rhThrombin) since developed
Chitosan-based agents	• Biocompatible polysaccharide extracted from freshly harvested shrimp shells • Natural wet-adhesion properties that firmly bind to mucosal tissue, red blood cells and platelets for control of bleeding • Provides a physical barrier to protect wound bed, dissolves in 48 hours

(*Continued*)

A Practical Approach to Special Care in Dentistry, First Edition. Edited by Pedro Diz Dios and Navdeep Kumar.

(Continued)

Topical agent	Characteristics
Bone wax	• Sterile mixture of beeswax and isopropyl palmitate (wax softening agent) that achieves local homeostasis of bone by acting as a mechanical barrier
Fibrin glues/sealants	• Derived from human and/or animal blood products, which imitate the final stages of the coagulation cascade in the formation of a fibrin clot • A combination of a freeze-dried clotting protein (primarily fibrinogen) and thrombin is contained in separate vials and interacts during application to form a stable clot • Hence the preparation and application are complicated; fibrinogen must be dissolved in sterile water, while thrombin must be dissolved in a dilute $CaCl_2$ solution. Subsequently, both solutions are loaded into a double-barrelled syringe that facilitates their combination as they are applied • Some sealants contain 2 additional ingredients: human blood factor XIII, which strengthens blood clots, and aprotinin, extracted from bovine lung, which inhibits the enzymes that degrade blood clots
Cyanoacrylate	• Also found in consumer products • Main surgical use has been to close skin incisions
Platelet-rich plasma (PRP) gel	• Autologous platelet-rich plasma is an advanced wound therapy used in hard to heal acute and chronic wounds • Derived from an individual's blood by centrifugation process • The gel consists of cytokines, growth factors, chemokine, and a fibrin scaffold derived from a patient's blood • The mechanism of action for PRP gel is thought to be the molecular and cellular induction of normal wound healing responses similar to that seen with platelet activation

Index

A Practical Approach to Special Care in Dentistry, First Edition. Edited by Pedro Diz Dios and Navdeep Kumar.

d